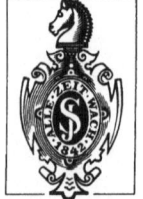

Otto G. Bier Wilmar Dias da Silva
Dietrich Götze Ivan Mota

Fundamentals of Immunology

Completely Revised Second Edition

With a Contribution by
Reinhard Burger

With 173 Figures

Springer-Verlag
Berlin Heidelberg New York
London Paris Tokyo

Dr. Otto G. Bier †
Laboratório Especial de Imunologia Aplicada
Instituto Butantan, São Paulo, SP., Brazil

Dr. Wilmar Dias da Silva
Instituto de Biôciencias, Departamento de Microbiologia e Imunologia
Cidade Universitária, São Paulo, SP., Brazil
Formerly Center for Blood Research, Boston, MA, USA

Dr. med. habil. Dietrich Götze
University Medical School, Heidelberg, FRG
Formerly Associate Professor of Immunology
The Wistar Institute – The University of Pennsylvania
Philadelphia, PA, USA

Dr. Ivan Mota
Centro de Imunologia da OMS/OPS, Instituto Butantan
CP. 65, São Paulo, SP., Brazil

Contributor:
Dr. med. habil. Reinhard Burger
University Medical School Heidelberg
Institut für Immunologie und Serologie
Im Neuenheimer Feld 305, Heidelberg, FRG

Cover page figure: schematic representation of the T cell antigen receptor (TAR) α and β chains in the cell membrane associated with the CD3 (γ, δ, ε) molecule

ISBN-13:978-3-540-15332-0   e-ISBN-13:978-3-642-70393-5
DOI: 10.1007/978-3-642-70393-5

Library of Congress Cataloging-in-Publication Data. Fundamentals of immunology. Includes
bibliographies and indexes. 1. Immunology. I. Bier, Otto, 1906–.
QR181.F85 1986   616.07'9   86-17881
ISBN-13:978-3-540-15332-0 (U.S.)

2127/3130-543210

Preface to the Second Edition

The good acceptance of this textbook is an indication that it has served its purpose. The present edition has been prepared in order to cover the main progress achieved in the five years that have elapsed since the first edition.

The structure of the book remains essentially the same but a considerable amount of new material has been introduced, particularly in certain areas such as the genetics of immunoglobulins and T cell receptor, the regulation of the immune response, hypersensitivity reactions, and cellular immunology.

Today, immunology is essential for biologists in general and in particular for physicians, veterinarians, and pathologists. The great progress and diversification that has taken place in the last few years is due to its enormous value both for the understanding of theoretical biology and for the practical resolution of biochemical, genetic, pathological, and biological problems. Greatly contributing to this progress have been relatively sophisticated techniques, such as immunofluorescence, radioimmune assay, transmission electron microscopy, scanning electron microscopy, isoelectric focusing, quantitative cytofluorimetry, affinity chromatography, and techniques that allow separation of the different lymphocyte subpopulations. A potentially fabulous field was recently opened with the development of techniques for obtaining monoclonal antibodies by fusion of immunologically active lymphocytes with myeloma cells. These hybrid cells produce large amounts of monoclonal antibodies or other lymphocyte factors. The establishment of this hybridoma technology, that is already routine in most laboratories, is being used in the resolution of general biology problems, particularly in the study of the various cell surface molecules. The production of monoclonal antibodies against cancer cell antigens, parasite antigens, virus antigens, or numerous clinically important antigens, like interferon, will have a large application in the near future. As a consequence of all these advances, immunology is today a science developing at the speed of a jet, or to be more accurate, at the speed of a rocket. All this makes it very hard to write an up-to-date immunology book. In the latent period between handing the manuscript to the editors and the selling of the book, symptoms of thymic involution already start appearing, as is particularly true for subjects like cellular immunology, where the acquisition of new knowledge is extremely fast.

This book is particularly dedicated to the young students, and we will be satisfied if it helps them in their way to immunocompetence.

June 1986   WILMAR DIAS DA SILVA
                                             DIETRICH GÖTZE
                                             IVAN MOTA

Preface to the First Edition

This textbook of basic and clinical immunology has been written primarily for medical and biology students who are receiving their first introduction to this fascinating field. Although we have presumed some knowledge of basic biology (particularly physiology and biochemistry), our primary intent has not been to cover in depth the latest research findings. Rather, we have sought to lay a firm foundation for subsequent reading in the laboratory and clinical sciences: internal medicine, pediatrics, microbiology, serology, physiology, cell biology, and genetics. Hence the first part of the text presents the various components of basic immunology, while the second shows how these elements interact under both normal physiologic and pathologic conditions.

To facilitate comprehension of the relationship between basic and clinical immunology, we have introduced cross-references throughout the book. A glossary of important terms has also been included. Selected references are provided with each chapter to guide the student to additional information on topics of special interest.

Throughout the book we have attempted to convey to new students of immunology some of the excitement which the subject has long held for us. If we have succeeded, the task of writing will have been worthwhile.

December 1980

OTTO G. BIER
WILMAR DIAS DA SILVA
DIETRICH GÖTZE
IVAN MOTA

Contents

Chapter 1   Tissue and Cells of the Immune System
            IVAN MOTA. With 18 Figures 1

Chapter 2   Activity of Immune Cells
            IVAN MOTA. With 9 Figures 35

Chapter 3   Antigens
            IVAN MOTA. With 4 Figures 63

Chapter 4   Antibodies
            OTTO G. BIER. With 23 Figures 73

Chapter 5   Complement
            WILMAR DIAS DA SILVA. With 9 Figures 115

Chapter 6   The Major Histocompatibility Complex
            DIETRICH GÖTZE and REINHARD BURGER.
            With 16 Figures 139

Chapter 7   Antigen-Antibody Interaction
            OTTO G. BIER. With 37 Figures 179

Chapter 8   Blood Groups
            OTTO G. BIER. With 5 Figures 227

Chapter 9   Hypersensitivity
            IVAN MOTA. With 19 Figures 243

Chapter 10 Transplantation
            DIETRICH GÖTZE and IVAN MOTA.
            With 4 Figures 297

Chapter 11 Immunity
            DIETRICH GÖTZE and WILMAR DIAS DA SILVA
            With 9 Figures 317

Chapter 12 Immunodeficiencies
            WILMAR DIAS DA SILVA and DIETRICH GÖTZE.
            With 5 Figures 359

Chapter 13   Autoimmunity
             WILMAR DIAS DA SILVA and DIETRICH GÖTZE.
             With 11 Figures 383

Chapter 14   Immunomodulation
             WILMAR DIAS DA SILVA. With 4 Figures 415

Brief History of Important Immunologic Discoveries
and Developments 439

Glossary of Immunologic Terms 445

Subject and Author Index 457

Chapter 1 Tissue and Cells of the Immune System

IVAN MOTA

Contents

Histology and Histogenesis
    of Lymphoid Tissue   1
    Lymph and Lymph Vessels   2
    Primary and Secondary Lymphoid Organs .   3
    Origin of the Lymphoid Cells
    of the Primary Lymphoid Organs   3
    Immunologic Dichotomy
    of the Lymphoid System   4
Cells of the Immune System   5
    Polymorphonuclear Cells   5
    Mast Cells   8
    Monocytes   9
    Lymphocytes   9
    Platelets 13
Immunologic Activity of the Primary
    Lymphoid Organs 15
    Thymus 15
    Bursa of Fabricius 22
Immunology Activity of the Secondary
    Lymphoid Organs 23
    Lymph Node System 23
    Spleen 27
    Other Lymphoid Structures 30
    Localization of the Antigen
    in the Lymphoid Organs 30
Phylogenic and Ontogenic Development
    of Immunologic Capacity 32
References 33

Histology and Histogenesis of Lymphoid Tissue

The immune system is formed by antigen-specific cells represented by thymus-dependent or T lymphocytes and by thymus independent or B lymphocytes (B from *bursa* in birds or *bone* marrow in mammals). Functionally closely associated with these cells are antigen non-specific cells such as macrophages, dendritic cells, and the epithelial cells of the primary lymphoid organs. The lymphocytes are part of a complex network of cells interacting with each other through recognition molecules (receptors) in order to keep the system in homeostasis. This autoreactivity seems to be essential for the function of the immune system. The introduction of a foreign substance or antigen (that must have some similarity with self molecules) into the organism pertubates the lymphocyte network homeostasis resulting in a transitory increase in the lymphocytes whose receptors fit the antigenic determinants (epitopes) of the foreign substance. Since these lymphocytes are part of the chain of interacting cells the whole system is pertubated. The assemblage of changes caused by the antigen constitutes the so-called immune response.

Lymphoid tissue is constructed of fibrillar reticulum whose networks contain free cells. This fibrillar reticulum is composed of reticular fibers, reticular cells, and fixed macrophages that are integral to the reticuloendothelial system. The majority of free cells are lymphocytes in different stages of differentiation plasma cells and macrophages. Two types of lymphoid tissues are recognized – loose lymphoid tissue in which reticulum cells predominate, and dense lymphoid tissue in which lymph cells predominate. The dense lymphoid tissue is capable of organizing nodular formations that constitute nodular lymphoid tissue.

Once localized in the primary lymphoid organs the primordial immature cells are subjected to the action of a number of differentiation and growth factors present in the hemopoietic-inducing microenvironment (HIM) of these organs. T lymphocytes differentiate in the HIM of the bursa of Fab-

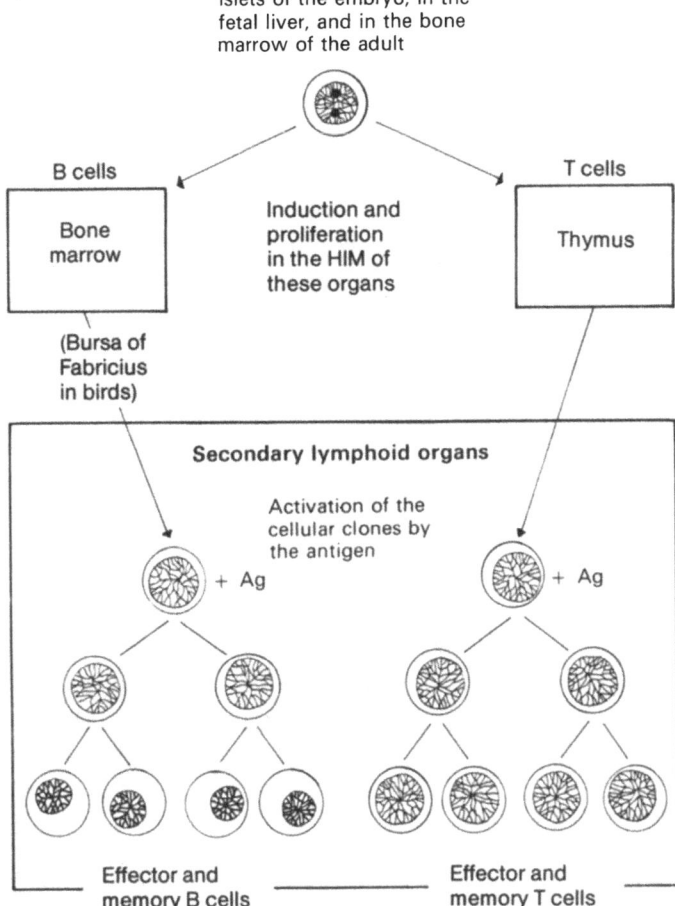

Undifferentiated immature cell
existing in the blood-forming
islets of the embryo, in the
fetal liver, and in the bone
marrow of the adult

B cells

Bone
marrow

Induction and
proliferation
in the HIM of
these organs

T cells

Thymus

(Bursa of
Fabricius
in birds)

Secondary lymphoid organs

Activation of the
cellular clones by
the antigen

+ Ag   + Ag

Effector and
memory B cells

Effector and
memory T cells

Fig. 1.1. Origin and differentiation of the lymphoid cells in the primary lymphoid organs

ricius in birds and probably in the bone marrow HIM in mammals. After differentiation, the lymphocytes migrate to the secondary lymphoid organs where they complete their differentiation. It is believed that after a few days in these organs the lymphocytes die unless they contact antigens. In meeting antigen these cells are activated and proliferate resulting in effector cells and memory cells (Fig. 1.1). Most of these cells then leave the secondary lymphoid organs and enter the circulatory pool of lymphocytes.

Lymph and Lymph Vessels

Lymph vessels originate in tissue as extremely fine lymph capillaries that communicate with each other and then anastomose, forming networks. These capillaries are of varying diameter and develop into the major lymphatic vessels. Their walls are composed of a layer of endothelial cells, outwardly surrounded by a loose reticular fibrous lattice. Lymphatic capillaries, unlike blood capillaries, do not possess basement membranes. This fact is probably responsible for the capacity exhibited by lymphatic capillaries to absorb macromolecules present in interstitial liquid and in inflammatory exudates. Lymph results from interstitial liquid that passes through the walls of lymphatic capillaries and is directed via these capillaries to the lymph nodes. The passage of lymph through the interstices of the meshwork of these organs allows intimate contact between substances or particles borne in the lymph and the macrophages, as well as immunologically competent cells of these organs. At the same time, the lymph receives cells originating from the lymph nodes. After passage through these organs, the lymph of the entire organism finally is delivered to venous circulation through the thoracic lymphatic ducts.

Primary and Secondary Lymphoid Organs

Lymphoid tissue is found concentrated in the lymphoid organs, which are divided functionally into primary and secondary organs. During phylogenetic evolution and embryogenesis, the first lymphoid organs to appear are the thymus and the bursa of Fabricius, together with the first lymphocytes. These organs are thus termed the primary lymphoid organs. From an embryologic point of view, the primary lymphoid organs are distinguished from other lymphoid structures by their points of origin – points at which there exists a direct contact between the ectoderm and the endoderm. This fact suggests that such areas may have special inductive properties in relation to those lymphoid elements that are formed in these organs.

The spleen, the lymph nodes, and the other lymphoid aggregates of the vertebrates whose lymphoid populations are dependent upon primary organs, constitute the secondary lymphoid organs. Lymphoid tissue appears first in the thymus and in the bursa of Fabricius, and only later in the other lymphoid organs. The thymus maintains a pure epithelial structure until the end of the second month of intrauterine life in man, when for the first time cells appear bearing lymphoid characteristics. In the bursa of Fabricius, which is found only in birds, the first lymphocytes appear on the fifteenth embryonic day. The abundance of lymphocytes in the thymus and bursa of Fabricius contrasts with the scarcity of these cells in the spleen, in the lymph nodes, in Peyer's patches, and in the serum during the embryonic stage of life. Lymphopoiesis becomes evi-

dent in these organs only after birth, possibly due to antigenic stimulus. In fact, animals born in sterile environments, despite having well-developed thymuses, possess poorly developed secondary lymphoid organs. In birds the development of secondary lymphoid organs is also accelerated by antigenic stimulus. However, this response of secondary organs to antigenic stimuli proceeds only in the presence of the thymus, thymectomized animals being incapable of such response. All these observations are compatible with the notion that most lymphocytes are differentiated in the thymus and in the bursa of Fabricius (or its equivalent in mammals), then migrate through the lymphatic circulation to the secondary lymphoid organs, where they localize and proliferate under antigenic stimulus.

Origin of the Lymphoid Cells of the Primary Lymphoid Organs

The origin of lymphocytes present in lymphoid organs has been extensively debated. Some have contended that these cells originated by differentiation of the embryonic epithelial reticulum of these organs, whereas others have held that lymphocytes of these organs were derived from undifferentiated mesenchymal cells that invaded the epithelial structures at an early stage. Although initially it was accepted that the lymphocytes of the thymus originated from the epithelium of the organ, more recent experiments with parabiosis and transfer of cells with labeled chromosomes to irradiated animals demonstrated that immature cells resembling hemocytoblasts migrate early to the blastema of the thymus and to the bursa of Fabricius, where they differentiate under the influence of the epithelium of these organs. The cells that migrate to these organs originate in the embryo, from the blood islands of the vitelline sac and from hematopoietic tissue of the liver and, in the adult, from the bone marrow.

Studies of regeneration of destroyed lymphoid tissue by transfusion of cells of diverse origins have shown that cells present in the bone marrow are responsible for the regeneration of lymphoid tissue. The morphology of this cell in the adult is not known. Thus, the repopulation of the primary lymphoid organs appears to depend upon undifferentiated cells that normally originate in the bone marrow and that either migrate to the thymus, where they differentiate and are transformed into immature T cells under the influence of the hormones produced by the epithelium of the organ, or mature in the bone marrow, are transformed into B cells, and migrate to the lymphatic system. It is thought that the cells that migrate from the bone marrow to the thymus are already specifically preconditioned to differentiate into T cells. Apparently, the cells of the bone marrow destined to be transformed into T cells have receptors for thymopoietine whereas the cells destined to differentiated into B cells do not.

Functional Properties of Primary Lymphoid Organs. The lymphoid cells of the primary organs are characterized by an intense proliferative activity that is independent of antigenic stimuli. For this reason, the mitotic activity of lymphoid populations of these organs is high even in the fetus and in animals born under aseptic conditions. This situation contrasts with that existing in secondary lymphoid organs, in which lymphopoiesis is practically nil in the fetus and even in the newborn, and continues as such in animals born and maintained in sterile environments. Furthermore, the cellular alterations that occur in secondary lymphoid organs in response to antigenic stimulus normally do not occur in primary lymphoid organs subjected to a stimulus of the same type. This, however, does not signify that the lymphoid cells of these organs are not modified in response to determined situations of antigenic stimulus. For example, thymic suppressor cells (i.e., cells, capable of specifically inhibiting the production of the antibody) can be obtained from the thymuses of hyperimmunized animals. The ablation of the primary lymphoid organs, if performed before they have an opportunity to promote the development of secondary lymphoid organs, prejudices the specific immunologic functions of the latter.

Immunologic Dichotomy of the Lymphoid System

In birds, there is a distinct dichotomy between the production of cells capable of evolving into antibody-producing cells – a process dependent on the bursa of Fabricius – and the production of cells capable of evolving into sensitized cells, which is a thymus-dependent process. Thus, bursectomized chicken do not exhibit primary or secondary responses (i.e., do not respond with formation of antibodies) after either a first or a second antigenic stimulus. However, cellular responses that depend upon the production of sensitized cells (e.g., the rejection of grafts) proceed normally because the development of cellular immunity depends upon the thymus. Removal of the thymus in birds, if performed just after hatching, leaves the immunoglobulin-producing system intact but seriously affects development of cellular immunity. In mammals, also, thymectomy diminishes the reactions of cellular immunity but has less impact on the antibody system. This finding indicates that a system corresponding to the bursa of Fabricius, i.e., one that regulates the development of antibody-producing cells, must develop in mammals. Certain syndromes of immunologic deficiency encountered in the clinic mimic, in man, the experimental surgical ablation of lymphoid organs in laboratory animals. In DiGeorge's syndrome, in which there is agenesis of the thymus, the cellular immunologic reactions are deficient, whereas the production of antibodies is practically normal. With other syndromes not associated with thymus anomalies, the opposite is true: One observes hypogammaglobulinemia, whereas the cellular immune reactions are normal. These clinical observations permit the deduction that in man there exists a thymus-dependent system that regulates the cell-based immunologic reactions, and another system whose function is similar to that of the bursa of Fabricius in birds, the components of which are unknown, and which regulates production of antibodies. It is probable that in mammals B lymphocytes originate and mature in the bone marrow leaving these organs directly to the secondary lymphoid organs where they settle and are activated and proliferate on contact with antigens.

Cells of the Immune System

Several types of cells participate in the defense system of organisms. In adults, they almost all originate, multiply and mature in the bone marrow, and are found in the mature stages in the blood, in which they either stay or from where they migrate into the tissue. Some of these cells act unspecifically and their activity is not altered by a first contact with antigen. These include granulocytes, monocytes, macrophages, platelets and mastocytes. Other cells act specifically and their activity is usually increased by a first contact with antigen. These are represented by the lymphocytes which are the immune cells *sensu strictu*, endowed with the capacity to recognize as well as to react specifically with foreign antigenic material via specific receptors.

Polymorphonuclear Cells

Metchnikoff, the great Russian zoologist, was the first to recognize a group of cells which played a major role in the defense of the organism against a great variety of extraneous invaders. Metchnikoff named the white cells of the blood microphages (now known as polymorphonuclear cells), believing them to be concerned solely with the defense of the organism against small microorganisms, i.e., bacteria, and designated as macrophages certain cells in the tissues because they phagocytozed large preys like parasites and other cells. The distinction is now known to be erroneous, since both cell types are capable of phagocytozing large and small particles.

The polymorphonuclear leukocytes constitute about 60%–70% of the total circulating leukocytes and are subdivided into three types, based on staining characteristics (Wright or Giemsa type stain): (1) neutrophils possess granules that do not stain intensively when viewed under the light microscope; (2) eosinophils have granules that stain a bright orange-red; and (3) basophils having granules that stain a dark blue-black. The normal range of total polymorphonuclear leukocytes is between 4,000 and 8,000 per mm³ of blood; the vast majority ($>90\%$) consist of the neutrophilic series.

All three lineages derive from a common pluripotent stem cell in the bone marrow (of adults) under the influence of granulopoietin probably identical to the "colony stimulating factor" (CSF); CSF has been partially characterized in serum and urine as a glycoprotein with a molecular weight of approximately 45,000. The earliest morphologically distinct *neutrophil* precursor is the myeloblast (Fig. 1.2), which has a large nucleus and very little cytoplasm. Granules begin to appear in the next, or promyelocyte stage and are very obvious in the myelocytes; because of their histochemical staining characteristics, the granules are referred to as azurophilic. They arise from the concave side of the Golgi-apparatus, are relatively large in size, and are electron dense. They contain acid hydrolases, lysozyme, myeloperoxidase, neutral proteases, cationic proteins with bactericidal activity and NADPH-oxidase.

As the cells continue to develop, the beginning of segmentation of the nucleus occurs in the metamyelocyte stage. At this stage, secondary or specific granules appear, which are smaller and less dense than azurophilic granules. The specific granules contain alkaline phosphatase, lysozyme, lactoferrin, and collagenase.

The band form and the mature neutrophil arise from the metamyelocyte stage and enter the circulation from the bone marrow (Fig. 1.3 A). The mature cells are virtually devoid of mitochondria. There is a large reserve of granulocyte precursors in the bone

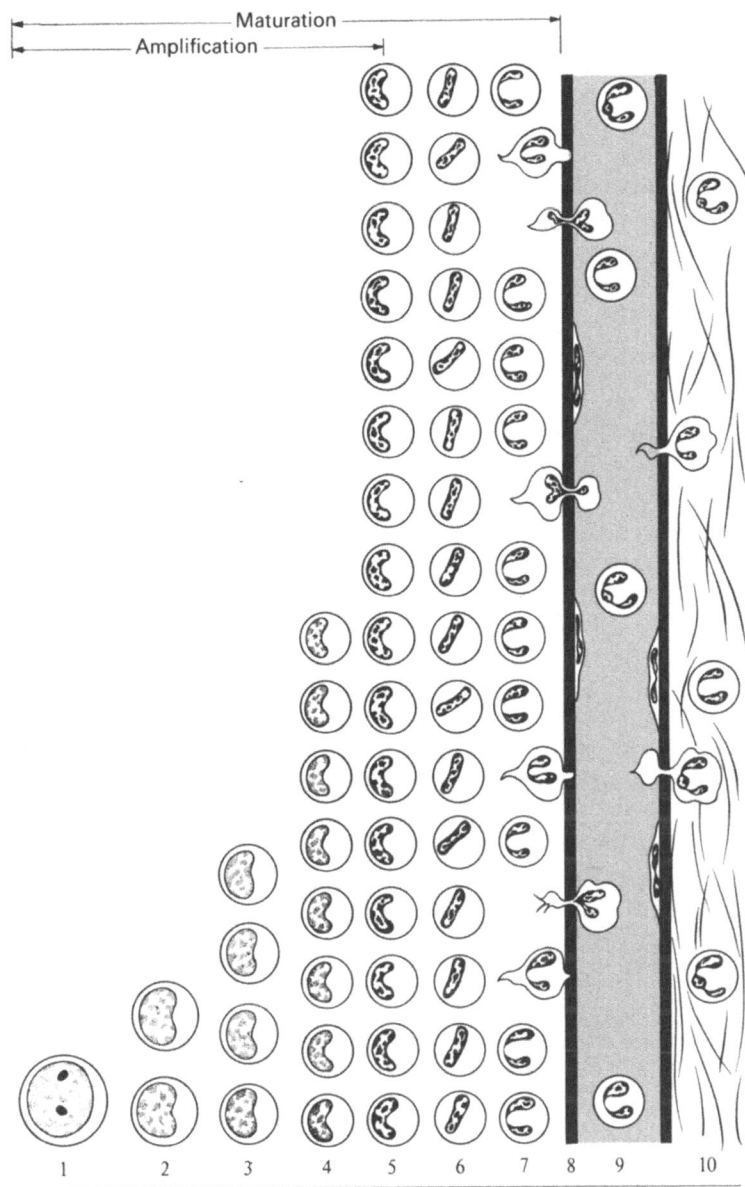

Maturation

Amplification

Fig. 1.2. Stages of granulocytopoesis. Left: bone marrow; middle: blood; right: tissue. *1* Myeloblast, *2* Promyelocyte, *3,4* Myelocyte, *5* Metamyelocyte, *6* Band, and *7–9* Segmented granulocyte. (Reproduced with permission from M. Bessis, 1977)

marrow; the complete maturation process requires approximately 9–11 days. Once in the circulation, however, the half-life of the mature neutrophil in the blood is only 6–8 h. This gives rise to an estimated neutrophil turnover of approximately 126 billion cells per day in a normal 70-kg individual. The largest number of granulocytes seem to be lost from the blood through the gastrointestinal tract. Granulocytes also pass from the blood vessels into the tissue, attracted by bacterial and other chemotactic substances, and die there quite rapidly. The death can occur by fragmentation or the cells may be phagocytized and rapidly digested by macrophages.

Neutrophils have a well developed capacity for locomotion when they are attached to a solid surface (endothelia). They extend a clear cytoplasmatic projection (protopod) in

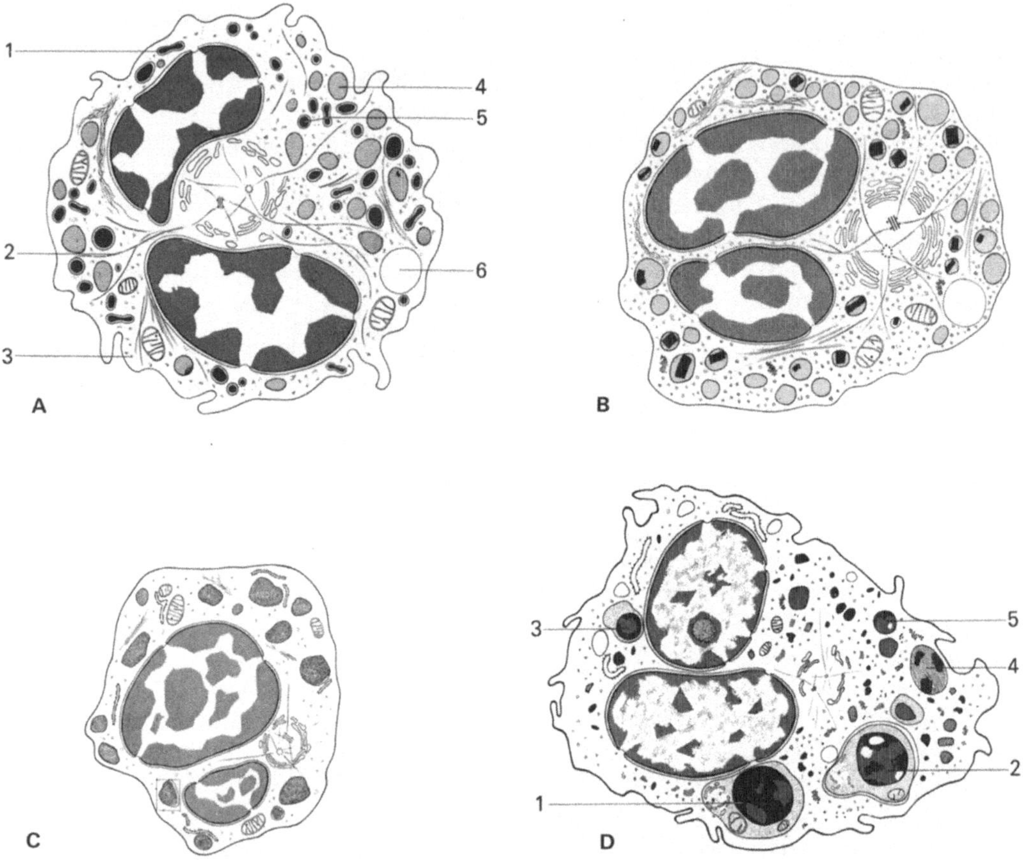

Fig. 1.3. Polymorphonuclear cells and monocyte. **A** Neutrophil PMN (band form); *1, 5*, neutrophilic granules; *2*, microtubules; *3*, glycogen particles; *4*, azurophilic granules; *6*, contractile vacuole. **B** Eosinophil; **C** Basophil; **D** Monocyte; 1–5 stages of digestion of phagocytized lymphocytes. (Reproduced with permission from M. Bessis, 1977)

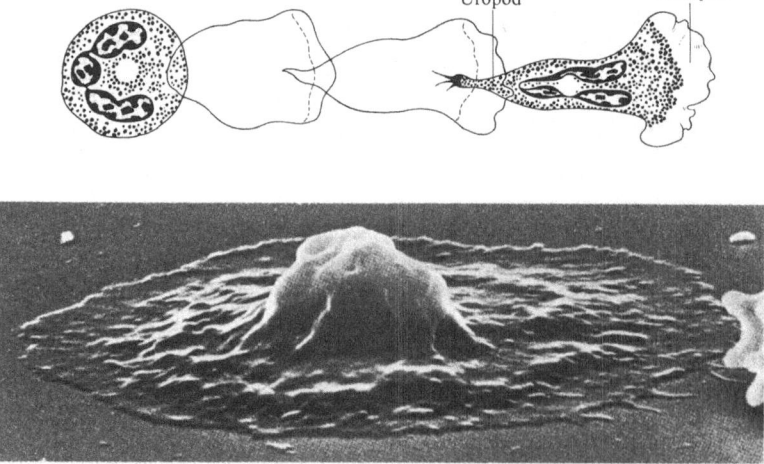

Fig. 1.4. Locomotion and spreading of a polymorphonuclear cell. (Reproduced with permission from M. Bessis, 1977)

the direction of locomotion, while the opposite end of the cell (uropod) is attached to the support by a number of filaments (Fig. 1.4). They easily adhere to surfaces, migrate into the tissue by diapedesis, and are able to phagocytoze microorganisms but also cells and inorganic substances of considerable size (erythrocytes, leukocytes, crystals).

Maturation of *eosinophils* parallels that of neutrophils, except that large eosinophilic granules take the place of neutrophilic granules in the myelocyte, in which the production of the secondary, specific granules starts. The granules are formed at the Golgi-complex in the same fashion as those of the neutrophils. Very recent findings suggest that the differentiation and maturation of eosinophils might be under control of their "own CSF", distinct from neutrophil CSF. The granules contain acid phosphatase, glycuronidase, cathepsin, ribonuclease, arylsulphatase, and other enzymes. Peroxidase is present but different from the myeloperoxidase of neutrophils. The eosine granules contain phospholipids as well as basic proteins (Fig. 1.3 B).

The mature eosinophils possess more and larger mitochondria than neutrophils, and their Golgi-apparatus is well developed. They have numerous glycogen particles.

The fate of eosinophils is unknown; some of them are phagocytized, others are probably eliminated through the intestinal tract and the lungs. The eosinophils respond to the same chemotactic stimuli as neutrophils, but particularly to soluble bacterial factors and antigen-antibody-complexes. They play a particular role in allergies and helminthic infections (see Chap. 11, p. 344).

The maturation of *basophils* runs a course very similar to the one of neutrophils and eosinophils, except that metachromatic granules are produced. The earliest identifiable granules are formed in the Golgi complex during the promyelocyte stage and contain abundant glycogen deposits in their cytoplasm. The mature basophil has numerous large and opaque granules masking the nucleus (Fig. 1.3 C). The granules contain acid mucopolysaccharides, histamine, and heparin in large quantities, and numerous enzymes, e.g. dehydrogenases, diaphorase, histidin-carboxylase, and peroxidases. The movement of basophils is ameboid and is similar to the movement of eosinophils though less active. The basophils have little phagocytic capability. They possess on their surface receptors for IgG and IgE as well as C 3 b. Nothing is known about life span and death.

Mast Cells

Mast cells are connective tissue cells which contain granules that stain metachromatically. The granules are rich in histamine and other pharmacologically active substances. In addition, these cells also contain heparin proteoglicans that serve to store preformed chemical mediators and are responsible for the metachromatic staining of the granules. Mast cells are widely distributed in the body but are particularly concentrated in places which are in contact with antigens such as the subepithelial connective tissue of the respiratory, intestinal and urinary systems. Free mast cells are found in the peritonial cavities of rats and mice. The free mast cells have been widely used in studying the mechanism of the anaphylactic histamine release. They provided the first evidence showing that the anaphylactic antibody-antigen (Ab-Ag) reaction occurs on the membrane of these cells (see Chap. 10). More recently, techniques have been developed for the isolation of the mast cells by enzymatic or mechanical dissociation of intact tissues such as the lungs.

Mammals contain two distinct types of mast cells that differ in their morphology, histochemical staining and location. One type, abundant in the normal connective tissue of most organs, can be obtained from the peritoneal cavity of rodents and forms the basis of our classical knowledge of mast cells. The other type is usually referred to as mucosal mast cells because in normal rats it has been observed only in mucosal tissue. Infection with helminth parasites induces an extensive accumulation of mast cells and eosinophils in the tissues. Parasites of the mucous surface, in particular, stimulate a rapid hyperplasia of mucosal mast cells. Both mucosal mast cells and connective tissue mast cells derive from a bone marrow precursor. However, unlike connective mast cells, mucosal mast cells require the thymus for differentiation. Apparently, progenitors of mucosal mast cells leave the bone marrow and locate in the intestinal mucosa where they proliferate and differentiate under the effect of a growth-stimulating factor produced in this tissue by T lymphocytes which have reached the place from mesenteric lymph nodes. IL-3, a lymphokine produced by activated T lymphocytes is a absolute requirement for the growth of a number of haemopoietic cell lines including the mast cell progeny. The role of mast cell in anaphylaxis is discussed in Chap. 10.

Monocytes

The monocyte lineage comprises a variety of phagocytic cells, related by origin and function, which include the blood monocyte, alveolar (lung) macrophages, peritoneal macrophages, Kupffer cells in the liver, free and fixed macrophages of the bone marrow (osteoclasts) and lymphatic tissue, and histiocytes in tissues. It is generally believed that all of these cells are derived from bone marrow monoblasts and promonocytes, that they enter the blood stream as monocytes, and later the tissue to develop into macrophages.

The precursor cell of the monocyte in the bone marrow is unknown, but most probably, it derives from a stem cell common with granulocytes and thrombocytes. Monocytes vary considerably in size, i.e., from 20 to 40 μm in diameter, they have a large, usually kidney-shaped nucleus. The chromatin appears pale and has lace-like or reticular appearance without compact chromatin blocks. The cytoplasm is ample, greyish-blue and has fine azurophilic granulations. Cytoplasmic vacuoles are quite common (Fig. 1.3 D).

Monocytes stay in the circulation between 15 and 30 h, after which they leave the blood randomly and regardless of age, by diapedesis, after they have become adherent. In sites of inflammation, they accumulate very rapidly. The daily monocyte turnover is approximately 7×10^6 cells per hour per kg body weight.

The life span of macrophages is long and can attain 75 days and more. The death of monocytes and histiocytes proceeds in an unknown manner, but it is known that the cells when damaged and particularly after intense phagocytosis can, in turn, be phagocytized by other macrophages.

Monocytes adhere very well to solid surfaces, have a locomotion similar, though more slow, to the one of PMN, possess a quite marked sensitivity for chemotactic stimuli, and are very actively phagocytic. They may ingest a variety of cells, including protozoa, bacilli, viruses as well as antigen-antibody complexes, and a variety of inorganic substances (carbon, silica, asbestos, a. o.). They are endowed with receptors for immunoglobulins (Fc receptors) and complement components (C 3 b receptor) (see Chap. 5).

Lymphocytes

The lymphocytic lineage consists of a succession of cells which, starting with the committed stem cell, leads to the production of the small lymphocyte. Morphologically, it comprises the lymphoblast, the large lymphocyte, and the small lymphocyte (Fig. 1.5 B and C). In stained blood smears (Wright or Giemsa staining), lymphoblasts (15–20 μm in size) have a round or oval nucleus. The cytoplasm is sharply delineated, scanty, and basophilic. Large lymphocytes (9–15 μm in size) have a large nucleus, usually eccentric, the cytoplasm is scant, moderately basophil, or a light blue, and contains azurophilic granules (lysosomes). Small lymphocytes (6–9 μm in size) have a round, indented nucleus, and scanty cytoplasm often barely visible.

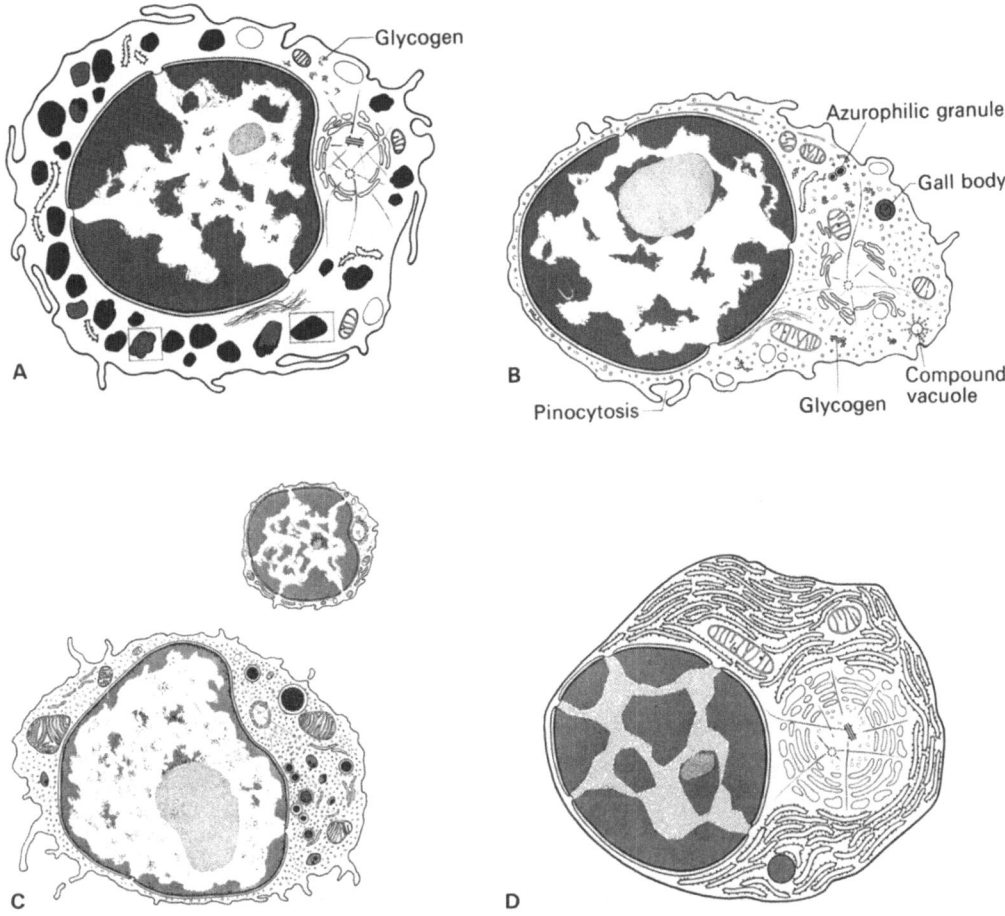

Fig. 1.5 A–D. Lymphocytes and mastocytes. **A** Mastocyte. **B** Lymphoblast. **C** Small lymphocytes with indentation of the nucleus caused by the centrosome and a transformed lymphocyte. **D** Plasmocyte (Reproduced with permission from M. Bessis, 1977)

The maturation and differentiation of lymphocytes diverges at the stage of pre-lymphoblasts or lymphoblasts into two sublineages, which are not distinguishable by morphological criteria: part of the lymphocytes differentiates in the thymus (thymus-derived, or T lymphocytes), the other part in the bone marrow (bone-marrow, or B lymphocytes).

T Lymphocytes. In the mouse embryo, lymphocytes originate in the fetal liver on about the eleventh day of gestation. These large basophilic blast-like cells gradually accumulate by migration into the thymus and begin to proliferate. Ultrastructurally, these basophilic cells are large and have the typical morphology of lymphoblasts, with copious dense cytoplasm filled with ribosomes but relatively few other organelles and a large nucleus that contains prominent nucleoli. The proliferation of these cells results in the production of typical small thymic cortical lymphocytes. By other than morphological studies, the intrathymic small lymphocytes can be subdivided into two populations: a major group accounts for about 90% of the total; they are small, dense, and short lived, located predominantly in the cortex, and express the TL antigen, high levels of Thy-1 antigen but low levels of H-2 antigens (these antigens are cell-surface markers which can be detected by serological methods and are explained in more detail in forthcoming chapters), and are cortisone sensitive. The minor population which appears to be the functionally active group, is also composed of small lymphocytes, though they are generally larger and less dense than the major group. This minor population, located mainly in the thymic medulla, is cortisone resistant and differs antigenically in being TL negative and expressing high levels of H-2 antigens but low levels of Thy-1 antigen.

The high rate of intrathymic mitotic activity and the differentiation of the stem cells are independent of antigenic stimuli and are probably under some as yet poorly understood thymic epithelial cell influence. There are indications that the induction of mitotic activity is in some way due to close contact between lymphocytes and cortical epithelial cells.

T Lymphocytes Alloantigens. *Thy-1* – One of the first alloantigens studied in the T lymphocytes was the Thy-1 (formerly Theta). This alloantigen was discovered during immunization of C3H mice with thymocytes from AKR mice. It was observed that the antiserum obtained reacted with AKR thymocytes but not with C3H thymocytes. Conversely, antiserum obtained by injecting C3H thymocytes into AKR mice reacted with C3H thymocytes but not with AKR thymocytes. These results showed that the thymocytes of these two strains had alloantigens. When thymocytes from other strains were tested with these antisera, it was observed that most of them reacted with anti-C3H serum (for instance DBA/2, B1O, BALB/c, CBA, and C57B1/6) and that only some of them reacted with the anti-AKR serum. This showed that there are two alleles controlling the expression of Thy-1. Some strains have the C3H allele and others have the AKR allele. This antigen is also present in the brain and in the cells of epidermis. Addition of an anti-Thy-1 serum plus complement to a suspension of lymphoid cells destroys the T lymphocytes leaving intact the B lymphocytes.

Lyt antigens – These alloantigens are present exclusively on T lymphocytes. There are three distinct Lyt loci, Lyt-1 on chromosome 19 and Lyt-2 and Lyt-3 on chromosome 6. Each of these loci has two alleles, and each allele codes for two alternate antigens designates 1 and 2. Lyt-1 and Lyt-2 alloantigens exists in two allelic forms: Lyt-1.1 and Lyt 1.2, and Lyt-2.1 and Lyt-2.2. All strains have the alloantigens Lyt-1, Lyt-2 and Lyt-3, but the allelic forms differ in different strains. All thymocytes and T lymphocytes present one allelic form of these antigens but each T lymphocyte does not present all of them. Cantor and Boyse found that 33% of the peripheral T lymphocytes are Lyt-1$^+$, 10% are Lyt-2,3$^+$ and 50% are Lyt-1$^+$, 2,3$^+$. Using antisera specific for these antigens (+complement) it was possible to destroy specifically functionally different T lymphocytes subpopulations. Thus T helper cells are Lyt-1$^+$, whereas suppressor and cytotoxic T lymphocytes are Lyt-2,3$^+$. During pre-natal life the first cells to appear are Lyt-1$^+$, 2,3^1 and only later appear Lyt-1$^+$ and Lyt-2,3$^+$ cells. In mice, there is a balance among these three subpopulation of T lymphocytes. The activity of the T suppressor and T cytotoxic cells would be controlled by the Lyt-1$^+$, 2,3$^+$ lymphocytes that would exert a regulatory effect on the two first subpopulations. An increase in the functional activity of the helper T lymphocytes would induce through a feed-back mechanism an increase of the T suppressor cells. Whereas an increase in T suppressor cells would result in an increase in the helper T cell activity.

Qa alloantigens – The series of mouse alloantigens designated Qa are coded for by five linked loci which are located between H-2D and Tla on chromosome 17. Qa1 and Qa2 are present on thymus cells as well as on peripheral T lymphocytes, whereas Qa3, Qa4 and Qa5 are present on peripheral T lymphocytes.

TL – This antigen was first detected in thymus leukemia. TL antigen is expressed on the thymocytes of only certain strains. It is a differentiation antigen which appears on the prothymocyte when it enters the thymus and dissappears from these cells when they leave the organ to the periphery. It then serves as a marker for thymocytes.

GIX – Some cell membrane associated viral glycoproteins in infected cells may mimic alloantigens. The most well known of these is GIX, a glycoprotein constitutent of the Gross leukemia virus which distributes in T lymphocytes similarly to TL.

B lymphocyte. In the mouse fetus, B lymphocytes arise in the liver at about 14 days of gestation (in adults in the bone marrow); these cells are larger than normal B lymphocytes, they divide rapidly and synthesize small amounts of monomeric IgM. These cells, called pre-B cells, contain cytoplasmic IgM but do not bear on their external surface the stable immunoglobulin receptors which characterize B lymphocytes. Pre-B cells lack most of the surface components characteristic of the majority of mature B lymphocytes: functional surface antibody receptors, Fc-receptors for IgG, and receptors for C3, a complement component. It is also unlikely that pre-B cells will be found to express surface receptors for T helper factors (see Chap. 6). The absence of these functional receptors serves to protect them from influences exerted by contact with antigens, antigen-antibody complexes, and activated C3. In this stage, clonal diversification has occured, i.e., selective expression of immunoglobulin genes present either on the paternal or on the maternal chromosomes, selective expression of either kappa (κ) or lambda (λ) light chains, and expression of different sets of genes encoding light- and heavy-chain variable regions (V_L and V_H). The expression of V gene products in pre-B cells implies that the genetic translocation event (see Chap. 4) has occured by this stage of differentiation. By this time, each small pre-B cell is ready to become on

sIgM$^+$ B lymphocyte, its antibody specificity is determined.

Expression of sIgM (secrete IgM) antibodies signals the onset of B lymphocyte differentiation. The gradual acquisition of receptors for activated C3 and IgG and of other classes of surface Ig appears.

Within a given clone of B lymphocytes, all cells are committed to the synthesis of antibodies of identical specificity, but some members become genetically programmed to convert from IgM antibody synthesis to synthesis of IgG, IgA, or IgE antibodies. At this stage, B lymphocytes express sIgD in addition to either IgM, IgA, or IgE. After mature sIgD$^+$ B lymphocytes are triggered by antigens (or mitogens), sIgD expression is rapidly reduced to low or undetectable levels (Fig. 1.6).

When B cells with all of these receptors are stimulated by the appropriate antigens and T helper cells, they may respond with division giving rise to memory B lymphocytes and with further differentiation into mature plasma cells. Thus memory cells are generated by antigen-driven expansion of B cell clones. Contrary to red blood cells and platelets (see below) whose entire functional life takes place in the blood, and unlike mature granulocytes, which leave the blood vessels without entering them again, lymphocytes leave the circulation and return to it many times in the course of their life. They leave the blood stream predominantly in the lymphoid spaces of the tissue, are taken up by the lymphatics, and after traversing one or more lymph nodes return to the blood stream by way of the thoracic duct.

The life span is believed to be 10–20 days for nonstimulated lymphocytes; committed lymphocytes may live several months or even years.

The peripheral blood of man contains about 3,000 lymphocytes per mm³, 70%–80% are T lymphocytes and 15%–20% are B lymphocytes, the rest being difficult to classify. About 85% of the lymphocytes in thoracic duct are T lymphocytes, about 80% in lymph nodes, and about 35% of the lymphocytes of the spleen are T cells.

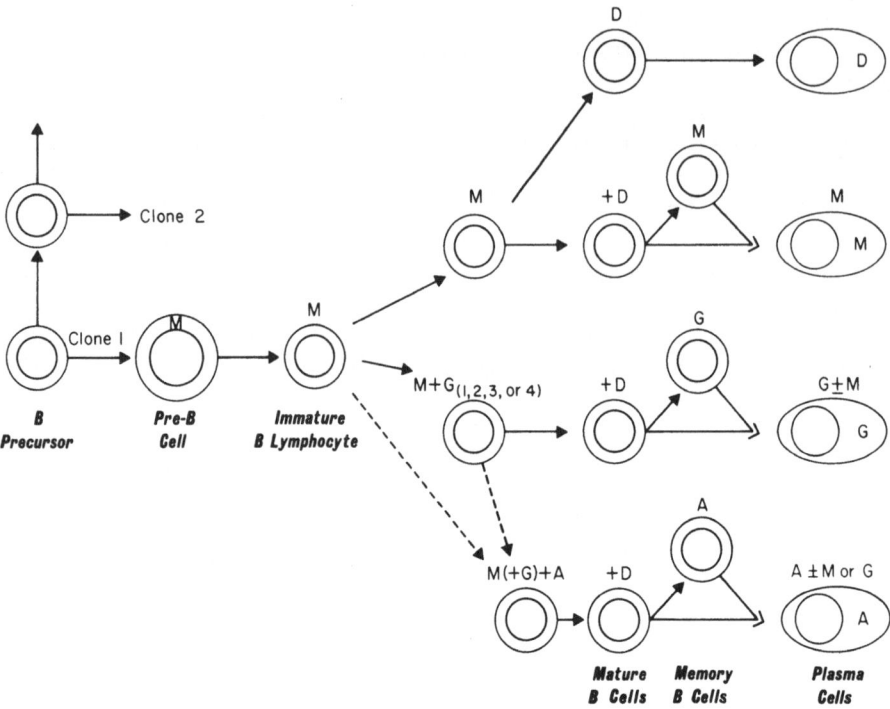

Fig. 1.6. Model illustrating some of the different stages in differentiation of a B cell clone. It outlines the present view of the intraclonal generation of immunoglobulin class or isotype diversity. The pivotal cell type in the switch is the immature surface IgM$^+$ lymphocyte which may mature to express other Ig classes. Each of the cell types depicted in this diagram represents multiple cells. For example, each maturing sIgM$^+$ cell that begins to express IgG makes only one of the four IgG subclasses (see Chap. 4). Thus there are multiple sublines of B cells within the clone which are capable of differentiation into mature plasma cells secreting the various subclasses of IgG antibodies. Two pathways leading from sIgM$^+$ to sIgA$^+$ expression are indicated by arrows since the available evidence suggests that both may be possible. sIgD is a late expression on all of the B cell sublines and, except for the subline of IgD producing cells, is lost after antigen or mitogen stimulation. (Reproduced with permission from Cooper et al., 1979)

Plasma cells. These are the final stage of fully differentiated B lymphocytes. They are usually oval, the nucleus is almost always situated at one pole. The arrangement of the chromatin is characteristic: the chromocenters from seven to nine large blocks of approximately polygonal outline, resembling a tortoise shell or a "cartwheel" picture. In stained smear preparations, the cytoplasma is intensely basophilic and its ultramarine colour identifies them immediately (Fig. 1.5D). Under normal conditions, they are rarely found in the blood. Lymph nodes and particularly their medullary cords are rich in plasmocytes, they are also present in the spleen, bone marrow, and the intestine.

Plasma cells develop from stimulated B lymphocytes within 2–3 days and probably die within a few days.

Platelets

Thrombocytes, or platelets, are non-nucleated cells liberated into the circulation from megakaryocytes in the bone marrow. Thrombocytic cells are derived from a committed stem cell susceptible to the action of thrombopoietin and, in turn, derived from a pluripotential cell. In contrast to other cell lineages in which multiplication (amplification) is accomplished by the successive duplication of DNA accompanied by cell divi-

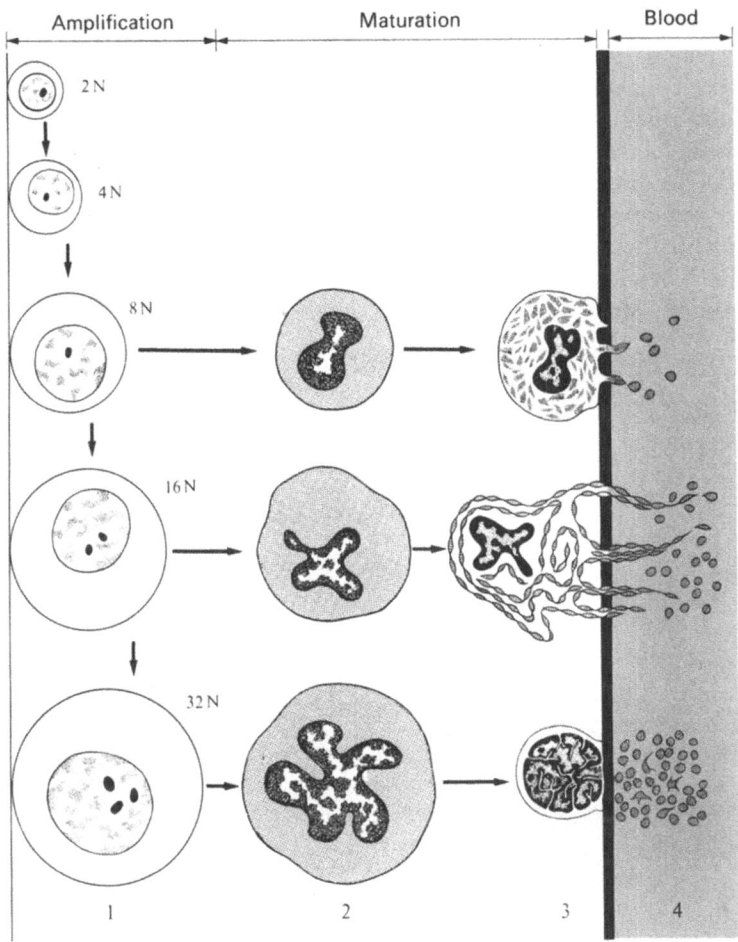

Fig. 1.7. Different stages of thrombopoesis. *1* Basophilic megakaryocytes (amplification=polyploidization 2 N to 32 N); *2* granular megakaryocyte; *3* platelet-forming megakaryocyte and liberation of platelets; *4* platelets in the circulation. Maturation starts after amplification has been completed. (Reproduced with permission from M. Bessis, 1977)

sion (see Fig. 1.2), megakaryocytes multiply their DNA (about four-times) without cytoplasmic division. Amplification thus consists of polyploidization of the cell. The cells enlarge during amplification but maturation takes place almost exclusively after amplification is completed (Fig. 1.7). Maturation includes lobulation of the nucleus, increase in cytoplasm, appearance of granules, and later, of platelet territories. Four stages of maturation can be distinguished: basophilic, granular and, platelet-producing megakaryocytes, and platelets. The total matura-

tion time is estimated to be 34 h. A 32 N megakaryocyte produces approximately 4,000 platelets.

Platelets measure 2–5 µm in diameter, they contain microtubules, microfilaments, granules, vacuoles, canaliculi, mitochondria, and inclusions (glycogen).

The granules are of several types: azurophilic granules, the content of which is still being debated. Dense granules are storage sites of serotonin (5-hydroxytryptamine) which is made by the enterochromaffin cells of the intestine and picked up by the circulating platelets from the plasma. The dense granules also contain calcium and nucleotides. Catalase has been identified in perioxisomes which are also small vesicles. Platelets secrete all of these substances as well as platelet factor 4 and fibrinogen during the "release" reaction (see below).

Platelets play a role in adhesion and aggregation. They are capable of endocytosis. Various stimuli, e.g. contact to foreign surfaces, but also thrombin, proteolytic enzymes, bacterial endotoxin, and collagen, can trigger the release of their granules.

Immunologic Activity of the Primary Lymphoid Organs

Thymus

The thymus is located in the thorax immediately behind the upper portion of the breastbone (sternum). Its two lobes are enveloped by a thin capsule of connective tissue that emits prolongations or septula that penetrate the organ and divide it into incomplete overlapping lobes. The peripheral part of each lobe, the cortex, is composed of dense lymphoid tissue, whereas the central portion or medulla is loosely arranged lymphoid tissue. The lobes may be considered a three-dimensional mesh of epithelial cells in whose networks are found lymphoid cells. These are much more numerous in the cortex than in the medulla. In the thymus, the lymphoid tissues do not form nodules as in other structures of this tissue. In the medulla are found Hassal's corpuscles, structures typical of this organ, formed by a central part containing concentric layers of epithelial cells (Fig. 1.8). The origin and nature of these corpuscles are unknown. The capillaries and small vessels of the thymus possess special structural features, including a thick basement membrane and an enveloping layer of epithelial cells, that is also supported by a basement membrane. Even though the epithelial membrane is not totally continuous, it acts as a barrier that impedes, but does not totally prevent, the passage of macromolecules present in the blood into the interior of the parenchyma and consequently into contact with the lymphocytes of the organ. The thymus does not possess lymphatic circulation – only efferent lymphatics that pass through the septula and upon leaving the organ lead to the lymph nodes of the mediastinum.

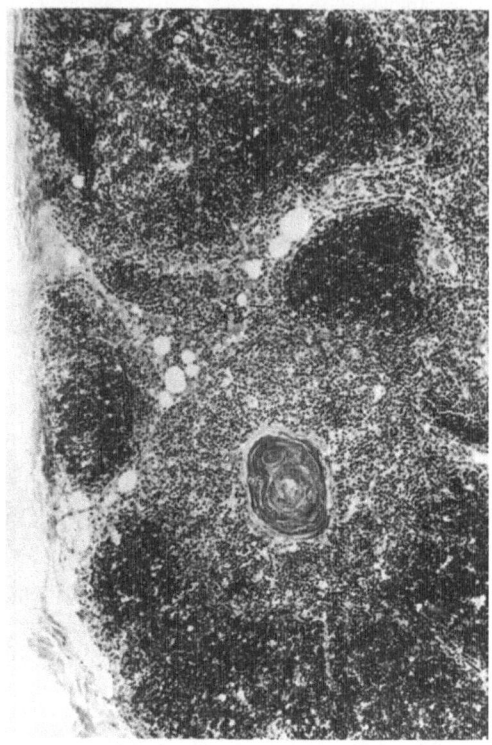

Fig. 1.8. Photomicrograph of human thymus, showing Hassal's corpuscles. (Courtesy of LC Junqueira and J Carneiro, Instituto de Ciências Biomédicas, Universidade de São Paulo)

Mitotic Activity of Lymphocytes of the Thymus. The intensity of production of lymphocytes in the thymus is much greater than that of the other lymphoid organs of the organism. It has been calculated that in the mouse 1 mg of thymic tissue produces approximately 1 million lymphocytes per day. The number of mitoses in this organ is five to ten times that in the lymph nodes or in the Peyer's patches. This mitotic activity is greater in the neonate, thereafter diminishing with age. The majority of the mitoses occur in the cortex, mitoses being rare in the medulla.

The proliferative activity of lymphoid cells of the thymus has been studied through the injection of tritiated thymidine. After a single dose of this substance, only labeled large lymphocytes appear initially; later labeled small lymphocytes appear in increasing numbers. The accumulation of labeled lymphocytes is, as would be expected, much greater in the thymus than in the other lymphoid structures. When observed over a period of time, the augmentation in the percentage of labeled lymphocytes follows a linear distribution. Since 50% of the lymphocytes are labeled within 2 days, the population of lymphocytes in the organ must therefore be substituted every 4 days. However, since the percentage of labeled cells present 4 days after the injection of tritiated thymidine is only 95%, it may be deduced that the remaining 5% must have a greater life span. Since the size of the thymus remains constant for periods in excess of 4 days, this rapid production of cells must be offset by a loss of equal magnitude, either through the destruction or the migration of these cells.

Destiny of Lymphocytes of the Thymus. The possibility that lymphocytes migrate from the thymus to other lymphoid organs was initially suggested by the observation of histologic preparations of this organ, which suggested diapedesis of these cells to the inside of the vessels. Furthermore, large numbers of lymphocytes were found in blood collected from the veins of this organ. In subsequent studies, tritiated thymidine was injected directly into the thymus in quantities adjusted so as to label just the cells of that organ. Later observations of histologic sections taken from other organs indicated that cells labeled with thymidine had migrated to the lymph nodes and to the spleen. However, the number of migrated cells was always small. The same results were obtained when mice thymectomized just after birth were subjected to thymic grafts from syngeneic newborn donor mice whose cells contained labeled chromo-

somes. In this case also, only a small number of donor cells were discovered in the lymph nodes and spleen of the recipient. These results, which indicate that only a small proportion of the thymic lymphocytes migrate to other lymphoid organs, imply that the great majority of lymphocytes generated in this organ is destroyed in situ. There is evidence that some of the lymphocytes leaving the thymus home to the spleen, whereas others home to the lymph nodes. The spleen-seeking lymphocytes are short-lived, cortisone sensitive cells that locate selectively in the red pulp; the lymph node-seeking lymphocytes are long-lived cortisone resistant cells that locate selectively in the thymus-dependent areas of the lymph nodes and spleen.

Effect of Thymectomy. Until 1961, when for the first time the effect of thymectomy was studied in newborn animals, numerous attempts to illuminate the functions of the thymus failed. Only then was it observed that removal of this organ in the first hours after birth resulted in noticeable diminution in the development and function of lymphoid tissue (Fig. 1.9). Thus, within 2–3 months following thymectomy, the quantity of circulating lymphocytes diminishes – particularly the small lymphocytes – and the lymphoid organs exhibit a significant reduction in volume. For example, the number of lymphocytes that may be drained from the thoracic duct of the rat in a 48-h period, though normally in the range of 100 million, falls to just 3 or 4 million following thymectomy. The intensity of these effects varies, however, with the degree of development of the lymphoid organs at birth – the less developed, the greater the effects of the thymectomy. In the mouse and in the rat, the organ must be removed no later than 48 h after birth, for after the third postnatal day, the effects of the thymectomy approximate those obtained in the adult, where only a slight depression in the number of lymphocytes occurs. Apparently, once stimulated by the functioning of the thymus, the secondary lymphoid organs under normal conditions

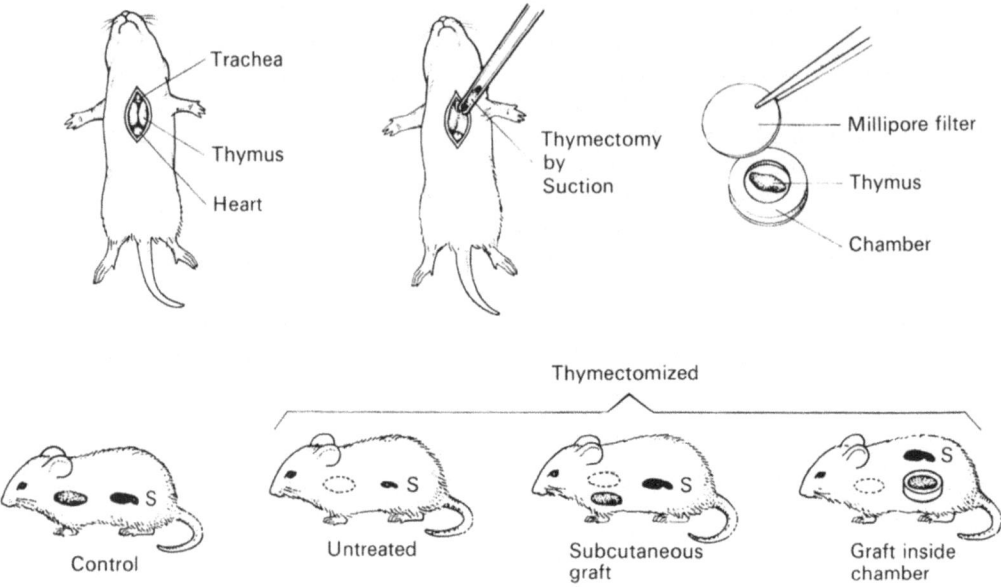

Fig. 1.9. Protocol of experiment showing thymectomy followed by reimplantation of the organ in a free state or enclosed within a Millipore chamber. The Millipore chamber permits the passage of macromolecules but not of cells. The experiments, performed with newborn mice, demonstrate that the presence of the thymus, even in conditions that make migration of cells to other organs impossible, permits the development of immunologic functions that are prejudiced by thymectomy. The development of the lymphoid organs is indicated by the size of the spleen (S) (Adapted from Levey RH (1964) The thymus hormone. Sc American 211:66)

become relatively self-sufficient. The thymus is the first lymphoid organ to appear during embryogenesis, whereas the spleen and the lymph nodes develop as lymphoid organs only later from cells that migrate from the thymus and the bone marrow to these organs.

In the lymphoid organs, the diminution in the lymphoid population induced by thymectomy occurs selectively in certain areas. For example, there is an accentuated diminution of lymphocytes in the paracortical areas of the lymph nodes (see section "Lymph Nodes" in this chapter) and in the periarterial sheaths of the spleen and of the diffuse lymphoid tissue of the Peyer's patches. Accordingly, such regions are termed *thymus dependent*. These are the areas through which the small lymphocytes circulate in their path from the blood to the lymph. As we have seen in the discussion of lymphocytes, all the experimental evidence favors the idea that the majority of circulat-

ing small lymphocytes constitutes a class of cells whose development depends upon the normal functioning of the thymus. On the other hand, the lymphoid nodules, the germinal centers of the spleen, and the lymph nodes are not altered by thymectomy, being composed of *thymus-independent* cells (B lymphocytes). The number of plasma cells present in these organs and in the connective tissue also ordinarily remains unaffected after thymectomy.

Importance of the Thymus in the Production of Antibodies. As we have seen, in animals thymectomized shortly after birth there is a cessation in the development of cellular immunity. Animals in this condition do not demonstrate delayed hypersensitivity of rejection of grafts; humoral immunity – reflected in the level of immunoglobulins and in the production of antibodies in response to some antigens – is normal. However, most antigens suffer a reduction in their immunogenic capacity in thymectomized mice. Antigens whose immunogenic capacity is impaired in thymectomized animals, are termed thymus-dependent antigens. The depression and restoration of the humoral response to these antigens, particularly to sheep erythrocytes in mice, became a model for the study of the immunologic functions of the thymus. The humoral response to these antigens requires the interaction of thymus-dependent cells with thymus-independent cells (see discussion of cooperation between T lymphocytes and B lymphocytes, Chaps. 2 and 6). This conclusion is based upon experiments in which mice incapable of forming antibodies against sheep erythrocytes after neonatal thymectomy evidence a restoration in the ability to produce antibodies after reimplantation of their thymus. An interaction between cells of the thymus and cells that are precursors of cells that form antibodies was first demonstrated by injecting thymectomized and irradiated mice with sheep erythrocytes mixed with cells of the thymus, the bone marrow, or of both. The humoral response of the mice infected with both types of cells always exceeded the sum of the responses induced by each of the individual cell types.

As we have seen, the cells that synthesize antibodies (B lymphocytes) develop independently of the thymus, generally speaking, whereas the cells responsible for the cell-based immune reaction require the thymus in order to develop immunologic competence. Nevertheless, both cell systems – T and B lymphocytes must work together in order to mount a mature, humoral immune response. This collaboration is discussed in greater detail elsewhere (see Chaps. 2 and 6).

Functions of the Thymus in the Adult. In man, the thymus continues to grow after birth and attains its maximum size at about 15 years of age, after which it slowly involutes. In the mouse, the organ continues to grow for 2 months after birth. Despite this, a thymectomy performed a few days after birth does not cause the dramatic effects produced when performed immediately after birth. Ordinarily, thymectomy in the adult produces only a slight drop in the number of lymphocytes and in the weight of the lymphoid organs. T lymphocytes represent long-lived cells that make up part of the pool of circulating lymphocytes; as a result, the effects of thymectomy appear only after a lengthy period of months in the mouse and of years in man. Accordingly, the thymectomized adults ordinarily do not sicken, but apparently remain in normal health. However, under certain conditions, harmful effects may be observed in the thymectomized adult. Thus, animals sublethally irradiated, in which a dramatic reduction in hematocytopoiesis occurs, do survive – recovering their immunologic activity within 2–3 weeks. Yet when the animal has been thymectomized prior to irradiation, it does not then fully recover its immunologic activity. Apparently, despite total regeneration of the bone marrow, undifferentiated cells, which normally migrate to the thymus, do not, in the absence of this organ, develop into mature lymphoid cells. This indicates that the thymus is necessary in the adult to compensate for attrition in the population of lymphocytes already immunologically differentiated. This attrition, which occurs slowly under normal conditions, may occur rapidly in exceptional circumstances. It should be noted that thymectomized adult mice, when observed for many months, reveal what is frequently verifiable as a noticeable diminution in their immune responses.

Effects of Thymic Grafts in Thymectomized Animals. Animals that are immunologically deficient due to thymectomy regain their immunologic functions upon receipt of a grafted thymus. The grafted organ functions the same even if it is allogeneic or if its lymphoid cells have been destroyed by irradiation. Regeneration of the grafted thymus occurs slowly; 1 or 2 days after the graft is performed, the transplanted organ consists of a necrotic central mass and a peripheral area of live tissue consisting of lymphoid and reticular cells. The central necrosis results from nutritional deficiency due to lack of circulation. The cells in the peripheral area remain viable, receiving nutrients locally available through diffusion of tissue fluid. From the third day on, the mitotic activity of the surviving tissue increases, and within 5–6 days the typical structure of the organ is regenerated, with its lobules and cortical and medullary areas totally regenerated.

It was thought initially that the transplanted thymus, once regenerated, dispatched its own cells to the secondary lymphoid organs, thus repopulating them. However, analysis of the contribution of the recipient of the engrafted thymus to the process of regeneration revealed that events transpire differently. Animals whose cells contained chromosomal markers were recipients of the grafts. It was shown that, although initially the cells that proliferated in the transplanted organ had originated exclusively in the donor, beginning with the third week, the proliferating population of the graft consisted of cells from the recipient. Moreover, the lymphoid cells that then appeared in the secondary lymphoid organs also originated from the recipient. When the lymphoid cells of the engrafted thymus were destroyed previously by irradiation, the initial phase of regeneration by donor cells failed to occur, but the graft functioned and the animal nevertheless recuperated immunologically. If, however, the recipient animal also had been irradiated previously, the graft endured only as an epithelial structure without ever becoming lymphoid in character.

Origin and Differentiation of Lymphocytes of the Thymus. Results of experiments that restore immunologic function in thymectomized animals, achieved through the engrafting of another thymus, are completely compatible with the notion that lymphoid cells do not originate from the epithelium of that organ. Rather, they originate from cells that migrate to this organ through the circulation. It now appears definitely established that during the embryonic stage undiffer-

entiated cells migrate from the yolk sac and from the liver (centers of myeloid hematopoiesis in the embryo) to the thymus. There, in contact with the epithelium of the organ, they proliferate and differentiate both functionally and structurally, acquire new antigens in their membranes, such as the TL and Thy-1 (theta, θ) antigens of mice.

The TL antigen is present only on the thymocytes and on thymus leukemia cells. The Thy-1 antigen is present on thymocytes and on the surfaces of lymphocytes originating from the thymus. The TL antigen is lost when the thymocytes leave the thymus. The Thy-1 antigen may thus serve as a marker for lymphocytes originating in the thymus but appearing in other lymphoid organs. Undifferentiated cells appear in the thymus of mice around the 11th day of embryonic life, at which point they still do not bear Thy-1 or TL antigens on their surfaces. About 8 days after this, these cells take on the aspect of lymphoid cells, from which point they have these antigens on their surfaces. Cell populations undergoing mitosis and lymphocytes are sensitive to radiation; thus, the hematopoietic cells of animals subjected to a lethal dose of X-rays are destroyed, including the lymphoid cells of the thymus. Lethally irradiated animals can be saved by transfusion of cells taken from the bone marrow of normal syngeneic donors. In such cases, not only the bone marrow is repopulated, but also the lymphoid cells of the thymus and the secondary lymphoid organs. Under the same conditions, other transfused lymphoid cells – whether obtained from the lymph, from the lymph nodes, or from the thymus – failed to repopulate. Myeloid cells of the donor proliferate initially in the bone marrow and the thymus and appear only later in the lymph nodes. Identical results were obtained through experiments involving transplantation of the thymus in which cells of this organ were rendered identifiable through chromosome markers. In this case, although the regeneration of the lymphoid population of the transplanted thymus initially takes place at the expense of its own cells, within a few days its cells are totally replaced with cells from the bone marrow of the recipient. If, however, the marrow of the recipient was previously destroyed by irradiation, repopulation of this organ does not proceed beyond the first few days, in which case repopulation of the organ occurs at the expense of its own cells. These experiments demonstrate (1) that the lymphoid population of the thymus originates from cells that migrate from the bone marrow to this organ and (2) that the lymphoid cells present in the thymus have a minimal capacity for autoregeneration.

Differentiation of T Lymphocytes in the Thymus. Intense modification of cell surface antigens characterize the different stages of T lymphocyte ontogeny in all mammalian species. These modifications occurs mostly within the thymus where cells can be segregated in two phases of differentiation, cortical and medular. Bone marrow derived cells migrate to the thymus where they locate initially in the outer cortex (subcapsular region), proliferate and move deeper in the cortical and later in the medulla. Along their pathway within the thymus the thymocyte proliferate, express differentiation antigens, acquire antigen specifity and become functionally committed to the different T lymphocyte subpopulation. In the mouse, most cortical thymocytes are functionally immature, cortisone-sensitive, present low levels of H-2 and high amounts of Thy-1 antigens, are Lyt-1,2,3$^+$ and bear receptors for peanut agglutinin. Conversely, most medular thymocytes are functionally competent, cortisone-resistant, have lower level of Thy-1 and higher H-2 content, have no receptor for peanut agglutinin and are now subdivided in functionally distinct subpopulations which bear different alloantigens. This differentiation step is antigen-independent and genetically predetermined. In mice the Lyt, Qa and I-J alloantigens distinguish the different T lymphocyte subpopulations whereas in humans this distinction is made with antigens detected with monoclonal antibodies (see p. 47 and 55).

Acquisition of Antigen Specificity in the Thymus. Arriving in the thymus, the T lymphocyte precursors proliferate and during their maturation acquire specificity for conventional antigens as well as for the antigens encoded by the Major Histocompatibility Complex (MHC, see pp. 168) of the species including self antigens. According to Benacerraf, in the first stage of their maturation in the thymus, T cells specific for self-MHC antigens are selected to proliferate and differentiate. Then, in a second stage only those cells with low affinity receptors for self-MHC antigens are allowed to mature and leave the thymus as functional T cells. These cells having low reactivity for self-MHC antigens have concomitantly high affinity for variants of self-MHC antigens. These variants seem to be the same or very similar to the allogeneic MHC antigens of the same species. Simultaneously and independently T lymphocytes develop receptors specific for conventional antigens. The high reactivity of T lymphocytes to alloantigens and the lower reactivity to xenogeneic MHC antigens may be accounted for by the fact that low affinity receptors for self-MHC antigens might be expected to react optimally with allogeneic antigens but much less so with xenogeneic antigens. This may explain the fact that the strongest T cells responses are not elicited by antigens further moved phylogenetically from the responder. Since the specificity of the T cell receptor for self-MHC is normally determined by the self MHC antigens of the thymus epithelium it would be expected that the T cell repertoire vary according to the MHC antigen of the thymus in which the T cell differenciates. Indeed, in chimera experiments in which (A × B)F1 bone marrow cells and grafted with thymus from either A or B parental, the T cells recognize as self the MHC of the grafted thymus. These experiments show that the environment in which the T cell develops determines the MHC restriction of the effector T cells. It must be pointed out, however, that the thymus environment does not extend the MHC restriction beyond the genetic potential of the cell.

Hormonal Activity of the Thymus. For many decades, numerous unfruitful attempts were made to demonstrate a hormonal function in the thymus. The subsequent demonstration of the effects of neonatal thymectomy and the observations that these effects could be eliminated by grafts of thymus enclosed in millipore chambers impermeable to cells, have renewed interest in the probable hormonal activity of the thymus and its influence in immunologic phenomena. This renewed interest resulted in the isolation of numerous substances from thymus extracts, some of which are listed in Table 1.1.

It is possible that some of the activities now attributed to different substances will subsequently be established as due to the same substance. Thymopoietine is an extremely active substance that induces the differentiation into thymocytes (immature T cells) of the immature cells of the bone marrow that migrate to the thymus. The addition of thymopoietine in vitro to mouse bone marrow or spleen cultures produces the appearance of cells with surface antigens typical of the T lymphocytes. Studies that culminated in the isolation of this substance resulted from investigations into the pathogenesis of myasthenia gravis, a disease characterized by symptoms of muscular weakness due to a defect in the mechanism of neuromuscular transmission, frequently in association with pathologic alterations of the thymus. The idea that the central cause of the disease might be autoimmune thymitis gave rise to a series of experiments that culminated in the isolation of two polypeptides (thymopoietine I and II) that are slightly different physicochemically but that behave functionally as the same substance. The thymopoietines apparently are produced by the epithelial cells of the thymus. In addition to inducing the differentiation of the cells originating in the bone marrow into T cells, they also impede the transmission of the neuromuscular impulse. Their neuromuscular effect appears only 18 h after the first injection of the hormone (in mice). The primary effect of thymopoetine is the transformation of "stem cells" into immature T cells.

Evidence suggests that adenosine $3',5'$-phosphate (cyclic AMP) is the intracellular mediator of the differentiation of prothymocytes and that the response of the prothymocytes can be induced or facilitated by substances that augment the intracellular level of cyclic AMP.

Wasting Disease. Animals thymectomized just after birth contract a disease characterized by weakness, discontinued growth, lethargy, bristling hair, loss of weight, periorbital edema, diarrhea, and death within a few weeks. This syndrome closely resembles runt disease, provoked by the graft-versus-host reaction, which occurs when mice are neonatally inoculated with allogeneic lymphoid cells. The cause of this syndrome is not well understood. However, the fact that wasting disease is prevented by treatment with constant doses of broadspectrum antibiotics or by maintenance of

Table 1.1. Active substances produced by the thymus

Designation	Composition	Mol Wt	Biologic Activity
Thymosine fraction	Protein	1,000–15,000	Lymphocytopoiesis + differentiation of T cells
Thymosine α_1	Protein	3,108	Induction of expression of Ly-1,2,3 phenotype and T-cell helper functions
Thymopoietine I	Protein	5,562	Induction of the appearance of specific antigens of the T cells + inhibition of neuromuscular transmission
Serum thymic factor (STF)	Polypeptide	857	Induction of specific antigens of T cells in vitro; induction of positive Thy-1 cells in nude mice
Thymic humoral factor (THF)	Polypeptide	3,000	Restoration of immunologic competence in vivo and in vitro

the thymectomized animals in sterile environments suggests that this syndrome is in some manner caused by multiple infections.

Bursa of Fabricius

Encountered in birds and located near the cloaca, this organ is structurally similar to the thymus (Fig. 1.10). In the chick, this organ appears on the tenth day of incubation as a diverticulum of the cloaca that originates from a region where there is intimate contact of the ectoderm with the endoderm. The organ is composed of numerous epithelial folds whose lamina propria contain numerous isolated groupings of dense lymphoid tissue that resolve into structures similar to the lobules of the thymus. At the time of hatching, the lobules are distinguish-able into cortical and medullary zones. Extirpation of the bursa of Fabricius, or bursectomy, when performed immediately after hatching, produces a diminution or even complete absence of the germinal centers and of plasma cells of the secondary lymphoid organs, accompanied by a considerable diminution in the formation of antibodies. However, the thymus and the thymus-dependent areas of the lymphoid organs are not altered, nor are the cell-based immunologic reactions affected. There thus exists in birds a clear dichotomy of the immunologic functions, which are governed either by the thymus or by the bursa of Fabricius. A structure equivalent to the bursa of Fabricius is unknown in mammals. Although the appendix, Peyer's patches, and the ton-

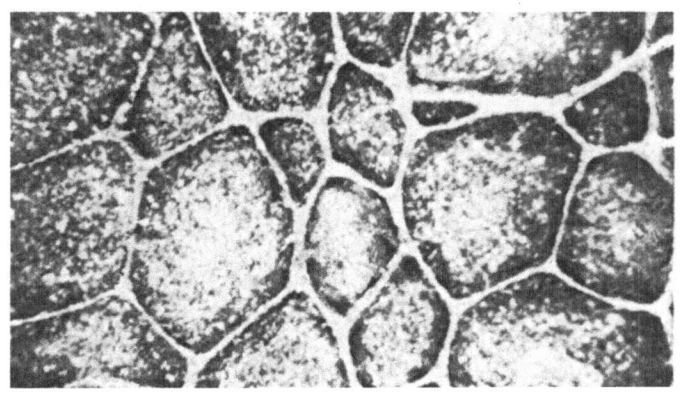

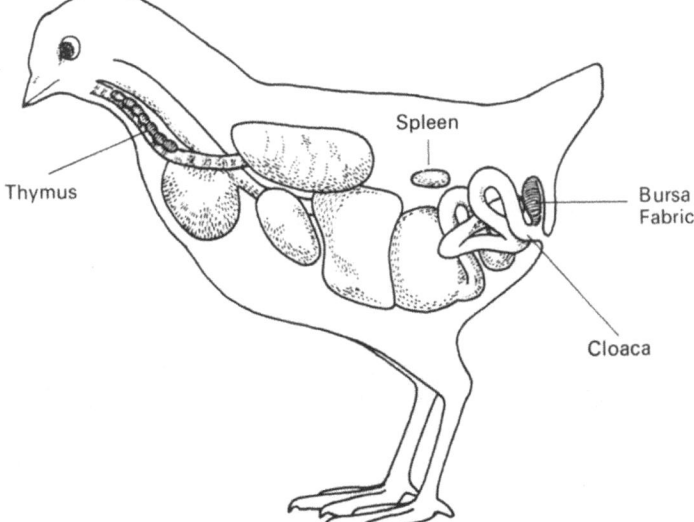

Fig. 1.10. Localization of the thymus and bursa of Fabricius in fowl. Photomicrograph of section through the bursa of Fabricius *(above)*. Note similarity to the thymus

sils have been suggested as organs capable of exercising the functions of the bursa in mammals, there is lack of definitive experimental data supporting these contentions.

Immunologic Activity
of the Secondary Lymphoid Organs

Lymph Node System

The secondary lymphoid organs are complex structures that possess mixed populations composed of thymus-dependent and bursa-dependent cells (thymus-independent in mammals). These cells occupy selectively determined areas in these organs. The terms thymus-dependent and thymus-independent merely signify that for their formation, these cellular zones are dependent upon the thymus. Once located in the secondary lymphoid organs, these cells do not depend for their functioning upon the thymus or the bursa of Fabricius (in birds). This explains why a normal immunologic response is obtained in animals thymectomized or bursectomized upon reaching adulthood (that is, after the secondary lymphoid organs have been populated by cells that have been conditioned by the primary lymphoid organs).

Lymphoid Nodules. The lymphoid nodules are irregular spherical formations of dense lymphoid tissue that measure 0.2 mm–1 mm in diameter. They are not permanent structures and may appear and disappear in a determined location. In neonates and in animals born in sterile environments, the nodules are scarce or even absent, which indicates that their presence may depend upon the existence of local antigenic stimuli. They exist isolated in the connective tissue of numerous organs (particularly in the lamina propria of the digestive tract, in the upper respiratory tract, and the urinary system), and are always present in normal secondary lymphoid organs, where they are usually termed "lymph follicles". They frequently exhibit a clearer central region called a germinal center, in which cells of an immature aspect appear, sometimes in intense proliferative activity. A single dose of tritiated thymidine results in a great number of labeled cells in these structures. Most of these cells are immature lymphocytes in differentiation, among which are found free macrophages and a network of dendritic reticular cells. The role of these lymphoid nodules in the immune response is discussed in conjunction with that of the lymph nodes.

Lymph Nodes. The lymph nodes are ovoid or reniform formations that measure from 1 mm to several centimeters in length and appear along the routes of the lymphatic vessels. On one border of a lymph node, there is a depression, or a hilus, where blood

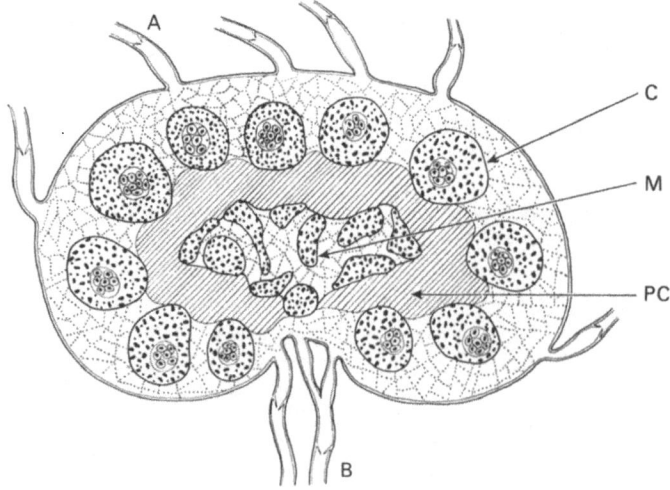

Fig. 1.11. Schematic structure of lymph node. *A*, afferent lymphatics; *B*, efferent lymphatics; *C*, cortical region with lymphoid nodules exhibiting germinal center; *PC*, paracortical region; *M*, medullary zone with medullary cords and sinuses. The cortical and medullary regions are thymus-independent, whereas the paracortical region is thymus-dependent

vessels enter and exit, and where the efferent lymphatics exit (Fig. 1.11). The afferent lymphatics enter the organ through diverse points along the border opposite the hilus. The lymph nodes are enveloped in a capsule of dense connective tissue and are composed of a delicate web of reticular fibers that support reticular cells and fixed macrophages. In the networks of this web, there are two lymphocytes populations: the thymus-dependent and thymus-independent.

Lymphoid tissue is distributed in the organ in three distinct regions that are recognizable as containing specific structures, but whose limits are imprecise: (1) There is a superficial, peripheral area termed the cortical region. The lymphocytes of this region are grouped in rounded or oval formations constituting the primary nodules or lymphoid follicles. In the central portions of the lymphoid follicles, germinal centers appear frequently that are rich in immature cells in the process of proliferation, in dendritic reticular cells, and in fixed macrophages. This region is thymus-independent and as such is not affected by thymectomy. (2) There is a central or medullary region in which dense lymphoid tissue is distributed in irregular formations that appear as trabeculae or threads, between which run the medullary sinuses. This region also is thymus-independent. (3) There is an intermediate zone called the paracortical region, situated imprecisely between the cortical and medullary zones. Situated under and between the follicles, it is composed of irregular masses of dense lymphoid tissue (Fig. 1.12). This region, also called the diffuse cortical area, hy-

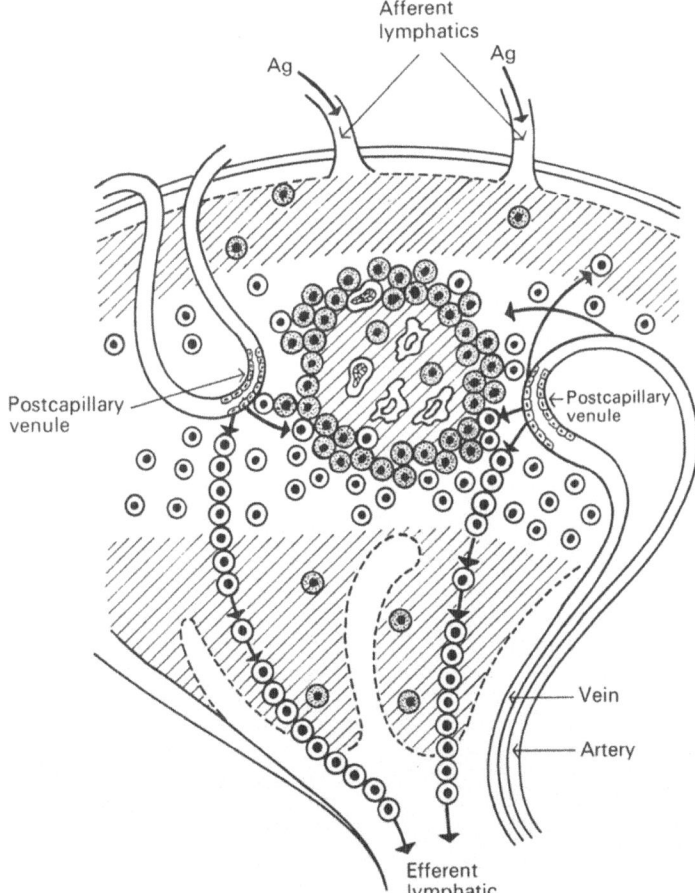

Fig. 1.12. Localization of the T and B lymphocytes in the lymph nodes. The thymus-dependent (*TD*) region is in *white;* the *shaded* area shows the thymus-independent (*TI*) regions. In the *TD* region, the majority of the cells are conditioned to react to the antigen with the production of sensitized cells; in the *TI* regions, the majority of the cells are antibody-forming cells when they come in contact with antigens. The T lymphocytes circulate constantly, passing from the postcapillary venule to the lymphatic parenchyma, where they enter into contact with the dendritic cells and the B lymphocytes. In passing through the lymph nodes, the T lymphocytes localize preferentially in the paracortical region (in *white*), from which they reach the medullary sinuses and gain access to the lymphatic circulation (Adapted from Cradock CG et al. (1971) Lymphocytes and the immune response. New Engl Med 285:378)

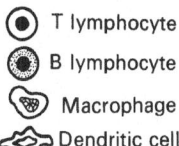

◉ T lymphocyte

◉ B lymphocyte

🐾 Macrophage

🪶 Dendritic cell

pertrophies considerably after antigenic stimuli that induce delayed hypersensitivity reactions. The lymphocytes of this region disappear after thymectomy and for this reason are considered thymus-dependent.

All formations of dense lymphoid tissue are permeated by loose lymphoid tissue constituting the subcapsular, perifollicular, and medullary sinuses through which the lymph travels in the direction of the efferent lymphatics. It is important to remember that all of the dense lymphoid tissue of the lymph node and of the lymphatic sinuses is continuous. The latter are not composed of vacant spaces separated by membranes; rather, they are an open meshwork of reticular tissue that constitutes the stroma of the organ. The lymph that enters the subcapsular sinus continues through the interfollicular sinuses

and, upon passing through the medullary sinuses, reaches the efferent lymphatics. In this fashion, contact is facilitated between the foreign particles of the lymph and the macrophages of the reticulum. It should be remembered that the retention capacity of the lymph nodes for foreign particles is greatly augmented during inflammatory processes.

Postcapillary Venules. Once it had been verified that the great majority of lymphocytes reaching the systemic circulation returned to the lymph, attention was focused upon tracing the return path of these cells, i.e., a precise determination of the structures through which the lymphocytes passed in penetrating the lymphatic circulation. Rats were inoculated with lymphocytes labeled with tri-

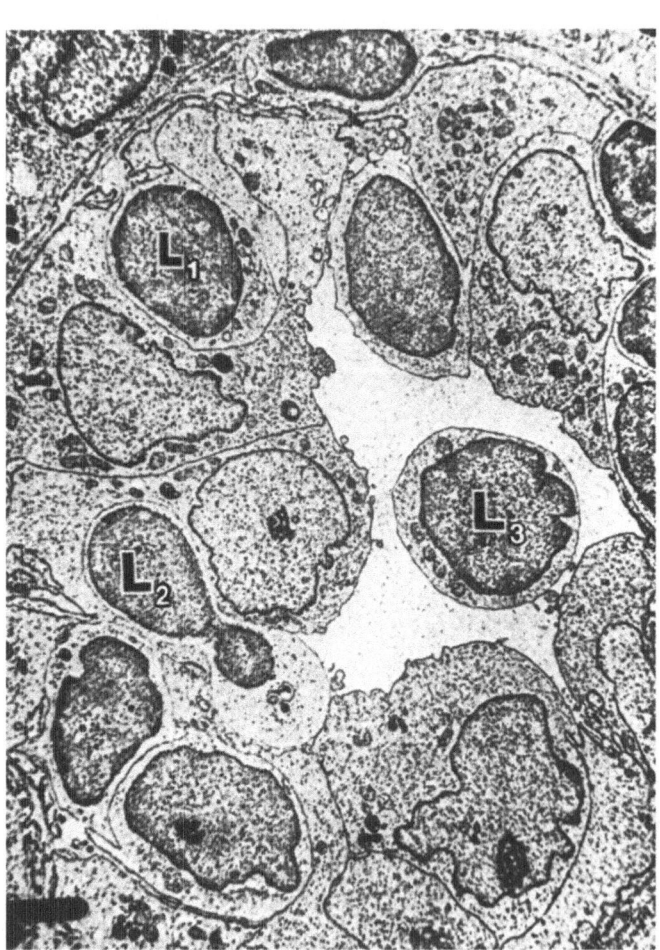

Fig. 1.13. Electron micrograph of postcapillary venule. Lymphocytes are observed within the cytoplasm of the cuboid epithelial cells (L_1 and L_2) and within the lumen of the vessel (L_3). Modified from Nossal GJV, Ada GL (1971) Antigens, lymphoid cells and the immune response. Academic Press, New York

tium (^{3}H) and were killed a few hours later. Autoradiographic examination of their organs indicated that the lymphocytes leave the blood through the so-called postcapillary venules (called Schulze venules in man), situated in the paracortical region of the lymph nodes. The venules are characterized by narrow central cavities constricted by an endothelium of cuboid cells, through which lymphocytes pass in their migration from the blood to the paracortical region of the lymph nodes (Fig. 1.13). Apparently, the passage of the lymphocytes through the endothelial cells is due to the presence of polysaccharides in the lymphocyte membranes for which specific receptors exist on the endothelial cells. Autoradiographs of lymph nodes reveal numerous labeled lymphocytes migrating through the endothelial cells of these venules. These lymphocytes are concentrated in the paracortical zone of the organ and later are encountered in the lymphatic sinuses, through which they return to the lymphatic circulation together with newly formed lymphocytes.

Lymphoid Follicles. These are represented fundamentally by groupings of lymphocytes and dendritic reticular cells that possess long cytoplasmic extremities, numerous and contorted, which form veritable labyrinths in which lymphocytes move about. Antigens are retained for long periods among these prolongations. Unlike the medullary macrophages, these cells do not phagocytize the antigens, but maintain them on their surfaces. Two types of follicles may be distinguished – primary follicles, which do not possess germinal centers, and secondary follicles, which possess a germinal center surrounded by a mantle of small lymphocytes in stained histological sections. Germinal centers appear as a light area in the internal portion of the follicle; they are composed of proliferating immature cells and, frequently, macrophages containing nuclear inclusions that apparently result from the phagocytosis of lymphocytes in degeneration. The germinal center appears in response to antigenic stimuli, and its development is a func-

tion of the intensity of such stimuli. When the antigenic stimulus is over, the germinative centers diminish their proliferative activity and resume the appearance of primary follicles, which in this case contain many macrophages with nuclear inclusions. Germfree animals possess only follicles without germinal centers.

Antigen-Induced Cellular Alterations in Lymphatic Organs. The cellular alterations that occur with a humoral reaction and cellular immunity are caused by antigen recognition, transformation of blasts, and proliferation of lymphocytic cells, particularly in the lymph nodes and spleen.
Early histologic changes consist primarily of an increase in T cells in the paracortical areas around the postcapillary venules in the lymph nodes and in the periarterial sheath in the spleen. Only later do plasmablasts appear in the lymph nodes and in the red pulp of the spleen. In most cases, antigens induce a mixed immune response with cellular modifications in both thymus-dependent and thymus-independent areas. Some antigens preferably give rise to cell alterations in only one area. Thus, pneumococcal polysaccharides cause changes only in thymus-independent areas, whereas, for example oxazolone induces changes in thymus-dependent areas.
Antigenic stimulation can result in a humoral reaction, with production of antibodies, or in a cellular hypersensitivity reaction, with production of sensitized cells. These reactions differ according to whether they are a primary or a secondary response. At the beginning of a primary reaction, the antigen is encountered in numerous macrophages in the medullary region and possibly later in a small but significant quantity of dendritic reticular cells of the germinal centers. When labeled antigen is used, it is noted that although the antigen present in the macrophages diminishes rapidly, that attached to the dendritic reticular cells persists for many weeks. Four to five days after contact with the antigen, moderate proliferations of immature cells can be observed

that, because of the difficulty in foreseeing their future proliferation, are designated immunoblasts. These cells appear principally in the medullary cords and rarely inside the lymphatic nodules. Most of these cells give origin to plasmablasts and plasma cells. In the primary response, the germinal centers usually exhibit discrete alterations, revealing minimal hypertrophy in the late phase (sixth day) of the response. However, these alterations can be more intense when the antigen used is highly immunogenic. After a second contact with the same antigen, i.e., in the secondary response, the immunoblasts appear not only in the medullary chords but also in the germinal follicles, which greatly increase in size. In the secondary response, the intervention of the germinal centers is much more accentuated and the plasma cells appear much more rapidly and in greater number than in the primary response. Moreover, the antigen is encountered not only in the macrophages of the medulla but also in a large portion of the dendritic reticular cells of the germinal centers, thereby coming in close contact with the lymphocytes. It is recognized that these cells represent a mechanism for retention of antigens that is particularly efficient in the secondary response. This situation, particularly due to the mobility of the lymphocytes, augments the contact of these cells with the antigens present in the dendritic macrophages. It is possible that the antigens remain on the surfaces of the dendritic reticular cells in the form of antigen-antibody complexes. The activity of the germinal centers result in the production of a large number of cells that differentiate into plasma cells or memory lymphocytes. A large number of these cells migrate to the medullary region, from which some of them reach the circulation. When an antigen is introduced into an organism for the first time, it induces not only the production of plasma cells but also a considerable increase in the number of cells capable of recognizing it. These recognition lymphocytes, which appear to originate in the germinal centers, are termed memory

cells and are responsible for the secondary response.

When the antigen is applied in order to excite a response of the delayed type, the alterations of the lymph nodes, which also become evident from the fourth day, consist of the appearance of numerous immunoblasts in the paracortical region. The percentage of these cells in this region, which under normal conditions is about 1%, rises to 8%–10%. Subsequently, these cells differentiate into lymphocytes. In this type of response, plasmablasts do not appear, nor do the nodules become involved.

The hypertrophied areas of the paracortical region sometimes assume a nodular appearance and are thus termed paracortical nodules. One characteristic peculiarity of this type of response is the obstruction of the medullary sinuses by agglomerations of small lymphocytes that disappear as soon as the reaction begins to diminish. The sinuses apparently represent the exit routes for lymphocytes from the paracortical region; these become temporarily obstructed by the great numbers of cells produced under these conditions. Often, there is simultaneous activation of the germinal center and the paracortical area of the lymph nodes, so that a picture arises of simultaneously occurring reactions of the immediate and delayed types.

Spleen

Histology. The spleen constitutes the major accumulation of lymphoid tissue interposed in the systemic circulation. Examination of sections of this organ reveals white-grey, rounded nodules dispersed in a dark red mass called the red pulp. The white-grey nodules are composed of dense lymphoid tissue (Fig. 1.14) termed white pulp. The capsula of the organ, formed of dense lymphoid tissue, emits trabeculae that divide the parenchyma or splenic pulp into incomplete compartments. Through these trabeculae run arteries that, upon attaining a diameter of 200 μm, penetrate the paren-

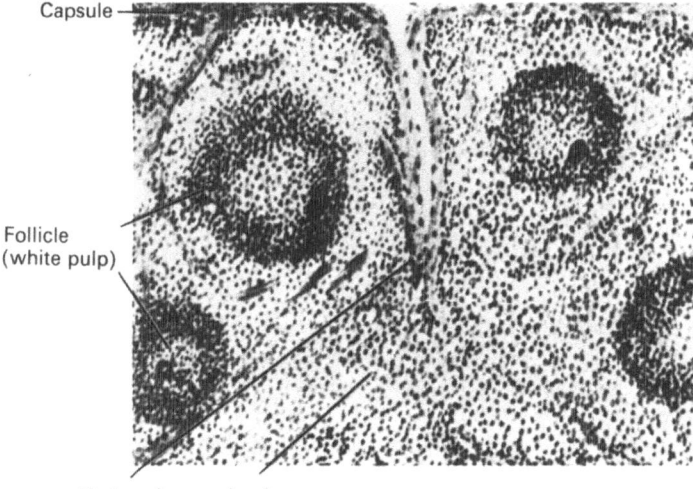

Capsule

Follicle
(white pulp)

Trabecula   red pulp

Fig. 1.14. Photomicrograph of the spleen showing the white pulp and the red pulp. Also seen are the capsula and a trabecula

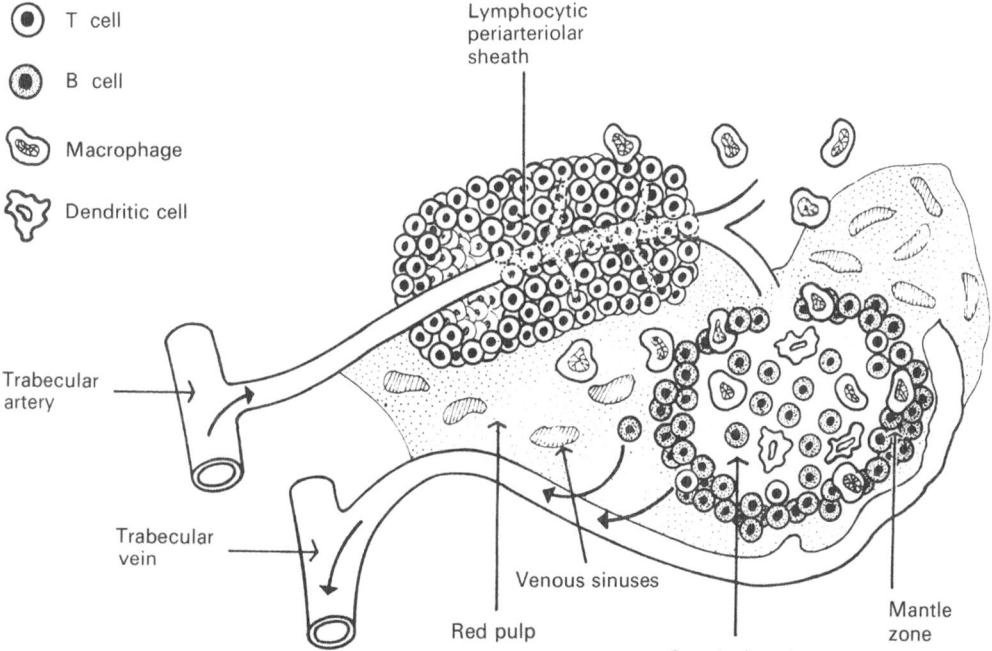

T cell

B cell

Macrophage

Dendritic cell

Lymphocytic periarteriolar sheath

Trabecular artery

Trabecular vein

Venous sinuses

Red pulp

Germinal center

Mantle zone

Fig. 1.15. Thymus-dependent (*TD*) and thymus-independent (*TI*) regions of the spleen. The lymphocytic periarteriolar sheath constitutes a *TD* region whereas the lymphoid follicles and adjacent lymphoid tissue represent the *TI* zone (Adapted from Cradock CG et al. (1971) Lymphocytes and the immune system. New Engl Med 285:378)

chyma of the organ where they are immediately enclosed in a sheath of dense lymphoid tissue. This tissue expands at certain points, forming lymphatic nodules or splenic follicles (Malpighian bodies). In this fashion, the white pulp becomes divided into a periarteriolar sheath of lymphoid tissue and into lymphoid nodules. The latter, together with the adjacent lymphoid tissues, constitute the thymus-independent zone of the organ, whereas the periarteriolar lymphoid tissue represents a thymus-de-

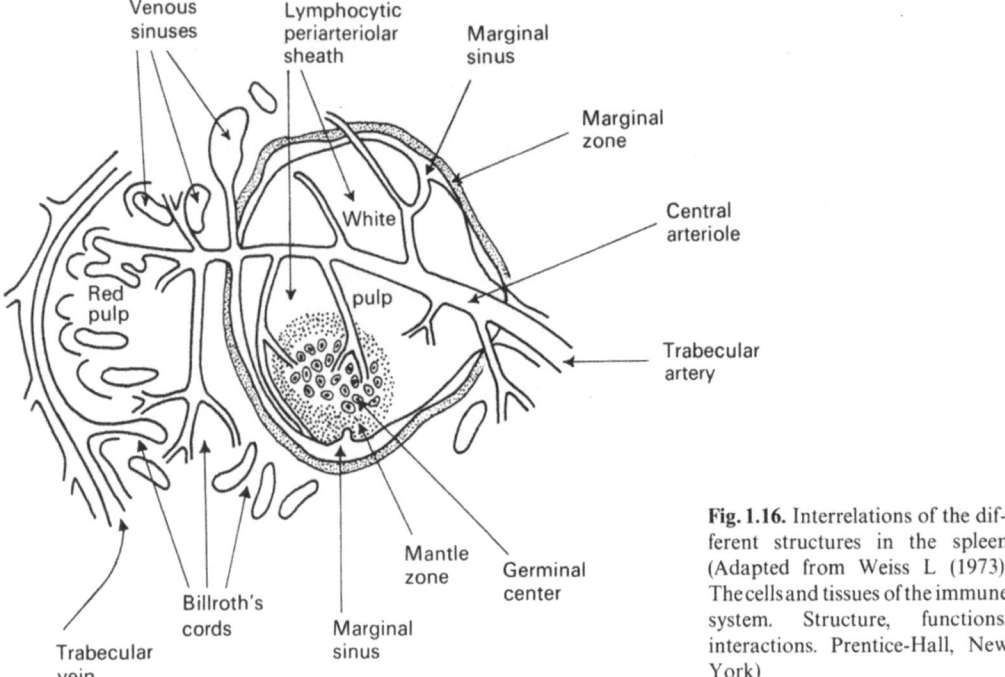

Venous sinuses

Lymphocytic periarteriolar sheath

Marginal sinus

Marginal zone

White

Central arteriole

Red pulp

pulp

Trabecular artery

Mantle zone

Germinal center

Billroth's cords

Marginal sinus

Trabecular vein

Fig. 1.16. Interrelations of the different structures in the spleen (Adapted from Weiss L (1973). The cells and tissues of the immune system. Structure, functions, interactions. Prentice-Hall, New York)

pendent zone. The relations between the thymus-dependent and thymus-independent zones of the white pulp are schematized in Fig. 1.15. The red pulp is made up of splenic cords and venous sinuses. The splenic cords are composed of cytofibrillar reticulum, itself composed of reticular fibers, reticular cells, and fixed macrophages, in whose meshes are found formed elements of the blood along with free macrophages and plasma cells. Among the cords appear venous sinuses, which are capillaries of irregular diameter coated with intensely phagocytic cells. Although these cells voraciously phagocytoze carbon particles, they phagocytoze only inefficiently numerous protein antigen. The spleen differs from the lymph nodes in that it is not involved in lymphatic circulation, in its erythrocatheretic function, and – in certain species – in its possession of myelopoietic capabilities. On the other hand, a series of splenic structures in this organ is similar to those of the lymph nodes: the lymphoid follicles, the lymphoid tissue of the periarteriolar sheath, which corresponds to the paracortical lymphoid tissue of the lymph nodes, and the cords of the red pulp, which correspond to the medullary cords of the lymph nodes. In addition, the spleen possesses an anatomic structure apparently without equivalent in the lymph nodes – the marginal sinuses. These structures result from anastomoses of the terminal capillaries of the white pulp, which are situated immediately inside the marginal zone (thus far, the marginal sinus has been described only in the rat). Common to many species, including the human, this structure consists of loose lymphoid tissue that possesses long, ramified prolongations constituting a network of mesh containing a small number of lymphocytes and macrophages. The limits between the marginal zone and the red pulp are not well defined. The relation between these splenic structures is shown in Fig. 1.16. The marginal zone is important immunologically, since it is the region where many of the antigens carried in the blood are retained. Radioactive protein antigens, after injection, are rapidly encountered along the surfaces of the cytoplasmic prolongations of the reticular cells of this region and only later in the interior of the lymphoid follicles.

Antigen-Induced Modifications of the Spleen. The cellular alterations of the spleen after antigen stimulus are similar to those that occur in the lymph nodes. One to four days after intravenous injection of antigen, immunoblasts appear in the white pulp, localizing in the periphery of the periarteriolar sheath and in the marginal zone. These cells proliferate and differentiate, originating a large number of plasmablasts and plasma cells, many of which invade the red pulp. Some of these cells also appear in the lymphoid follicles of the white pulp. After 5–6 days, the plasma cells rapidly disappear; it is supposed that they move from this organ into the blood. In the secondary reaction, there is, in addition to these alterations, intense proliferative activity in the lymphoid follicles, resulting in the presence of numerous plasma cells situated in the periphery of the follicles and principally in the red pulp.

Other Lymphoid Structures

Agglomerations of lymphoid nodules appear along the respiratory and digestive systems in close association with the epithelium of the region. In man, these organs are represented by the palatine, lingual, and pharyngeal tonsils, whose lymphoid tissue is associated with the epithelial crypts of these structures; by Peyer's patches, agglomerations of lymphoid nodules localized in the wall of the small intestine; and by the appendix vermiformis, whose follicles form dense agglomerations in the submucosa of the organ. The lymphoid follicles of these structures behave as thymus-independent zones whereas the interfollicular tissue corresponds to the thymus-dependent paracortical zones of the lymph nodes. The alterations induced by antigens are similar to those induced in the lymph nodes.

Trapping of Lymphocytes. Trapping or retention of the lymphocytes occurs on lymphoid organs 24 hours after contact with antigen. When ^{51}Cr labeled lymphocytes are injected intravenously or intraperitoneally into antigen-stimulated syngeneic mice, the lymphocytes are found trapped in the spleen; after subcutaneous administration or after grafting of non-syngeneic skin they are trapped in lymph nodes. Apparently the lymphocytes enter the lymphoid organs but their exit is prevented by an unknown mechanism. 48 hours to 5 days later occurs an increase in the number of lymphocytes leaving the lymphoid organs. During this time, a larger number of lymphocytes pass from blood to lymphoid tissue and the mechanism preventing their exit is no more operative. The lymphocytes specific to the pertinent antigen disappears from circulation during this period probably retained in the lymphoid organs. After a week the number of lymphocytes leaving the lymphoid organs becomes normal, whereas the antigen-specifically activated lymphocytes leave the lymphoid organs and through the circulation spread the immune response throughout the organism.

Localization of the Antigen in the Lymphoid Organs

Knowledge regarding the localization of antigens in the tissues has resulted from the injection of fluorescent antigens or of antigens labeled with radioactive isotopes (particularly ^{3}H, ^{131}I, and ^{125}I) into the organism, followed by the study of sections or smears of lymphoid organs through fluorescence microscopy or autoradiography.

The entrance of antigens into the internal medium of an organism appears to constitute a threat to its integrity even for the most primitive forms of life. This perhaps is the explanation for the phylogenic observation that the means for the elimination of foreign substances that penetrate an organism have appeared well before the capacity to produce an immune response. In fact, most antigens that penetrate the organism are eliminated without having a chance to activate the immune system. Possibly for this reason, the locations in which antigens have been detected after introduction into an organism do not always represent the region where immunologic reactivity occurs. Actually, it is usual to observe antibody-producing cells in areas of lymphoid tissue that are practically free from concentrations of antigens; conversely, concentrations of antigens may occur in areas where antibody-forming cells do not exist.

It is now accepted as certain that the first event that stimulates an organism to demonstrate its immunologic potential is the encounter of the antigen with receptors existing on the surfaces of immunologically competent cells. Where and how the antigens enter into contact with these cells depends upon the manner in which they gain entrance into the organism. Generally, antigens that penetrate the epithelia move to the lymph nodes that drain the region, where they localize in the macrophages of the medullary region and in the dendritic cells of the lymphoid follicles; antigens that penetrate directly into the blood circulation are captured principally by the cells of the marginal zone and dendritic cells of the spleen. When the antigen is injected subcutaneously, it reaches the satellite lymph node through the afferent lymphatic vessels, enters into the marginal sinus, and is encountered about 1 min after injection in the medullary sinuses. Within 5 min, it is encountered in the macrophages of the medullary cords. One to two hours later, the antigen concentration in the medullary region reaches its peak; the antigen may disappear within days or may persist for monthes, depending upon the nature and the quantity of the antigen. In the medullary sinuses as well as in the medullary cords, macrophages containing antigen are occasionally found enclosed in a layer of lymphocytes.

This fact seems to be functionally significant (passage of information regarding the nature of the antigen from the macrophage to the lymphocyte). The localization of antigen in the dendritic cells of the lymphoid follicles occurs later than in the medullary macrophages and is really only significant in the secondary response or in animal previously injected with antibodies specific for the antigen in question. In this respect, it is important to consider the observation that the localization of antigens in animals born and kept in sterile environments is minimal. In immunized animals, the antigen combined with the antibody penetrates rapidly into the cortex, and within 15 min after injection is encountered among the lymphocytes of the superficial region of the lymphoid follicles. Autoradiographs of lymph nodes 1 h after injection of antigen into immunized animals frequently reveals a crown of antigens in the perifollicular regions (Fig. 1.17). Subsequently, the antigen is encountered within the sec-

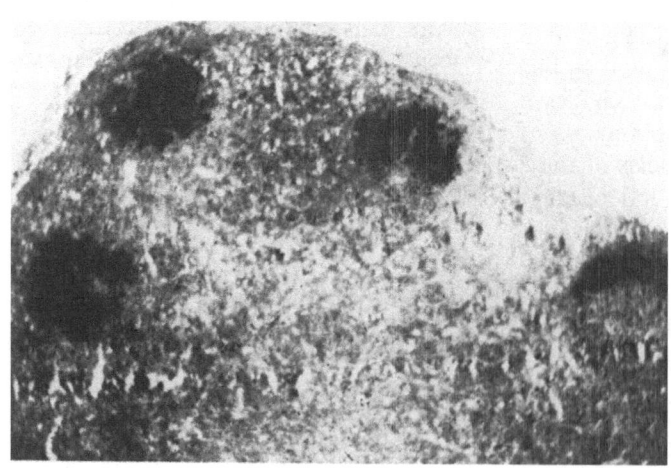

Fig. 1.17. Autoradiograph of lymph node taken 1 h after injection of radioactive antigen. Note location of the antigen in the follicles. Photograph by courtesy of A Szenberg, WHO, Geneva

ondary follicles and, more diffusely, in the primary follicles. In the dendritic cells, the antigen becomes localized on the surfaces of its cytoplasmic prolongations. Thus, the function of the dendritic cells appears to be that of concentrating the anttigen in a locale that is strategically favorable to the establishment of contact with immunocompetent cells.

In the spleen, the antigen is encountered initially in the marginal zone, associated with the cytoplasmic prolongations of reticular cells found therein. Autoradiographs of spleens of animals killed at different intervals following injection of antigen appear to indicate a continuous flow of antigen from the marginal zone to the white pulp, where the antigen is retained in the follicles for long periods. For many antigens, the lymphoid follicles represent the only site of retention in this organ, whereas the marginal zone appears to be an important region for a transitory concentration of antigen. The localization of antigens in the other lymphoid structures is similar to that described for the lymph nodes.

Phylogenic and Ontogenic Development of Immunologic Capacity

Knowledge of the phylogeny of the immune response is still scanty. Some invertebrates such as the annelids and, perhaps, the tunicates may have an immune response, albeit primitive (such as refection of grafts, which in these invertebrates requires a considerably longer period of time than in the vertebrates). These animals do not possess a thymus, and the cells present in cellular infiltrate in the graft area are purely histiocytic in character. There are as yet no data that suggest the production of humoral antibodies by any species of invertebrate. The first species to exhibit immunologic activity, including both humoral and cellular responses, is found among the agnates. The hagfish and the lamprey are capable of rejecting grafts and or responding with production of antibodies when stimulated with

particulate or soluble antigens. The antibodies produced, however, appear to be of a single class, similar to IgM in vertebrates. Little if anything is known regarding the cellular mechanism of the immune response in this species – save merely the fact that adult specimens examined have neither a thymus vor lymphoid aggregates. It should be noted, however, that cells similar to lymphocytes, present in the peripheral blood of hagfish immunized with sheep erythrocytes, exhibit specific immunofluorescence when incubated together with antigen: possibly, these cells are totally or partially responsible for the production of antibodies. In more highly developed vertebrates, such as sharks and rays, there is already a central lymphatic system in the form of a thymus-primordium, lymphoid cell follicles in the spleen, and circulating lymphocytes; however, lymph nodes are still absent. In these animals – which also have the capability to reject grafts and to exhibit distinct humoral responses – the antibodies produced are still predominantly of the IgM type. In the teleosts, two different classes of antibodies appear for the first time – IgG and IgM. The pulmonate fish of Australia appears to be the first vertebrate with two well-defined classes of immunoglobulins. The amphibians also exhibit two well-defined classes of antibodies and, although they possess no lymph nodes, they have lymphatic agglomerates responsible for the production of antibodies. In these vertebrates B and T lymphocytes functions are first plainly demonstrated. For instance, thymectomy in toads reduces T lymphocyte activity abolishing the ability to reject allografts but keeps B lymphocyte functions preserved. Reptiles have a well differentiated lymphoid system and present T lymphocytes with regulatory and helper activities. Its B system is well developed and an IgD-like immunoglobulin has been described on tortoise B lymphocytes. The highest point in the evolution of the immune system is attained in birds and mammals, in which there are five isotopes of functionally and antigenically different immunoglobulins. In

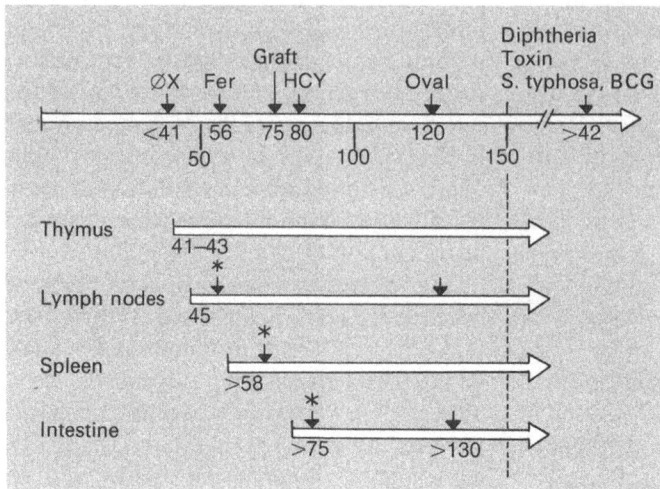

Fig. 1.18. Comparison of the appearance of the immune response and the development of the lymphoid system in the sheep. The *numbers* represent the elapsed time of gestation. ∅, bacteriophage; *Fer,* ferritin; *HCY,* hemocyanin; and *Oval,* ovalbumin. From Silverstein AM, Prendergast RA (1971) The maturation of lymphoid tissue structure and function in ontogeny. In: Lindahl-Kiessling K, Ada GL, Hanna MJ, Jr (eds) Morphological and functional aspects of immunity. Plenum, New York

birds there is full establishment of a dichotomy of the lymphoid system with the appearance of the bursa of Fabricius. In mammals, in spite of the absence of the bursa or an equivalent organ, the T and B systems are plainly distinct both functionally and phenotypically (see Chap. 2).

During ontogenesis, the capacity of the developing vertebrate to exhibit an immunologic response coincides, generally speaking, with the appearance of the thymus and the first lymphocytes. In tadpoles, for example, the capacity to reject skin grafts is established only when the first lymphocytes appear; in the opossum, the capacity for the production of antibodies appears simultaneously with the first lymphocytes. In sheep, the capacity to respond to antigenic stimulus appears gradually during embryogenesis – apparently as a series of isolated occurrences (Fig. 1.1.8). As shown, from the 75th day of gestation, the fetus is capable of rejecting grafts, whereas the capacity to respond with the formation of antibodies against bacteriophages can be induced after 41 days of gestation, against ferritin after 56 days, against hemocyanin after 80 days, and against hemocyanin after 120 days of gestation (in sheep the period of gestation is 150 days). It is interesting to compare these data with the development

of lymphoid tissue in this species. The first lymphocytes are seen in the rudiments of the thymus from the 41st day of gestation and later in the lymph nodes (45th day), in the spleen (58th day), and in Peyer's patches (130th day).

References

Baum SJ, Ledney GD (eds) (1979) Experimental Hematology Today, 1979, Springer-Verlag, New York-Heidelberg

Bessis M (1977) Blood smears Reinterpreted. Springer-Verlag, New York-Heidelberg

Cooper MD, Lawton AR, Preud'homme JL, Seligmann M (1979) Primary Antibody Deficiencies. In: Cooper MD, Lawton AR, Miescher PS, Müller-Eberhard HJ (eds) Immune Deficiency. Springer Verlag, New York-Heidelberg

DeChatelet LR (1979) Phagocytosis by human neutrophils. In: Gadebusch HH (ed) Phagocytes and cellular immunity. CRC Press. Boca Raton, Florida

Friedman H (1975) Thymus factors in immunity. New York Academy of Science, New York

Hildemann WH (1974) Some new concepts in immunologic phylogeny. Nature 250:116

Jarret EE, Haig DM (1984) Mucosal mast cells *in vivo* and *in vitro.* Immunol Today 5:1

Low TLK, Goldstein AL (1980) Thymosin and other thymic hormones and their synthetic analogues. In: Chedid L, Miescher PA, Müller-Eberhard HJ (eds) Immunostimulation. Springer Verlag, Heidelberg-New York, pp 129–146

Marchalonis JS, Cone RE (1973) The phylogenetic emergence of vertebrate immunity. Aust J Exp Biol Med Sc 51:461

Moretta L, Webb SR, Grossi CE, Lydyard PM, Cooper MD (1977) Functional analysis of two human T cell subpopulations: Help and suppression of B cell responses by T cells bearing receptors for IgM (T_M) and IgG (T_G). J Exp Med 146:184

Owen JJ (1971) The origins and development of lymphocyte populations. Ontogeny of acquired immunity. Excerpta Medica, Amsterdam

Sprent J (1977) Recirculating lymphocytes. In: Marchalonis JJ (ed) The Lymphocyte, part I. Dekker, New York

Walford RL (1974) The immunologic theory of aging: current status. Fed Proc 33:2020

Chapter 2   Activity of Immune Cells

IVAN MOTA

Contents

Lymphocytes   35
    T Lymphocytes   40
    B Lymphocytes   48
Differences Between B and T Lymphocytes . .   54
The Antigen Receptors in
    B and T Lymphocytes   56
Cooperation Between B and T Lymphocytes. .   57
Macrophages   59
    Role of Adherent Cells
    in T-B Cell Cooperation   60
    Role of Macrophages in Humoral
    Immune Response   60
    Role of Macrophages in Cellular Immunity .   61
Dendritic Reticular Cells   61
References   62

Lymphocytes

Lymphocytes originate from an undifferentiated cell and, through a series of divisions and differenciations, transform as follows: lymphoblasts→prolymphocytes→large lymphocytes→small lymphocytes. It is estimated that 6–9 mitoses occur during this process. The lymphocyte percursor cells exist in the liver and in the bone marrow in the fetus, but only in the bone marrow in the adult. In the intrauterine state as well as in adults, these cells migrate from the bone marrow to the thymus and other lymphoid organs where they proliferate and produce the lymphoid cell populations of these organs.

Usually, the cells are resting. *In vitro,* however, they are extremely mobile, with a particular tendency to slide about the surfaces of other cells, including macrophages. The small lymphocytes were for many years defined solely in negative terms, or as cells with little cytoplasm, containing few organelles, and were considered terminal cells. However, even some of the early researchers, such as Maximow, considered the lymphocyte a cell endowed with great capacity for differentiation – a totipotential cell. Since then, numerous experimental data have definitely demonstrated that small lymphocytes are not terminal cells, although they are presented morphologically by a homogeneous population, functionally, they represent an extremely heterogeneous population. Moreover, there are significant variations in size (6–12 μm), in the density of components (separable into at least four fractions of different densities), in longevity (several days to years), and, most importantly, in function.

Migration of Lymphocytes. Together, lymphocytes represent nearly 1% of total body weight and are distributed among the so-called lymphoid organs, represented in mammals by the thymus, peripheral lymphoid organs (spleen, lymph nodes, and lymphoid aggregates), and by the pool of circulating lymphocytes. In the lymphoid organs, lymphocytes do not constitute a static population; on the contrary, they recirculate actively, passing through the blood and through the lymph – eventually to return to the lymphoid compartments (Fig. 2.1). The cellular migratory currents thus produced (Fig. 2.2) have been established by experiments involving transfusion of labeled lymphocytes to normal or irradiated recipient animals. It is recognized, moreover, that cells from the bone marrow migrate to the secondary lymphoid organs, with some of these cells passing first through the thymus, where they multiply and differentiate, acquiring special properties.

These migratory currents constitute what Yoffey called the fourth circulation. The lymphocytes present in the blood and lymphatic circulation represent cells in transit among diverse organs. The existence of these migratory patterns of lymphocytes explains why immunologic reactions always acquire a systemic character, in other words, why contact of the antigen with a restricted part of an organism produces a generalized immunologic response. The migratory patterns of lymphocytes are schematized in Fig. 2.2.

Ecotaxis. When labeled T and B lymphocytes are re-injected into a syngeneic animal, these cells locate selectively in areas in

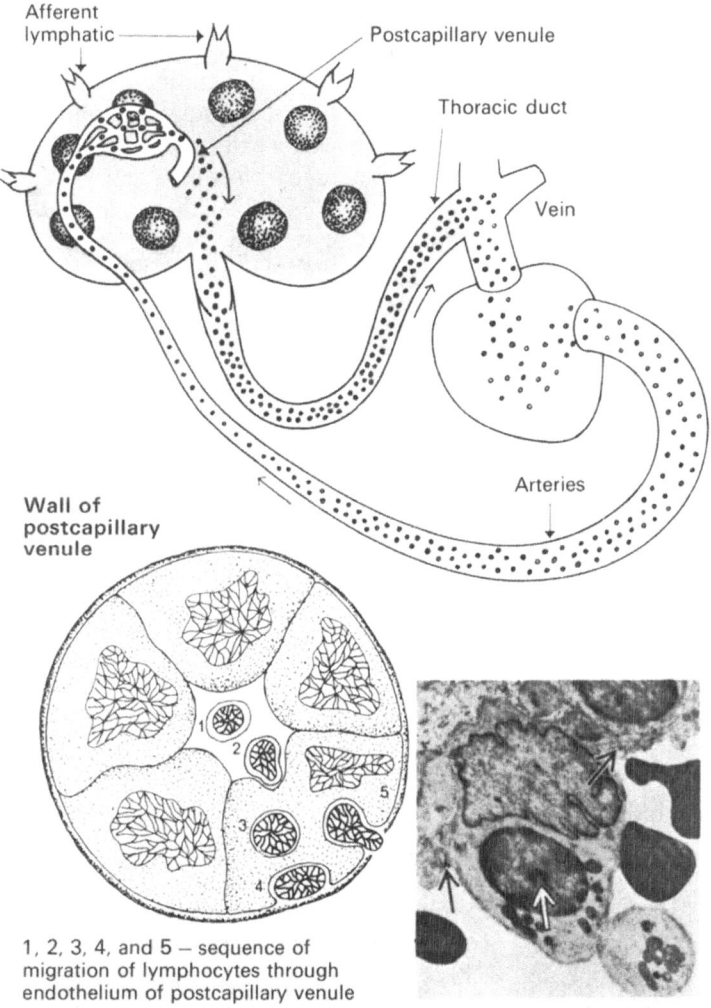

1, 2, 3, 4, and 5 — sequence of migration of lymphocytes through endothelium of postcapillary venule

Fig. 2.1. Path followed by the lymphocyte in passing from the lymph node to the lymph, thence to the blood, and then returning to the lymph node. The electron photomicrograph *(lower right)* shows a lymphocyte *(white arrow)* passing through the endothelium of the postcapillary vein. At the junction of the two cells, intact endothelia are indicated by the *black arrows*. (Modified from Gowans, 1971)

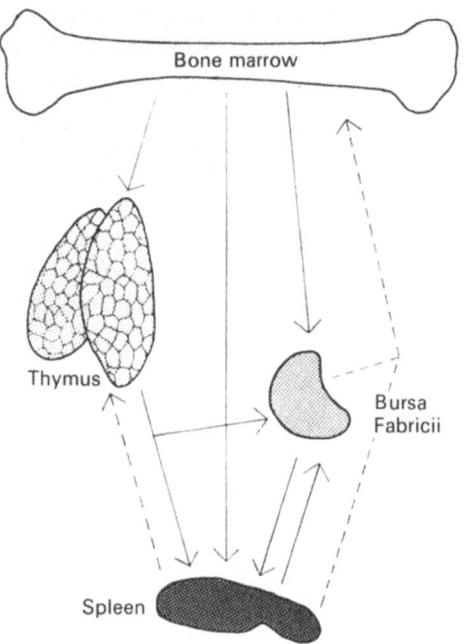

Fig. 2.2. Migration of the lymphocytes among the different lymphoid compartments. The *broken lines* indicate less certain migratory pathways

which they are normally found. Thus, T lymphocytes migrate to the paracortical areas of lymph nodes and the periarteriolar sheet of the spleen, whereas B lymphocytes locate themselves in the lymphoid follicles. This ability of the lymphocytes to recognize specifically certain areas of the lymphoid organs is called ecotaxis (from the greek "oikos" meaning house and "tassein" meaning movement). This lymphocyte property is probably due to recognizing molecules present in their membrane (homing receptors).

Long-lived and Short-lived Lymphocytes. Experiments concerning the incorporation and persistence of thymidine labeling have demonstrated the existence of two populations of lymphocytes – one consisting of long-lived cells and one of short-lived cells. The first experiments on this subject were performed by injecting components containing radioactive phosphorus into pa-

tients, then following over time the radioactivity of the circulating lymphocytes. Using this method, it has been calculated that approximately 80% of lymphocytes have an average life span of 100–200 days. In later experiments, the percentage of labeled lymphocytes after either fleeting or prolonged contact with tritiated thymidine was determined by means of autoradiography. In both humans and various laboratory animals, it was soon verified that the majority of lymphocytes are of the long-lived sort, for only a small number of these became radioactive after short contact with thymidine. In the rat, for example, after continuous injection of thymidine over a 12-h period, only 1% of the small lymphocytes of the thoracic duct exhibited radioactivity. In other experiments in which the organism remained in contact with tritiated thymidine for up to 200 days in order to quarantee that all recently formed cells became radioactive, only 10% of the small lymphocytes of the blood had not been labeled. This means that 10% of the cells had been formed before the thymidine was administered – about 7 months earlier. Autoradiographic studies indicated that the percentage of long-lived lymphocytes in the different lymphoid sectors of the rat varies widely – 90% in the toracic duct, 66% in the peripheral blood, 75% in the lymph nodes, and 25% in the spleen. In humans, there is evidence that some small lymphocytes survive without division for about 10 years. This finding was possible because of observations on lymphocytes obtained from patients subjected to X-ray therapy approximately 10 years earlier. When mitosis was induced in these lymphocytes by the addition of phytohemagglutinin *in vitro*, chromosomal alterations incompatible with the survival of postmitotic cells were observed. This finding led to the conclusion that the observed mitoses were the first undergone by these lymphocytes since the moment the patients had last been irradiated – about 10 years earlier. It is now known that both types of lymphocyte populations (T and B) possess long-lived cells.

Immunocompetence of Lymphocytes. The technique of draining lymph from the thoracic duct was used to demonstrate that small lymphocytes function as immunologically competent cells. Animals thus treated were unable to respond to a primary antigenic stimulus with the production of antibodies – even to antigens extremely immunogenic to the control animals. However, the capacity to respond to these stimuli was rapidly restored by inoculation of small lymphocytes obtained from syngeneic animals. Moreover, lymphocytes obtained from an immunized animal and injected into a normal syngeneic recipient transferred to the latter the capacity to mount a secondary response. In other experiments, the specifity of the immunologic response transferred by the lymphocytes was demonstrated by the injection of small lympho-

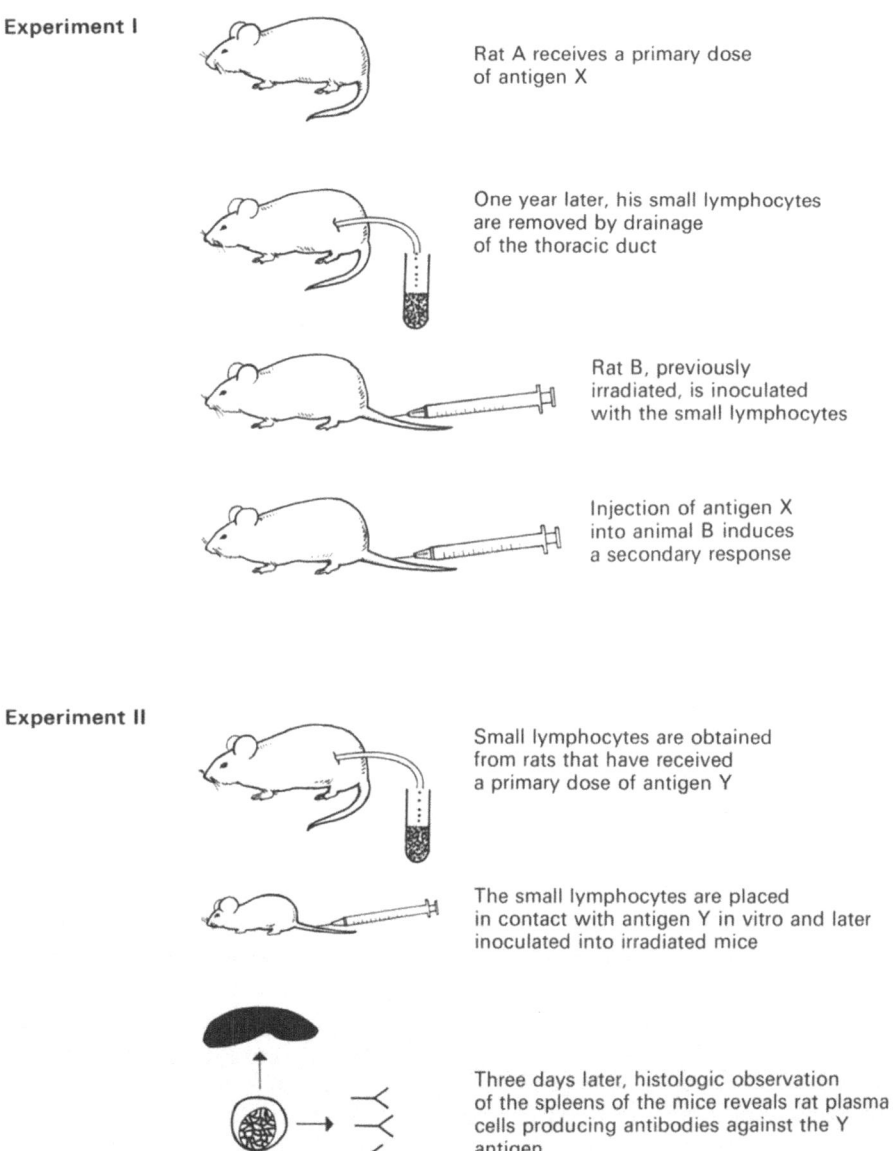

Experiment I

Rat A receives a primary dose of antigen X

One year later, his small lymphocytes are removed by drainage of the thoracic duct

Rat B, previously irradiated, is inoculated with the small lymphocytes

Injection of antigen X into animal B induces a secondary response

Experiment II

Small lymphocytes are obtained from rats that have received a primary dose of antigen Y

The small lymphocytes are placed in contact with antigen Y in vitro and later inoculated into irradiated mice

Three days later, histologic observation of the spleens of the mice reveals rat plasma cells producing antibodies against the Y antigen

Fig. 2.3. Experiment showing the existence of immunologic memory cells among small lymphocytes

cytes taken from animals tolerant to sheep erythrocytes. Under such conditions, the recipient animal demonstrated incapacity to react to the sheep erythrocytes, yet responded normally to other immunogenic stimuli.

The small lymphocytes also include cells responsible for the rejection of grafts and for delayed hypersensitivity reactions, since these also are restored by transfusion of small lymphocytes. In all these experiments, special methods were utilized that made it possible to obtain cellular suspensions extremely rich in small lymphocytes. One particularly recommended technique that permits collections of a practically pure sample of small lymphocytes consists of draining lymph from the thoracic duct and incubating it at 37 °C for 24 h with light shaking. This procedure destroys large and medium-sized lymphocytes, leaving just the small lymphocytes. However, the lymph obtained after 4–5 days of continuous drainage of the thoracic duct contains almost exclusive large and medium-sized lymphocytes that, unlike small lymphocytes, are incapable of restoring immunologic capacity to animals deprived of their small lymphocytes.

Memory Cells. The immunologic memory is specific and long-lasting and results from the first contact of immunologically competent cells with the antigen. This contact leads to an increase in such lymphocytes, which carry on their membranes to receptor specific for the antigen. As shown in the experiments reproduced in Fig. 2.3, the small lymphocytes are responsible for immunologic memory. Because both B and T cells have antigen specificity, both types of cells are capable of expressing immunologic memory. The following experiments have proved the existence of T and B memory cells:

1. *The production of antibodies* against a protein-hapten complex depends on the cooperation of carrier-specific T cells with hapten-specific B cells (see below). The first contact with the carrier protein (through which the activation of carrier-specific T cells is induced) enhances the formation of hapten-specific antibodies, when the body is subsequently stimulated with the protein-hapten conjugate. These results are indicative of the presence of T memory cells.

2. *Lymphocytes treated with anti-Thy-1 serum* (Thy-1 antigen, formerly θ antigen), is specific for T cells (p. 11) whereby almost all T cells are destroyed, lose the capability to transmit a secondary response *in vivo* as well as *in vitro*.

3. *Lymphocytes treated with an anti-B-cell serum* lose the capacity to transmit passively a secondary antibody response. The addition of B cells to this cell population restores this capacity.

The induction of memory cells is dose-dependent. T memory cells appear quickly following a small dose of antigen; B cells appear slowly and only after a relatively large dose of antigen. It is thought that B memory cells originate in the germinal center.

Thymus-Dependent and Thymus-Independent Lymphocytes. Extensive data obtained from experiments with laboratory animals, particularly mice, suggest that in mammals, cells obtained from the bone marrow mature into two populations of lymphocytes, the T lymphocytes and B lymphocytes. Both populations circulate, yet they pass through different areas within the lymphoid organs. After leaving the thymus, the T lymphocytes enter the paracortical areas of the lymph nodes and the periarterial sheaths of the lymphoid follicles of the spleen. From these organs, the T lymphocytes pass via the blood through the efferent lymphatics and possibly also through the blood vessels of the spleen, thereupon to return again to the lymphoid compartments. One characteristic of the T lymphocyte is the ability, upon contact with antigen, to form a "blast," from which the small, sensitized lymphocytes originate. These lymphocytes are responsible for cell mediated reactions such as delayed hypersensitivity and the rejection of grafts. The T lymphocytes do not produce antibodies in the classic

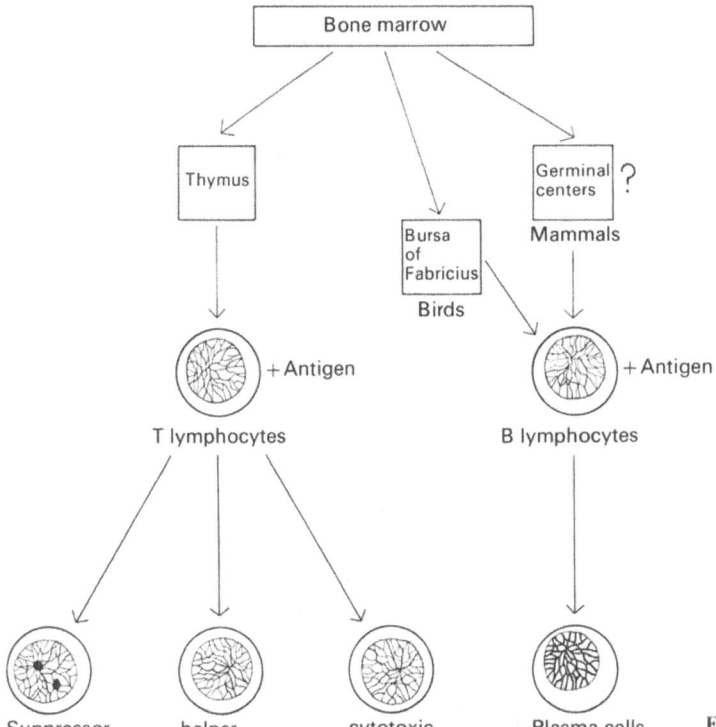

Suppressor   helper   cytotoxic   Plasma cells   **Fig. 2.4.** Origin and destiny of T
(and memory)   (and memory)   (and memory)   (and memory)   and B lymphocytes

sense – that of molecules of immunoglobulin being secreted in the serum. However, they possess antigen-reecognizing receptors on their surfaces. The thymus is considered a source of T lymphocytes uncontaminated with B lymphocytes. When T lymphocytes of the thymus are injected into previously irradiated recipient animals, a portion of these cells migrate to the spleen where they acquire new characteristics, the most notable of which is a greater efficiency in collaborating with the B lymphocytes in the immune response.

Adult thymectomized mice, lethally irradiated and then protected through transfusion of bone marrow cells, possess a lymphoid population composed almost exclusively of B lymphocytes. The life cycle of B lymphocytes is not well understood. It is recognized that these cells also originate from cells proceeding from the marrow that may be influenced in some extrathymic lymphoid compartment – perhaps in the

germinal center of the lymph nodes. Actually, the immature cells present in these center divide frequently and are unaffected by thymectomy. It is possible that they represent those B lymphocytes that, once stimulated by antigen, yield antibody-producing cells. The possible origins and destinies of this type of lymphocyte are schematized in Fig. 2.4.

T Lymphocytes

The importance of lymphocytes derived from the thymus (T lymphocytes) in the genesis of immunologic competence has only been recognized in the last few years because T lymphocytes are involved only indirectly in the formation of antibodies – therefore their activities can be analyzed only by complex methods involving analysis of the function of the cells rather than simple measurement of antibody quantities. Even so, description of the functions of the lymphoid system is impossible without an adequate comprehension of the function of T lymphocytes.

The thymus lymphocytes originate from primordial cells (stem cells) present in the fetal liver and, later on, also in the bone marrow. These cells migrate to the interior of the thymus and, probably under hormonal influences, enter into a process of differentiative proliferation. The thymus is impermeable to the majority of the blood cells, and the mechanism by which the stem cells are admitted to the thymus is unknown.

Stem cells initially transform into large pyroninophilic blasts in the cortex of the thymus and undergo a series of divisions during which the size of the cells diminishes and they acquire the morphology of lymphocytes. These are different lymphocytes, called thymocytes, which possess on their cell membrane alloantigens that are not found on stem cells or B lymphocytes. These alloantigens are termed Thy-1 (formerly theta), TLa, Gv-1, Ly-1, Ly-2, Ly-3, and Ly-5. Moreover, the thymocytes also differ from mature T lymphocytes, which are formed in the medulla of the thymus. For example, when compared with T lymphocytes, the thymocytes bear less histocompatibility antigens on their surface and are more sensitive to destruction by corticosteroids and radiation than T lymphocytes. During maturation the T lymphocytes lose the TLa antigens, lose some Thy-1 antigens, and gain histocompatitbility antigens, acquiring the membrane conformation typical of the recirculating T lymphocytes. There is evidence that the thymic environment is not indispensable for the differentiation of stem cells into thymocytes. Thus, when a suspension of peripheral cells, e.g. spleen cells, from athymic mice (mutant mice congenitally without thymuses) is exposed in vitro to hormonal substances extracted from the thymus (thymopoitin), it is possible to detect the rapid appearance of cells expressing the alloantigens TLa and Thy-1, typically expressed by thymocytes. More significantly, these antigens can be expressed even in the absence of thymopoietin, when the cells are exposed to mitogens such as concanavalin A or even endotoxins. Under normal conditions, obviously, this differentiation occurs in the thymus, but these observations are important in that they indicate that the stem cells can be stimulated to differentiate in the absence of the thymus.

With maturation completed, the T lymphocytes leave the thymus for the circulation where they remain for very long periods, stopping for various intervals in the "thymus-dependent" areas of the spleen, the lymph nodes, and other lymphoid structures. Large concentrations of T lymphocytes are encountered in the lymph of the thoracic duct and in the blood; they are more abundant in the lymph nodes than in the spleen and are relatively rare in the bone marrow.

T Lymphocyte Subpopulations. The genetic program of T lymphocytes combines information for the synthesis and expression of an unique pattern of surface glycoproteins which serve as markers for identification of the different T lymphocyte subpopulations. With the use of specific antisera to these markers (plus complement), it is possible to eliminate each of these T cell population separately and thus study the contribution of each one of them to the regulation of the immune system. This experimental approach has identified the existence of three major populations of T lymphocytes in mice: $Lyt-1^+$, $2,3^+$, $Lyt-1^+$, $2,3^-$ and $Lyt-1^-$, $2,3^+$. The $Lyt-1^+$ cells are mostly T helper cells (Th), the $Lyt-2,3^+$ cells include T suppressor (Ts) and T cytotoxic (Tc) cells, whereas the $Lyt-1,2,3^+$ cells contain the precursors of the $Lyt-2,3^+$ cells (see Table 2.1).

T Helper Cells. The T cells that express the $Lyt-1^+$ phenotype are inducer or helper T cells. They induce B cells to make antibodies, induce the precursors of the delayed type hypersensitivity cell and of the cytotoxic cell to develop into effector cells, in-

Table 2.1. Subpopulations of T lymphocytes (mouse)

Inductor T lymphocytes	Th of B lymphocytes	$\begin{cases} \text{Lyt-}1^+2^-; \text{ I-J}^-, \text{ Qa}^+ \\ \text{Lyt-}1^+2^-; \text{ I-J}^-, \text{ Qa}^- \end{cases}$
	Th of Ts	Lyt-1^+2^-; I-J$^+$, Qa$^+$
	Th of Tc	Lyt-1^+2^-; I-J$^-$, Qa$^-$
	Th of T$_{DH}$	Lyt-1^+2^-; I-J$^-$, Qa$^-$
Effector T lymphocytes	Ts	Lyt-1^-2^+; I-J$^-$, Qa$^+$
	Tc	Lyt-1^-2^+; I-J$^-$, Qa?
	T$_{DH}$	Lyt-1^+2^-; I-J$^-$, Qa$^-$
Regulator T lymphocytes	of Th	Lyt-1^+2^+; I-J$^-$, Qa$^+$
	of Ts	Lyt-1^+2^+; I-J$^+$, Qa$^+$

duce macrophages and other non-specific cells to engage in delayed reactions and they induce suppressor T cells to express optimal suppressing activity.

It seems certain that these different helper functions are mediated by different populations of helper T cells. For instance, the Lyt-1^+ cell that induces Ts cells is 1^+, 2^+ contrasting with the Lyt-1^+ cell that induces B cells, which ist 1^+, 2^-. Further, Lyt-1^+ that induces B cell proliferation, but no antibody secretion are Qa-1^-, whereas Lyt-1^+ cells that help antibody secretion but no proliferation are Qa-1^+ (see Table 2.1).

T-Suppressor Cell. In addition to helper T cells, there is a second category of T cells with regulatory activity, the T suppressor cell (Ts). These cells play a very important role in the regulation of the immune system. Their suppressive activity is exerted on B lymphocytes, other T lymphocytes and macrophages. For example, in certain situations of T-cell deficiency (thymectomy, injection of antilymphocyte serum), the production of antibodies is enhanced, whereas when an excess of T cells is present, the production of certain antibodies is diminished or halted. The existence of suppressor cells has been elegantly demonstrated by Judith Kapp after it had been postulated by Gershon and his collaborators many years before. There are strains of mice which are phenotypically unable to produce an antibody response to the haptenic terpolymer GAT (glutamine-alanine-tyrosine) coupled to bovine serum albumin (BSA). She immunized one group (1) of mice of this strain with GAT, another group (2) remained untreated. After several days, the spleen cells of mice of these two groups were prepared and half of the cells of each group were mixed and seeded into agar which contained BSA-GAT to induce a response in cells of group 2, and red blood cells coated with GAT as indicator. The remaining half of spleen cells of group 1 mice having received initially GAT was treated with anti-Thy-1 serum to eliminate T cells, and was then mixed with the remaining half of spleen cells of the other group (2) of mice. This mixture was seeded as the first cell mixture in agar containing BSA-GAT and indicator red blood cells. After the secreted antibodies had beed allowed to diffuse and to bind the red blood cell bound GAT, the agar plates were incubated with anti-mouse immunoglobulin antibodies and complement. Lysis of red blood cells was observed only in the agar plate of the second, anti-T cell treated mixture, indicating that T cells of GAT primed animals suppressed the normal response (Fig. 2.5).

There are two types of Ts cells, those that suppress an immune response against all antigens and thus are antigen-nonspecific, and those that are antigen-specific suppressing the immune response only to a single antigen. The former has specificity for idiotypes on antibody and on T and B receptors, whereas the latter reacts with

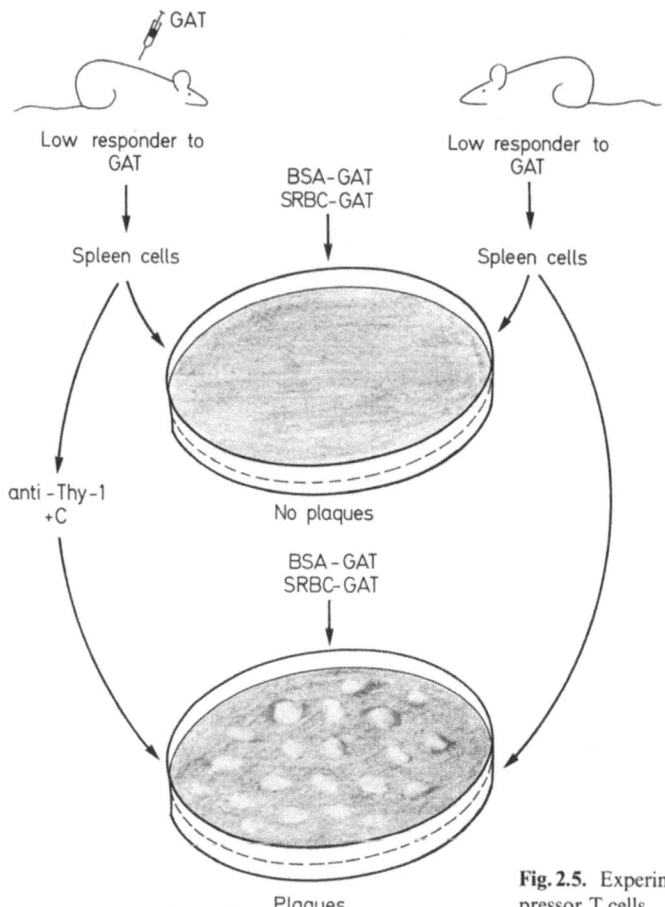

GAT

Low responder to
GAT

BSA-GAT
SRBC-GAT

Spleen cells

Low responder to
GAT

Spleen cells

anti - Thy-1
+C

No plaques

BSA - GAT
SRBC-GAT

Plaques

Fig. 2.5. Experiment showing the existence of suppressor T cells

antigen. According to Gershon, there exists a suppressor circuit that includes an inducer cells (Lyt-1⁻, 2,3⁺; I-J⁺), a precursor cell (Lyt-1, 2,3⁺), an amplifier cell (Lyt-1⁺, 2,3⁻; J-J⁺), and an effector cell (Lyt-1⁻, 2,3⁺; I-J⁻). The mechanism of induction of Ts cell is highly heterogeneous. The cells of this circuit communicate between themselves by direct contact or apparently more frequently through soluble suppressor factors. The final effector Ts cell regulates the activity of the immune system through its action on B lymphocytes, macrophages and even other T cell populations. Many suppressor factors produced by Ts cells are composed of two molecules, one of which have inhibitory activity, and another that binds to the former and focuses it to its target cell. Each of these molecules alone cannot produce the suppressor activity, the combination of the two molecules being necessary for the suppressive activity. Thus, suppressor factors are constituted by two molecules one of which serves as a functional chain (the I-J⁻ molecule) and another that serves as a carrier chain (the I-J⁺ molecule). Two different suppressor systems have been well studied. One involving the suppression of a primary *in vitro* response to sheep red blood cells, and another involving the suppression of an adoptive transfer of delayed hypersensitivity. In the first system, a Ts1 inducer cell produces an antigen-specific factor (Ts1F) which acts on a precursor cell transforming it into an effector Ts2 cell. The Ts1F is composed of two separate molecules, one of which binds to antigen and confers the antigen specificity to the factor and another that is antigen-nonspecific, I-J$^+$ and is the source of the IgH-V region-linked genetic restriction exhibited by the factor in its interaction with the acceptor cell. This cell now produces a Ts2F that has effector function and can directly suppress the PFC formation by spleen cells depleted of all Lyt-2,3$^+$ cells. In contrast to TslF, the Ts2F is composed by a single molecule that binds to antigen, has no MHC-linked genetic markers and exhibits a MHC-linked genetic restriction in its interaction with the target cell. However, like the TslF, the final suppressive signal is given (in this system to helper T cell) by Ts2F plus an I-J$^+$ antigen nonspecific molecule from the Lyt-1$^+$ inducer cell that confer an IgH-V region restriction to this factor. This second I-J$^+$ molecule required for Ts2F activity is supplied by an Lyt-1$^+$ I-J$^+$ cell in the assay system which, if removed, completely abolishes the suppressive activity of the Ts2F.

The effector system operative in delayed hypersensitivity is slightly different and permitted the study of idiotypic markers on the cells of the suppressor circuit. Here, the Tsl inducer cell produces a factor, TslF, which has an idiotype and reacts with a second Ts2 cell that has an anti-idiotype on its membrane. This cell then produces a factor, Ts2F, that induces a third Ts3 cell which has an idiotype to suppress the activity of the effector Ts cell.

Regulatory Circuits. The immune system is self-regulated. This means that the system is kept in an homeostatic balance whose disturbance leads to immunopathology. Two immunoregulatory systems are recognized, the idiotype-anti-idiotype network and the T cell regulatory circuit. The network concept of Jerne (see also pp. 110) deals primarily with the mutual recognition of idiotypes present on antibodies and on B and T cell antigen receptors, whereas the T cell circuit concerns the selective interactions of different cell types regardless of the structures used in their mutual recognition. The network of idiotypes-anti-idiotypes admits

that the antigen-recognizing receptor of B and T cells has both a distinct idiotype and an anti-idiotypic activity. T and B lymphocyte subpopulations recognize each other through idiotype-anti-idiotype reactions and this results in positive (stimulation) or negative (suppression) responses. Interactions between idiotypes and anti-idiotypes would normally keep the immune system in homeostasis. This is clearly observed in the humoral responses, when an antigen is naturally or experimentally introduced in the organism. Mice immunized with pneumococcal vaccine produce antibodies to phosphorylcholine (PC). When the amount of anti-PC antibodies diminishes with time, other antibodies appear that react with the idiotype of the anti-PC antibody. One admits that the anti-anti-PC antibody was elicited by the increase of the anti-PC antibody and that it suppresses further production of the anti-PC antibody. In addition, a third antibody against the anti-anti-PC antibody is also elicited and this may be repeated over and over increasing the size and complexity of the network. It must be pointed out, however, that the idiotype-anti-idiotype network has some degree of finity. Thus, due to degeneracy of the antigen recognizing receptors, the lastly induced anti-idiotype receptors start reacting with the first ones as if the system starts to bite its tail.

Superimposed on the idiotype network there is a T cell regulatory circuit concerned with selective interactions between different cell populations regardless of the structures used in their recognition. This cellular circuit is probably interconnected with the idiotypic network but exactly how is not yet known. The cellular regulatory circuits works basically on a series of positive and negative feedback reactions. For example, the positive effect of helper T cells to induce B lymphocytes to produce antibodies results in a feedback regulatory effect that sends in signals transmitted to the Lyt-1, 2, 3$^+$ cells leading to the development of Ts cells that neutralizes the helper effect. Although both Lyt-1$^+$Qa$^-$ and Lyt-1$^+$Qa$^-$

are involved in the helper effect only the first population is able to induce the suppressive signals. This suggests that the balance between these two populations of Lyt-1^+ cells can influence the size of the antibody response.

The Ts cell circuit works in a similar way. Thus, an increase in Ts effector cells produces feedback signals transmitted to the Lyt-1,2,3$^+$, that results in the development of a Lyt-2,3$^+$; I-J$^+$ cells that inhibit the activity of the Ts cells. These last cells have been designated contra-suppressor cells.

Cytotoxic T Lymphocytes. A third subset of T lymphocytes was described at the end of the sixties, capable of specific destruction of allogeneic cells against which the animal had been primed usually by transplanting cells of tissue. They may also be generated in vitro by incubating lymphocytes from a normal or presensitized individual for a few days with lymphocytes from another individual, differing from the former in its major histocompatibility antigens (see Chap. 6). This type of immunization in vitro by mixed lymphocyte culture (MLC) has made it possible to elucidate the cytolytic T lymphocyte (CTL) system in detail. In brief, when exposed to foreign antigen on the surface of the stimulator cells, some small lymphocytes of T-lineage will start to differentiate and to proliferate. Inition of this process may require participation of macrophages and perhaps also some other regulatory T-cells (see below, and Chap. 6). Proliferation leads to the development of highly cytotoxic, medium- to large-sized lymphocytes called early CTL. Upon further maturation, these cells revert to small-sized lymphocytes called memory CTL. When exposed to the same antigen at a later occasion, these memory cells will again transform into larger cytotoxic effector cells now called secondary CTL. These secondary CTL will again proliferate and revert to small memory cells and this cycle may be repeated many times. It is easily seen how these cyclic processes will result in an enlargement of the pool of lymphocytes

adapted to react with the antigen involved in the initial process of immunization.

The CTL-system has very exquisite specificity requirements. Thus, CTL lyse allogeneic cells carrying H-2 (or HLA, see Chap. 6) antigens different from their own. However, CTL also attack syngeneic cells, i.e., MHC-identical cells, but modified in their surface by a virus (see Chap. 6), by tumor transformation, or by introduction of a hapten. CTL recognize target cell antigens by means of specific receptors apparently synthesized by the cells which carry them. Each individual has many different clones of such T cells, each clone with receptors for a given specificity. The CTL-receptors are not conventional antibodies of immuno-globulin-type, and the reaction with the target cells does not require complement but direct contact between the cytolytic T cell and its target. There are some indications that only the contact-reaction is antigen-specific, but the subsequent killing reaction is an independent and nonspecific step. Nothing is known about the mechanism(s) of killing by cytologic T lymphocytes. These cells possess membrane markers similar to those found on T suppressor cells, Ly-1$^-$, 2$^+$, 3$^+$, but apparently they lack Ly-5 present on the membrane of suppressor cells (see Table 2.1). A more detailed account of the reaction mediated by these cells and their specificity is given in Chaps. 6 and 9.

Killer and Natural Killer Cells. Two additional sets of lymphocytes with the capacity for lytic activity have been described: Killer (K) cells and Natural Killer (NK) cells. The lineage of these cells, whether T or B cells, is not known, and the distinction between these two sets of cells is not sharp.

Killer Cell – The cytotoxic reaction mediated by K-cells is experimentally studied by mixing lymphocytes from normal ("non-immune") donors with target cells in the presence of antibodies against some surface antigens on the latter. This reaction is, therefore, called antibody-dependent cell-mediated cytotoxicity (ADCC) (see

Chaps. 6 and 9). The antibody serving as recognition factor for the initiation of cytotoxicity is not made by the K cells themselves. K cells and CTLs are distinct lymphocytes: (1) K cells have receptors for IgG antibodies which mediate the cytotoxic reaction. These Fc-receptors are proteins with low affinity for monomeric IgG, but they have high affinity for aggregated IgG of most subclasses or for IgG which has reacted with antigen, e.g., after having formed immune complexes on the surface of the target cells (2) K cells are a heterogeneous population in regard to their surface characteristics: about 40% of them possess a T cell specific marker, the receptor for sheep red blood cells in addition to Fc-receptors for IgG; these cells may belong to the subset of peripheral T cells in an immature stage. Another 40% lack this T cell marker as well as surface-bound immunoglobulin M and/or D (S-Ig), a marker of B cells, but they possess receptors for activated complement (C3b, see Chap. 5). The remaining 20% of K cells lacking these markers may include cells of nonlymphocytic lineage.

K cell-mediated target cell lysis is an extremely sensitive reaction; under optimal conditions, a few hundred molecules or less of antibody per target cell are enough to lyse 50% of the target cells in an incubation mixture. The lytic process appears to be identical to that of CTL (see above).

Natural Killer Cell – Natural cell mediated cytotoxicity refers to the lytic activity of lymphocytes from apparently healthy, not deliberately immunized donors against a variety of antigens. Obviously, this definition is ambiguouts since it is difficult to know whether or not a "normal" donor has previously in life been immunized, perhaps by exposure to microorganisms carrying antigens which crossreact with antigens on the target cell surface. In most instances these natural cytotoxic reactions are selective, i.e., some target cells are susceptible to the action of lymphocytes from a given donor while others are not. This pattern will often be different when the cytotoxicity

of the lymphocytes from different individuals is compared. In other words, the reactions are "specific." However, since we usually do not know the antigens which are involved and since we even do not know whether or not this phenomenon has an immunological basis in a strict sense, the term selective rather than specific is commonly applied in this context. Natural killer cells are the least well defined population of cytotoxic cells, and may resemble in part K cells. The effector cells are lymphocytes of unknown lineage, but believed to be (at least in their majority) pre-T cells originating from preprogrammed precursor cells in the bone marrow; they are found in the blood and the spleen. The generation and activity is thymus-independent, and they are found in high numbers in young individuals. Part of their activity can be inhibited by purified Fab-fragments of rabbit antibodies to immunoglobulin, suggesting that NK cell-mediated cytotoxicity is not known; it might be produced by contaminating B cells and taken up by NK cells, or NK cells may have the IG absorbed to their surface when removed from the donor. On the other hand, when lymphocytes from healthy donors are added to target cells the surface of which has been modified by an acute or persistent virus infection, natural cytotoxicity is strongly enhanced. This enhancement is a common phenomenon which is obtained with lymphocytes from practically every healthy donor. The phenomenon is distinct from CTL mediated cytotoxicity. It seems to be non-specific and to be unrelated to the possible presence of anti-viral antibodies in the lymphocyte donor's serum. It is obtained with a great variety of viruses. The effector cells in this virus dependent "natural" cytotoxicity have Fc-receptors for IgG but no surface-bound immunoglobulin. On the basis of surface marker analysis, 30%–40% may be T cells, distinct from the majority of the human blood T cells. However, this enhanced natural cytotoxicity is not an antibody-dependent reaction since it is not inhibited by anti-immunoglobulin. There is evidence that factors such as interferon (see Chap. 11) or similar substances are involved in the cytotoxic reaction in an unspecific manner.

The NK-system is believed to protect the organism against growth of certain tumors, particularly those of the lymphatic system itself. It may also have a general regulatory role on the normal function of the entire hemopoietic system. Hence, the role of this NK-system would be similar to that of the CTL system. However, while the CTL system requires the presence of a functioning thymus, the NK system does not. Therefore, the two systems seem to complement each other in their biological function.

Human T Cell Subpopulations. Functional and phenotypic heterogeneity of human T lymphocytes is now well established. Two

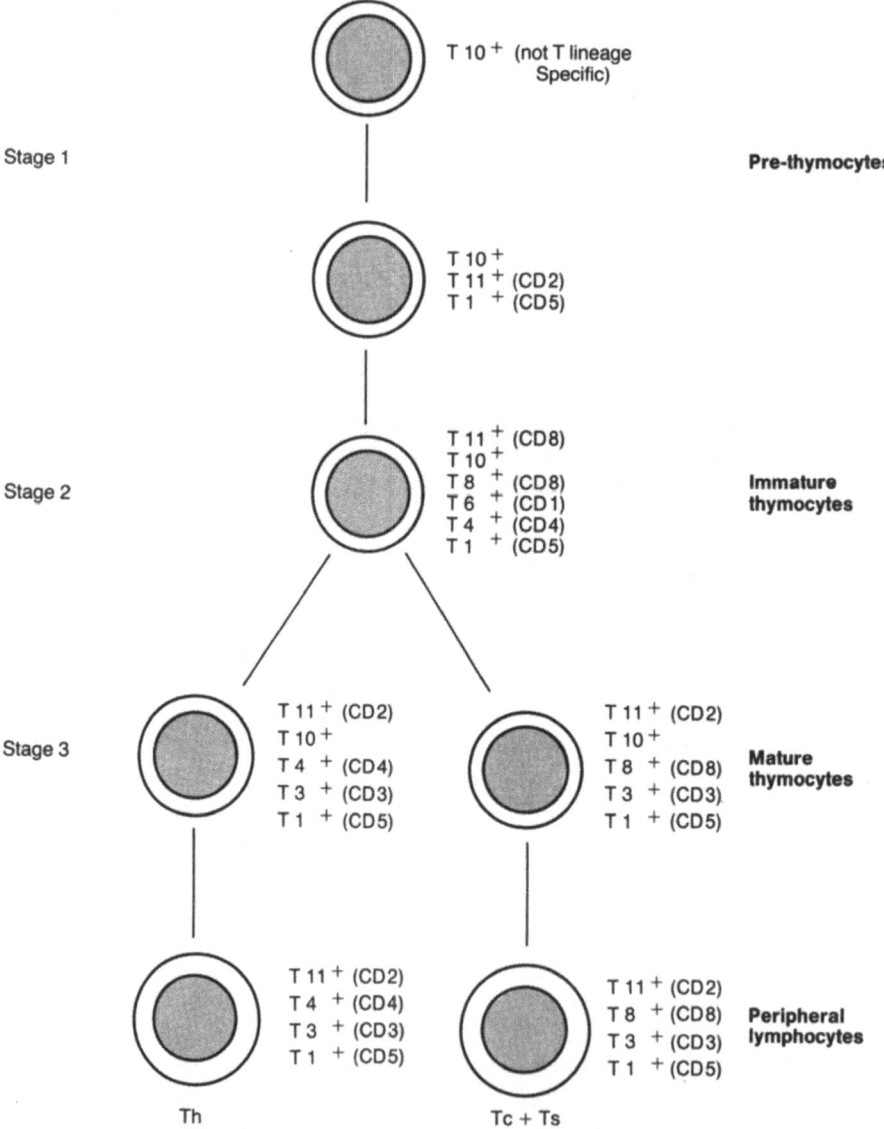

Stage 1 — T 10$^+$ (not T lineage Specific) — Pre-thymocytes

T 10$^+$
T 11$^+$ (CD2)
T 1 $^+$ (CD5)

Stage 2 — Immature thymocytes

T 11$^+$ (CD8)
T 10$^+$
T 8 $^+$ (CD8)
T 6 $^+$ (CD1)
T 4 $^+$ (CD4)
T 1 $^+$ (CD5)

Stage 3 — Mature thymocytes

T 11$^+$ (CD2)
T 10$^+$
T 4 $^+$ (CD4)
T 3 $^+$ (CD3)
T 1 $^+$ (CD5)

T 11$^+$ (CD2)
T 10$^+$
T 8 $^+$ (CD8)
T 3 $^+$ (CD3)
T 1 $^+$ (CD5)

Peripheral lymphocytes

T 11$^+$ (CD2)
T 4 $^+$ (CD4)
T 3 $^+$ (CD3)
T 1 $^+$ (CD5)

T 11$^+$ (CD2)
T 8 $^+$ (CD8)
T 3 $^+$ (CD3)
T 1 $^+$ (CD5)

Th

Tc + Ts

Fig. 2.6. Differentiation of human T lymphocyte. The antigens expressed during differentiation were defined with monoclonal antibodies. See text for details. According to Reinhertz and Schlossman (1980) New Eng J Medicine 303:370 (Th, T helper cell; Tc, cytotoxic T cell; Ts, suppressor T cell)

major subpopulations have been defined, namely effector T cells that mediate cellular immunity and regulator T cells containing helper and suppressor T lymphocytes. These two subpopulations have been defined with heteroantisera, autoantibodies and monoclonal antibodies directed at cell-surface antigens. They are both programmed for their respective functions during intrathymic differentiation. The earliest human lymphoid cells within the thymus have antigens shared by some myeloid cells but lack mature T lymphocyte antigens. These cells representing approximately 10% of thymic lymphocytes, are strongly reactive with two monoclonal antibodies, anti-T11 (CD2) and anti-T10 and react slightly with T1 (CD5). During maturation these cells loose T11 (CD2), retain T10 and acquire 3 new antigens defined by anti-T4 (CD4), anti-T8 (CD8) and anti-T6 (CD1). The thymocytes expressing T10, T6 (CD1), T8 (CD8) and T4 (CD4) represent about 70% of the thymic cell population. With further maturation, the thymocytes loose T6 (CD1), acquire T3 (CD3) and then segregate into two subpopulations that express either T4 (CD4) or T8 (CD8) antigen (see Fig. 2.6). Immunologic competence is acquired at this stage but is not completely developed until thymic lymphocytes migrate outside the thymus. In contrast with the majority of thymocytes, circulating T lymphocytes are $T1^+$ ($CD5^+$) and $T3^+$ ($CD3^+$). The T4 (CD4) antigen is present on approximately 55–65% of peripheral T lymphocytes, whereas the T8 (CD8) antigen is expressed on 20–30%. These two subpopulations correspond to helper, and to suppressor and cytotoxic T cells, respectively. The $T4^+$ ($CD4^+$) lymphocytes provide inducer function in T–T, T–B and T–M0 interactions. Although $T4^+$ ($CD4^+$) lymphocytes are not cytotoxic, they are required for optimal development of cytotoxicity by the $T8^+$ ($CD8^+$) effector cell. Thus, $T4^+$ ($CD4^+$) lymphocytes provide helper function in T–T interactions. $T4^+$ ($CD4^+$) lymphocytes are also necessary to induce B lymphocytes to differentiate into plasma cells. The regulatory activity of the $T4^+$ ($CD4^+$) lymphocytes are not restricted to lymphoid cells. On reactions with antigen, T lymphocytes produce helper factors that modulate erythroid stem-cell production *in vitro* and it is probable that the $T4^+$ ($CD4^+$) subpopulation is important in hematopoietic differentiation. In addition to its cytotoxic activity, the $T8^+$ ($CD8^+$) subpopulation contains T lymphocytes with suppressor functions. After activation with ConA, it suppresses the proliferative response to alloantigens. Thus, the $T4^+$ ($CD4^+$) subpopulation appears to be similar to the murine $Lyt-1^+$ lymphocytes that have helper functions, whereas the $T6^+$ ($CD1^+$) subpopulation is analogous to the murine $Lyt-2,3^+$ which mediates cytotoxic and suppressor functions. T3 (CD3) is expressed at low density on cortical lymphocytes and is linked to the antigen-specific receptor. Removal of T3 (CD3) from the lymphocytes is followed by loss of T cell receptor activity; this suggests that the T3 (CD3) antigen is associated with the receptor.

B Lymphocytes

B lymphocytes are cells that migrate to thymus-independent areas (areas not affected by thymectomy, see Chap. 1) of the secondary lymphoid organs: the follicles and medulla of the lymph nodes, the peripheral regions of the white pulp of the spleen, and follicles of the lymphoid tissue associated with the intestine. The majority of these cells are sedentary: once they have reached the secondary lymphoid organs, they survive there for about 10 days, not having been stimulated by antigen.

Each of the B lymphocytes express on its membrane about one hundred thousand antibody molecules with the same specificity. Two types of antibodies apparently can be concomitantly expressed on the membrane: IgD molecules and monomeric IgM, different from the pentameric form normally encountered in the circulatory system (see Fig. 1.6). These two types of membrane antibodies can execute different functions when they come in contact with the specific antigen. It has been calculated that each organism possesses between 10^6 and 10^7 different types of B lymphocytes in its lymphoid tissue and that any particular antigen is able to bind to 10 million B lymphocytes when injected into the organism. This cell population, which binds antigen, includes cells of many different clones of B lymphocytes, expressing antibodies of different specificities. In some cases, the antibodies bind the antigen with great affinity; in other cases, the linkage may be loose and insufficient to activate the cell. Depending upon the antigen dose, the activated population is either comprised exclusively of more avid cells (low antigen dose) or contains both highly avid and weakly avid cells (high antigen dose). The activation of the B lymphocytes induces the cell to enlarge and to divide. The transformation (blast transformation) can be measured biochemically by incorporation of DNA precursors such as thymidine, of morphologically. The blasts are large (15–20 μm) cells with abundant basophilic (pyroninophilic) cytoplasm, large nuclei with prominent nucleoli – quite different from lymphocytes in the resting phase. The blasts divide repeatedly and differentiate during each division, each time generating a greater number of small cells more adapted to the synthesis of antibodies. The final cell, known as plasma cell, does not resemble either a blast or a lymphocyte. Plasma cells are small, and have eccentric nuclei, with the chromatin arranged as in a cartwheel and with endoplasmatic reticulum and well-developed Golgi apparatus in the cytoplasm (see p. 10, and Fig. 1.5 D).

Activation of B Lymphocytes. During the humoral immune response to T dependent antigens, three distinct cell populations cooperate in the induction of antibody synthesis but only one of them produces antibody, the B lymphocyte. The other two cells are the T helper lymphocyte and the macrophage that do not produce antibodies but collaborate for their production. After

antigen penetrates the organism it is taken up by macrophages; macrophages digest the antigen (antigen processing) and in this degraded form it reappears on the membrane of these cells associated with products of the MHC (class II MHC antigens, see Chap. 6) and is presented to and recognized by the T lymphocytes.

When antigen is presented by the macrophages associated with Ia both the helper T lymphocytes and the macrophages produce monokines and lymphokines that regulate the differentiation and proliferation of various hemopoietic cell lineages including the T and B lymphocytes. Macrophages produce interleukin-1 (IL-1) that acts on antigen-activated T lymphocytes inducing them to proliferate and to produce interleukin-2 (IL-2). Thus, IL-1 aids in the differentiation of antigen-activated IL-2 producer T lymphocytes. As a consequence of antigen stimulation, T cells acquire the capacity to react to IL-2 by expressing receptors for this factor. IL-2 then acts on T lymphocytes stimulating their proliferation. Both IL-1 and IL-2 are able to restore the *in vitro* responsiveness of athymic mouse spleen cells to heterologous erythrocytes. Recent investigations suggest that IL-1 can act directly on B cells to enhance both proliferation and maturation on these cells. Factors that induce proliferation of B lymphocytes seem to be different from those able to induce maturation and both seem different from the colony-stimulating factors and from IL-2. These factors can be divided into three classes: B-cell growth factors; B-cell differentiation factors (T-replacing factor) and those that promote both growth and differentiation. These factors seem to act on different target cells and on different cell stages during the process of differentiation. It is not clear how many different molecules are involved in the control of B cell proliferation and maturation and the relationship between them is difficult to determine due to the variety of the *in vitro* assay methods used. It is clear, however, that activation of T helper cells and macrophages by antigen results in the production of antigen nonspecific polyclonally acting lymphokines. One problem is how the activation of every lymphocyte is prevented once recognition of antigen has induced the production of lymphokines. The answer seems to be that resting T lymphocytes with specificities for other antigen not present in the system remain resting because they do not have receptors for IL-2 and resting B lymphocytes with specifities to other antigens remain resting because they are insensitive to the action of B cell growth and maturation factors.

An additional important mechanism of B cell activation is the help of T lymphocytes through antigen specific factors produced by these cells. Although these factors are generally considered to act in the process of binding antigen to cells, it is not exactly known how these factors interact with B cells. They possess idiotypic determinants and have Ia antigens, that seems to be responsible for the MHC restricted activity of some of these factors (see Chap. 6). These specific factors though responsible for specific B cell clonal expansion, are insufficient to induce B cell differentiation and require the collaboration of antigen nonspecific factors (B cell growth and maturation factors). Activation of B lymphocytes by antigen has two consequences: proliferation that results in clonal expansion, and differentiation that results in antibody-secreting cells. In the first situation the B lymphocyte goes from the resting G_0 stage into the S stage. The proliferative response of B lymphocytes is not unique for antigen but may be induced by many different agents such as anti-IgM, anti-IgG, anti-IgD, anti-idiotype, calcium-ionophores etc. In the case of thymus-dependent antigens direct contact between T helper cells and B lymphocytes brought about by a bridge in which the carrier is bound to T cell and the hapten to B cell seems to be a probable initiation signal for B lymphocyte activation. A question not yet solved is whether interaction between T and B lymphocyte is MHC restricted. Considering, that T cells see antigen complexed to Ia molecules, one would assume that this interaction must be MHC restricted. However, there is some evidence that B cells in different stages of differentiation may respond to different activation factors and that subpopulations of B cells may exist that are or are not MHC restricted in their interaction with T lymphocytes.

In summary, there seems to be different pathways of B cell activations: direct contact between B and T cells which is MHC restricted; activation of B cells by T cell soluble factors that does not require direct cell contact. Anyway, when B lymphocytes that bind T-dependent antigens are exposed to T lymphocytes also capable of recognizing the antigen, the proliferation of B lymphocytes is greatly amplified, IgM antibodies are formed in greater quantities, and more characteristically, they differentiate into plasma cells that synthesize IgG, IgA, and IgE. Furthermore, the level of reactivity to the antigen is augmented, and memory cells appear that permit secondary responses to greatly reduced doses of antigen.

The differentiation signal given by T lymphocytes to B lymphocytes drastically modifies the activation sequence of these cells. During clonal expansion, a portion of the activated cells revert to a B lymphocyte morphology instead of differentiating progressively into plasma cells. However, these are different B lymphocytes. They survive for months and not merely a few days. They are recirculating rather than sedentary cells. In the event of new contacts with the antigen, they are capable of differentiating rapidly for the synthesis of IgG, IgA, and IgE – not being limited to IgM synthesis. It has been suggested that the antibodies expressed on the membranes of these "memory" B cells are different from those expressed by the original B cells. The original B cells express only monomeric IgM on their membranes; the memory B cells have a mixture of monomeric IgM and IgD on their membranes or even have IgG, IgA, or IgE. The mechanism of B cell activation by thymus-independent antigens is discussed in Chap. 3.

Localization of the Immunoglobulin on the B Lymphocyte Membrane. It is calculated that the number of immunoglobulin molecules on the B lymphocyte surface varies from 50,000 to 150,000 and averages 100,000. The immunoglobulin molecules are apparently distributed randomly over the surfaces of the B lymphocytes. Exactly how they are bound to the membrane is not known; presumably, however, the Fab fragments of the molecule are exposed, since the immunoglobulin on the lymphocyte surface can combine with the antigen. Some of the Fc fragments also must be exposed to explain the fact that the antibodies specific for the heavy chains react with the immunoglobulins on the cell surface. The localization of the immunoglobulin molecules on the lymphocyte surfaces has been studied principally with the use of fluorescein or ferritin-conjugated anti-immunoglobulin antibodies.

The fist observations with this technique revealed two types of labeling: (1) diffuse distribution of immunoglobulin over the cell surface, which microscopically resembled a ring-like pattern, or (2) a polar position giving the appearance of polar "caps" (see Chap. 6). It was soon verified that this difference in localization was due to a redistribution of the immunoglobulin molecules induced by their interaction with the anti-immunoglobulin. Electron-microscopic observation of the lymphocytes incubated with anti-immunoglobulin conjugated with ferritin showed that lymphocytes treated at 4 °C exhibited diffuse distribution of immunoglobulins, whereas those treated at 20 °C exhibited polar-capping distribution. Under the light microscope, the direct redistribution of the immunoglobulin molecules was observed by permitting the lymphocytes to react with the fluorescent anti-immunoglobulin at 4 °C and then observing the behavior of the cells as the temperature was increased 37 °C, the immunoglobulin molecules assumed a polar distribution. After 5 min at 37 °C, the fluorescent material was localized within the lymphocytes. These lymphocytes no longer reacted with the anti-immunoglobulin, showing that the redistribution of the surface immunoglobulin is followed by pinocytosis and disappearance of the majority of the membrane immunoglobulin molecules. These observations suggest that the redistribution of the molecules of the receptor immunoglobulins may be an important phenomenon in the activation of lymphocytes by the antigen.

When the lymphocytes that had lost their surface immunoglobulin were maintained in culture, there was a gradual reappearance of the surface immunoglobulins, which showed up initially at one pole of the cells and then later diffused over the entire surface. The kinetics of the appearance and disappearance of the lymphocyte surface immunoglobulin molecules is roughly similar to that of the change of immunoglobulin in untreated lymphocytes and to the turnover of cell membrane components in general, suggesting that this phenomenon constitutes a general cellular phenomenon.

Plasma Cells. The plasma cell is the cell responsible for the production of the immunoglobulins. The search for the location of antibody production in the organism led, at an early date, to the lymphoid organs as the structures responsible for the synthesis of these proteins. Pfeiffer and Marx (1898) appear to have been the first to perform the experiments demonstrating that the spleen, the lymph nodes, to a lesser degree the bone marrow, and possibly the lungs were the organs responsible for the production of the major portion on the antibodies. Some years later, McMaster and Hudack (1935) showed that injections of antigen into the footpaths of rabbits gave rise to the production of antibodies, first in the peripheral lymph nodes and then in the other lymphoid organs. Furthermore, they showed that if different antigens were injected into each one of the paws, the antibody concentration in the lymph node was much greater for the antigen injected into the region directly drained by that lymph node than in the central lateral nodes. Since a major percentage of the antigens frequently had been found in the macrophages, it was natural at first to suppose that these cells were those responsible for the antibodies produced by these organs. Later, the observation of a considerable increase in the lymphocyte population of the lymph nodes and of the spleen after antigenic stimulus led to affirmation of the fact that the lymphocytes and not the macrophages were the cells directly responsible for the production of antibodies.

Although some turn-of the century histologists had implicated a basophilic cell with an eccentric nucleus in the production of antibodies, only much later did convincing data begin to appear pointing to plasma cells as producers of antibodies. One of the first favorable indications in this regard was the observation that patients with hyperglobulinemia possessed an increased concentration of plasma cells in their tissues. Almost simultaneously, Bjorneboe and colleagues in Scandinavia, showed that hymperimmunization of rabbits caused a considerable increase of immunoglobulins in the serum accompanied by an increase in the number of plasma cells in the tissues. In the meantime, Fagraeus studied the correlation between the histologic alterations of the spleen and the production of antibodies and definitely showed the relationship between plasma cells and antibodies. Fagraeus studied the cell types that appeared in the red pulp of the spleen in response to an antigenic stimulus. The first cells to increase in number were large immature cells indistinguishable from similar cells normally existing in this organ. Subsequently, the relative ribonucleic acid (RNA) content of the cytoplasm of these cells increased, as indicated by the increased pyroninophilia, whereas the nucleus simultaneously diminished in size, condensed its chromatin, and became eccentric, thus acquiring the characteristics of the plasmatic series. Furthermore, simultaneous determination of the level of antibodies in the blood showed a clear correlation between antibody levels and the quantity of plasma cells in the spleen.

After the studies of Fagraeus, numerous other techniques were used to study this problem, giving rise to a more direct demonstration of the production of antibodies by plasma cells. One of the first such demonstrations utilized the phenomenon of bacterial adherence: Bacteria incubated with cells obtained from the lymph nodes of animals previously immunized with the same bacteria adhered specifically and exclusively to the plasma cells. Subsequently, Coons, employing the immunofluorescence technique, arrived at the same conclusion. The most commonly used method is the so-called sandwich technique: Histologic cuttings or cell smears obtained from lymphoid organs of an immunized animal are immersed in an antigen solution that combines with the antibody present in the cells. The preparation is then carefully washed to remove all of the uncombined antigen and only then immersed in a fluorescent antibody solution that combined with the antigen fixed by cells that contain antibodies. Under such conditions, practically all the cells that turn fluorescent are plasma cells; a few weakly fluorescent cells are lymphocytes. The same result is obtained when radioactive antigen and autoradiography are employed.

The intense production and secretion of immunoglobulins by plasma cells is in accord with the ultrastructure of these cells, which possess in their cytoplasm the organelles necesssary for the synthesis and secretion of proteins, such as endoplasmatic reticulum, ribosomes, and well-developed Golgi complexes (Fig. 2.7). Notably, these same structures are present in other protein-producing cells such as acinar cells of the pancreas. However, the exact mechanism by which the secretion of immunoglobulins proceeds in plasma cells is not known. It may occur by plasmacytosis, i.e., the loss of small portions of cytoplasm. Experimental data from different laboratories using different techniques indicate that each plasma cell synthesized immunoglobulins of an unique class and subclass, as well as a unique type of heavy (H) and light (L) chain. For ex-

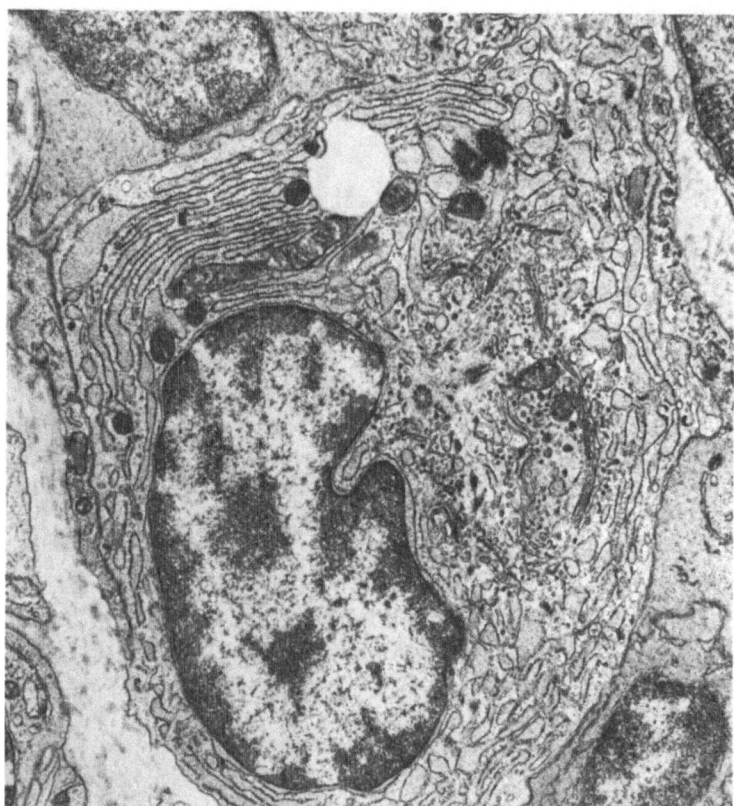

Fig. 2.7. Monkey *(Callithrix)* plasma cell. Note the abundant granular endoplasmic reticulum. A Golgi zone is seen at the *right* of the nucleus. Courtesy of LC Junqueira, Instituto de Ciências Biomédicas, Universidade de Sao Paulo (× 21,000)

ample, in individuals heterozygous for a specific allotype of immunoglobulin, even though both the allotypes coexist in the serum, the plasma cells show allelic exclusion; i.e., each cell produces only one allotype and not both. This findings suggests that during the differentiation of immunocompetent cells a somatic mechanism enters into action in such a way that one of the allotypic genes is suppressed. In short, each plasma cell produces only immunoglobulins of the same isotype, allotype and idiotype. In the same manner, numerous experiments show that the plasma cells synthesize antibodies of a single specifity. Thus, in animals immunized simultaneously with various antigens, or as usually happens, with an antigen containing diverse antigenic determinants in the same molecule, each plasma cell forms antibodies specific for just one of these determinants.

A possible exception to the rule that each plasma cell forms immunoglobulins of a unique class comes from the observation that frequently in a primary response, the synthesis of one immunoglobulin class (IgM) is followed shortly by the synthesis of another (IgG). Examination of plasma cells at the point in time where synthesis of IgG reveals that a significant minority of plasma cells produces both classes of immunoglobulins simultaneously. This elicited the hypothesis that some cells synthesize IgM to IgG is related to the "maturing of the immune response" through the reciprocal action of T-helper cells under whose influence antigen-stimulated B cells differentiate into antibody-secreting plasma cells and memory cells.

While the lymph nodes are in a resting state, only a small number of plasmocytic cells are present (about 1%–3%); after an antigenic stimulus, their number increases significantly. The origin of these cells has been studied in two ways. According to one method, tritiated thymidine is given to an unimmunized animal for a short time followed by an antigenic stimulus. After 3–4 days, labeled plasma cells appear. Such results suggest that the plasma cells originate from immature lymphoid cells ready to divide – lymphoblasts – that exist in lymphoid organs and that differentiate into plasma cells when stimulated by the antigen. With the other methods populations of small lymphocytes, obtained by cannulation of the thoracic duct, exhibited the capability to restore the capacity for production of antibodies in irradiated animals. These results suggest that the small lymphocyte might be able to differentiate into plasma cells after antigenic stimulation.

Other experimental results support the first alternative. For example, the transformation of lymphocytes into large pyroninophilic cells has been observed in cultures. In addition, it has been verified that lymph node specimens obtained from animals previously immunized with antigens A and B lose the capacity to form antibodies in vitro against antigen A when subjected simultaneously to the presence of this antigen and to 5-bromodeoxyuridine (a substance that blocks cellular division of incorporated in sufficient quantity into the DNA); yet the capacity to form anti-B antibodies is retained. Taken together, these observations suggest that the plasma cells may originate from the small lymphocytes that, under antigenic stimulus, revert to the condition of an immature cell, synthesize DNA, enter rapidly into division, and differentiate into plasma cells. In addition, some small lymphocyted do transform into memory cells.

Differences Between B and T Lymphocytes

The scanning electron microscope was used to detect morphologic differences between B and T lymphocytes. B cells are rich in microvilli whereas T cells tend to be smoother, having fewer and shorter villi. However, such differences are relative: Some cells cannot be classified by these criteria. The B lymphocytes can be differentiated from T lymphocytes by a series of membrane markers:

1. The *B lymphocytes* possess a high concentration of membrane immunoglobulin; these immunoglobulins are homogeneous in each B cell in terms of their immunologic specifity. The classes expressed are IgM (monomeric), IgD, or both.

2. In addition, to expressing on its membrane self-synthesized immunoglobulins, the B lymphocyte also possesses *receptors for the Fc* parts of other immunoglobulins bound in this way belong to a specific IgG subclass (in mice, IgG_1) and are not restricted in specificity. The physiologic function of these receptors is not known, but they can function as an accessory process in the concentration of antigens on the B lymphocyte membrane.

3. In addition to immunoglobulin receptors, B lymphocytes express on their membranes *receptors for C3b,* which is the active form of the third component of the complement system. These receptors make possible the concentration on the B lymphocyte membrane of soluble antigen-antibody complexes that have fixed complement.

4. B lymphocytes express on their membranes *alloantigens* not represented in T lymphocytes. Some of these antigens are also expressed on other cell types such as plasma cells and stem cells. They include antigens defined by heterologous antisera (e.g., rabbit antimouse) such as mouse-specific B-lymphocyte antigen (MBLa), as well as other which can be detected by alloantisera (e.g., mouse antimouse) such as Ly-4 and the Ia antigens (cf. Chap. 6).

B and T cells also differ in characteristics that depend upon the structure of the cell membrane.

5. They differ in their *response to lectins.* Lectins are products of plant or bacterial origin that, for unknown reasons, are capable of inducing activation in lymphocytes when exposed to the latter in vitro. B lymphocytes are relatively insensitive to the ac-

tion of certain lectins (phytohemagglutinin, concanavalin A) which are highly effective in the activation of T lymphocytes. On the other hand, B lymphocytes can be strongly activated by mitogens such as lipopolysaccharides (endotoxin) of *Escherichia coli* (T-independent antigen) that do not act upon T lymphocytes. Furthermore, B lymphocytes can be activated by anti-immunoglobulin antibodies that link to their membrane immunoglobulins; this does not occur with T lymphocytes.

6. The fractionation of cell suspensions of lymphocytes indicated that B lymphocytes are slightly smaller and less dense than T lymphocytes. Thus, these cells can be separated, according to their sedimentation rate, in gravitational or centrifugal fields.

Furthermore, B lymphocytes adhere more strongly to surfaces such as glass or nylon than do T lymphocytes; thus, when lymphoid cell suspensions are passed through columns containing nylon fibers, the population that passes through the column is enriched in T lymphocytes.

The *T lymphocytes* of certain species are capable of fixing heterologous erythrocytes on their surfaces, forming rosettes. Although the mechanism of the phenomenon is unknown, the formation of rosettes with sheep erythrocytes by human T lymphocytes is a routine test for identification of these cells in humans. The differences between T and B lymphocytes are summarized in Table 2.2.

Table 2.2. Differential membrane markers of T and B lymphocytes, and macrophages

Marker	T lymphocytes			B lymphocytes	Macrophages
	Helper cells	Suppressor cells	Cytotoxic cells		
Surface Ig[a, b]	−	−	−	+	−
Receptor for IgG-Fc[a]	−	+(Tγ)	.	+	+
Receptor for monomeric IgM[a]	+(Tμ)	−	.	.	.
C3b-receptor[a, b]	−	−	−	+	+
Ia/DR antigen[a, b]	−	+[b]	−	+	+
Thy-1[b]	+	+	+	−	−
Ly-1[b, c]	+	−	−	−	−
Ly-2, 3[b, c]	−	+	+	−	−
Ly-4[b]	−	−	−	+	−
Ly-5[b]	−	+	−	−	−
Receptor for SRBC[a, d]		+		−	−
CD antigens[e] in man	T4 (CD4)	T8 (CD8)	T8 (CD8)		CD9 CD11

− Absent; + present; · not known
[a] In human
[b] In mice
[c] Recently, Nagy and colleagues have provided some indications that the Ly-phenotype may not correlate to the differentiated *function* of lymphocytes (helper, suppressor, cytotoxic cell) but rather to the *restricting structures* (see Chap. 6), i.e., T cells recognizing antigens in association with K molecules assume the Ly-1^{-2+}, those recognizing antigens in association with A molecules are Ly-1^{+}2^{-}, and those recognizing antigens in association with E molecules are Ly-1−2^{+}
[d] Sheep red blood cells; it is not known which subsets of T cells are involved in the rosette formation with sheep red blood cells
[e] Human lymphocyte antigens defined with monoclonal antibodies; CD, cluster of differentiation
  Additional antigens are: TL (CD1) on thymocytes
  T11 (CD2) on E-rosette forming T cells
  T3 (CD3) on most peripheral blood T lymphocytes; CD7 on all T lymphocytes
  T1 (CD5) and CD6 on all T lymphocytes and some B lymphocytes

7. T and B lymphocytes recognize antigen in a different way. B lymphocytes can recognize either free antigen or antigen bound to an immunabsorbent but T lymphocytes respond to antigen only when it is on a cell membrane. Indeed, the T lymphocyte recognizes antigen mostly in the context of MHC molecules of the antigen-presenting cell (see Chap. 6). Thus, when a suspension of lymphocytes are passed through a column of immunabsorbent containing antigen, the specific B cells are bound to the column, whereas specific T cell pass freely through the column and can be recovered in the eluate (with the exception of T suppressor cells). In order to isolate specific T lymphocytes, a suspension of these cells obtained from a immunized animal is allowed to contact a monolayer of fibroblasts containing antigen in their membranes. In this condition the specific T lymphocytes adsorb to the fibroblasts from which they can be isolated by gentle treatment with trypsin. It has been shown that the recovered lymphocytes are specific for the antigen bound to the fibroblasts.

The Antigen Receptors in B and T Lymphocytes

Both T and B lymphocytes have antigen specific receptors. It has been known for many years that the B lymphocyte receptor is an immunoglobulin molecule whose specificity is clonally distributed (for details, see Chap. 4). However, the nature of the T cell receptor remained unknown until recently. The first indication that it had some similarity with the variable region of the immunoglobulin was the demonstration by Binz and Wigzell of the presence of idiotopic determinants on the antigen-binding T cell receptor. Since then much was learned through the use of specific antisera and monoclonal antibodies that recognize clone-specific proteins on the surface of T-cell clones, hybridomas or T-cell lymphomas. The first glimpse of the receptor came when protein dimers that seemed essential

for T lymphocyte activation by antigen was precipitated with monoclonal antibodies specific for individual T lymphocyte clones. These studies suggested that the portion of the receptor responsible for specificity is a heterodimeric glycoprotein having a molecular weight of about 90 K and consisting of two subunits, an α-subunit with 40–45 K and a β-subunit with 42–44 K (see Fig. 2.8). Analysis of peptide fingerprints suggested that both subunits are composed of a variable and a constant region similar to the heavy and light chains of the immunoglobulins. Recently, two research groups have succeeded in isolating T lymphocyte-specific cDNA clones of mouse and human origin which show significant homology with

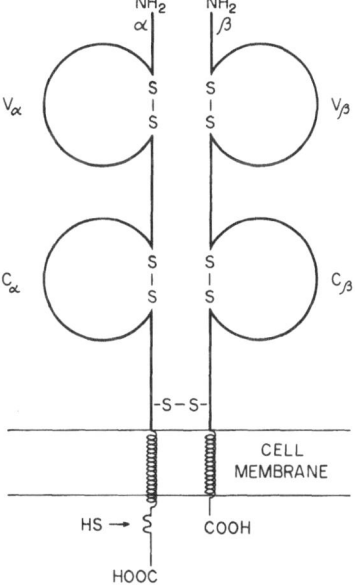

Fig. 2.8. Proposed structure of the T cell receptor. The receptor is probably composed by two polypeptide chains, α and β, each having two extra-cellular immunoglobulin-like domains, an amino-terminal variable and a carboxy-terminal constant domain. These domains are stabilized by an S-S bridge. Both chains are glycosylated and are held together by a single interchain S-S bond located close to the cell membrane. A short carboxy-terminal peptide rich in cationic residues penetrates in the cytoplasm from each chain. The SH group present in the cytoplasmic segment of the α-chain may interact with a membrane or cytoplasmic protein and may be important for the cell's effector function. (Adapted from Saito et al. 1984)

immunoglobulin genes. It was also shown that the cDNA encoded a protein made up of a variable amino-terminal segment and a constant-terminal segment. Afterwards, the genomic sequence for the α- and β-subunit was reported. These studies showed that like the immunoblobulin genes, the α- and β-subunits genes are split into segments in the germ line and that the segments are brought together in mature T lymphocytes to compose a functional gene. Of course, since each gene segment is present in a number of forms that can be assorted at random, an enormous number of different receptors can be encoded. The receptor's structure suggested by Saito and colleagues looks very much like two immunoglobulin chains both anchored in the T cell membrane by a stretch of hydrophobic amino-acids such as it happens with the membrane immunoglobulin. Each subunit has two domains on the external surface of the membrane, one constant and one variable with the variable region at the amino-terminal segment of the chain. Between the constant domain and the cell membrane there is a short segment that contains an S-S bridge that connects the two subunits. Studies are now in progress comparing receptor molecules from different T lymphocytes clones (see also Chap. 6 and cover).

Cooperation Between B and T Lymphocytes

B and T lymphocytes exhibit a collaborative effect in their immune response against T-cell-dependent antigen. For example, the capacity of irradiated mice to respond with the production of antibodies to the presence of sheep erythrocytes is not reestablished by the transfer of thymic cells alone or by that of bone marrow cells alone, yet it is easily resorted by the transfer of both cell types. In the immunologic response to hapten-carrier antigen (hapten-protein conjugate), it has been verified that the T lymphocytes respond specifically to the carrier protein, whereas the B lymphocytes react specifi-

cally to the hapten. The immune response to almost all antigens requires the cooperation of the two types of lymphocytes. This can be clearly shown in an experiment using bovine serum albumin as antigen. In this experiment, lethally irradiated mice were inoculated with thymus and bone marrow cell mixtures in varying proportions and were inoculated quickly thereafter with the antigen. About 1 month later, the level of antibodies present in the serum was determined, permitting verification that for a constant dose of thymus cells, the antibody level diminished with decreasing doses of marrow cells; for a constant dose of marrow cells, the antibody level diminished with decreasing doses of thymus cells. These results clearly indicate cooperation between the two types of lymphocytes in the immune response. The phenomenon also has been observed in cell culture, where a primary response to erythrocytes are present. Thus, although spleen-cell cultures obtained from mice thymectomized shortly after birth (containing only B lymphocytes) or thymus-cell cultures (containing only T lymphocytes) do not produce antibodies against sheep erythrocytes, a culture-containing both types of cells produces hemolytic antibodies. It appears that T lymphocytes assume a helper function in the immune responses of the B lymphocytes. In the experiments, shown in Fig. 2.9, irradiated mice were divided into three groups – A, B, and C. In group A, the animals were inoculated with the thymus cells, in group B, with thymus cells plus antigen; and in group C, only with the antigen. Six days later, the animals of the three groups were killed and, from each group, suspensions added to bone marrow cells and the antigen under study. The immune responses of these animals were then compared. The experiment demonstrated considerable augmentation of the immune response in the animals of group E, which had received spleen cells of the mice from group B, which in turn initially had been injected with thymus cells plus the specific antigen. These results show that the T lym-

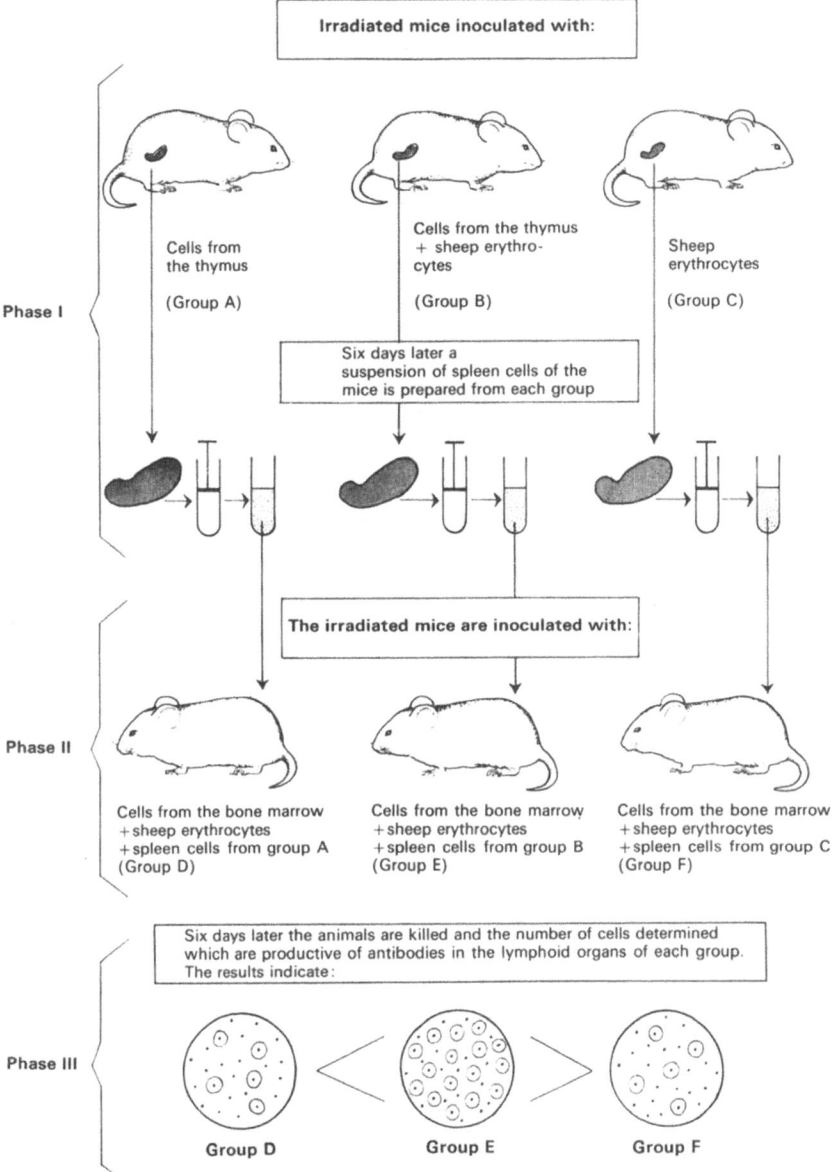

Fig. 2.9. Protocol of experiments showing the conditioning of T lymphocytes by antigen

phocytes of the group B animals were con-ditioned by prior contact with the antigen. Because cooperation between these two types of cells is not necessary for all antigens, one differentiates between thy-mus-dependent antigens and thymus-inde-pendent antigens.

T-T Lymphocyte Cooperation. The basic ex-periments used to demonstrate cellular co-operation consist in looking for a synergis-tic effect when 2 different cell populations are mixed. For instance, in cellular cooper-ation for antibody production, the mixture of T and B lymphocytes results in an anti-body response well above that expected from the simple sum of the antibody production by each one of these cell populations alone. Using this observation it was possible to demonstrate that different T lymphocyte populations cooperate in T cell mediated responses. For instance, the generation of cytotoxic lymphocytes requires cooperation between T Lyt-1$^+$ and Lyt-2,3$^+$. The elimination of each one of these lymphocyte population by pre-treatment with specific anti-Lyt-1$^+$ or anti-Lyt-2,3$^+$ prevents the full generation of cytotoxic lymphocytes. T-T lymphocyte cooperation is also required in delayed type hpyersensitivity and other cell mediated responses.

Macrophages

The term macrophage is generally applied to phagocytic cells encountered in the connective tissue that are capable of ingesting bacteria, cellular remains, and foreign substances generally present in the tissues. The prefix "macro-" distinguishes these cells from other smaller phagocytic cells existing in the blood and tissues, the polymorphonuclear neutrophils.

In lymphoid tissue, the macrophages may be of the fixed variety, reticuloendothelial cells that border the lymphatic sinuses and sinusoids; or they may be mobile, like the free phagocytes that move actively in the tissues. The form of the macrophage depends upon its functional status and localization. Fixed macrophages are star-shaped or spindle-shaped, possessing nuclei of delicate chromatin with one or two nucleoli and slightly basophilic cytoplasm. The mobile macrophage is usually round or oval, with a kidney-shaped nucleus. Both types of macrophages posseess irregular cytoplasmic membranes with numerous prolongations and entry points that are related to the mechanism of phagocytosis.

Macrophages originate from precursor cells in the bone marrow and pass into the blood as monocytes. They remain in the circulation for some hours (6–12 h in the mouse) after which they migrate into the tissues, and transform to macrophages. They ac-

quire greater phagocytic activity, more cytoplasm and more cytoplasmic organelles such as lysosomes, microtubules, microfilaments, and Golgi membranes. In addition, the nucleus becomes more irregular and acquires one or two nucleoli. Functionally, the monocytes and macrophages make up part of a system of highly phagocytic mononuclear cells, the mononuclear phagocyte system. The dendritic cells of the fillicles of the spleen and lymph nodes, although capable or retaining antigens of their surfaces, are not considered as belonging to this system. The macrophages customarily migrate to the peritoneal cavity and to other serous cavities, the red pulp of the spleen and the lymph node medullae. Fixed macrophages such as the Kupffer cells of the liver probably also originate from monocytes. Epithelioid cells and giant multinucleated cells result from the fusion and transformation of the macrophages.

Monocytes and macrophages are characterized by intense phagocytic activity and by the capacity of adherence to certain materials such as glass. Many techniques for isolationg these cells takc advantage of these properties.

The process of phagocytosis can be divided into two phases: the adherence of the particle to the surface of the cell and the ingestion of the particle.

Monocytes as well as macrophages possess receptors for the Fc pieces of the immunoglobulins and for the complement system (C3b). The adherence phase of the particles is mediated by andibodies of by antibodies plus complement. The time during which the particle is coated with IgM plus C3 corresponds to the first phase, the adherence phase; if IgG is bound to the particle, ingestion of the particle occurs even in the absence of C3. Adherence also can be facilitated by other serum factors that in some cases have been identified as immunoglobulins. Apparently, some types of particles can adhere to the macrophages without the intervention of the serum factors. Phagocytosis mediated by immunoglobulin with or without complement is called immune phagocytosis. The monocytes and macrophages that possess receptors for immunoglobulin and for complement on their cell membranes can be considered "professionel" pagocytes such as fibroblasts, reticular cells, and endothelial cells, which probably do not possess such receptors but rather ingest the particles independently of the antibodies and complement.

Role of Adherent Cells
in T-B Cell Cooperation

In the experiments to study cellular cooperation both lymphocyte suspensions (thymic and bone-marrow) contained adherent cells. The adherent cells can be separated through their capacity to adhere to glass or plastic surfaces. Thus, when one leaves a splenic cell suspension for a few hours in a Petri dish and then removes the supernatant, the non-adherent cells (mostly B and T lymphocytes) are removed with the suspension medium, whereas adherent cells (mostly macrophages) are left on the Petri dish. It has been observed that when antigen is added to a culture containing only adherent or non-adherent cells no antibody is produced whereas a culture containing both types of cells produces antibodies. Therefore, for antibody production cooperation is necessary among three different types of cells: non-adherent antigen-specific cells (T and B lymphocytes) and adherent antigen-non specific cells (macrophages). As we will see in the following sections, all immune responses require the presence of macrophages which are necessary for antigen presentation to T lymphocytes (T lymphocytes recognize antigens associated with MHC products in the macrophage membrane), for the proliferative T lymphocyte response induced by either antigen or mitogens (phytohemmagglutinin and concanavalin A) as well as for the generation of cytotoxic T lymphocytes and of T lymphocytes involved in delayed type hypersensitivity. In all these interactions macrophages and lymphocytes must share membrane molecules coded for the MHC of the species, in order to be able to interact (see Chap. 6).

Role of Macrophages
in Humoral Immune Response

Evidence that the macrophages are important in induction of the immune response originated from early studies on the immune response to several different antigens. It was then well known that particular antigens as red cells, bacteria and viruses were strongly immunogenic, whereas soluble proteins were weak antigens. However, polymerization of soluble proteins converted them in good immunogens. These results suggested that antigens that are more efficiently taken up by macrophages induce a better immune response. Several experiment have shown that antigens associated with live macrophages are more immunogenic. Macrophages obtained from peritoneal exudates were incubated for a brief period with radiolabeled proteins, washed and transferred to syngeneic recipients which were later tested for antibody production. The results of these experiments showed that antigen bound to live macrophages were highly immunogenic.

Further, *in vitro* experiments showed that when T and B lymphocytes were cultured with small numbers of macrophages containing antigen or with free soluble antigen, the immunogenicity of antigen associated with the macrophages was considerably superior. These results indicated interactions between T and B lymphocytes and macrophages. Later studies have suggested that the primary interaction is between T lymphocyte and macrophage, this event allowing effective interactions between T and B lymphocyte for antibody production. The importance of antigen presentation by macrophages is emphasized by experiments showing that when antigen is presented directly to T lymphocytes no helper cell develops, but instead T suppressor cells develops and block the response to antigen.

It is now firmly established that the presentation of antigen by macrophages is essential for the specificity of the activated T lymphocyte and that this is the mediated by the Ia molecule on the macrophage membrane (see Chap. 6). In this regard, it has been shown that macrophages can be divided into two types, on bearing and the other lacking Ia molecules. Although both types take up the antigen only those having Ia molecules are able to cooperate with the T lymphocyte.

It has been shown that primed T lymphocytes from two inbred strains that differed only by their Ia molecules responded *in vitro* with proliferation only when the antigen was presented on the syngeneic macrophage. These results indicated that T lymphocytes recognize the antigen on the surface of the macrophage in association with Ia molecules and that the specificity of the activated T lymphocyte is directed at both the foreign antigen and the macrophage Ia molecule. It seems that the role of the Ia molecules of the macrophage is to control in some way recognition of foreign antigens by T lymphocytes.

Role of Macrophages in Cellular Immunity

Many infectious agents are able to survive and multiply within the macrophages after having been phagocytized (Mycobacterium tuberculosis, Listeria monocytogenes, Candida albicans, Trypanosoma cruzi etc.). However, macrophages from immune individuals are able to kill these pathogens provided they are activated by soluble mediators produced by immune T lymphocytes on interaction with the specific antigen. These mediators are able to recruit and activate macrophages to a state of high cytocidal activity. It has been shown that the activated macrophages have the power to stop the growth of intracellular bacteria or parasites. The activated macrophage acts nonspecifically, i.e., it will kill any infectious agent regardless of the organism that stimulated the immune T lymphocyte.

The specificity of the T lymphocyte was demonstrated by cell transfer experiments.

Thus, normal mice that were inoculated with lymphocytes obtained from mice immune to Listeria monocytogenes were protected from a lethal challenge with Listeria, but not from a lethal challenge with Mycobacterium tuberculosis. Nothwithstanding, these animals could resist infection with Listeria. The T lymphocytes immune to Listeria were able to activate the macrophage only on specific challenge with Listeria, but not with M. tuberculosis to which there was no immune T lymphocyte, yet the activated macrophages protected against the M. tuberculosis (as they would do against any bystander pathogen). Activated macrophages show an enhanced synthesis of several enzymes, but this fact does not necessarily correlate with their increased cytocidal activity. In addition, activated macrophages show an increased metabolism and secrete oxygen-derived products as superoxide anion and hydrogen peroxide. Recently, it has been postulated that these products may be involved in the cytocidal activity of the macrophages. The role of macrophages in delayed hypersensitivity is considered in Chap. 10.

Langerhans Cells. Recent observations showing that epidermal Langerhans cells express Ia molecules and receptors for the Fc portion of IgG and for C3b suggest that these cells may represent an epidermal equivalent of the macrophage. Indeed, *in vitro* studies showed that antigen bearing Langerhans cells are able to induce a proliferative response in immune T cells and that the two cells have to be syngeneic to interact. These observations have important clinical implications regarding to the function of Langerhans cells in cutaneus delayed hypersensitivity.

Dendritic Reticular Cells

These are cells encountered principally in the germinative centers of the lymph nodes. Their profuse cytoplasmic prolongations are so intricate and extensive as to be suggestive of a three-dimensional spider's web. Ulike macrophages, these cells do not phagocytose antigens, but retain on their surfaces for considerable periods of time. This retention is accentuated particularly in the secondary response and appears to depend upon the presence of antibodies. Some authors consider these cells a special type of reticular cells, whereas others hold them to be a particular type of macrophage, termed dendritic macrophages. The function of these cells in the immune response is discussed in relation to the response of the lymph nodes to antigenic stimulus.

Allogeneic Effect. In experiments to study T-B cooperation, it was observed that addition of non-adherent cells taken from neonatally thymectomized mice restaured the ability of these cells to produce antibodies. This was expected since non-adherent cells contain T lymphocytes. Surprisingly, it was observed that if adherent allogeneic cells were used instead of adherent syngeneic cells, the antibody production was increased. Similar observation was made with the carrier-specificity effect. As we know, animals immunized with an hapten-protein A conjugate do not present a secondary response to the hapten when challenged with the hapten conjugated to a different carrier protein B. However, if a few days before the challenge with the hapten-heterologous protein B, the animals are injected with allogeneic cells, one obtains a secondary antibody response against the hapten. This phenomenon is termed "allogeneic effect." The allogeneic effect depends essentially upon a graft-versus-host reaction and consequently requires T lymphocytes alive and metabolically viable. The allogeneic effect can also be induced *in vitro*. For that, one cultivates *in vitro* lymphoid cells from an F1 individual with lymphoid cells from a parental individual. The parental cells react against the F1 cells and produce a graft-versus-host reaction *in vitro*. In this situation it is possible to obtain in the culture supernatant a factor able to reproduce the allogeneic effect (allogeneic effect factor). The

factor that has no antigen-specificity, is a heat sensitive glycoprotein probably constituted by two polypeptide chain, a heavy and a light chain. It has been established that the allogeneic factor is a product of the I region of the H-2 complex. It is possible that the allogeneic factor may act as a helper factor.

References

Cantor H, Boyse EA (1976) Functional subclasses of T lymphocytes bearing Ly antigens. I. The generation of functionally distinct T-cell subclasses is a differentiative process independent of antigen. J Exp Med 141:1376

Cantor H, Boyse EA (1976) Functional subclasses of T lymphocytes bearing Ly antigens. II. Cooperation between subclasses of Ly^+ cells in the generation of killer activity. J exp Med 141:1390

Greenwalt TJ, Jamieson GA (eds) (1977) The granulocytes: Function and clinical utilization. Liss, New York

Gupta S, Good RA (eds) (1979) Cellular, molecular, and clinical aspects of allergic disorders. Plenum, New York

Howie S, Mcbride WH (1982) Cellular interactions in thymus-dependent antibody responses. Immunology today 3:273

Kapp JA, Pierce CW, Schlossman S, Benacerraf B (1974) Genetic control of immune response in vitro. V. Stimulation of suppressor T cells in nonresponder mice by the terpolymer L-glutamic acid^{60}-L-alanine^{30}-L-tyrosine^{10} (GAT). J Exp Med 140:648

Katz DH (1977) Lymphocyte differentiation, recognition, and regulation. Academic, New York

Melchers F, Andersson J (1984) B cell activation: three steps and their variation. Cell 37:715

Möller G (ed) (1980) Unresponsiveness to haptenated self molecule. Immunol Rev Vol 50. Munksgaard, Copenhagen

Moretta L, Ferrarini M, Cooper MD (1978) Characterization of human T cell subpopulations as defined by specific receptors of immunoglobulins. Contemp Top Immunobiol 8:19

Nelson DS (ed) (1976) Immunobiology of the macrophage. Academic, New York

Perlmann P (1979) The cytotoxic effector function of lymphocytes. Behring Inst Res Comm 63:7

Reinherz EL, Haynes BF, Bernstein ID (1985) Leukocyte Typing II. Springer New York

Saito H, Kranz DM, Takagaki Y, Hayday AC, Eisen HW, Tonegawa S (1984) Complete primary structure of a heterodimeric T-cell receptor deduced from cDNA sequences. Nature 309:757

Winchester G (1984) The T-cell receptor completed. Nature 309:750

Chapter 3   Antigens

IVAN MOTA

Contents

Antigens   63
Chemical Basis of Antigenicity.   64
   Synthetic Antigen Conjugates   64
   Specific Determinants of the Natural Antigens   65
   Antigenic Determinants of Polysaccharides .   66
   Antigenic Determinants and Cross-Reactions .   67
   Conformation and Antigenic Specificity . . .   68
Chemical Basis of Immunogenicity   68
   Importance of the External Groupings
     of the Antigen in Immunogenicity   70
   Adjuvanticity   70
Thymus Independent Antigens.   72
References   72

Antigens

Classical immunology defines antigen (from greek *"anti"* – "against"; and *gen*, from *"gignomai"* – "to generate") as complex molecules recognized as foreign (nonself) by the immunologically competent cells. However, more recent developments support a different concept of antigen. According to the network theory of Jerne, the immune system is an auto-regulated, self-contained network of complementary T and B receptors (idiotype-anti-idiotype network) that are constantly reacting against themselves to keep the homeostasis of the system (see p. 110). This chain of reactions goes on under physiological conditions independently of external stimuli. However, the specificity of the self-recognition receptors is degenerate and some of them cross-react with molecules of the external environment as if the receptor confuses these external molecules as self. In this sense antigens are not foreign molecules (nonself) but on the contrary are molecules that have some similarity with self and are rec-

ognized by the immune system as such. Thus, the clones of immunocompetent cells that are stimulated by antigen are not primarily designed to react with antigen but rather with the endogenous components of the network that Jerne designates as the internal image of the antigen (antigen represents the external image of the idiotype). Since in natural conditions the organism is in constant contact with molecules coming from the external milieu, the organization of the idiotypic network reflects at every moment an unbalanced state caused by the constant antigenic stimulation. The final consequence of antigen stimulation is an increase in the level of antibodies and of cells able to specifically react with that antigen. This expansion in the population of antibodies and specific cells diminishes with time after antigenic stimulation. However, in most situations the system is not completely brought back to the initial basal level, as it is shown by the quicker and higher level of the immune response to a later contact with the same antigen (secondary response). At this point it is important to emphasize that the assertion of the classical immunology that only under exceptional circumstances there is a formation of antibodies (or cells) capable of reacting with constituents of the own organism, is no more valid. On the contrary, auto-recognition is a physiological and essential mechanism of the immune system. The autorecognition, however, is kept under strict control by not well known mechanisms whose unbalance leads to immune diseases (see Chap. 12).

Antigens are usually complex and large molecules though even small molecules

(<1,000 mw) can function as antigens. However, molecules of less than 10,000 mw are usually not able to function as antigen. To act as an antigen it is not enough that a substance is macromolecular. Synthetic polymers such as nylon, teflon, polysterene, polyacrylamide, etc., possess bulky molecules and yet are devoid of immunogenic activity. Apparently they are too different from self molecules to evoke an immune response.

Lipids apparently are not immunogenic, yet they may function as haptens when mixed the human of porcine serum. In this manner, antibodies have been obtained against cholestero, cephalin, and lecithin. The operative mechanism of the serum is unknown, but it is thought to function as a carrier or Schlepper protein. An important lipid from the serologic point of view is cardiolipin, used in the serodiagnosis of syphilis. Two discrete properties are exhibited by antigens: (1) the capacity to induce the formation of antibodies, or immunogenicity, and (2) the capacity to react with antibodies, or antigenicity. Only complete antigens, i.e., complex macromolecules possess both properties. There are substances that are not immunogenic but are antigenic. These substances are too simple to be capable of inducing an immune response. However, when they are part integral of a larger molecule (carrier), they be-

come immunogenic and able to induce the formation of antibodies with which they react, even if isolated from the carrier. When these non-immunogenic but antigenic molecules are part of natural molecule, they are designated antigenic determinants of epitopes, whereas when they are artificially introduced in a molecule, they are designated haptens.

Chemical Basis of Antigenicity

Synthetic Antigen Conjugates

Karl Landsteiner performed a series of brilliant investigations with artificial antigen conjugates that led to an understanding of the chemical basis of antigenic specificity. Landsteiner made use of the observation that the antibodies against a conjugated protein (a carrier protein plus a hapten) react and form precipitates with other proteins when conjugated with the same hapten. In experiments with protein conjugates, the antigen used for obtaining the antisera and those used in reactions in vitro, must be prepared through conjugates of the hapten to different proteins (e.g., serum albumin and gamma globulin) in order to eliminate reactions due to the determinants belonging to the carrier proteins. The method used most by Landsteiner to unite haptens to proteins and obtain artificial antigen conjugates

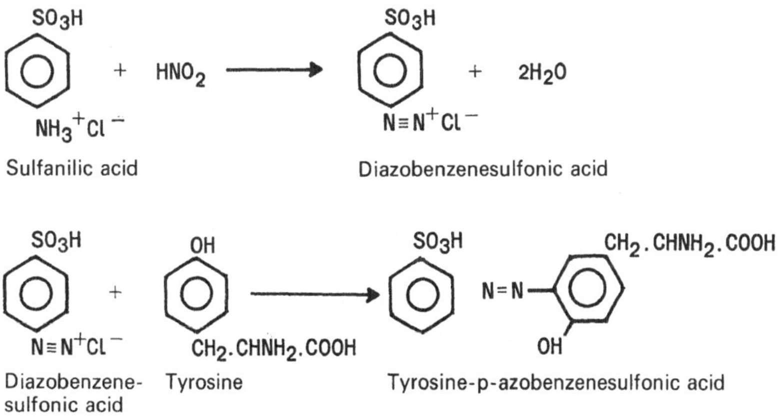

Fig. 3.1. Diazotization reaction used by Landsteiner for preparation of hapten–protein conjugates by diazotization with the tyrosyl residues of a natural protein

was that of diazotization. This method, applicable in cases in which the hapten is an aromatic amine (arylamine), consists of transforming the hapten into the respective diazo salt in order to couple it with a protein (residues of tyrosine, histidine, lysine) via an -N-N- linkage (Fig. 3.1).

The indicated reaction is run for the first time in acid medium at 0 °C, and for the second time in alkaline medium. A typical result of an experiment of this type is exemplified in Table 3.1.

Table 3.1. Precipitation tests with proteins conjugated by diazotization to sulfanilamide and to sulfapyridine

Antigens	Precipitation with Anti-	
	BSA-azosulfanilamide	BSA-azosulfapyridine
BGG-azosulfanilamide	+ +	−
BGG-azosulfapyridine	−	+ +
BSA	+ +	+ +
BGG	−	−

BSA = bovine serum albumin; BGG = bovine gamma globulin

Utilizing the methodology to be described in the following remarks, Landsteiner investigated the importance of different factors in the determination of the specificity of antigen conjugates. DNP conjugates are other frequently used synthetic antigen(s) that can be preserved by nucleophilic substitution through halogen derivatives, e.g., 2,4-dinitrofluorobenzoyl. The coupling can be made over the α- or the ε-NH$_2$ group, as is illustrated with α,ε-DNP lysin:

DNP-HN
$\diagdown$
    CH–CH$_2$–CH$_2$–CH$_2$–CH$_2$–NH-DNP
HO–C$\diagup$
    $\|$
    O

Spatial Configuration. The influence of this factor can be illustrated by studying the serologic specificity of the proteins conju-

Table 3.2. Serologic specificities of the tartaric acids

Antigens	Antisera		
	Levo	Dextro	Meso
Levo	+ + +	±	+
Dextro	0	+ + +	+
Meso	±	0	+ + +

gated to isomers of levo-, dextro-, and meso-tartaric acid (Table 3.2).

As indicated in Table 3.2, each antiserum reacts strongly with its homologous antigen without there being appreciable cross-reaction between the levo- and dextrotartaric acids; however, as one could anticipate, the serum against the mesotartaric acid exhibits conspicuous cross-reaction with the levo- and dextro-forms.

Another good example of the influence of isomerism in antigenic specificity is the capacity of antibodies to distinguish specifically between glucose and galactose, which differ only by the inversion of the position between a hydrogen atom and a hydroxyl group linked to the same carbon atom.

Polar Groups. The radicals that exhibit electrostatic charges of contrary signs and that act as dipoles are highly active as determinant groups of antigenic specificity. This can be verified, for example, in the reaction between the antisera produced to meta-aminobenzoic and meta-aminobenzenesulfonic acid, in the presence of the following antigens whose formulas are reproduced, in the order indicated, in the horizontal column of Table 3.3: aniline, para-aminobenzoic acid, meta-aminobenzoic acid, a methylated derivative of the preceding substance, and meta-aminobenzenesulfinic acid.

Specific Determinants
of the Natural Antigens

What part of the antigenic molecule participates in immunologic specificity? The classic investigations of Obermayer and Pick (1904) demonstrated that proteins treated with io-

Table 3.3. Importance of the polar groups and of their positions in the specificity of antibodies

Antiserum against	Haptens used in the precipitation reaction				
	NH_2 (ring)	NH_2 (ring) $COOH$	H_3C (ring) NH_2 $COOH$	NH_2 (ring) $COOH$	NH_2 (ring) SO_3H
NH_2 (ring) $COOH$	0	0	+++	+++	+
NH_2 (ring) SO_3H	0	0	0	0	+++

In this table the following is clearly verified:
1. The determinant action of the polar groupings $COOH$ and SO_3H
2. The influence of the position (meta or para) of the $COOH$ radical
3. The lack of action of the CH_3 radical
4. The co-reactivity of the $COOH$ and SO_3H groups when they occupy the same position

dine lost their original specificity (species-specificity) but acquired a new specificity (chemical), becoming reactive with the iodo-proteins of other species. The same is true, to a certain extent, with the azoproteins; however, in this case the original species specificity does not disappear.

The secondary and tertiary structures of the protein molecule are also important, i.e., the manner in which the peptide helices are coiled so as to constitute a three-dimensional protein molecule. Depending upon such structure, miniscule reactive areas on the surface of the globular molecule are exposed. The antibodies attach themselves to these areas, which correspond to the determinant groups of antigenic specificity.

The determinant groups are numerous (the number rising as the molecular weight increases), and not all of them are alike: To each determinant of distinct specificity there corresponds a homologous antibody. This fact was demonstrated elegantly by La-presle (1955) in immunoelectrophoresis experiments with human serum albumin fragmented by means of a cathepsin.

As with a key fitting a lock, immunologic specificity evidently depends upon the perfection with which the determinant matches the cavity of the antibody. If the fit is perfect (homologous reactions), the antigen and the antibody come within sufficient proximity for effectual action of the short-reaching secondary valence forces (Coulomb forces, Van der Waals forces, and hydrogen bonds) and the stabilization of the union. The same does not occur, however, in the case of cross-reactions, in which the fit is imperfect and thus does not foster a firm union of the components involved.

In agreement with the theory of clonal selection, one lymphoid cell, carrying one specific combining site, corresponds to each antigenic determinant. Lymphocytes are able to recognize the substitution of a single amino acid (the minimum size of one determinant has been measured to be about 6 amino acids) in the antigenic determinant, which leads to a shift in the specificity of the respective antibody.

Antigenic Determinants of Polysaccharides

The most simple polysaccharide antigens are represented by homopolymers of glucose, among which the most studied from the immunologic point of view is dextran, which is composed of principal chains of polyglucose

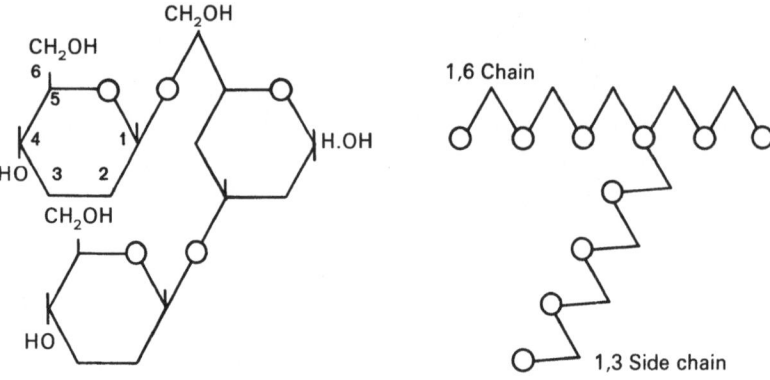

Fig. 3.2. α-1,6 and α-1,3 glucose chains of dextran

in an α-1,6 linkage and secondary chains in an α-1,3 linkage (Fig. 3.2).

As that synthesized by certain microorganisms (e.g., *Leuconostoc mesenteroides*), native dextran has a high molecular weight (10^7–10^8 daltons), whereas clinical dextran, used as a plasma substitute, is partially hydrolyzed so as to reduce its molecular weight to about 75,000 daltons. Even so, clinical dextran still is capable of producing antibodies in man – sometimes in high titers.

A more prolonged hydrolysis of dextran yields oligosaccharides, of which those with two to seven glucose molecules (isomaltose and isomaltose triose, pentose, hexose, and heptose) are of particular interest.

Pioneering studies by Kabat on the quantitative inhibition of the dextran-antidextran reaction by the oligosaccharides permitted measurement of the maximum size of binding site of the antibody. Evidently, this size must correspond to that of the oligosaccharide capable of producing maximum inhibition; this was found to be hexose or heptose. The maximum size of the antibody binding was therefore estimated in terms of the dimensions of the distended isomaltose hexose molecule, i.e., $34 \times 12 \times 7$ Å

Aside from this, the study of various human antidextran antisera has yielded different inhibition curves for the various oligosaccharides, which came to demonstrate the heterogeneity of the antibodies with respect to the size of the combining sites, i.e., from two to six or seven glucose molecules.

Data obtained later with other systems, in particular with synthetic polypeptides, confirmed the maximum size established with the dextran oligosaccharides – five to six amino acid residues.

Antigenic Determinants and Cross-Reactions

When two antigens possess common or structurally similar antigenic determinants, the antibodies obtained to one of these antigens tend to react with the other antigen. These reactions are called cross-reactions. The antigen used as the immunogen is usually termed the homologous antigen, whereas the antigen that cross-reacts is called heterologous. Cross-reactions occur not only between phylogenically related antigens, but also between substances of phylogenically remote origins – or even between substances that bear no known relationship. In the first case, known cross-reactions occur between the ovalbumins of different fowl and between the serum albumins of different species. A typical example of the cross-reaction between phylogenically unrelated antigens is that of the Forssman antigen, which is a substance encountered in many animal species and in diverse bacteria. Rabbits immunized with sheep erythrocytes form two types of hemolytic antibodies: isophilic, which are species-specific (recognizing only the antigenic determinants of the species) and heterophilic, which are specific for the Forssman antigen. The Forssman antigen is but one example; there are many other examples distributed among phylogenically distant species that can cause totally unexpected cross-reactions. Antigens of this type are called heterophilic antigens.

Conformation and Antigenic Specificity

Numerous observations have evidenced the importance of steric conformation in antigenic specificity. In natural protein antigens and in synthetic polypeptides, it is possible to distinguish determinants whose specificity is due to the sequence of amino acids (sequential determinants) and determinants whose specificity depends on the conformation of the molecule (conformational determinants). Antibodies produced against a sequential determinant react with other determinants of a similar sequence, whereas antibodies of a specificity directed against a conformational determinant cannot react with a determinant that exhibits the same sequence of amino acids but does not possess the original steric conformation of the immunogen. For example, it is possible to digest a lysozyme molecule and thus to isolate a polypeptide composed of 20 amino acids that, in the molecule as a whole, form a "loop" united to the former by a disulfide bridge, situated between the cysteines that occupy positions 64 and 80. Antisera prepared in rabbits using as antigen the intact peptide conjugated to lysine are capable of reacting with the isolated "loop" as well as with the entire lysozyme molecule (in this case, evidently, through the loop region), but not with the peptide "loop" opened by the rupture of the disulfide bridge through reduction and alkylation. Similarly, antibodies produced against pancreatic ribonuclease do not react with it after denaturation and rupture of its disulfide bridges.

Myoglobulin is an even better example: Not only is its primary structure known, but its tertiary structure as well – established by Kendrew through crystallographic diffraction studies with x-rays. As with hemoglobin, myoglobin is a heme molecule where the heme is lodged in a "cavity" of the protein molecule, bound to the Fe^{2+} by hydrogen bridges to two histidines that occupy positions 64 and 93. These linkages ensure that the metamyoglobin will have a conformation different from the apomyoglobin.

In inhibition studies of the precipitation of antiapomyoglobin by apo- or metamyoglobin in the presence of six chemotryptic peptides, it was verified that two of them (A 2 and A 4) were producing the same degree of inhibition, even though the A 2 contained 15 amino acids and A 4 contained 19 amino acids. The four additional amino acids in A 4 corresponded, however, to amino acids "buried" in the myoglobin molecule and therefore not participating in the antigenic determinant.

A third peptide (B 1), composed of amino acids 56–69, was capable of inhibiting the reaction with apomyoglobin but not that with metamyoglobin, showing that the union through the heme of the 64 and 93 histidines creates a conformational specificity (Fig. 3.3).

Of the remaining peptides studied, D 1 and D 2 were active and included external amino acids; D 3, being inactive, contained only internal amino acids.

It is possible that the antigenic specificity of the globular proteins and even of some fibrillar proteins such as collagen is principally of the conformational type.

Chemical Basis of Immunogenicity

The chemical basis of immunogenicity is not understood as fully as that of antigenic specificity.

It has been known for a long time that certain proteins are potent antigens whereas others are weak, and that, generally speaking, this difference is related to molecular size. However, other characteristics undoubtedly participate in immunogenic capacity – in particular, the nature of the amino acids that make up the immunogenic determinant (but not necessarily that of the

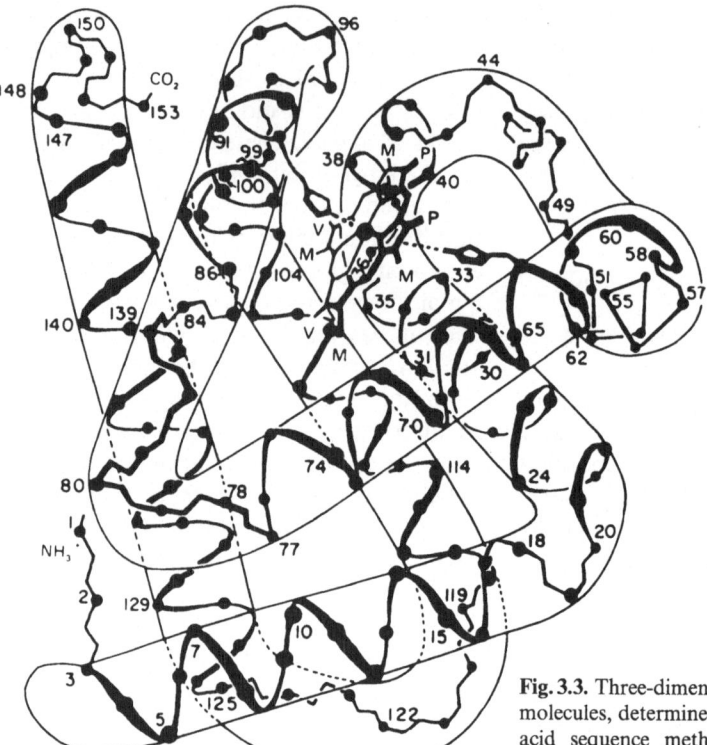

Fig. 3.3. Three-dimensional structure of the myoglobin molecules, determined by crystallographic and amino-acid sequence methods (Reproduced from Kabat, 1976)

specificity) and also the accessibility of this determinant. An example is that of gelatin, a fibrillar protein obtained by boiling collagen in water or in acid; its lack of immunogenicity has been imputed to a deficiency in aromatic amino acids (tryptophan, tyrosine). Although other factors cannot be excluded, there is no doubt that the addition of a small quantity of tyrosine, under certain experimental conditions, can enhance the immunogenicity of gelatin, notwithstanding the nonparticipation of this amino acid in the antigenic specificity. The weak immunogenicity of gelatin, meanwhile, appears to be due to its strong constitutional similarity to collagen in various species; the substitution of only a few amino acids renders it barely distinguishable for various organisms.

An enormous impetus to the study of the chemical determination of immunogenicity was imparted by the investigations undertaken with synthetic polypeptides, in particular by Sela and associates, in Israel. The synthetic polypeptides are polymers of α-amino acids prepared by the polymerization of monomeric amino-acid derivatives, usually carboxyanhydrides, which can be prepared with either ramified or linear chains. Such polymers offer, with respect to the proteins, a great advantage in that at the will of the experimenter the nature and the positions of the amino acids that constitute them can be varied to facilitate their study relative to immunogenic capacity.

Investigations with such polymers permitted a considerable advance in the understanding of immunogenicity. For example, it has been verified that the homopolymers (polymers composed of a single amino acid) such as polylysine (PLL) usually are not immunogenic in rabbits; however, when conjugated to proteins or simply precipitated by oppositely charged proteins, they can induce an immune response. On the other hand, many copolymers (polymers of differing amino acids) of two amino acids are immunogenic principally when they contain a cyclic amino acid. These copolymers frequently are immunogenic only for some individuals or for some isogeneic strains. For example, whereas the polymers of glutamic acid and alanine are not immunogenic for strain 13 guinea pigs, they are immunogenic for strain 2; at the same time, the polymers of glutamic acid and tyrosine, although nonimmunogenic for strain 2, are immunogenic for strain 13. When "outbred" guinea pigs are immunized with these polymers, some react with strain 2, others with strain 13, and others behave as hybrids by responding to both polymers. Copolymers of three or more amino acids are immunogenic for all animal species.

Importance of the External Groupings of the Antigen in Immunogenicity

The immunogenicity of the antigen depends upon the groupings present on its surface and not upon those localized in the interior of the molecule. For example, polymers composed of an axial skeleton with internal groupings of DL-alanine (nonimmunogenic) and external groupings of tyrosine-glutamic

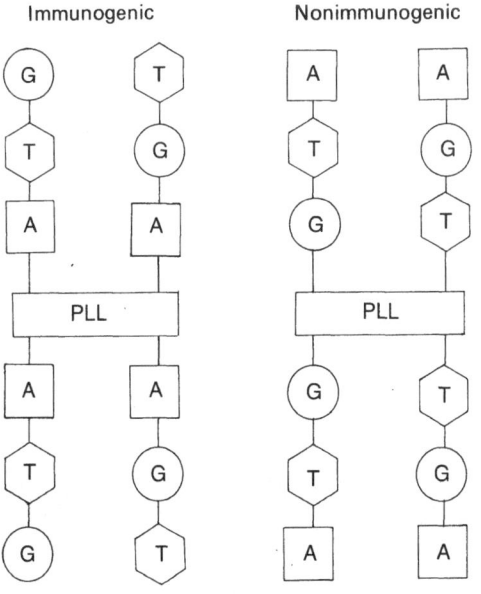

Fig. 3.4. External grouping of the antigen molecule in immunogenicity. *T*, tyrosine; *G*, glutamic acid; and *A*, DL-alanine

acid (immunogenic) are in fact immunogenic; however, when the order of the grouping is inverted – by placing the nonimmunogenic DL-alanine grouping on the surface – the polymer becomes nonimmunogenic (Fig. 3.4).

Experiments with polymers of D-amino acids, which are poorly immunogenic, also confirm the importance of the accessibility of the immunogenic groupings: ramified polymers with 95% L-amino acids (which are immunogenic), and 5% D-amino acids (which are nonimmunogenic) on their surfaces are as poorly immunogenic as polymers that contain 100% D-amino acids; on the other hand, polymers with 95% D-amino acids and with 5% L-amino acids on the molecule exterior are as immunogenic as those with 100% L-amino acids.

Adjuvanticity

Substances or treatments that augment the immunogenicity of antigens are termed adjuvants (Latin *adjuvans*, aiding). The observation that certain substances potentiate the production of antibodies when applied simultaneously with the antigen (though not necessarily mixed with it) was made about 45 years ago, some decades after the discovery of antibodies. Ramon was one of the first to note this phenomenon. He observed that the production of antitoxoid antibodies in horses was greatly increased when these substances were injected adsorbed to a particulate substance rather than in their pure state. The adjuvant concept also originated from the use of toxoid-associated vaccines plus bacterial vaccines, e.g., the so-called triple vaccine, in which it was observed that one of the components reinforced the humoral response to the other. Currently, many heterogeneous substances are known to be capable of augmenting immunogenicity: alum, aluminum phosphate, aluminum hydroxide, beryllium sulfate, saponin, alginate of calcium, guanidine silica, mineral oil emulsions, double-helix synthetic nucleic acids such as the complexes of polyadenylic (poly A) and polyuridylic (poly U) acids and of polyinosinic (poly I) and polycytidylic (poly C) acids, and lipopolysaccharides obtained from numerous gram-negative bacteria such as *S. typhi*, *B. pertussis*, and *E. coli*. Although the operative mechanism of the adjuvants is poorly understood, it is accepted that they augment the production of antibodies in three ways: (1) by continuous and gradual liberation of the antigen (depot effect), (b) by stimulation of phagocytosis, and (c) by activation (nonspecific) of the lymphocytes (mitogenicity).

One frequently used adjuvant mixture is Freund's adjuvant. It is composed of a mixture of a mineral oil (Bayol F), an emulsifying agent (Aquafor, Falba, Arlacel), and an aqueous antigen solution. This mixture is prepared to obtain a water–oil emulsion. In this manner, the antigen is dispersed with the finest fat droplets, from which it is slowly liberated. In the so-called complete Freund's adjuvant, the mixture also contains dead mycobacteria in suspension (*M. tuberculosis* or *M. butyricum*); the adjuvant without mycobacteria is called incomplete adjuvant. The operative mechanism of Freund's adjuvant has three principal effects: (1) a depositing action that retards the systemic absorption of the antigen, (2) local formation of a granuloma rich in macrophages and immunocompetent cells, and (3) farther-reaching action in the lymphoid organs (there is an almost immediate dissemination of the emulsion droplets through the lymphatics to the lymph nodes). With the complete adjuvant, the addition of mycobacteria is indispensable for production of a state of delayed hypersensitivity. Complete adjuvant is therefore essential for the production of the experimental autoallergic diseases such as encephalomyelitis, thyroiditis, arthritis, and others (see Chap. 13).

Cytologic examination of the lymph of the efferent lymphatic vessels of the granuloma produced by the injection of the Freund's adjuvant into the tissues has revealed an intense outpouring of lymphocytes. This fact and the older observations that the injection of antigen into a tuberculous granuloma induces a state of delayed hypyersen-sitivity for the injected antigen, suggests that the encounter of the antigen with the immunocompetent cells within or near the granuloma is important for the establishment of a hypersensitivity state.

The adjuvant activity of the mycobacteria has been attributed to various substances extracted from them – particularly to wax D (peptidoglycolipid composed of mycolic acid esters with different polysaccharides, united by an amide linkage to a heptapeptide) and also to ribonucleic acid.

The strong adjuvant effect of the gram-negative bacteria appears due in large part to the endotoxin contained in these bacteria. The term endotoxin is applied to complex, high-molecular-weight substances existing in the cell walls of many bacteria; they are extremely toxic, pyrogenic, immunogenic, and produce an adjuvant effect. These complexes are composed of polysaccharides, lipids, and proteins. The biologic activity of the endotoxins is present in a smaller molecule, a lipopolysaccharide (LPS), that is free of proteins. There appears to be a direct relation between the toxic effect of LPS and its adjuvant effect. For example, rabbits that have been made tolerant to LPS simultaneously become refractory to the adjuvant effect of this substance. The lipopolysaccharide, in addition to being a thymus-independent antigen, is also a specific mitogen of the B lymphocytes that stimulates the proliferation of specific cellular clones in the absence of the antigenic stimulus. It is possible that the adjuvant effect of LPS is related to its mitogenic effect upon the B cells.

Certain adjuvants appear to favor specific classes of antibodies to the detriment of others: Guinea pigs immunized with ovalbumin and complete Freund's adjuvant produce preferentially antibodies of the IgG_2 type, whereas under the same conditions, incomplete adjuvant induces a greater production of IgG_1. The adjuvant effect of *B. pertussis* gives rise to the preferential production of IgE-class antibodies in rats, mice, and guinea pigs. In the first two species, the preferential formation of IgE appears to be due to the histamine-sensitizing factor

(HSF), whereas in the guinea pig, the adjuvant effect is directly associated with the LPS. It is probable that the adjuvants act particularly at the cellular level and that the type of cell affected determines the class of antibody predominating in the humoral response.

Curiously, many immunosuppressive agents also possess adjuvant activity when applied at the right moment in relation to contact with the antigen. These agents include, among others, X and gamma rays, 6-mercaptopurine, 5-fluorouracil, and 5-fluorodeoxyuridine (see Chap. 14).

Thymus Independent Antigens

Most antigens require help from T lymphocytes to be able to induce antibody synthesis whereas some other antigens can induce antibody synthesis without T cell cooperation. The former type of antigens are termed thymus-independent antigens (TD) and the latter thymus-independent (TI). The tyhmus-independent antigens have a series of properties in common: they have high molecular weight, repeated antigenic determinants, are slowly metabolized, are easily tolerogenic, generate a restricted antibody response, usually only IgM (plus IgG3 in mice), and induce weak or no secondary response. In addition, some of them are polyclonal activators and some other activate the alternate complement pathway. There are some indications that thymus-independent antigens can be divided in two groups, TI-1 and TI-2 that act on different B cell populations. TI-1 antigens would act on less differentiated B cells whereas TI-2 would act on more nature B cells. Thymus-independent antigens of type 2 present the antigenic determinants in repetitive form to the B lymphocyte. Cross-linking of membrane bound Ig on B lymphocyte is probably involved in B cell activation. High concentrations of these substances does not stimulate B lymphocytes polyclonally. On the other hand, thymus-independent antigens of type 1 at high concentrations are polycolonal B lymphocyte activators. In this case they seem to circumvent the binding to Ig and use other unknown membrane receptors. When concentration lower than the polyclonally activating level is used, binding of these antigens to B cells occurs via antigen-specific Ig that in fact locally concentrates the polyclonal activator on the antigen-specific resting B cell and thereby activates it. Although earlier studies indicate that macrophages were not required for activation of B cell for thymus-independent antigen, more recent and more efficient techniques of macrophage depletion have shown that activation of B cells by thymus-independent antigens do require macrophages. These cells probably act by producing activating factors required for complete B cell activation (see B cell growth and maturation factors, p. 49).

References

Borek FF (1972) Immunogenicity. Physico-chemical and biological aspects. North-Holland, Amsterdam

Kabat EA (1976) Structural concepts in immunology and immunochemistry, 2nd edn. Holt, Rinehart & Winston, New York, Chap. 2

Landsteiner K (1962) The specificity of serological reactions. Bover, New York

Sela M (1965) Immunological studies with synthetic polypeptides. Adv Immunol 5:29

Sela M (ed) (1973) The antigen, vol I. Academic, New York

Staub AM, Raynaud M (1971) Cours d'Immunologie générale et de Sérologie de l'Institut Pasteur, vol I. C.D.U., Paris

WHO Scientific Group on Immunological Adjuvants (1973) Report Series No 595. World Health Organization, Geneva

Chapter 4   Antibodies

Otto G. Bier

Contents

Antibody Formation at the Level
of the Organism 73
Preparation of Immune Sera 73
Dynamics of Antibody Formation 74
Antibody Formation at the Cellular Level . . . 76
Jerne Plaque Technique 76
Rosette Technique 77
Microdrop Technique 78
Hybridomas 78
Antibody Formation at the Protein Level . . . 80
Purification of Antibodies 81
Nature and Heterogeneity of Antibodies . . 84
Immunoglobulin Structure 85
Enzymatic Fragmentation 87
Classes and Subclasses of Human
Immunoglobulins 92
Classes and Subclasses of Animal
Immunoglobulins 97
Genetic Markers of the Immunoglobulins:
Allotypes and Idiotypes 97
Electron-Microscopic Studies of the
Antibody 100
Antibody Formation at the Gene Level 100
Organization of Immunoglobulin Genes and
Their Expression 101
Regulation of Antibody Formation 105
Factors Relating to the Antigen 105
Factors Relating to the Organism 108
Factors Inherent to the Immune System . . 109
References 113

Antibody Formation at the Level of the Organism

Preparation of Immune Sera

A prerequisite to the study of antigens (from Greek *anti* = against, and *gen* = gignomai, to create, see Chap. 3) and antibodies is the production of antisera (immune sera), i.e., of sera that react specifically with antigens. In laboratory experiments, small animals, usually the rabbit, are used for the production of antisera. However, when it is necessary to produce therapeutic or diagnostic antisera on a large scale, larger animals are used – primarily the horse.

Antisera produced by injecting animals with antigens obtained from a different species are termed xenoantisera (from Greek *xenos* = foreign), e.g., rabbit anti-chicken ovalbumin serum, or horse anti-diphtheria toxin serum. On the other hand, antisera may be raised to detect lesser antigenic differences, for example, the Rh antigens on human erythrocytes. In this case, it is advisable to utilize an animal of the same species that does not possess the antigen in question. Thus, if a rabbit is immunized with Rh^+ human erythrocytes, antibodies are produced against other predominant human erythrocytic antigens, thereby masking or impeding the formation of anti-Rh antibodies. If, however, an Rh person is immunized with blood from an Rh^+ individual, both sharing the same ABO antigens, the species-shared erythrocytic antigens are ignored and only anti-Rh antibodies are produced. This intraspecies immunization is termed alloimmunization (from Greek *allos* = the other), and the antiserum obtained is called alloantiserum.

Immunization Schedules. The techniques for immunization, largely empirical, vary according to the nature of the antigen. Particulate antigens such as bacteria or cells usually do not require adjuvants, which, on the contrary, are of great advantage in the case of soluble protein antigens.

Examples of the first kind are the immunization schedules to obtain hemolytic or antibacterial antibodies (antipneumococcic or antisalmonella sera). For the preparation of hemolysin (anti-Forssman antibody) a good schedule consists in a series of daily intravenous injections of increasing doses of boiled sheep erythrocyte stromata, e.g., 1×0.5 ml, 5×1 ml, and 5×2 ml of a suspension standardized to contain 1 mg N/ml. In the case of salmonella antisera 1, 2, 4, and 6 billion organisms are injected intravenously at intervals of 4 days. Rabbits are bled 4–6 days after the last inoculation. For the production of precipitating antibodies against soluble proteins such as ovalbumin or bovine gammaglobulin, two methods may be used:

1. Method I consists of a series of intravenous injections of alum-precipitated protein at the rate of 4 per week in the course of 4 weeks: 4×1 mg, 4×2 mg, 4×3 mg, and 4×4 mg, totalling 40 mg per animal at the end of the fourth week. A sample of blood is taken 4–5 days after the last inoculation and if a sufficient titer of antibody is obtained a large bleeding (50–60 ml) is drawn on the 5–7th day. After a period of rest of one to three weeks a second series of injections following the same schedule may be started.

2. Method II involves one single subcutaneous injection of 1–2 mg of protein emulsified in Freund's complete adjuvant (see p. 67) at four or five points (0.2 ml per site) in the back of the neck or into footpads. Usually, this single injection is sufficient to yield satisfactory titers within 4–6 weeks. If an even higher titer is desired, an intravenous or intraperitoneal booster injection of 2–5 mg of alum-precipitated antigen can be administered.

Methods I and II may be combined, as for example in the production of anti-lymphocytic serum.

The antisera obtained in final bleedings are separated under aseptic conditions and kept frozen at -20 °C or preferably below, without any preservative. Alternatively, a suitable bacteriostatic agent may be added, such as thiomerosal (merthiolate) 1:10,000 or sodium azide 1:1,000, and the antiserum is kept at refrigerator temperatures (0–5 °C).

Two fundamental rules must be remembered in the preparation of antisera: (1) Before starting the immunization, a sample of serum must be collected to verify the possible pre-existence of antibodies reacting with the antigen in question.

(2) Because the responses of individual animals vary, it is advisable to assay the antisera individually. Making mixtures or pools of antisera before assaying them may result in the loss of important information available from an individual antiserum.

Dynamics of Antibody Formation

The dynamics of the formation of antibodies in the organism is expressed by two types of immune response: primary and secondary.

Primary Response. The name primary response is given to the reaction observed to the first antigen stimulus. This reaction occurs only after a determined latent period (days to weeks), the duration of which varies with the animal immunized and with the immunizing antigen.

In rabbits, appreciable titers of antibodies against red blood cells, bacteria, and other particulate antigens can be observed after 5 days, whereas antibodies against diphtheria toxin are first detectable 2–3 weeks after injection of the toxoid.

In any case, the curve representing the production of antibodies after a primary antigenic stimulation inclined toward a maximum, remains at a plateau for a long period of time, and then declines at varying speeds, depending upon the balance between the catabolism and the biosynthesis of the antibody (Fig. 4.1). Accordingly, the disappearance of the antibodies from the blood requires periods ranging from several weeks to several years, depending upon the antigen involved.

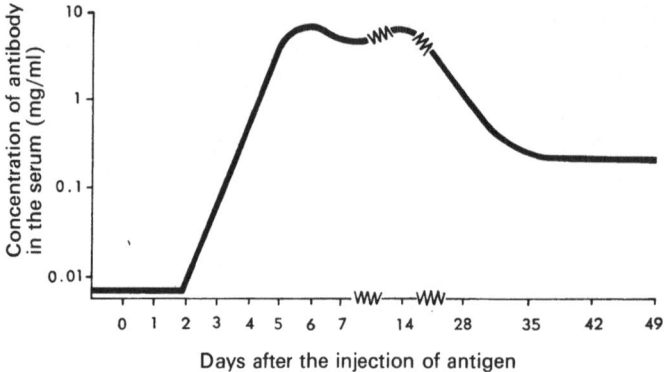

Fig. 4.1. Time course of specific antibody activity (concentration) after a single injection of antigen: primary response

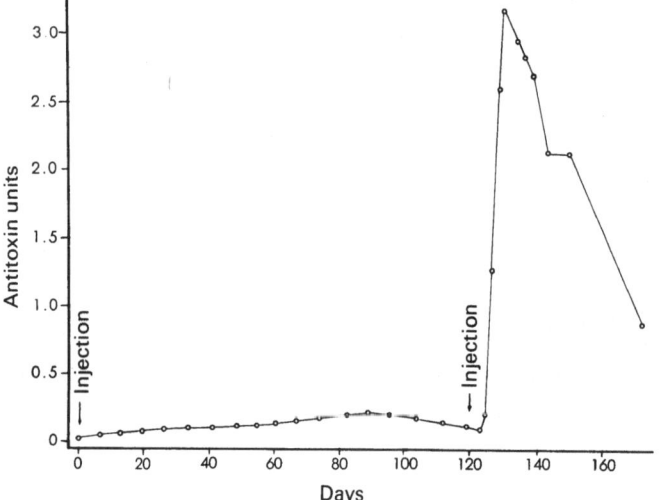

Fig. 4.2. Time course of antibody activity (concentration) specific for diphtheria toxin in the horse after booster injection: secondary response

The persistence of the antigenic stimulus and the rate of catabolic destruction are the determining factors in the decline of the antibody titer. Particulate (insoluble) antigens produce a more prolonged stimulus than to soluble antigens, and for this reason give rise to elevated antibody levels that persist over long periods. The same occurs with the polysaccharides, e.g., the pneumococcic polysaccharides, which are poorly attacked by enzymes in the organism. Proteins, on the other hand, are destroyed in vivo with relative rapidity.

Secondary Response. In an animal previously sensitized by a primary stimulus, a second dose, or booster, produces an accelerated and more elevated response than that associated with the first dose (Fig. 4.2). The secondary response, also called the anamnestic response, is attributed to what has been termed immunologic memory, i.e., part of the cells stimulated by the first antigen stimulation differentiate and proliferate not to become plasma cells but to become "memory cells" which after restimulation with the same antigen immediately turn into plasma cells.

Adopting the terminology introduced by Sercarz and Coons, using X to indicate the immunocompetent (sensitive to antigen) cell, Y to indicate the primed or memory cells, and Z for the antibody forming cell, we can schematically follow the primary and secondary responses:

$$X \frac{\text{Antigen}}{\substack{\text{Primary} \\ \text{Stimulus}}} \rightarrow Y \frac{\text{Antigen}}{\substack{\text{Secondary} \\ \text{Stimulus}}} \rightarrow Z$$

In both the primary and secondary responses, the phase during which the antibodies increase is logarithmic in relation to time; this strongly suggests a multiplication of the cells that form antibodies – more rapid in the case of the secondary response by virtue of the prior accumulation of memory cells.

Antibody Formation at the Cellular Level

For the study of antibody formation at the cellular level and its cytodynamics several methods have been utilized: (1) the Jerne plaque technique, (2) the rosette technique, (3) the microdrop technique, and (4) the hybridization of plasma cells with myeloma cells.

Jerne Plaque Technique

In the Jerne plaque technique, a suspension of lymphoid cells of the immunized animal is mixed homogeneously with an adequate quantity of melted agar, and red cells bearing the same antigen used for immunization are added to the culture medium. Once the mixture is solidified, complement is added. The antibodies diffuse radially from the cells that synthesize them, and produce circular plaques of hemolysis in the layer of agar (Fig. 4.3).

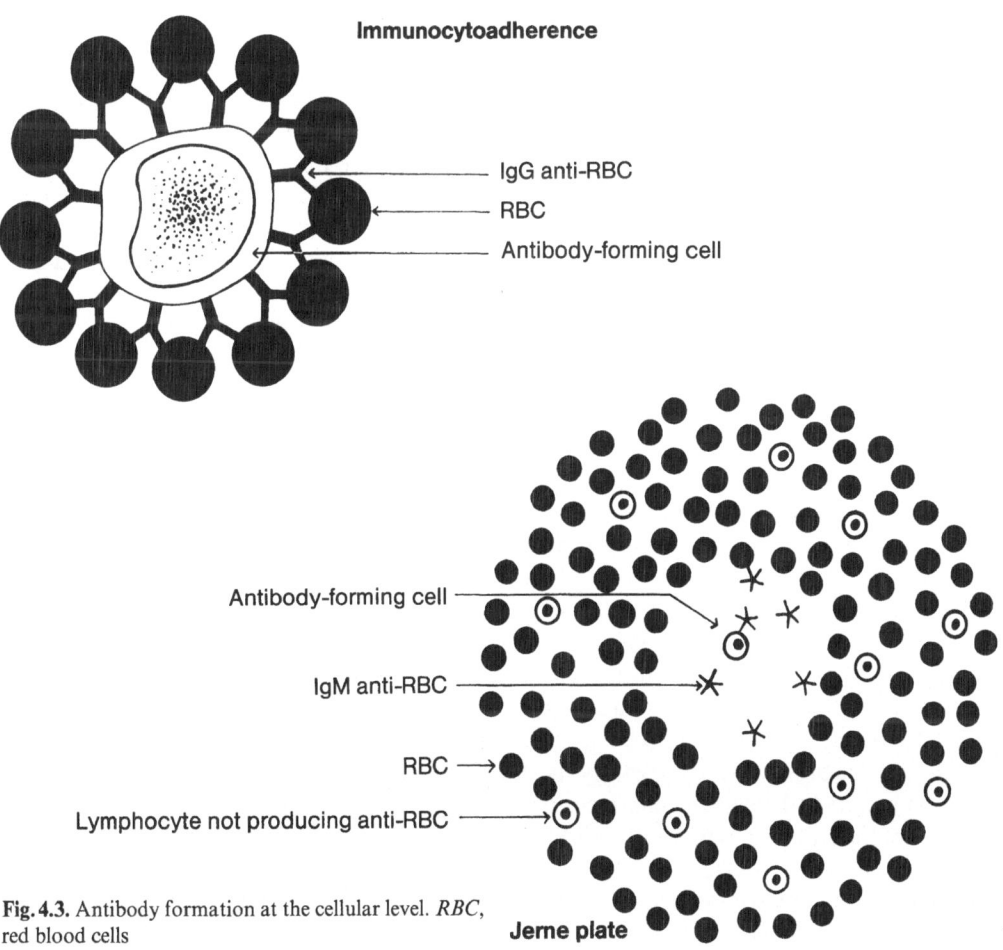

Fig. 4.3. Antibody formation at the cellular level. *RBC*, red blood cells

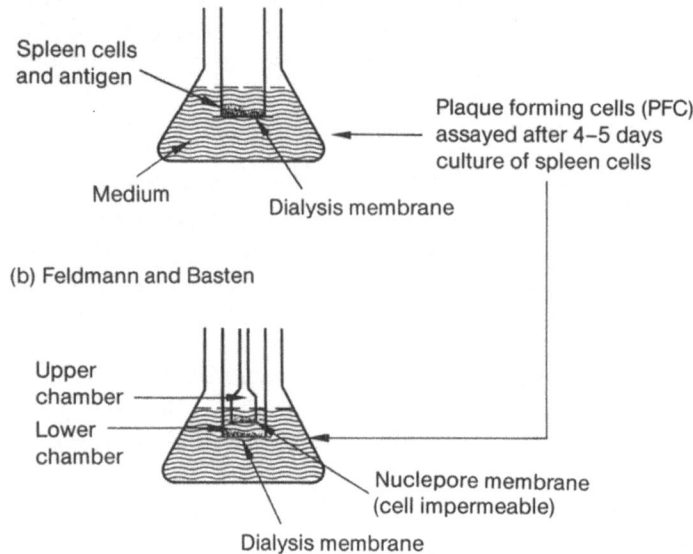

(a) Marbrook

Spleen cells
and antigen

Plaque forming cells (PFC)
assayed after 4–5 days
culture of spleen cells

Medium

Dialysis membrane

(b) Feldmann and Basten

Upper
chamber

Lower
chamber

Nuclepore membrane
(cell impermeable)

Dialysis membrane

Fig. 4.4. Chambers for *in vitro* studies of antibody formation

The plaque-forming cells (PEC) are generally plasma cells, and the antibodies revealed by the described technique are of the IgM type (see below). To detect IgG antibodies that do not fix complement, the addition of complement must be preceded by the addition of anti-IgG serum. In this manner, both IgG and IgM types of antibodies can be detected – the first being distinguishable by noting the differene in relation to the plaque test done without antiglobulin serum.

Such as described, the Jerne plaque assay permits only the detection of antibodies to red blood cells. However, by using antigen-coated erythrocytes, one may also detect by passive hemolysis the formation of antibodies to soluble antigens.

Lymphoid cells may also be cultivated in the presence of antigen for 4–5 days and then be assayed by the hemolytic plaque technique. Marbrook has successfully used a system in which the spleen cells are separated from the culture medium by a dialysis membrane, in order to avoid dilution of the macromolecular environment of the cells, and Feldman and Basten has modified this

technique by the use of a double chamber separated by a nucleopore membrane, thus allowing free diffusion of macromolecules, but keeping cells scpaprate (Fig. 4.4). T cells may be placed in the upper chamber and B cells in the lowe chamber, providing a useful model for the analysis of the mechanism of T-B cooperation (see p. 56).

Rosette Technique

Also called immunocytoadherence, the rosette method was developed by Biozzi and his colleagues. It consists in the microscopic verification of the formation of rosettes of erythrocytes (Fig. 4.3) in a suspension of lymphoid cells from immunized animals and of red cells bearing the antigen used for immunization. For the same suspension of lymphoid cells and the same erythrocytes, the number of PFCs is much smaller than the number of rosettes, because the latter technique is capable of revealing much smaller quantities of both classes of antibodies, IgG and IgM. Almost all cells that form rosettes are lymphocytes, but rosettes may also be encountered around plasma cells, blasts, and even macrophages that have absorbed cytophilic antibodies.

Microdrop Technique

This method, utilized extensively by Nossal and his colleagues, requires separation of microdrops that contain single lymphocytes, and involves a search in these for bacteria-immobilizing antibodies (by direct microscopic observation) or phage-neutralizing antibodies (by observation of areas of lysis in agar). With the help of these methods it was possible to establish that lymphoid cells are capable or producing immunoglobulins of a single specificity only, and at a given time produce only one class of immunoglobulin. From this, it was concluded that all plasma cells derive from one stem cell, which itself does not form antibodies, but has the capacity to generate as many differentiated plasma cell clones as there are different antibody specificities (Fig. 4.5).

Since antigens in general are complex molecules, they possess several structural "patches" which are recognized by specific receptors on lymphocytes; these patches are called antigenic determinants or epitopes (see Chap. 3, p. 64). From this, it follows that immunization with any antigen, even highly purified, will lead to the stimulation of several clones, each recognizing a different or only partially identical epitope on the same antigen molecule, i.e., immune sera are polyclonal and therefore, heterogeneous in respect to specificity and immunoglobulin class of single antibodies. Attempts to obtain oligoclonal antisera, or monoclonal antibodies of known antigen or epitope specificity have been made. For this, very simple antigens, for example synthetic polypeptides (see Chap. 3, p. 64) or certain bacterial polysaccharides, have been used as antigens, and indeed have produced rather homogeneous antisera.

Hybridomas

A new approach to obtain specific monoclonal antibodies became possible in 1975 after Köhler and Milstein succeeded in demonstrating that, when fused with plasma cells from immunized donors, plasmocytoma cells growing in vitro secreted the specific antibody of that plasma cell in addition to their own. Such specific antibody-producing hybrid cells derived after fusion of a myeloma cell with a plasma cell are called *hybridomas (hybrid myeloma)*. The procedure for obtaining such hybridoma lines is shown in Fig. 4.6. The mycloma cell lines (derived from BALB/c mouse plasmocytomas) used for the production of monoclo-

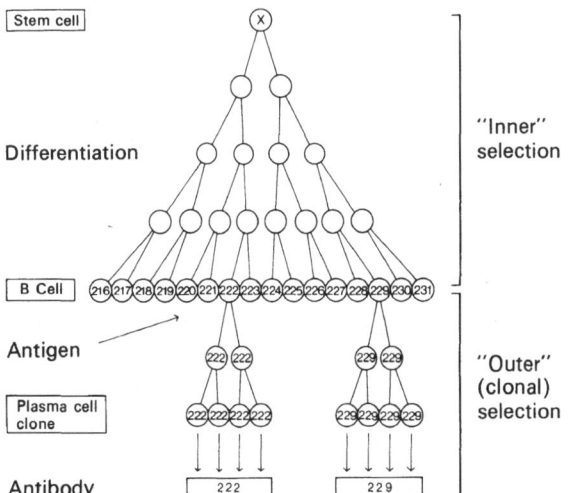

Fig. 4.5. Differentiation of antibody-forming cells. The undifferentiated stem cell is multipotent. It has the ability to generate approximately 10^6 different, antigen-specific B cells. Each B cell is only "unipotent" (monopotent). After contact with an antigen, the corresponding B cell differentiates to a plasma-cell clone with only one specific antibody

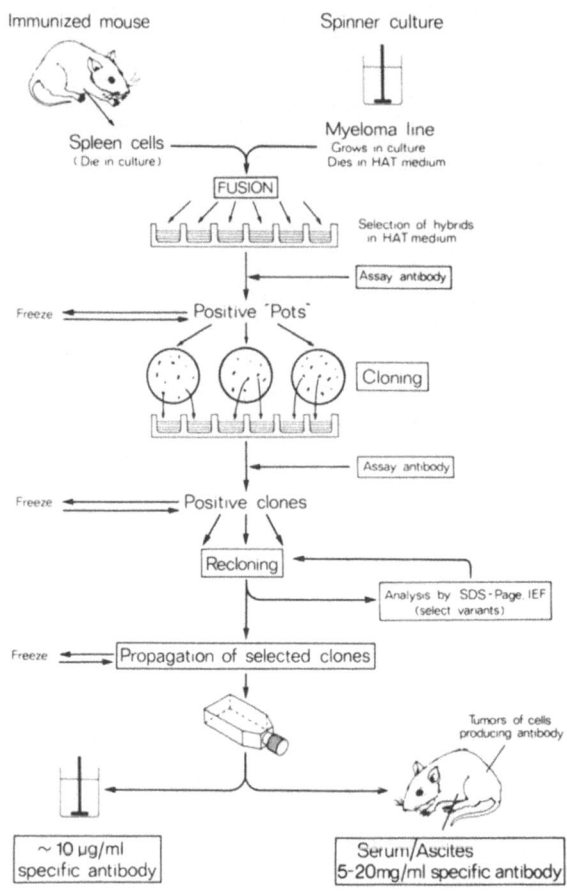

Fig. 4.6. Procedure for the production of monoclonal antibodies by fusion of primed spleen cells with myeloma cells, and selection of specific antibody-producing cell hybrid clones. (With permission reproduced from Milstein and Lennox 1980)

nal antibodies were selected for thymidine-kinase (TK) and/or hypoxynthine-guanine-phosphoribosyl-transferase (HGPRT) deficiency. Neither of these enzymes is needed by the cells under normal culture conditions. However, if the main pathway for the synthesis of pyrimidine and purine is blocked by the folic acid antagonist aminopterin (or methotrexate), the cells die. Normal plasma cells that are not TK or HGPRT deficient compensate this deficiency by complementation when fused with the myeloma cell, and the hybrid cells can grow, provided that the culture medium contains Hypoxanthine and Thymidine in addition to Aminopterin (HAT-medium) (nonfused normal spleen cells die naturally in culture). The fusion is performed with plasma cells from the spleens of immunized

donors 3–4 days after the last intravenous antigen injection, and myeloma cells in a ratio of 2 to 5:10.

Polyethylenglycol (PEG, mol.wt. 1,000–4,000) in a concentration of 35%–50% (v/v)

$$HO-\underset{\underset{H}{|}}{\overset{\overset{H}{|}}{C}}-\underset{\underset{H}{|}}{\overset{\overset{H}{|}}{C}}-O-(\underset{\underset{H}{|}}{\overset{\overset{H}{|}}{C}}-\underset{\underset{H}{|}}{\overset{\overset{H}{|}}{C}}-O)_x-\underset{\underset{H}{|}}{\overset{\overset{H}{|}}{C}}-\underset{\underset{H}{|}}{\overset{\overset{H}{|}}{C}}-OH$$

$x = 25$ for mw. of 1,000

is used as a fusion reagent. The plasma cell-myeloma cell mixture is incubated for 1–8 min with 0.2–0.5 ml of PEG, the PEG is then diluted out with about 30 ml medium, the cells are washed and placed in wells of microtiter plates, and then incubated in

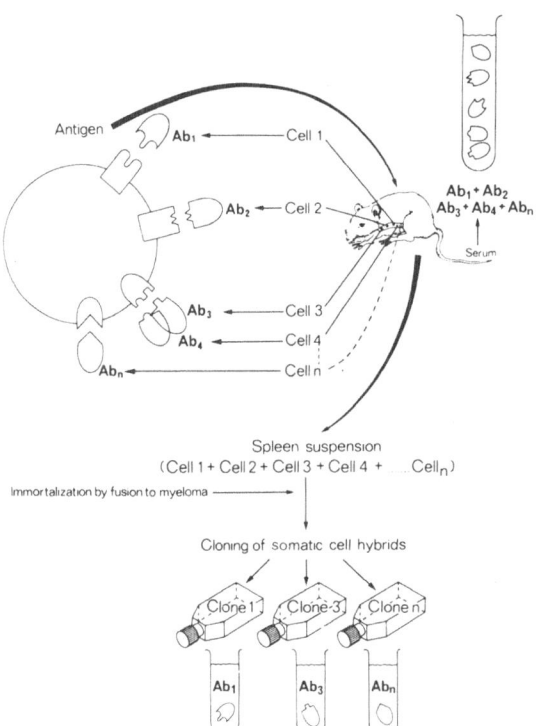

Fig. 4.7. Production of pure antibodies from impure antigens. Different antigenic determinants on a cell surface are recognized by B cells producing different antibodies. Single determinants can be recognized by different antibodies (Ab$_3$ and Ab$_4$), and the overlap in the antigenic determinants could be such that *different* antibody molecules recognize exactly the *same* determinant. Each antibody is made by a cell but the products are all mixed in the serum, so that the antiserum of an immune animal is a very heterogeneous mixture of antibody molecules. The hybrid myeloma method permits the separation of each antibody molecule by cloning the antibody-producing cell (with permission reproduced from Milstein and Lennox, 1980)

HAT-medium. After 5–7 days, the medium is exchanged, and 5–7 days later the supernatants of growing cultures are tested for antibody activity (binding test, hemagglutination, complement-dependent cytotoxicity, see Chap. 7).

The positive cultures are then cloned by limiting dilution; the cloned cultures are (a) propagated to produce mass cultures, (b) injected into BALB/c mice to obtain ascites, (c) recloned, and (d) frozen for storage in liquid nitrogen. The monoclonality of the produced antibody is proven by isoelectric focussing (IEF). This technique allows production of specific antibodies even when highly complex antigens such as cells are used or whenever the antigen of interest cannot be purified from contaminating substances (Fig. 4.7). Moreover, the production of monoclonal antibodies has proven to be highly valuable, particularly as a diagnostic tool and for research purposes, e.g., in the estimation of specific repertoire, classification of biological systems, etc.

Antibody Formation at the Protein Level

The production of antibodies at the molecular level has been studied in vitro using extracts of myelomas capable of producing large quantities of immunoglobulins (up to 40% of the total quantity of protein). Such extracts are much more convenient for studies of this nature than are those obtained from normal lymphoid organs, because the latter exhibit a high degree of heterogeneity of the synthesized immunoglobulins.

Myeloma cell extracts were incubated with labeled amino acids (along with those not labeled) to determine the time required for the heavy and light chains (see below, p. 85) to appear in the supernatant and in the sediment after sucrose-gradient centrifugation. The results indicated that the light chains appear in the ribosome fraction which sediments at 190 S after only 30 s, whereas the heavy chains associated with polyribosomes, which are considerably larger (250 S), do so only after 60 s. The times indicated (30 and 60 s) correspond to peaks in the formation of the respective chains. Before and after, the counts of labeled isotope fall considerably, indicating either that the chains were still being synthesized at the level of the polyribosomes, or that they were already being "excreted" in the liquid phase. It is important to mention that the fraction with the sedimentation coefficient of 250 S was found to obtain, in addition to heavy chains, small quantities of light chains, suggesting that the assembly of the immunoglobulin halfmolecule takes place at the level of the polyribosome arrays.

Purification of Antibodies

For the determination of antibody structure as well as for medical application in prophylaxis, diagnosis, and therapy, antibodies must be isolated and purified from other contaminating serum proteins. They can be purified by nonspecific or specific methods. The former are based on the physical or physico-chemical characteristics of immunoglobulins, and do not allow separation of the normal gamma globulins from the antibodies. Specific methods, on the other hand, are based on the dissociation or elution of immune complexes, thus permitting the isolation of antibodies to a high degree of purity, free of nonspecific immunoglobulins. Specific methods are used chiefly for experimental studies; they cannot be applied to therapeutic antisera because of the low yield inherent in the purification process. Without entering into detailed techniques, we might examine some representative examples of the different methods of purification, as outlined below:

1. Nonspecific methods
   (a) Precipitation with neutral salts ("salting out")
   (b) Chromatographic fractionation
   (c) Ethanol fractionation
   (d) Enzymatic digestion

2. Specific methods
   (a) Dissociation with 15% NaCl (antipolysaccharides)
   (b) Dissociation in acid pH (antiproteins)
   (c) Dissociation by means of haptens
   (d) Immunoadsorbents.

Nonspecific Methods. Precipitation with neutral salts (salting out) is a frequently used method employing ammonium sulfate and sodium sulfate as the preferred salts. When the aim is to precipitate the total globulin fraction, ammonium sulfate at 50% saturation or sodium sulfate in a 22% concentration (at 37 °C) can be added to the serum. Sometimes, however, there is an advantage in separating only the fraction that precipitates between 33% and 50% saturation; this is easily obtained in the following manner: (1) Add to 2 volumes of serum, 1 volume of saturated ammonium sulfate solution (hence 33% saturated) centrifuge. The precipitate contains the fraction called "euglobulin," insoluble in distilled water and composed predominantly of gamma globulin (IgG). (2) To the supernatant (approximately 3 volumes), add 1 additional volume of saturated ammonium sulfate to produce a 50%-saturated solution. The "33%–50%" precipitate contains significant quantities of gamma globulins plus most of the beta globulins (IgA, IgM).

In the sera of horses hyperimmunized with toxins, the antitoxins are concentrated principally in the "33%–50%" fraction, which can also be obtained by precipitation with semisaturated ammonium sulfate, followed by dialysis of the precipitate against distilled water. Under these conditions, the "euglobulins" precipitate, leaving only the "pseudoglobulins" in solution. Salting out does not permit satisfactory separation of the different globulins identified by electrophoresis. However, although the fractions obtained by salting out may indeed be impure and reveal numerous components upon electrophoresis, there is relative puri-

Table 4.1. Human serum fractions obtained by "salting out" and their relation to components identified by immunoelectrophoresis

Ammonium sulfate, % saturated	Sodium sulfate, % saturated	Characteristic components	% of total proteins	g/ml plasma
25	10	Fibrinogen	3	0.2
34	15	γ globulins	20	1.4
40	19	γ, β	15	1.0
50	27	α, β, A	14	1.0
70	–	Albumin	46	3.4

fication, for certain components predominate (Table 4.1).

Higher purification is achieved through chromatography in diethylaminoethyl (DEAE) cellulose. If the serum, or the serum fraction obtained through salting out, is eluted with 0.02 M phosphate buffer, pH 8.0, the IgG can be obtained in a nearly pure form.

In alkaline pH, the ionization of DEAE cellulose decreases and the ionized proteins (Pr-COO$^-$) are eluted in ascending order of their electrophoretic mobilities (γ, β, α and albumin).

$$RN^+H(C_2H_5)_2 \cdot Pr\!-\!COO^- \xrightarrow{\text{NaOH}}$$
$$(DEAE^+)$$
$$\qquad\qquad RN(C_2H_5)_2 + Pr\!-\!COO^-Na^+$$
$$\qquad\qquad (DEAE)$$

Among the chromatographic methods, we might also mention gel filtration and affinity chromatography.

In gel filtration, dextran (Sephadex) agarose (Sepharose) or polyacrylamide (Biogel) is used.

The Sephadex beads are obtained from fractions of dextran with different degrees of cross linkages and a proportional capacity to swell, i.e., to take up more or less water.

The grains of the swollen gel act as a molecular sieve, the loosely cross-linked having larger pores than the thightly cross-linked polymers, thus permitting the separation of molecules of different sizes.

Beads are prepared with varying porosities, from G 10 to G 200. The former have an imbition capacity of 1 ml/g and are penetrated only by molecules below 700 daltons; the G 200 beads absorb 20 ml/g and allow penetration of molecules up to 800,000 daltons.

For column chromatography, the Sephadex grains are first swollen in water and then, under appropriate pressure (without provoking the formation of air bubbles) are poured into the column. The large molecules pass directly into the liquid surrounding the beads (void volume, V_0), whereas the beads (inner volume V_i). The large molecules must only traverse V_0, whereas the small molecules penetrate through elution volume of the small molecules is equivalent to the sum of $V_0 + V_i$. Therefore, the molecules are eluted in the reverse order of their size. However, this observation is true only for gel particles that completely exclude or completely absorb a substance, i.e., when the molecules are dispersed either completely within the beads (dispersion coefficient $K_d = 0$) or outside ($K_d = 1$) them. Because K_d can vary from 0 to 1, the general equation for the elution volume is $V_e = V_0 + V_i \times K_d$. A gel with small pores, e.g., G 10 or G 25, is particularly suitable for the exclusion of electrolytes (substituting for dialysis), whereas G 100 to G 200 permit the separation of macromolecules, e.g., IgG and IgM. Gel filtration and ion-exchange chromatography can be combined, e.g., with DEAE-Sephadex or CM (carboxymethyl)-Sephadex.

Sepharose is used principally for the separation of large molecules such as DNA, RNA, viruses, and polysaccharide polymers, and is also useful as a matrix for the immobilization of ligands through chemical groupings that are coupled on the dextran beads, such as cyanogen bromide, 6-aminohexanoic acid, and others. The preparation called "Sepharose 4 B activated with CNBr" is particularly useful for the direct coupling of proteins or of other molecules that contain amino groups. After the coupling of an antigen, it is possible through affinity chromatography to bind the corresponding antibody and to isolate it by elution, and vice versa.

Fractionation with ethanol, introduced by Cohn and associates (1940) for the separation of the human plasma proteins, is performed through gradual addition of ethyl alcohol in varying concentrations and pH levels, and at a temperature close to that of the freezing point of the mixtures, in order to avoid the denaturation of the proteins (Table 4.2). Cohn's method is commonly used for fractionating proteins on an industrial scale to obtain two fractions of great therapeutic importance: albumin (fraction V) and gamma globulin (fractions II, III). In the latter case, fractionation by ethanol is especially advantageous because it permits elimination or inactivation of hepatitis B virus. Only those donors should be chosen who are proved free from HB antigen.

Deutsch described a variant technique for alcohol fractionation on a laboratory scale: The serum, diluted ¼ in distilled water and then chilled to 0 °C, is combined with a 50% solution of ethanol previously chilled to −20°, under slow but continuous agitation, to a concentration of 20%, in order to maintain the mixture at a temperature near the freezing point (−5 to −6 °C). The immunoglobulin precipitate (precipitate A) is resuspended in a buffer of 0.01 ionic strength, pH 5.1; ethanol at a concentration of 15% is then added. The IgA and IgM fractions remain soluble; the IgG fraction is precipitated with a yield of about 65% and a purity of 90%–98%.

The technique of enzymatic digestion was developed empirically by Parfentjev (1936) and by Pope (1939); today it is utilized only

Table 4.2. Fractionation of the plasma proteins by Cohn's method 6

Ethanol (%)	pH	Fraction	Principal components
8	7.2	I	Fibrinogen
25	6.8	II + III	β and α
40	4.8	V	Albumin

for the purification of antitoxins destined for therapeutic use. It consists essentially of the partial digestion of plasma with pepsin at pH 3.2, followed by thermocoagulation of the inert proteins (at 56 °C, pH 4.2) and by isolation of the digested antibody through precipitation with ammonium sulfate.

Specific Methods. The fact that the amount of antibody precipitated by pneumococcic polysaccharide was smaller when the reaction was carried out in 1.8 M NaCl than in 0.15 M NaCl, led Heidelberger and Kendall in 1936 to dissociate pneumococcic antibody through the extraction of the specific precipitate with 15% NaCl. Antibody solutions with a purity of 80%–100%, which were homogeneous after electrophoresis and ultracentrifugation, could be obtained by this method – sometimes in relatively high yields (30% for horse antisera). The same method was also applied to the purification of the anticardiolipin of syphilitic sera. Dissociation in 15% NaCl, however, does not permit the purification of antiprotein antibodies. In this case, other eluents are utilized, particularly acid buffers at pH 3.0.

Special reference must be made to the elution of antibodies by haptens, exemplified by the purification of antidinitrophenyl (DNP) antibodies by means of DNP-OH. In its general outlines, this method of purification, developed by Eisen, consists of the following steps:

1. *Precipitation* of the antibody by the hapten linked to a support protein different from that used to prepare the conjugate uti-

lized in the immunization, e.g., anti-DNP prepared by immunization with DNP-BGG is precipitated with DNP-BSA.

2. *Dissociation* of the anti-DNP/DNP-BSA complex with DNP-OH, pH 5.0, in the presence of streptomycin. The DNP-BSA molecules, dislocated from their combination with anti-DNP by the competitive action of an excess of DNP-OH, because of their negative charge, are precipitated by the basic streptomycin molecule.

3. *Dialysis* to remove the DNP-OH.

4. *Passage through* a column of Dowex 1-RX ion-exchange resin, which permits removal of the remaining DNP-OH or DNP-BSA, leaving the anti-DNP antibody in a free state.

Most recently, immunoadsorbents have been successfully used for the purification of antibodies. This method was first utilized by Campbell in the conjugation of diazotized proteins to p-aminobenzylcellulose. The antigen is bound to the insoluble immunoadsorbent-column and later eluted with an acid buffer. Identical results are obtained with protein antigens coupled by diazotization to polyaminostyrene or with insoluble polymers of protein obtained with ethyl chloroformate or glutaraldehyde.

Nature and Heterogeneity of Antibodies

Although it had long been known that the antibodies were contained in the globulin fraction of the serum, it was not until 1939 that Tiselius and Kabat identified them conclusively as gamma globulins:

1. In the serum of hyperimmunized animals, the electrophoretic peak corresponding to the gamma globulins exhibits abnormal elevation, being reduced to normal proportions in the supernatant of the antiserum after precipitation with the specific antigen (Fig. 4.8).

2. Antibodies purified by specific methods behave under electrophoresis in a similar fashion to the slow protein of the serum that Tiselius had previously termed gamma globulin.

Two years earlier, Heidelberger and Pedersen had studied the sedimentation rates of antibodies purified by ultracentrifugation and had established that certain antibodies, e.g., the pneumococcal antibodies of horses, cattle, and swine, sedimented rapidly (sedimentation constant 19 S, mol.wt. close to 900,000); others, however, such as human and rabbit pneumococcal antibodies, exhibited a 7 S sedimentation constant with a molecular weight of about 160,000. The former were identified as slow beta globulins (β_2), and the latter were called slow gamma globulins (γ_2).

Twenty years later, with the advent of immunoelectrophoresis, Grabar and associates demonstrated that what until then had been called gamma globulin in reality corre-

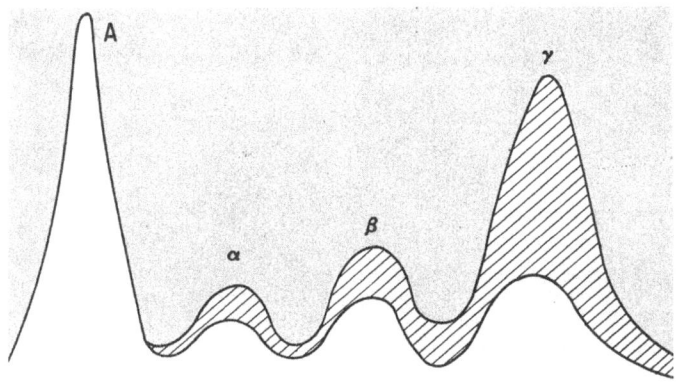

Fig. 4.8. Electrophoretic profile of an anti-ovalbumin rabbit serum before and after absorption of the antibody

sponded to a family of molecules that, although antigenically identical, possessed extremely diverse charges, imparting to them anodic mobility in alkaline pH (8.6), in a broad band that extended from the slow gamma (γ_2) to the slow alpha (α_2) region. They furthermore found that two other globulins, antigenically related but not identical to the gamma globulins, exhibited antibody activity. These two globulins, which under immunoelectrophoresis appeared as distinct arcs of precipitation, were at first called β_{2A} and β_{2M}, and were later changed to γ_A and γ_M, with the γ_G designation being used for the classic gamma globulin.

Following the suggestion of Heremans, all proteins that exhibit antibody activity or that are antigenically related to the antibody molecules are collectively called immunoglobulins; as proposed by a group of experts of the World Health Organization, they are designated by the Ig abbreviation, e.g. IgG, IgA, IgM, IgD, and IgE.

Immunoglobulin Structure

The modern era of antibody research began in 1959 when investigations conducted independently by Porter and by Edelman (Nobel Prize, 1972) showed that the immunoglobulin molecule was made up of four

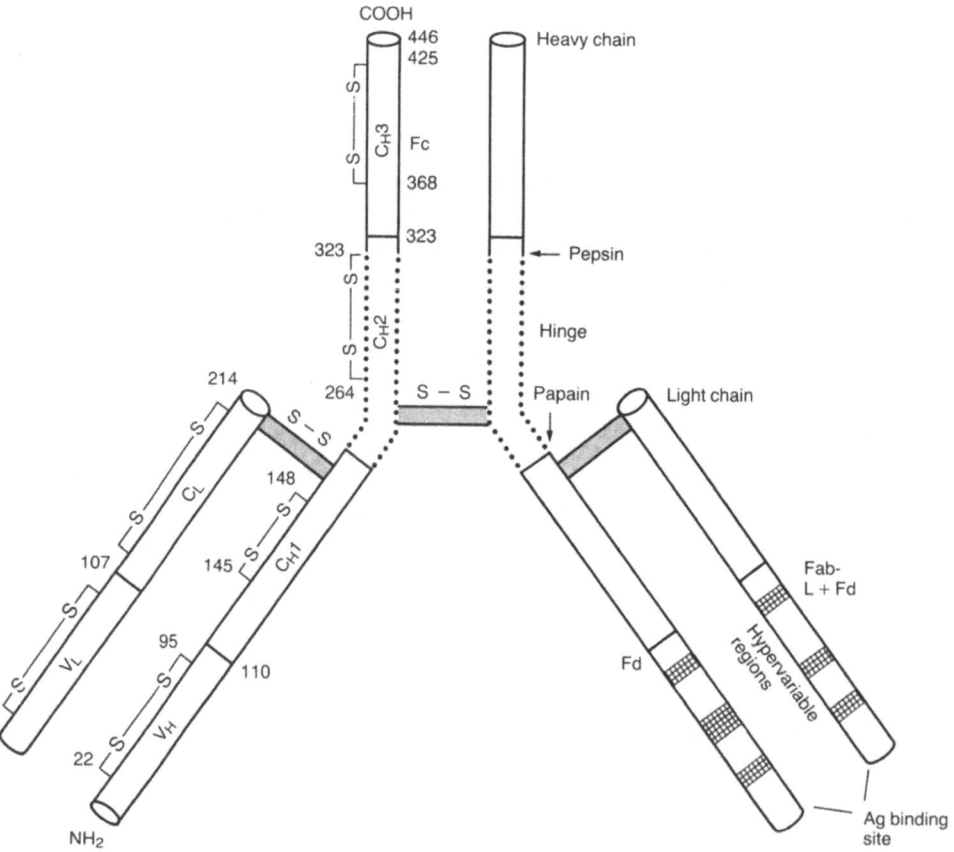

Fig. 4.9. Diagramatic model showing the four-chain structure of an IgG molecule (Human IgG1$_\kappa$). Chain L has 214 and chain H 446 amino acids. Numbers 107, 110, 220, and 341 correspond to transition limits between domains. Intrachain -SS- bonds and hypervariable regions (shaded areas in V_L and V_H are indicated). The hinge region in which the H chains are linked by two -SS- bridges [corresponding to sequence -Cys-Pro-Pro-Cys-(226 to 229)] is also approximately given. The points of attack of papain and pepsin are on positions 224 and 234, respectively. Carbohydrate is attached to residue 297

polypeptide chains. The basic anatomy of the IgG molecule was then established according to a four-chain model: two heavy (H) chains (mol.wt. 50,000) and two light (L) chains (mol.wt. 25,000), held together by non-covalent forces, such as hydrophobic and electrostatic forces, as well as by S-S bridges (Fig. 4.9).

Two lines of research led to this conclusion: a) separation of the chains by reducing agents; b) digestion of the immunoglobulin molecule by proteolytic enzymes (papain, pepsin).

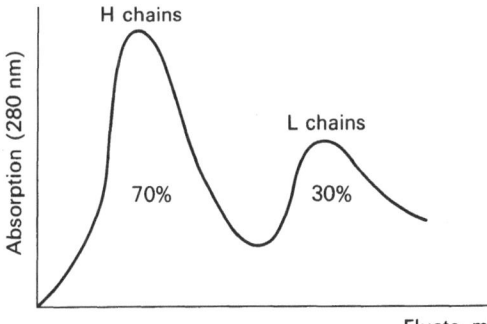

Fig. 4.10. Separation of H and L chains by Sephadex G 75 gel filtration. The gel was equilibrated with 1.0 M propionic acid. The protein was reduced and alkylated before being applied to the column

Separation of the Chains. In 1950, Porter investigated the number and the identity of the N-terminal amino acids in the 7 S immunoglobulin of the rabbit using the reaction with dinitrofluorobenzene and encountered only one N-terminal residue of alanine per molecule. Consequently, he concluded that the molecule was composed of a single polypeptide chain. However, when the same technique was applied to the immunoglobulins of other species, different results were obtained (2 N-terminal residues for human immunoglobulin and 4–5 for the horse immunoglobulin, for example), suggesting that in the rabbit the N-terminal ends of the other chains were blocked, perhaps by acetylation.

This caused Edelman and associates to attempt a technique for determining the number of peptide chains of the immuoglobulin molecule based on the reduction of the S-S bridges that covalently united the polypeptide subunits in numerous proteins. Under these circumstances, they showed that the molecular weight of the immunoglobulin fell from 150,000 to 50,000; furthermore, chromatography of the reduced material revealed another subcomponent of lower molecular weight (25,000). Such a finding strongly suggested that in the rabbit immunoglobulin molecule there were four polypeptide chains: two with a molecular weight of 50,000 each, and two with a molecular weight of 25,000 each.

The experiments of Edelman and his associates were conducted in the presence of urea

or guanidine. These substances acted as a denaturant, promoting the uncoiling of the peptide chain and the exposure of the intrachain S-S bridges; as a result, insoluble products that lacked any biologic activity were formed.

This inconvenience was overcome by Fleischman, Pain, and Porter by reduction with mercaptoethanol at pH 8.2, followed by alkylation with idoacetamide in order to avoid the reoxidation of the SH groupings, and by acidification with organic acids (acetic or propionic acid) to prevent the hydrophobic linkages and to confer positive charges upon the chains to impede their reassociation. Under these conditions, filtration in dextran gel (Sephadex G 75) equilibrated with acetic or propionic acid resulted in the distinct separation of two peaks – the former corresponding to the heavy chains and the latter to the light chains (Fig. 4.10).

Under the experimental conditions used by Porter and others, the secondary structure of the chains is preserved because the mild conditions under which the reaction proceeds permit reduction of only four or five of the 20–25 S-S bridges that exist in the immunoglobulin molecule. Thus, only S-S bridges between the chains are attacked; those within the chains are not.

Since there was almost complete recovery of the heavy and light chains, with approximately 70% in the first peak (H chain) and

30% in the second peak (L chain), it was possible to conclude by simple arithmetic that of the total molecular weight of the immunoglobulin, about 100,000 daltons corresponded to the heavy chain, and 50,000 daltons to the light chain. Moreover, since ultracentrifugation disclosed that the heavy chain had a molecular weight of 50,000 and the light chain a molecular weight of 25,000, it was concluded that the IgG molecule possessed two heavy chains and two light chains.

The manner in which these four chains are associated in the molecule was solved by enzymatic fragmentation experiments.

Enzymatic Fragmentation

In 1959, Porter subjected rabbit IgG to papain digestion in the presence of cysteine

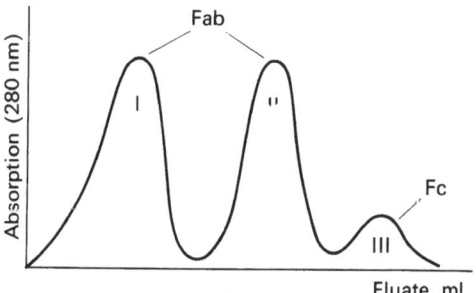

Fig. 4.11. Chromatographic separation in CM-cellulose of papain-digested rabbit IgG. Elution with acetate buffer, pH 5.5, gradient from 0.1 to 0.9 M. The Fc fragments crystallize when dialyzed against a low-ionic strength buffer. Two-thirds of the total IgG correspond to the Fab, and one-third to the Fc

and verified that the sedimentation constant of the digested material fell from 7 S to 3.5 S, indicating a cleavage into fragments of about 50,000 daltons. When the digested material was dialyzed against a phosphate buffer at pH 7 and passed through a column of carboxymethylcellulose at pH 5.2, three peaks were separated. In the order of their elution (using a pH 5.2 acetate buffer gradient) they were designated fragments I, II, and III (Fig. 4.11). Fractions I and II possessed the activity of monovalent antibody, for they inhibited precipitation by the complete antibody; fraction III was biologically inactive. Upon dialysis of the digested product against a buffer of low ionic strength, fragment III crystallized. Fragments I and II were antigenically identical and came from IgG molecules with different mobilities, thus appearing in separate peaks. These are now called Fab (antigen-binding) fragments because of their ability to combine with antigens. Fragment III is designated Fc (crystallizable fraction). The antigenic relationships among fragments I, II, and III are illustrated in Fig. 4.12.

Nisonoff and his associates, by digesting rabbit IgG with pepsin instead of papain, and in the absence of cysteine, showed that the molecular weight of the digested product dropped to just 100,000 (5 S), with the capacity for precipitation being preserved, which is a property of the bivalent antibody. If, in a second phase, cysteine was

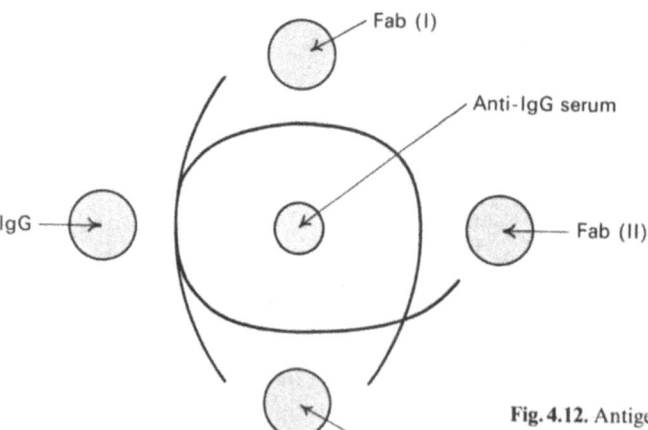

Fig. 4.12. Antigenic relationships among IgG, Fab (I or II), and Fc as revealed by gel precipitation

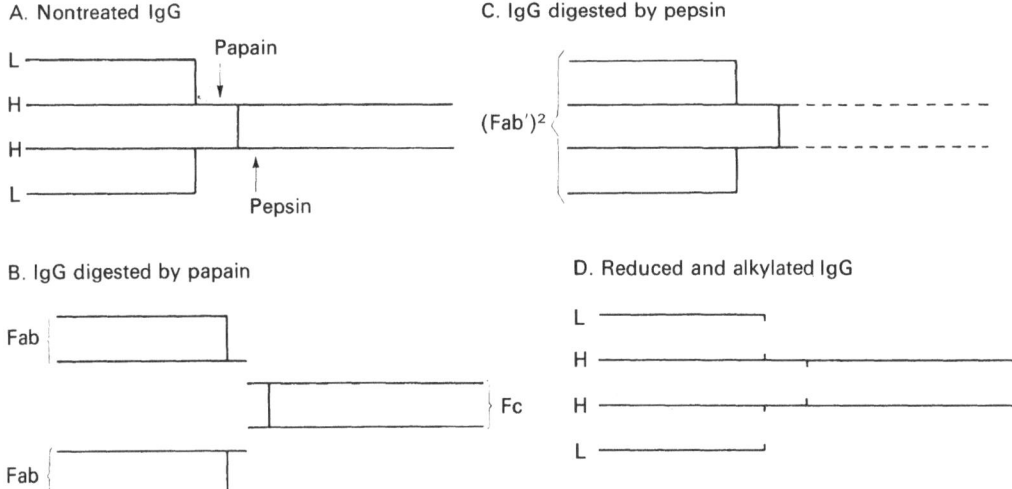

Fig. 4.13. Fragmentation of the immunoglobulin G molecule. IgG (mol.wt. 150,000), when digested by papain, produces three fragments of approximately 50,000 daltons each (2 Fab + 1 Fc). Digestion by pepsin leads to the destruction of Fc, leaving a divalent fragment (mol.wt. close to 100,000) designated (Fab')₂. If the S-S bridges between the chains of IgG are reduced and the SH-groups are stabilized by alkylation, 2 L chains (mol.wt. 25,000) and 2 H chains (mol.wt. 50,000) are separated

added, the molecular weight fell to 50,000 and precipitation no longer occurred, only inhibition of precipitation (monovalent fragment).

The monovalent pepsin fragments have a molecular weight slightly greater than that of the Fab fragment and thus ware termed Fab' fragments. Prior to the cysteine reduction, the two Fab' fragments are united by an S-S bridge, forming a bivalent 5 S fragment called the F(ab')₂ fragment. The Fc fragment is not recovered by pepsin digestion because it is digested into smaller fragments.

The results of digestion by papain and pepsin led to the conclusion that the points of attack of the two enzymes were situated, respectively, above and below the S-S bridge(s) that unite the heavy chains, at the special region called the *hinge* (cf. Figs. 4.9 and 4.13).

Relation Between Chains and Fragments. The relationship between the fractions obtained via reduction and the enzymatic fragments, which led to the currently accepted molecular model for the 7 S immu-

Table 4.3. Reaction of anti-Fab and of anti-Fc with H and L chains

Antisera	H chain	L chain
Anti-Fab	+	+
Anti-Fc	+	−

noglobulins (see Fig. 4.12), was elucidated through gel precipitation experiments between anti-Fab sera or anti-Fc sera and the heavy and light chains of the immunoglobulin (Table 4.3).

The results shown in Table 4.3 clearly demonstrate that the Fab fragment is composed of part of the heavy chain plus the light chain, where as the Fc fragment is made up of the other part of the heavy chain not included in the Fab, i.e., not associated with the light chain. The segment of the heavy chain in the Fab fragment is known as Fd.

Functions of the Fragments. The Fab fragments of the immunoglobulin molecule provide the combining sites that enable the antibody to unite to the antigen as a bivalent ligand. These must necessarily possess a large variety of configurations to cope with the many antigenic determinants that come into contact with the organism.

Most of the biological activities of the immunoglobulins, however, seem to be associated with Fc:

1. Complement Fixation. The activation of the complement system by the "classical" pathway (see Chap. 5) is initiated by the binding of C1q to the C_H2 region of IgG or IgM, the exposure of the reactive sites depending on previous interaction of the antigen with Fab. It should be noted, however, that the fragment (Fab')$_2$ of certain IgGs can trigger complement activation by the alternative pathway.

2. Transfer Across Membranes. The passage of immunoglobulins across epithelial membranes is extremely important for the protection of the newborn against environmental pathogenic microorganisms. This includes the transfer of IgA to external secretions (cf. Fig. 4.18) and the passage of maternal IgG through the placenta or to the colostrum (in ruminants). It is believed that these transfer processes depend on the structure of the heavy chain, because: a) it involves a certain degree of sub-class specificity; b) pepsin digested IgG is unable to cross the placenta, indicating that a specific site on Fc determines the passage by some active process.

3. Cell Binding. The fixation of homocytotropic antibodies (see p. 248) to the membrane of mastocytes is mediated by Fc receptors, as well as the attachment of opsonized particles to the surface of phagocytes.

4. Catabolism. The catabolic index, which controls the blood level of immunoglobulins is also a feature of Fc.

Domains. Edelman suggested the subdivision of the immunoglobulin molecule into domains, on the basis of homologous regions. According to this hypothesis, the antibody molecule consists of homologous compact loops or domains formed by ca. 60–70 amino acids held together by intrachain S-S bridges and separated by

Table 4.4. Functions of the domains of the immunoglobulin-G molecule

Domain	Verified or probable function
$V_H + V_L$	Antigen recognition (antigen combining site)
$C_H1 + C_2$	Noncovalent bond between L and H chains; S-S bridges between the distal Fd- and Fc ends
C_H2	Binding of $C1_q$ and control of catabolism
C_H3	Cytotropy for macrophages, lymphocytes, and mast cells. Noncovalent bond between the H chains

"spacer" regions of about 50 amino acids. There are two domains in the L chain (V_L and C_L) and four or five in the H chain (V_H, C_H1, C_H2, C_H3, and C_H4), as shown in Fig. 4.9. Table 4.4 summarizes the different functions ascribed to the domains of IgG. The domain hypothesis offers a theoretical concept on which an understanding of structural and functional characteristics of immunoglobulin can be based.

Heterogeneity and Structure of the Chains. Simple immunoelectrophoretic analysis demonstrates that the immunoglobulins are composed of heterogenous populations of molecules with highly different mobilities that, in the case of IgG, extend from the gamma region to that of the alpha-2 globulins (see Fig. 4.9).

This heterogeneity, typically observed with normal immunoglobulins, is much less evident in the pathologic proteins that appear in the serum of patients with myeloma-tumors of monoclonal plasma cells that produce immunoglobulins that are relatively homogenous.

In cases of myeloma, special proteins called Bence-Jones proteins appear in the urina as fragments of the same pathologic proteins encountered in the serum[1]. Since these pro-

---

1 Described in 1847 by Dr. H. Bence-Jones in the urine of a patient with myeloma, these proteins are characterized by the fact that they coagulate at 50°–60 °C at pH 4–pH 6; these proteins dissolve upon further heating, only to precipitate again upon cooling

teins occur in such large quantities, they are particularly useful for the study of the light chains, because they are composed of dimerized light chains with molecular weights of approximately 45,000.

The Bence-Jones proteins differ from one individual to another, yet when studied immunologically with rabbit antisera they have been found to fall into two groups, originally designated I (or B) and II (or A). Today, they are called "K" and "L", after the initials of the authors who studied them (Korngold and Lipari, respectively). The light chains that correspond to these two classes of proteins are termed κ (kappa) and λ (lambda). In the immunoglobulin molecule, the light chains can be either κ or λ, there being no hybrid molecules. In normal human serum, about two-thirds of the G immunoglobulins carry the κ chains, with the remaining one third bearing λ chains.

The structure of the immunoglobulin chains can be analyzed by gel electrophoresis in starch or acrylamide gel. Under these conditions, the heavy chains normally produce a single, diffuse, slow band; the light chains are resolved into a number (7–10) or relatively rapid bands. Myeloma and Bence Jones proteins are relatively homogenous, exhibiting a small number of light-chain bands.

The intrinsic heterogeneity of the normal immunoglobulins renders simple amino acid analysis even in purified preparations impossible. For this reason, the best approach to the solution of this problem is the use of monoclonal myeloma proteins or affinity-chromatographically purified antibodies or their fragments to determine the amino acid sequence. Studies of this sort have been undertaken principally with the Bence-Jones proteins of humans and mice. Of the 214 amino acids that constitute the light chains, the N-terminal half is variable (V_L), whereas the C-terminal half is constant (C_L), as exemplified in the following words:

$$V_L \quad C_L$$
PHYSI OLOGY
GYNEC OLOGY
IMMUN OLOGY

In these words, the first five letters represent the V_L region and the last five the C_L region.

Similarly, in the heavy chains, the first 110 N-terminal amino acid residues are variable (V_H), whereas the rest of the chain (ca. 3 or 4×110 residues, see below) is composed of constant segments (domains) – as represented in Fig. 4.14. The δ, γ, and α chains have three such segments, C_H1, C_H2, and C_H3, and the μ and ε chains, four, C_H1, C_H2, C_H3 and C_H4. Structural studies and comparisons with the immunoglobulins of primitive fish suggest that the "primordial" C chain corresponds to the present-day μ chain with four homologous segments (domains); the shorter δ and α chains arose through the loss of the C_H2 (μ) domain during phylogenic development. The homologous areas of the V_L and V_H regions suggest the doubling of an ancestral gene during evolution, and that subsequent mutations led to the variable regions with antibody function and species-specific residues in the constant regions of the L and H chains.

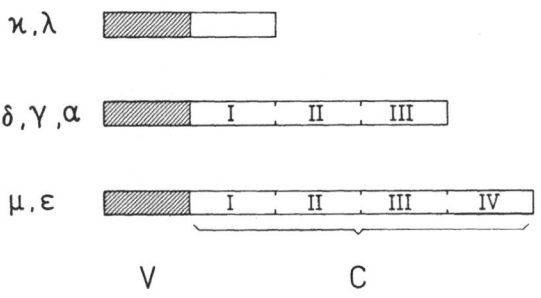

$$V \qquad\qquad C$$

Fig. 4.14. Length of different Ig chains. The variable *(V)* regions or all types of chains have about 110 amino acids and approximately the same length. The constant region of the L chain consists of 1, the constant regions of the γ, α, and δ heavy chains of 3, and the constant regions of the μ and ε heavy chains of 4 homologous segments (domains), each consisting of about 110 amino acid residues. (Reproduced with permission from Hilschmann et al., 1978)

Chemical Structure of the Combining Site.
By integrating inferences derived from sequence and affinity labelling data with the high resolution X-ray crystallographic findings, it is now possible not only to define the chemical structure of the antibody combining site, but also its spatial configuration (for details of these important studies, see Kabat, E.A., "Structural Concepts in Immunology and Immunochemistry", 2nd Ed., 1976, cf. p. 305).

We shall restrict us here to data concerning the maximum size and the hypervariable regions of the combining site.

1. The maximum size of the combining site may be inferred from its accommodation of molecules with the dimensions of a hexasaccharide or a hexapeptide; this approximates a molecular size similar to that of the molecule of the lysozyme substrate. In these molecules, 15–20 "contact amino acids" have been identified, and the same presumably holds true for the antibody combining site. If any residue can occupy one of these 15–20 positions, the possible number of variations is extremely large.

2. Both H and L chains have variable regions at their N-termini (V_H and V_L) but similar sequences in the C-domains. It is noteworthy, however, that V-domains, even in different species (man, mouse), also have constant portions known as *framework regions* (FR) which like the C-regions remained remarkably preserved during evolution.

Only three restricted areas of V_H and V_L called *hypervariable regions* participate directly in the formation of the combining site, by providing the contact aminoacids (5–10 for each hypervariable region) for the binding of the antigen.

In human V_K the hypervariable regions correspond approximately to positions 24–34, 45–56, and 89–98 (cf. Fig. 4.15), inserted between FR1 to FR4 (1–23, 35–49, 57–88, and 98–107) (Fig. 4.9). In human V_H, homologous hypervariable regions were shown at positions 31–35, 50–65, and 95–102. The sequences of each FR are grouped into different sets of 1–18 residues and the same set of FR1, for example, can be associated with different sets of FR2, FR3, and FR4. This

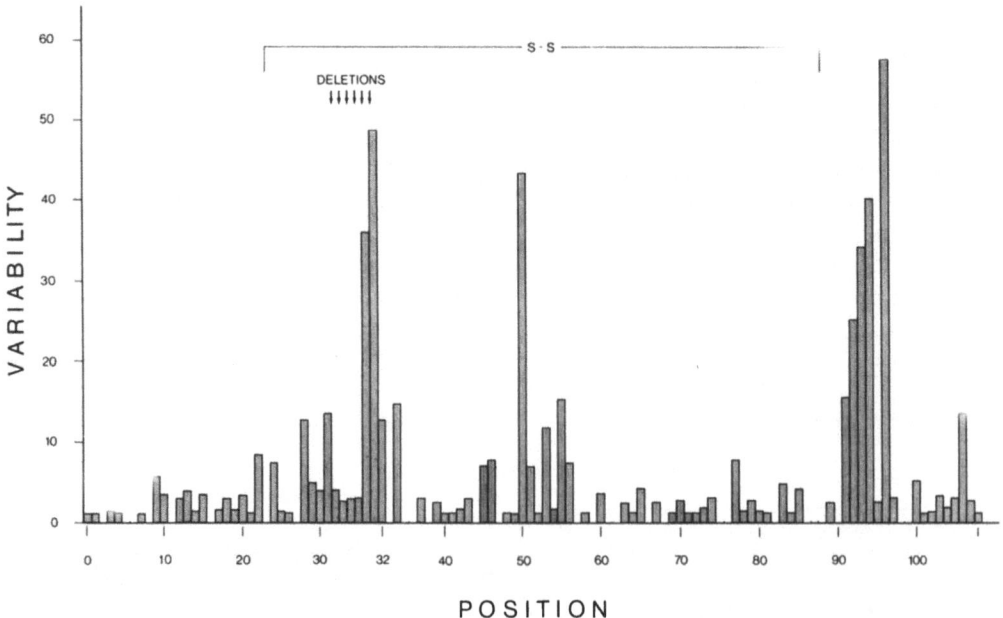

Fig. 4.15. Histogram of the variability of the V-domain. Three hypervariable sections can be recognized between the positions 28–34, 45–56, and 91–98. (Reproduced with permission from Hilschmann et al., 1978)

led Kabat to the stimulating hypothesis that the complete framework for the L and H chains V-regions is assembled during ontogeny from sets of minigenes for each FR segment. A considerable degree of diversity could be generated by this assembly of FR pieces from different FR segments and if we consider further that the positions corresponding to the hypervariable CDR's may be occupied by any one of 20 possible amino acids, the number of resulting specificities would be largely sufficient to cope with the epitopic universe.

Affinity-Labeling Technique. The so-called affinity-labeling technique is particularly suitable for defining the structure of the combining site. With this technique, a labeled, chemically modified hapten, which through an additional reactive group (e.g., diazonium-, bromacetyl-, or arylnitro-bindings) is capable of forming a covalent bond on or near the combining site, is added to the antibody. Then the amount of labeled hapten in the peptides, which is maintained through hydrolysis of the antibody (H and L chains), is determined. Finally, the amino acid sequence of the labeled peptide is determined.

The principle of the method can be shown schematically as follows:

$$B(y) + H^*(x) \rightarrow B \cdot y - x \cdot H^*,$$

in which B is the antibody combining site, H^*, the labeled hapten, y and x are the structures that lie in or near B or H^* and that from a stable $B \cdot y - x \cdot H^*$ complex through a covalent bond.

Certain controls must be considered: (1) the absence of labeled haptens in nonspecific immunoglobulins and (2) inhibition of labeling through previous administration of unmarked haptens.

The total results of such experiments with different antibodies and labeling agents support the hypothesis that tyrosine and lysine residues in the hypervariable regions of the V_H and V_L domains play a primary role in the specific binding of the antigen.

Classes and Subclasses of Human Immunoglobulins

The human immunoglobulins are presently divided into five classes, designated IgG, IgA, IgM, IgD, and IgE (Fig. 4.16). They are characterized by specific antigenic determinants in their heavy chains, respectively designated by the Greek letters γ (gamma), α (alpha), μ (mu), δ (delta), and ε (epsilon). The light chains are identical in all classes; κ (kappa) and λ (lambda).

Since the immunoglobulin molecules possess two heavy chains and two light chains, IgG is expressed as $\gamma_2\lambda_2$, or $\gamma_2\kappa_2$, and IgA as $\alpha_2\kappa_2$ or $\alpha_2\lambda_2$, and so on.

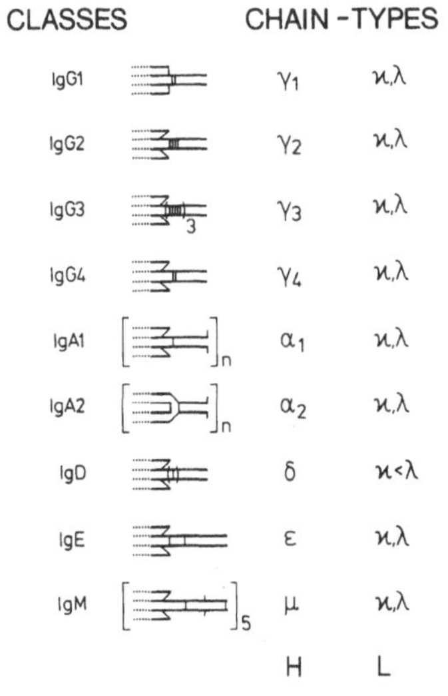

CLASSES		CHAIN-TYPES	
IgG1		γ_1	κ,λ
IgG2		γ_2	κ,λ
IgG3		γ_3	κ,λ
IgG4		γ_4	κ,λ
IgA1		α_1	κ,λ
IgA2		α_2	κ,λ
IgD		δ	$\kappa<\lambda$
IgE		ε	κ,λ
IgM		μ	κ,λ
		H	L

Fig. 4.16. Immunoglobulin classes and subclasses. The class or subclass of an antibody molecule is determined by the nature of the H chain. The different H chain types are distinguishable by their amino acid sequences and by the number of their interpeptidal disulfide bridges (vertical lines). L chains can be of λ- or κ-type. The complete structure of IgG, IgM, IgA₁, and IgE is known. The other molecules represent tentative structures which are sometimes only based on the analyses of disulfide-containing peptides. In one allotype of the IgA₂ subclass, the L chains are not covalently linked to the H chains but are linked to each other. The specificity is determined by the V parts (– – – –). (Reproduced with permission from Hilschmann et al., 1978)

To differentiate the classes, rabbit antisera are used that have been absorbed with immunoglobulins of classes different from those used for immunization, e.g. anti-IgG antiserum absorbed with IgM (specific for the γ determinant); or vice versa, anti-IgM absorbed with IgG (specific for the μ determinant).

IgG. Immunoglobulin G, which is quantitatively the major serum immunoglobulin (ca. 1,300 mg % compared to 160 or 90 mg % for IgA and IgM, respectively), has one of four "subdeterminants" on its Fc part (1, 2, 3, and 4) that characterize four subclasses (IgG$_1$, IgG$_2$, IgG$_3$, and IgG$_4$). Rabbit antiserum used to differentiate these subclasses is produced with a myeloma-G antigen and is absorbed with other IgG myeloma proteins. The chief characteristics of the differ-

ent classes of human immunoglobulins and the particulars of the IgG subclasses are summarized in Tables 4.5 and 4.6.

IgG (with the exception of IgG$_4$) and IgM, but not the other immunoglobulins, have the ability to fix C1q – a binding that appears to occur on the C$_H$2 domain. Except for IgG$_2$, IgG can also bind to heterologous skin, thereby inducing the anaphylactic reaction. Only IgG can pass through the placenta and bind to macrophages. This binding occurs in the middle of the C$_H$3 domain and, in contrasts to the binding of opsonizing and C-fixing IgG and IgM antibodies, it is independent of any previous antigen binding.

IgM. IgM (M stands for macroglobulin) consists of a pentamer whose 7 S units are held together by a peptide of about 25,000

Table 4.5. Physicochemical and biologic properties of the different classes of human immunoglobulins

Properties	IgG	IgA	IgM	IgD	IgE
Average concentration in serum mg/ml[a]	13.1	1.6	0.9	0.12	0.33×10^{-3}
Sedimentation coefficient (S)	7	7	19	7	8
Mol. wt. 10^3	160	170[b]	900	185	185
Carbohydrate (%)	2.9	7.5	11.8	13	12
J chain	−	+	+	−	−
Lability at 56 °C	−	−	−	−	+
Mercaptoethanol resistance	+ +	±	−	+ +	−
Isotypic determinants	γ1, γ2, γ3, γ4	α1, α2	μ	δ	ε
Allotypic determinants					
Gm (H chains)	+	−	−		
Inv (L chains)	+	+	+		
Synthesis (mg/kg/day)	28	8–10	5–8	0.4	
Catabolism (%/day)	3	12	14		2.5
Half-life (days)	23	5.8	5.1	2.8	2.5
Agglutinating activity	1	−	100		
Fixation of complement	+	−	+	−	−
Transplacental passage	+	−	−	−	−
Binding to macrophages	+	−	−	−	−
Binding to mast cells[c]	−	−	−	−	+
Reaction with staphylococcus A protein	+	−	−	−	−
Reaction with rheumatoid factor	+	−	−	−	−

[a] According to Johansson, 1967

[b] Secretory IgA is a dimer and is associated with a secretory piece. Secretory IgA has a molecular weight of ca. 390,000, that is, the sum $(2 \times 170,000) + 58,000$ (secretory piece)

[c] IgG$_1$, IgG$_3$, and IgG$_4$ bind to xenogeneic skin (see Table 4.6)

Property	IgG	IgG$_2$	IgG$_3$	IgG$_4$
% Total IgG	67	24	6	3
% in IgG myeloma	77	14	6	3
Half-life (days)	23	23	8	23
Fixation of complement	+ +	+	+ + +	0
Placental passage	+	+	+	+
Hetero-PCA (guinea pigs)	+	0	+	+
Homo-PCA	0	0	0	0
Macrophage cytophilia	+	0	+	0
S-S bridge between H chains	2	4	5	2
Reactivity with staphylococcus A protein	+	+	0	+
Gm allotypes	Many	Many	1 (No. 23)	0

Table 4.6. Principal properties of human IgG subclasses

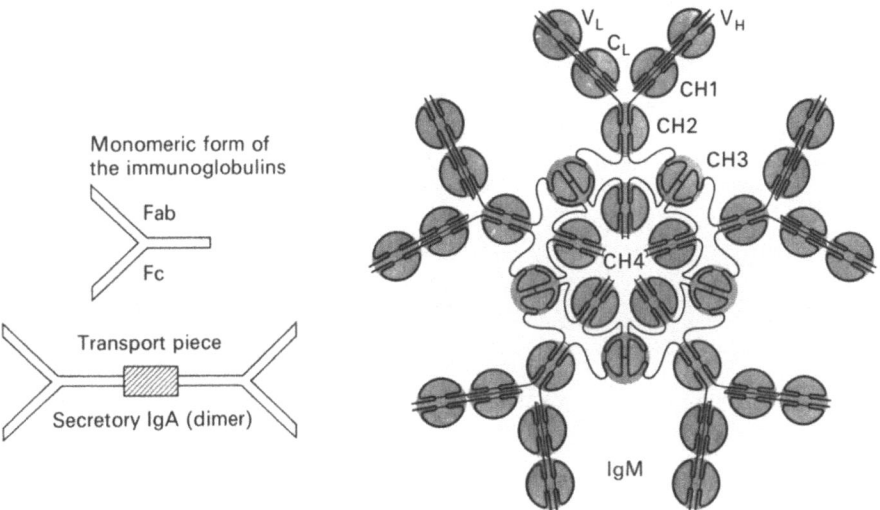

Fig. 4.17. Structural forms of immunoglobulins: IgG is monomeric; IgA exists in mono-, di-, tri-, and tetrameric forms; and IgM is pentameric. (IgM is reproduced from Hilschmann et al., 1978)

daltons, called the "J" (junction) chain. This peptide consists of a single amino-acid chain with a high content of cysteine (12 residues) and asparagine, and is also involved in the formation of IgA polymers by an as yet unknown mechanism.

Immunoglobulin M has a molecular weight of about 900,000 and a somewhat greater electrophoretic mobility than IgA, IgD, and IgE. The heavy chains composed of four homologous segments (domains): $C_\mu 3$ has a cysteine in position 102 that mediates the binding of the IgM subunits to pentamers (Fig. 4.17). IgM is much more active than IgG in the Clq binding; a single mole-

cule suffices for the sensitization of an erythrocyte.

Theoretically, IgM should have a valence of 10. However, this occurs only with small hapten molecules such as DNP. In most cases, for stereochemical reasons, only five antigen molecules can be bound (steric hindrance).

IgA. Immunoglobulin A usually circulates in monomeric (7 S) and dimeric (9 S) forms, but also occurs as 11 S and 13 S polymers. The units of this chain are connected by the J chain. Like the other immunoglobulins, IgA also has a carbohydrate part that is

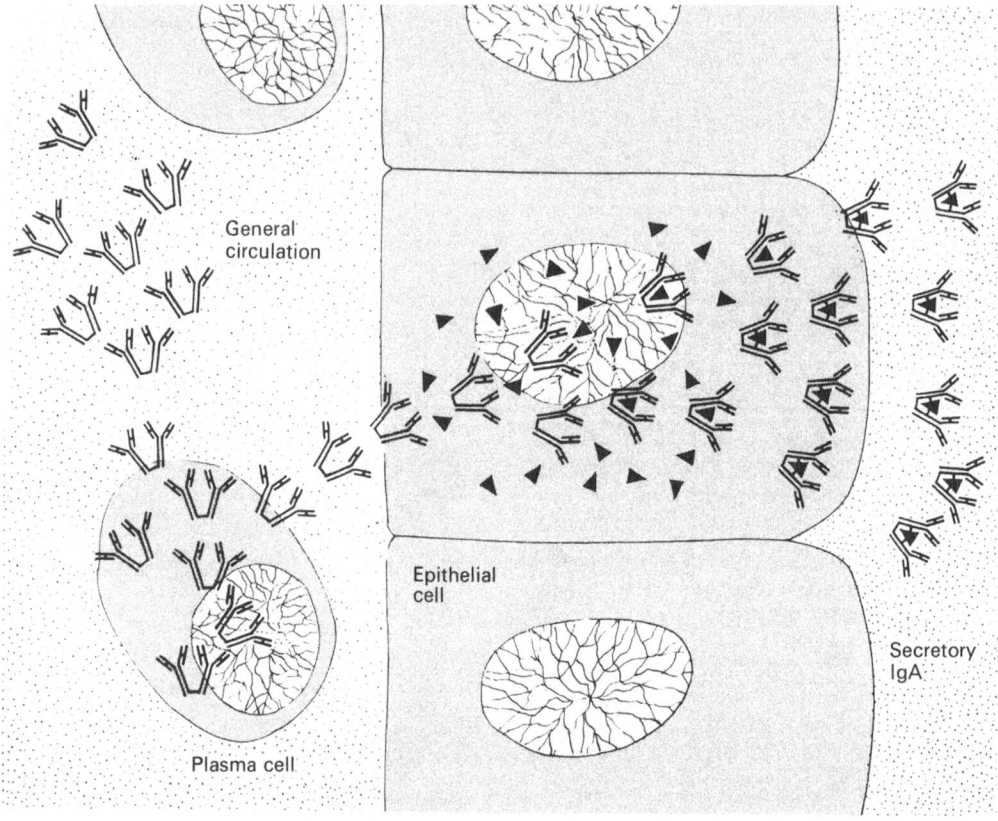

Fig. 4.18. Synthesis and transport of secretory IgA. (Adapted from Tomasi, 1970)

about three to four times larger than that on the IgG.

IgG and IgM are found in small quantities in secretions, e.g., saliva, tears, intestinal secretions, and colostrum; however, IgA, particularly IgA_1, is the predominant immunoglobulin in these secretions. Secretion IgA has a molecular weight of approximately 390,000 daltons. In 1963, Tomasi showed that two 7 S units are held together by an additional glycoprotein, mol.wt. 58,000, the "secretion piece" or "transport piece." This component is excreted from epithelial cells of the mucosa or from exocrine glands. Apparently, it confers a protection against proteolytic enzymes and assures the passage of secretory IgA synthesized in subepithelial regions to the surface of the mucous membranes (Fig. 4.18).

Although IgA does not bind complement and has no bactericidal effect, it is thought to play an important role in the localization of certain infectious agents (e.g., influenza and polio viruses on the mucous membranes of the intestine or the nose) and in the neutralization of some bacteria toxins.

IgD. This immunoglobulin was discovered in 1965 in the serum of a myeloma patient; because of the low serum concentration, it had remained undiscovered. The discovery of IgD-myelomas made possible the isolation of a large enough quantity of the immunoglobulin to make a physicochemical characterization. It is a 7 S immunoglobulin with a high carbohydrate content, whose H chain has a molecular weight of about 70,000 daltons and is bound by a single disulfide bridge. No antibody activity can be assigned to this immunoglobulin. New findings concerning IgD specificities against specific antigens (nucleoproteins, insulin) are questionable. It should be emphasized that IgM as well as IgD is found on the surface of lymphocytes, particularly in cases of lymphatic leukemia (see p. 13).

IgE. IgE corresponds to the reaginic antibody responsible for the PK test. It was identified as a distinct immunoglobulin in ingenious studies performed by Ishizaka and associates (1966): Rabbits were immunized with the serum of a patient sensitive to ragweed pollen. The antisera obtained were absorbed with immunoglobulins G, A, M, and D. The "empty" antiserum could contain only antibodies against immunoglobulins not belonging to these four classes, presumably against the immunoglobulins associated with the reaginic activity (later called IgE).

When the "empty" antiserum was mixed with a reaginic-rich serum (R), the supernatant lost the capacity to give a positive PK test – which had been strongly positive with the untreated R serum.

Furthermore, if a mixture of "empty" (anti-IgE) antisera plus labeled antigen (^{131}I) was located in the central well of an Ouchterlony plate, and IgG, IgA, IgM, IgD, and R were placed in the peripheral wells, a line of precipitation developed only between the anti-IgE and the R wells (Fig. 4.19). After careful washing of the plate and subjecting it to autoradiographic examination, the radioactivity was located on the line of precipitation.

The three facts just mentioned (specific immunoprecipitation, inactivation of PK activity in the supernatant after precipitation,

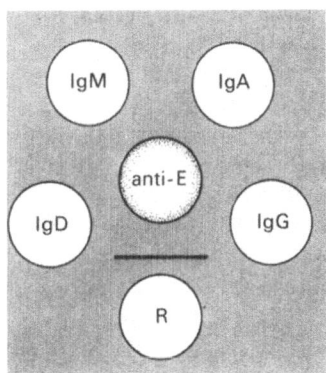
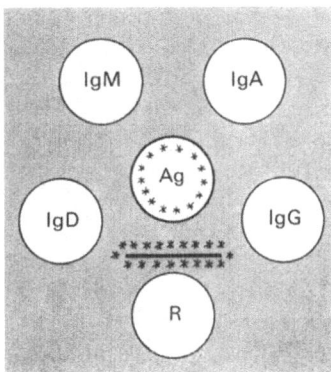

Fig. 4.19. Demonstration of the reaginic (IgE) antibody by gel precipitation and autoradiography

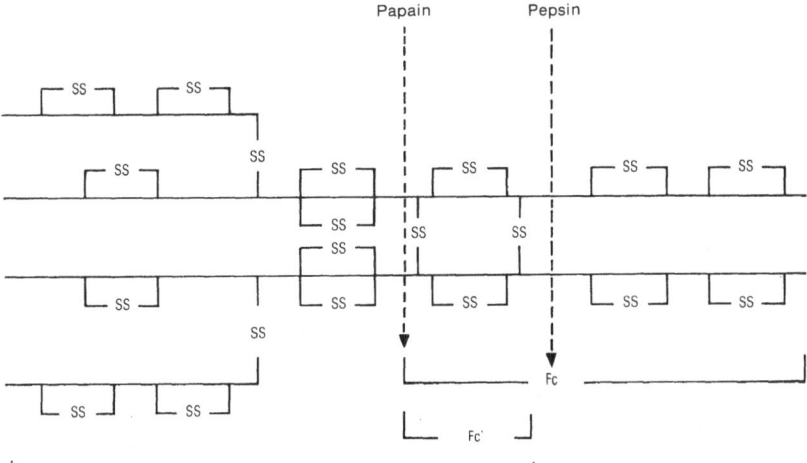

Fig. 4.20. Structure of the IgE molecule

and localization of radioactivity in the precipitation line) led Ishizaka and his associates to postulate that the reaginic antibodies were identical to a new immunoglobulin class (IgE) and not with IgA, as previously thought.

The later discovery of an atypical IgE-producing myeloma permitted the physicochemical study of the immunoglobulin and the elucidation of its structural characteristics (Fig. 4.20): (1) a molecular weight of approximately 200,000 daltons and not 50,000 daltons as with IgG, because, like the Hμ chain, they have four C domains; (2) a sedimentation constant of 8 S; (3) an abundance of carbohydrate (11%), methionine, and SH groups; and (4) thermolability at 56 °C after 4 h, probably due to destruction of a structure contained in the Fc part, which ensures fixation of the immunoglobulin into the mastocyte surfaces (C$_H$4 domain). Its serum level is low (like that of IgD) and its activity is revealed by the PK test. Because its serum concentration in most cases lies in the range of picograms to nanograms, it can be proved by precipitation only in exceptional cases. To determine its presence, the PK test or special methods are used.

Classes and Subclasses of Animal Immunoglobulins

Horse. In the sera of horses immunized with bacterial exotoxins (diphteria, tetanus) or snake venoms (*Crotalus, Bothrops*), two major types of antibodies have been identified: the usual IgG of a slow β_2 mobility (α_2 or β_1), termed the T component or IgG(T) (cf. p. 211). The main antibody in horse an-

tipneumococcal sera is of the IgM type, but on continued immunization IgA and IgG(T), as well as slow IgG are also found. Equine anti-LAC(lactosyl) antibodies could be separated chromatographically on DEAE-cellulose into six distinct immunoglobulins: IgGa, -b, -c, IgA, IgM and a 10 S protein moving in the fast gamma region.

Rodents. Benacerraf et al. have identified in guinea pig and mouse antibodies to DNP-proteins two fractions termed γ_1 and γ_2, the former migrating more rapidly in immunoelectrophoresis. These two fractions are designated as IgG$_1$ and IgG$_2$ in the guinea pig, and as IgG$_1$ and IgG$_{2a}$ in the mouse. They differ in biological properties in regard to complement fixation (γ_1-, γ_2+) and to passive sensitization of homologous skin (γ_1+, γ_2-) (cf. Chap. 10). Studies on the mouse immunoglobulins have been greatly facilitated by the availability of myeloma proteins produced by the intraperitoneal injection of mineral oil in BALB/c animals.

With these myeloma globulins it was possible to prepare antisera that allowed the identification of two additional subclasses of mouse IgG: IgG$_{2b}$ and IgG$_3$.

In the rat and in the rabbit there are also two subclasses of IgG and, as in guinea pigs and mice, also IgM, IgA, and IgE (cf. Table 4.7).

Genetic Markers of the Immunoglobulins: Allotypes and Idiotypes

It was long believed that the immunoglobulins possessed only isotopic antigenic speci-

Table 4.7 Nomenclature of animal immunoglobulins

Species	Classes or subclasses of immunoglobulin						
Horse	IgM	IgA	IgG a	IgG b	IgG c	IgG (T)	
Mouse	IgM	IgA	IgF (IgG$_1$)	IgG (IgG$_{2a}$)	IgH (IgG$_{2b}$)	IgI (IgG$_3$)	IgE
Guinea pig	IgM	IgA	IgG$_1$	IgG$_2$			IgE
Rat	IgM	IgA	IgG$_1$	IgG$_2$			IgE
Rabbit	IgM	IgA	IgG	IgG$_2$			IgE

ficities, i.e., specificities common to their own species.

In 1956, however, Oudin showed that specificities, termed allotypes, could be identified with the help of alloantisera produced by immunization of one rabbit with immunocomplexes or immunoglobulins of another rabbit. These allotypic determinants from protein molecules (not necessarily immunoglobulins) were inherited according to simple Mendelian rules. With minor differences, they correlate in the amino acid sequences.

In the rabbit at least five systems of allotypic markers are recognized, – a (H chain, variable region), b (χ chain, variable region), c (λ chain, variable region), d (γ chain, hinge), and e (γ chain, C_H3 domain):

V_H $\quad$ a_1 $\quad$ a_2 $\quad$ a_3

V_κ $\quad$ b_4 $\quad$ b_5 $\quad$ b_6 $\quad$ b_9

V_λ $\quad$ c_7 $\quad$ c_{21}

Hinge $\quad$ d_{11} $\quad$ d_{12}

C_H3 $\quad$ e_{14} $\quad$ e_{15}

Each system is determined through multiple alleles of different loci, e.g., a^1, a^2, b^4, b^5, and each animal shows a minimum of two, and a maximum of four, allotypic specificities. At the molecular level, however, only two alleles are expressed, so that both H and L chains always carry the same allotype (allotypic restriction). If the animal is a homozygote, e.g., $a^1a^1b^4b^4$, only molecules of allotypes a^1b^4 are synthesized. However, if it is a heterozygote, molecules of different allotypes can be synthesized, e.g., for the genotype $a^1a^2b^4b^5$, the allotypes a^1b^4, a^1b^5, a^2b^4, and a^2b^5, so that four allotypic specificities can be found in the serum.

Identical allotypes were found in the V regions of rabbit immunoglobulins of different classes, such as IgG and IgM (Todd phenomenon), and this led to postulate that separate V and C genes were translocated to form a cistron coding for the entire polypeptide chain.

Human Allotypes. Concomitantly with Oudin's discovery, Grubb has described allo-typic markers in human immunoglobulins (Gm for gamma globulin). Subsequently, two other systems of markers were described by Ropartz, namely the Km (kappa marker) or InV (In from inhibitor and V from the patient's initial) [2] allotype and the ISF (San Francisco) marker. A fourth human allotype, Am, was identified by Fudenberg in human IgA.

The identification of Gm and Km allotypes is made by the inhibition by immunoglobulins or fragments therefrom of the hemagglutination of red cells coated with the same allotype, as illustrated in Fig. 4.21. In Grubb's original observation, Rh+ human red cells were coated with incomplete Rh antibody and showed hemagglutination when tested with the sera of certain patients with rheumatoid arthritis. Since this agglutination could be inhibited by the sera of certain individuals but not of others, it was concluded that the agglutinating serum was Gm(a−) and contained anti-Gm(a+), i.e., antibodies against the allotype of the inhibiting serum.

Besides, rheumatoid sera which contain autoantibodies to their IgG (Rheumatoid Agglutinins or *Ragg*), normal sera (*SNagg*) having specific anti-Gm's, xenoantisera produced in rabbits or in monkeys against selected myeloma proteins, as well as human alloantibodies resulting from multiple transfusions or from incompatible pregnancies may also be used in the hemmaglutination inhibition reaction. As a matter of fact, the recognition of the Gm specificities is a difficult task and requires the use of a uniform nomenclature and the exchange of reagents among the investigators specialized in the field. In this regard, the cooper-

---

2 There are three kinds of InV determinants, whose specificity depends on the amino acid that occupies the position 191 in the kappa chain: leucine for InV 1, valine for InV 3, and serine for the chains having no InV allotype.

Human lambda chains show two isotypic differences related to positions 154 and 190, termed Kern and Oz, respectively. In Kern+, position 154 is occupied by glycine and in Kern− by serine; Oz+ have lysine at position 190, while for Oz− the amino acid is arginine

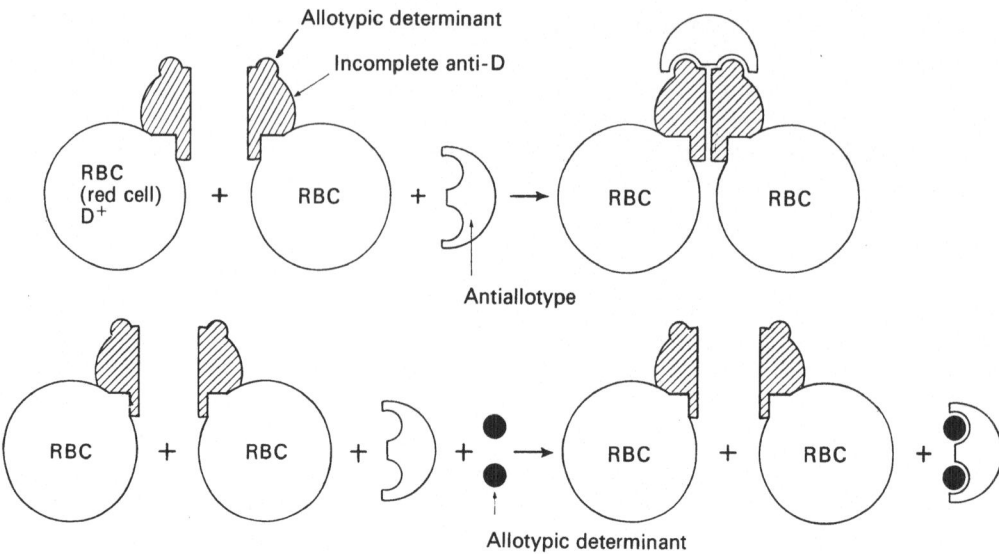

Fig. 4.21. Method for detecting human IgG allotypes

ation of the World Health Organization has been especially valuable.

Am markers are identified by passive hemagglutination with red cells coated with the allotype by the chromium chloride method.

Today at least 23 specificities are recognized in the Gm system and are designated by Gm1 through Gm25. The localization of these specificities in the Fc or Fd fragments of the IgG molecule, in subclasses IgG1, IgG2, and IgG3 is given in Table 4.8. No allotype has been so far identified in IgG4.

The system Am comprises only two allotypic specificities located in the Fc fragment of IgA2. As to Km allotypes, they localize in kappa chains of any immunoglobulin class.

Table 4.8. Distribution of Gm allotypes in human IgG

IgG subclass	Fc fragment	Fd fragment
IgG1	Gm 1, 2, 7, 18, 20, 22. ISF	(3=4), 17[a]
IgG2	Gm 8, 9, 23	
IgG3	Gm (5=12), 6, (10=13) 11, 12, 14, 15, 16, 21, 25	

[a] The pairs 3–4, 5–12, and 10–13 represents identical allotypes

Idiotypes. In addition to the allotypes, Oudin demonstrated that specific individual determinants (idiotypes) exist in the rabbit. While the allotypes are encountered in normal immunoglobulins and in certain groups of individuals, the specificities termed idiotypes can only be demonstrated in the antibodies of certain individuals, as evidenced in experiments with inbred strains of mice. The idiotypic specificities persist even after repeated absorption with immunoglobulins of the same subclass and allotype, appearing thus to have an unique relation to the hypervariable sequences and to the quaternary structure of the combining site. For example, the ability of the isomaltose series of oligosaccharides to inhibit precipitation by dextran parallels closely their capacity to inhibit the reaction of antidextran with its anti-idiotypic antibody.

To produce anti-idiotypic antibodies rabbits are immunized with antibodies to a particular antigen raised in another rabbit (donor). If the donor is genetically identical to the anti-idiotype producer rabbit, the response will be restricted to the structure of the antibody combining site. If, however, the two rabbits are genetically dissimilar, the anti-idiotypic serum has to be thoroughly absorbed with the immunoglobulins of the donor to render it specific to the idiotypic determinant.

Electron-Microscopic Studies of the Antibody

Valentine and Green verified that the soluble complexes formed by rabbit IgG from antidinitrophenyl (DNP) with di-DNP-octamethylendiamine [DNP-NH-(CH$_2$)$_8$-NH-DNP], when examined under the electron microscope, exhibit predominantly triangular or rhomboidal designs with lateral extensions at their corners (see Fig. 7.21). The length of the sides of these geometric figures is about 120 Å, i.e., twice the length of the Fab fragment (the antigen is disregarded because of its extremely small size and its position within a cavity of the antibody). The lateral extensions are interpreted as Fc fragments: They do not appear in antigen-antibody complexes digested by pepsin. The flexibility provided by the hinge region permits considerable variation in the angle between the two Fab fragments connected to the same Fc fragment, permitting the formation of trimers, tetramers, and pentamers.

IgM antibodies, because of their relatively large dimensions, can be observed directly with the electron microscope in purified and concentrated preparations. They appear in the form of stars with a central "wheel" of 100 Å and five lateral "arms" of 125 Å. After reduction and alkylation, the star-shaped structure disappears. Excellent electron photomicrographs have been obtained of IgM antibodies attached to viral particles (phages, polio viruses) or to the surfaces of erythrocytes.

Antibody Formation at the Gene Level

Antibodies are proteins with specific binding sites for any antigens, be they cells, bacteria, viruses, proteins, carbohydrates, in fact, almost all natural substances, provided they are macromolecules (see Chap. 3), and they are foreign or "non self" to the organism (see Chaps. 6, 10, and 13).

Where does the information for the millions of antibodies which one individual can synthesize come from? This question has been fundamental since the foundation of modern immunology. The first theory proposed for the formation of antibodies was the "side-chain" theory (1900) by Paul Ehrlich. He developed the idea that antibodies are preformed constituents of the cell surface which multiply under the influence of the antigen and are finally secreted into the blood plasma. This predetermination hypothesis was practically the only theory of antibody formation until the 1930s. Under the influence of the work of Landsteiner, who demonstrated that antibodies can arise even against antigens which normally do not exist in nature, an "instructive theory" became more and more accepted; according to this theory, the antigens act as a mold, or template, at some stage of the antibody formation. This theory reigned for about 25 years until Burnet, inspired by the ideas of Jerne (1955), formulated a new selection theory – the "clonal selection" theory – the essentials of which can be summarized thus: (1) mesenchymal cells, precursors of the cells that form antibodies, are made up of innumerable clones; (2) the clones capable of reacting with "self" components are eliminated (or suppressed) in the prenatal period; (3) the not-eliminated (or suppressed) clones specific for foreign substances react with the antigen fitting to the receptor, which leads to the proliferation of the clone (Fig. 4.5).

According to the theory of clonal selection, the sequence of the amino acids in antibodies of different specificities would be determined by the sequence of the nucleotides in the messenger RNA of the respective clone, which accordingly could form antibodies of a single specificity only. Experiments with isolated cells from animals immunized against three or four antigens have effectively shown that, indeed, single cells were capable of producing antibodies of only a single specificity (see p. 77).

The greatest problem for proponents of the clonal selection theory (as for any other previously formulated theory about antibody formation) was how to explain the extreme diversity of immunologically competent cells, i.e., the generation of diversity (see below).

Organization of Immunoglobulin Genes and Their Expression

The capacity of the organism to form antibodies with a practically unlimited number of specificities presupposes the existence of a similarly unrestricted mechanism for the recognition of the respective immunogen. The differentiation of the lymphoid cells that leads to immunologic competence must at the same time generate a mechanism through which each immunologically competent cell becomes capable, when stimulated by the antigen, of forming immunoglobulins of the corresponding specificity.

There is evidence that this mechanism of diversification – which operates not only in relation to specificity of the combining site of the antibody – is genetically controlled. As a matter of fact, the genetic mechanism of diversification was postulatd in relation to the L and H subgroup chains as soon as sequence studies of myeloma globulins and Bence Jones proteins indicated the existence of a constant and a variable region in both chains, long before it became clear how these mechanisms accounted for the diversity of antigen-binding sites. It was then hypothesized that separate genes are responsible for the coding of the V and C regions and that by a process of translocation these genes unit to build a cistron[3] that transcribed a single m-RNA coding for the amino acid sequence of the entire polypeptide chain. DNA cloning and sequence studies have now confirmed this hypothesis (see below).

3 "Cistron" is defined as functional unit made from different structural genes, which codes for the entire amino-acid sequence of a polypeptide chain

Table 4.9. System for genes important in coding for human immunoglobulin

Translocon	V subgroup gene	C gene
κ	V_κ I–III	C_κ
λ	V_λ I–V	C_λ Kern$^-$ O_{z+}
		C_λ Kern$^+$ O_{z-}
		C_λ Kern$^-$ O_{z-}
H	V_H I–IV	C_γ 1–4
		C_χ 1, 2
		C_μ
		C_δ
		C_ε

Table 4.10. Chromosomal location of immunoglobulin genes

Genes	Human chromosomes	Mouse
$V_\kappa C_\kappa$	2	6
$V_\lambda C_\lambda$	22	16
$V_H C_H$	14	12

The cistrons for the H chains of human IgG, IgM, IgD, IgA, and IgE are represented by $C_\gamma V_H$, $C_\mu V_H$, $C_\delta V_H$, $C_\alpha V_H$, and $C_\varepsilon V_H$; the cistrons for the kappa and lambda chains are termed $C_\kappa V_\kappa$ and $C_\lambda V_\lambda$, respectively. The "translocon" areas are not linked, they are on separate chromosomes (Table 4.10).

Individual B cells are monospecific – i.e., they make antibodies with only one type of H chain, one type of L chain and one single combining site. Since B lymphocytes, like any other somatic cell, are diploid, they must possess three pairs (one of each parent) of gene pools corresponding to the H, κ, and λ chains. There is evidence that successive choices are made along the development of the B cell, starting with the choice of H from one of the parents, and followed by the choice of κ or λ. This choice of either a maternal or a paternal allele is called *allelic exclusion*. In order to maintain monospecificity B cells cannot make κ and λ chains, otherwise the two chains having almost always different V regions would create more than on kind of antigen-binding site.

The first direct demonstration of a DNA rearrangement (translocation) during B-cell development was given by Hozumi and Tonegawa (1976) by experiments in which DNA extracted from mouse embryonic cells unable to make antibodies was compared with DNA from mouse myeloma cells encoding a specific myeloma λ chain. The two kinds of DNA were digested with a restriction nuclease and electrophoretically separated fragments carrying the V and C sequences were hybridized to a radioactive DNA sequence obtained by copying the V-region sequence of m-RNA molecules specifying the specific myeloma λ chain. Autoradiography showed that the V and C genes were on the same fragment in the case of myeloma cell DNA but in separate fragments in the DNA extracted from the embryo or from a different myeoloma tumor making a different light chain.

Lambda Chain Translocon. In contrast to the more complex κ and H systems (see below), the mouse lambda translocon contains only one or very few germline V genes separated from the C gene by a rather large DNA segment of about 4.5 kilobase (kb) pairs and preceded by a leader sequence (L). As shown by Tonegawa et al. in 1978, the mouse embryo V_{λ} gene, instead of coding for all 108 amino acids of the polypep-

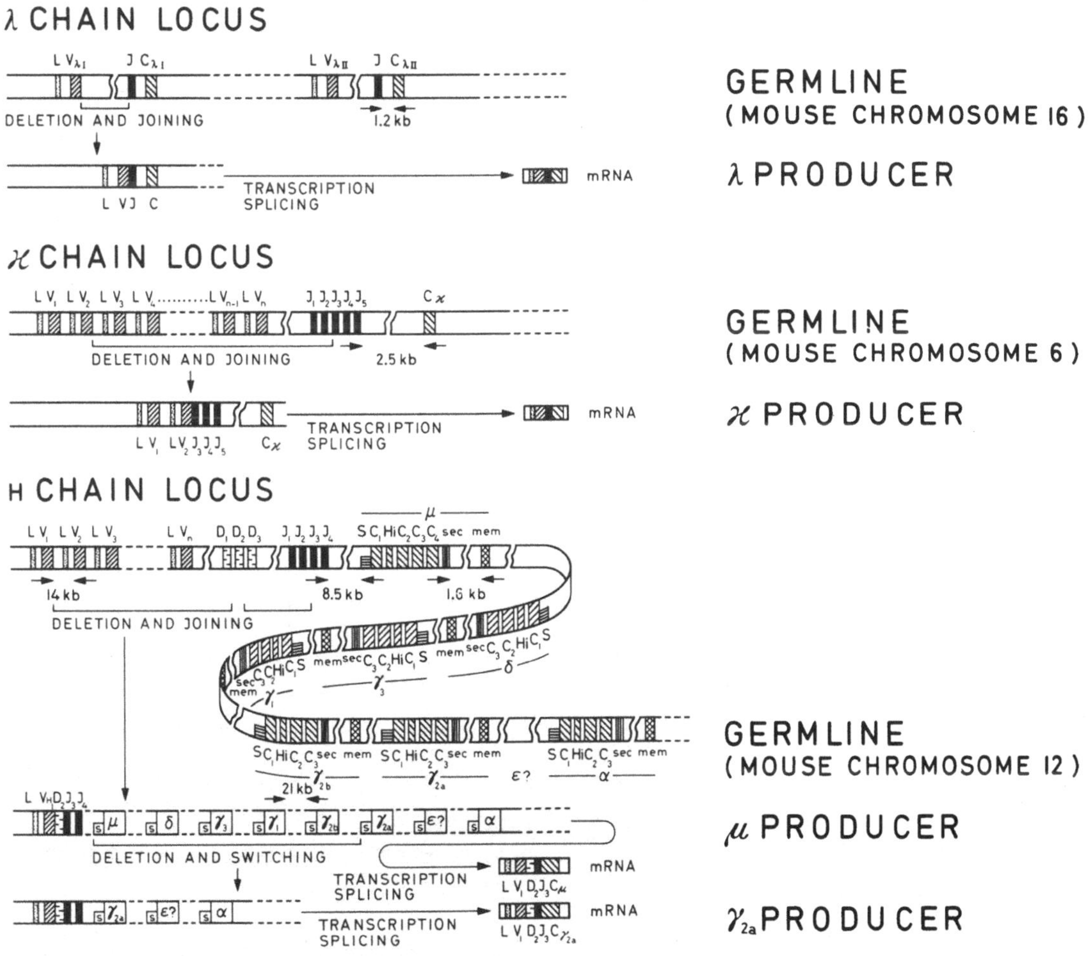

Fig. 4.22. Formation of active immunoglobulin genes from germline DNA by somatic recombination and deletion

tide chain, it encodes only the 95 N-terminal amino acids; the remaining 13 (96–108) are encoded by a separate region, called the joining (J) region, about 1.2 kb pairs "upstream" from the C region.

It is reasonable to suppose that the scarcity of lambda chains (5%) among mouse immunoglobulins is related to the very small number of V_λ genes.

Kappa Chain Translocon. There is strong evidence from V_κ hybridization experiments and cloning of V_κ genes that there are up to 600 (or more) V_κ genes. It appears that there are several distinct subsets of V_κ, with V_κ genes more similar within subsets than between them; whether or not the gene subsets correspond to the subgroups defined from N-terminal amino acid sequences of polypeptides remains to be seen. The available data indicate that each V_κ gene is separated from the next by an intervening noncoding DNA sequence (intron) of about 14 kb pairs. Each V_κ gene is also preceded by a leader (L) sequence.

Cloning and subsequent sequencing of segments of embryonic DNA which included the kappa C gene and 4.5 kb pairs upstream from the C gene revealed five J segments. The J segments are in a cluster, separated from each other by about 300 base pairs; the nearest to the C gene is about 2.5 kb from it. Of the five J segments, examples of four can be found in known kappa protein sequences; the J_3 sequence is not found in any known protein.

V-C Joining. During lymphocyte maturation, DNA undergoes somatic rearrangement (translocation) which brings the V gene but leaves the J-C intervening sequence intact (Fig. 4.22). Findings on nuclear precursor RNA suggest that the entire V-J-C genomic sequence is transcribed and the intervening sequences excised and deleted from the nuclear precursor RNA by RNA splicing, leaving a messenger RNA (mRNA) in which V, J, and C are continuous. The intervening sequence within the leader peptide sequence preceding the V re-

gion is also removed by splicing. The exact mechanism of VJ recombination is not yet clear. However, DNA sequence analysis revealed that it involves deletion of the introns, and that two short conserved sequences 5' to each germline J_κ gene are inverse complements of sequences 3' to germline V_κ genes close to the point of recombination. These structures are thought to be recognized by joining enzymes.

Apparently, in the case of the kappa genes, any V_κ can reassort with any of the J segments (except maybe J_3); this increases the variability of the variable region at least fourfold since the J segment encodes part of the third hypervariable region of the light chain (see p. 91, Fig. 4.15). Furthermore, additional variation is introduced into the first J_κ codon (amino-acid residue 96): by adjusting the point of recombination within the three nucleotides which follow the V coding sequence and the three nucleotides of residue 96 in the five J segments, one can generate all residue 96 amino acids known in mouse myeloma kappa proteins. This is exemplified by the myeloma MOPC-41 V segment and J_1:

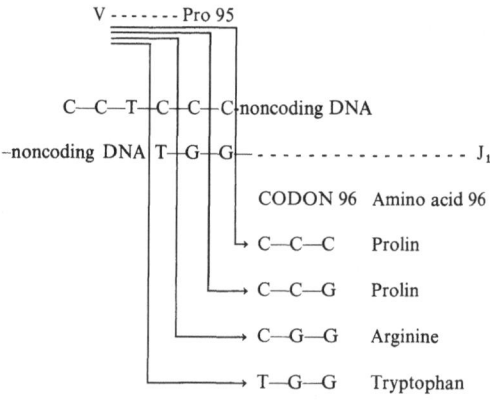

Since amino acid residue 96 is near or even at the antigen combining site, it is safe to assume that, in some cases at least, diversity generated by V-J joining can alter the antigen binding properties of immunoglobulins.

H Chain Translocon. The translocon for the H chains harbors the V_H as well as the C_H

genes of all immunoglobulin classes and subclasses, although the localization of C_ε relative to the other C genes is not known. Here too, cloning of V_H genes lends strong support to the idea that there are at least 400 V_H genes arranged in tandem arrays, and again grouped into subsets; the V_H are separated by noncoding sequences of at least 14 kb, and preceded by a leader sequence. Comparison between the DNA sequence of a germline V_H gene and the corresponding rearranged sequence expressed in a myeloma has shown that the germline V_H segment ends at the sequence coding for the third hypervariable region before the end of the expressed V_H sequence. This suggested that the missing sequence should be found in J segments near the C_μ gene, which is first expressed during B-cell ontogeny. Indeed, the J segments were found about 8 kb upstream from C_μ, although they did not account for all of the third hypervariable region. This suggested that the missing residues are separately encoded in yet another set of genes termed D segments (or diversity). How many D segments exist is not known, but there are at least three. At least four J_H segments have been identified. Whether or not heavy chain diversity is fully accounted for by random combination of V, D, and J segments and codon variation at the joins of these segments $(>400\ V_H \times 3\ D \times 4\ J_H = >4,800)$ is controversial. Further diversity may arise from point mutations at the other two hypervariable regions during the differentiation of B lymphocytes, although one might also expect separate sets of sequences for these two regions.

The heavy chain constant region genes are aligned in the order μ (C_1, hinge, C_2, C_3, C_4), δ, γ_3, γ_1, γ_{2b}, γ_{2a}, ε, and α – for C_ε, see above –, C_μ being the first about 8.3 kb downstream from J_4. Each C_1 gene is preceded by a small sequence (S) involved in the switching mechanism (see below), and each gene for the terminal C domain is followed by two sequences separated by about 1.6 kb, the one coding for a piece of polypeptide typical of secreted proteins, and the

other typical of membrane immunoglobulins.

Heavy Chain Switches. Unlike the light chains, for which there is only one C-region gene for each set of V regions, each heavy-chain V gene (V_H gene) may be expressed with any of eight different heavy-chain constant genes which define the different classes of immunoglobulin molecules. All V_H regions are first expressed with C_μ, but upon differentiation of lymphocytes into plasma cells the same V_H region may associate with any of the other C genes (heavy-chain class switch). Several hypotheses have been proposed to explain the mechanism of this switch, but the deletion model of Honjo and Kataoka now seems to be the most likely explanation, as evidenced by hybridization kinetics and gene counting with cloned probes. These investigations suggest that V-D-J first alignes with S-C_μ and then the intervening sequence is deleted; recombination between a switch site within the J-S element and one within the 5' flanking sequence of another C_H gene relocates the active V-D-J gene, together with much of the J-S element, to a site near the C_H gene to be expressed next. It is not known whether a clone can switch more than once. The deletion mechanism for V/J joining and C_H switching has strong implications for immunoglobulin expression as it is an irreversible process. Therefore, the order of C_H gene expression becomes tied to the linear gene order.

In general, there is no simultaneous expression of two types of immunoglobulins, with the exception of IgM and IgD. In order to explain this in accordance with the deletion mechanism, one may expect to find that C_μ and C_δ are jointly transcribed and spliced in two different ways to generate μ and δ mRNAs with the same V_H region. The problem of allelic exclusion, i.e., that only the genes of one chromosome are expressed, cannot be explained yet.

The question of the generation of membrane-bound and secreted immunoglobulins which differ in the end portion of their terminal C domain has been resolved recently by showing that two chemically and functionally distinct mRNAs can be derived from a single C gene, apparently by alternative modes of RNA splicing.

Generation of Diversity. Some years ago, the problem of antibody diversity was so obscure that it was put in "immunotheological" terms, by postulating that once during evolution a segment of DNA emerged that provided positive or negative signals to the V_L and V_H genes. This DNA segment was called "Generator of diversity" and, because it acted in an entirely unscrutable way, the abbreviation G.O.D. was considered appropriate for it.

Valuable theoretical contributions such as Jerne's network theory (see below) and Kabat's framework hypothesis (see p. 91) have certainly helped to elucidate the ways of GOD, but these began really to be unveiled thanks to the work of Suzuma Tonegawa and his collaborators on the somatic reorganization of immunoglobulin genes in the course of B lymphocyte differentiation.

Specific cleavage of DNA by restriction nucleases followed by nucleic acid hybridization makes it possible to identify specific sequences by their ability to bind a complementary nucleic acid sequence and the construction of restriction maps that show the location of each DNA cutting with its neighbours. Studies of this kind led to the establishment of the first nucleotide sequence of an immunoglobulin gene.

As indicated before, there are at least 600 V_κ and 4 J_κ combinations which can be associated with a minimum of 4,800 V_H combinations, resulting in more than 1.15×10^7 combining sites. By taking into account the somatic mutations which have been shown to occur in and around V-region genes the number of antigen-binding sites may be increased by a factor of 10–100.

In conclusion, the information for the antibody specificity is genetically determined and encoded in several hundreds of V genes which are linked to but separated from single C genes in the germline and stem cells. When multipotent stem cells possessing all genetic information for the synthesis of all specific anttibodies divide and differentiate, translocation and fusion of V and C genes occurs. Probably, all V genes have an equal chance of fusing with their corresponding C gene. This differentiation process is antigen-in dependent and irreversible, an "inner" selection process which results in a differentiated and committed "virgin" B cell with a newly recombined DNA and the synthesis of one type of antibody with one specificity which is incorporated as receptor into the cell membrane (see Fig. 4.5; p. 78). There are as many different "virgin" B cell clones as there are antibody structures.

From the enormous number of different possibilities, the antigen selects that particular B cell which carries the corresponding receptor ("outer", clonal selection). The contact of the antigen with the receptor stimulates this cell; proliferation then leads to the formation of a clone of cells bearing the same determinant (clonal expansion). Finally, part of the B cells are transformed into plasma cells, which no longer have receptors but secrete antibodies. Some of the B cells undergo persistent multiplication and develop to "memory cells" which, at a second contact with the antigen, give rise to a stronger and faster immune reaction.

Regulation of Antibody Formation

The production of antibodies is modulated and regulated by the interaction of a series of factors associated with the immunizing antigen, the immunized organism, and the immune system itself.

Factors Relating to the Antigen

The nature of the antigen, its dosage, and the manner of administration, have a definite influence on the formation of antibodies, not only in connection with the quantity and type of the immunoglobulin produced, but also in respect to its affinity for the binding.

Influence of the Antigen on the Magnitude of the Immune Response. Under standardized experimental conditions, it is possible to determine the relative immunologic potency of different antigens. If one uses as a reference antigen a single 100 pμg dose of bovine serum albumin (BSA) that produces a threshold immunogenic effect and compares it to the minimum doses necessary to achieve the same effect with other antigens, one sees that 10 μg bovine gamma globulin, 10^{-2} μg polymerized flagellin, and 10^{-9} μg Salmonella "O" antigen, respectively, have immunogenic potencies that are 10, 10^4, and 10^{11} times greater than that of BSA.

The principal parameters to which one might attribute these differences are molecular size, host capacity of the lymphoid system, and phylogenetic distance between the origin of the antigenic material and the reacting organism.

Molecular Size. Molecules below 10,000 daltons, such as glucagon (mol.wt. 2,500), insulin (mol.wt. 5,700), and protamines and histones (mol.wt. 6,000) are weakly immunogenic. The smallest known immunogen is hepta-L lysine coupled by its α-amino group to a dinitrophenyl (DNP) group. Similar compounds with fewer than seven lysine residues are not immunogenic. At above 10,000 daltons, the protein molecules begin to exhibit distinct immunogenic activity that increases with the rise in molecular weight (Table 4.11).

Polysaccharides are less potent immunogens than are proteins unless polymerized to higher molecular weights. A typical example is dextran: in its native polydispersed form, with a molecular weight of tens of millions of daltons, dextran possesses immunogenic power about 3.5 times greater than that of clinical dextran (mol.wt. $75,000 \pm 25,000$ daltons). Preparations degraded by mild acid hydrolysis that contain molecules from 35,000 to 50,000

Table 4.11. Approximate molecular weight of protein antigens

Protein	Molecular weight
Ribonuclease	14,000
Myoglobin	17,000
TMV peptide[a]	17,000
Crotoxin[b]	30,000
Flagellin[c]	40,000
Ovalbumin	45,000
Diphtheria toxin	62,000
Serum albumin	69,000
γ-Globulin (IgG)	160,000
Octopus hemocyanin	2,800,000

[a] Tobacco mosaic virus protein
[b] Primary component of the Brasilian rattlesnake poison
[c] Monomeric form

daltons were only weakly immunogenic. When the molecular weight fell below 10,000 daltons, the immunogenic capacity was totally abolished.

Similarly, the menigococcic A and C polysaccharides used in prophylaxis of meningococcic meningitis only exhibit immunogenic activity when polymerized to a molecular weight of 150,000 daltons or more.

Ability to Lodge in the Lymphoid Organs. The capacity of localize in strategic regions of the lymphoid organs where they could be recognized by the immunocompetent lymphocytes, also constitutes an important characteristic of antigens. Factors favoring this localization are, for example, the particulate nature of the antigen (erythrocytes, bacteria, viruses, grains of pollen, etc.), and the existence in the organism of antibodies arising from previous immunization with the same antigen or with cross-reacting antigens.

Phylogenic Distance. Finally, the phylogenic distance between the antigen and the constituents of the immunized organism – or the degree of foreignness – is a characteristic with direct bearing on the antigen's immunogenicity. An organism is immunologically tolerant to its own constituents and, by extension, to those that are similar to them. For this reason, antigenic variants of the constituents of the organism that are present in different individuals of the same species (isoantigenic variations) are recognized as "self" and usually exercise only weak antigenic activity. An exception should be made only for certain antigens that control the transplantation of tissues (transplantation antigens) such as those determined by the *H-2* locus in mice, or by the HLA region in man (cf. Chap. 6).

Influence of the Antigen on the Type of Immune Response. Aside from influencing the magnitude of the immune response, the antigen also determines the type of the response (cellular or humoral), and the type of immunoglobulin produced. Although the majority of antigens possess determinants capable of interacting with both T and B lymphocytes, certain antigens activate almost exclusively one or the other of these types of cells. Accordingly, pneumococcic polysaccharides stimulate only B lymphocytes, and consequently induce the formation of antibodies and the development of anaphylactic reaction of the immediate type, but not delayed-type hypersensitivity reactions. Conversely, oxasolone stimulates only T lymphocytes, inducing delayed hypersensitivity but not the formation of antibodies.

When referring to the preferential production of immunoglobulins, a discussion of the problem of successive synthesis of the immunoglobulins IgM and IgG is pertinent. Although the simultaneous presence of IgM and IgG in the same plasma cell is possible and can be shown by immunofluorescense, plasma cells usually do not synthesize the two concomtantly. From all indications, during immunization, a signal derived from T helper cells diverts the process of synthesis from the production of IgM to that of IgG. The particulate antigens, such as erythrocytes, trypanosomes (not Trypanosoma cruzi), or the plasmodia of malaria, induce preferentially

the synthesis of IgM, resulting in prolonged 19-S-antibody production. The antigens from helminths or from pollens, on the other hand, selectively stimulate the production of IgE. In respiratory virus infections, IgA antibodies are produced that appear in appreciable concentrations in the mucus in which they are secreted, but not in the blood.

Other examples suggestive of the influences of the antigen in relation to the type of immunoglobulin produced are the following: (1) The guinea pig, when immunized with the majority of antigens, produces varying quantities of IgG_1 and IgG_2, depending upon the adjuvant utilized and the manner of immunization. However, when immunized with the lipopolysaccharide of Escherichia coli, it produces only IgG_2. (2) Also in the guinea pig, the anti-DNP antibodies, which appear late in the course of immunization, carry only χ chains. (3) In guinea pigs, the antibodies against dextran and against teichoic acid belong predominantly to the IgG_2 subclass.

The interpretation of these facts remains problematic; yet the evidence suggests that certain antigens might selectively stimulate different subpopulations of lymphocytes involved in the syntheses of the different types of chains, from which the molecules of the different classes and subclasses of immunoglobulins are integrated.

Influence of the Antigen Dose on the Specificity and Affinity of Antibodies. Antisera produced after long periods of immunization contain a heterogeneous population of antibodies having specificities directed towards different antigenic determinants, and also having different affinities. These facts can be interpreted as a consequence of the simultaneous stimulation of distinct lymphocyte clones that correspond to different antigenic determinants – the later possessing varying degrees of affinity.

This problem can be analyzed with greater clarity by considering the production of antibodies against a small dose of one monovalent immunogen, e.g., a hapten conjugate: Such an experiment shows that the antibodies formed constitute a relatively homogeneous population of immunoglobulins of high affinity ("perfect fit"), even though the quantity of antibody produced may be small. However, if we were to inject repeated doses of the same antigen over a long period of immunization, the affinity mediated by the antibodies, measured in terms of the occupation of 50%, of the combining sites, would decline considerably. In complex antigens, e.g., large molecules carrying many antigenic determinants, the phenomenon is masked by the multiple uniting bridges provided by the antibodies directed against each determinant, which results in the formation of antigen-antibody (Ag-Ab) complexes that dissociate only with difficulty.

A mechanism of regulation exists, however, that permits the formation of antibodies of high affinity even after repeated antigenic stimulation. As immunization runs its course, the antigen, in addition to suffering excretion and metabolic elimination; this occurs as the same antibodies formed in response to the antigen compete with the antigen in relation to the lymphocyte receptors. Because the quantity of antigen diminishes considerably, there is a concomitant increase in the availability of lymphocytes with high-affinity receptors – thus reestablishing conditions conducive to the formation of antibodies of heightened affinity. This mechanism is sometimes referred to as "the maturation of the immune response."

Factors Relating to the Organism

Of special note are age, nutritional state, and genetic factors.

Age. Generally speaking, young animals immunize poorly. This may be attributed to the immunologic incompetence of the lymphoid tissues not yet sufficiently differentiated, or it might be attributed to a deficiency in those mechanisms for capture and processing of antigens at the level of the dendritic and macrpohage cells of the sec-

ondary lymphoid organs – particularly of the spleen and the lymph nodes (cf. Chaps. 2 and 11).

Highly elucidating results in relation to the ontogeny of immunologically competent cells were obtained in sheep fetuses that had been immunized in utero. In this animal species, whose gestation period is 150 days, immunization of the fetus at 40 days only elicited production of antibodies against phages (detectable in minimum quantities). At 80 days, the animals began to demonstrate the capacity for rejecting allografts; and at 120 days, there was formation of antibodies against ovalbumin. For certain antigens, however, such as the flagellar antigen Salmonella typhi, antibodies were formed only when the immunization was performed after birth (cf. Chap. 1 and Fig. 1.18).

Similar observations were made in human-newborns, including premature individuals, in whom immunization even during the first day of extrauterine life provoked the formation of antibodies against the flagellar antigen S. typhi, but not against the flagellar antigens S. paratyphi A and B. The antibody produced was of the 19-S type, so as to exclude passive maternal transmission, which is found only with 7-S antibodies. Prophylactic immunization of infants is common within the first trimester of life (see Chap. 11).

Nutritional State. Clinical and experimental observations indicate that even in cases of grave nutritional deficiency, the production of immunoglobulins does not diminish. This has been verified, for example, in Kwashiorkor, a syndrome observed in children with deficiencies in protein and certain amino acids, particularly methionine. Such children can have extremely low levels of albumin in their serum yet have normal or even augmented levels of immunoglobulins. From all indications, the diminished resistance to infections associated with nutritional deficiencies depends upon biochemical processes that affect nonspecific defense mechanism, but not the specific mechanisms involved in the synthesis of immuno-globulins.

Genetic Factors. Hereditary characteristics can significantly affect the production of antibodies, as demonstrated experimentally in many animals, and as observed naturally in man (see Chaps. 6 and 13). In man, the influence of heredity can be exemplified by a condition known as atopy – by the incidence of certain allergic ailments due to a state of immediate hypersensitivity to inhalable antigens, foods, etc., associated with a particular class of immunoglobulins (see Chap. 9).

Experimental evidence accumulated over the last two decades clearly demonstrates that the production of antibodies (but also the generation of specific effector cells), or in other words, the recognition of antigens, depends upon genetic factors (see Chap. 6). The first evidence derived from experiments by Benacerraf in guinea pigs with polylysine as antigen (*PLL* gene); his observations were extended by McDevitt using another synthetic polypeptide as antigen in the mouse (*Ir-gene*). This genetic control of antigen recognition is regulated by the genes and their products of the major histocompatibility complex (*MHC*), and will be described in detail in Chap. 6.

Factors Inherent to the Immune System

Immunologic Memory. Previous immunologic stimulations is without doubt among the most relevant factors in determining the magnitude and speed of the immune response. As a consequence of previous immunization, the number of cells in the lymphoid system capable of being stimulated by the antigen (memory cells) increases. Thus the secondary response sets in with greater rapidity and intensity, even in response to weaker concentrations of antigen. This phenomenon constitutes the basis for the "booster" immunization utilized routinely in immunoprophylaxis of toxic-infectious illnesses (cf. Tables 11.19 and 11.20).

Because memory cells include lymphocytes with considerable longevity (more than 1 year in the rat and more than 10 years in man), immunologic memory is frequently demonstrated after long periods of time.

With regard to specificity, immunologic memory can manifest itself among macromolecules that are carriers of common antigenic determinants or among immunogens of similar configurations. In the first case, antibodies are produced only in relation to the common determinants, and, consequently, intensity of production varies according to the number of these determinants; the secondary response elicited by the determinants of similar configuration can result in the formation of antibodies against the original antigenic stimulus that is more intense than against the antigen used in the second immunization.

In antigen conjugates (see Chap. 3), immunologic memory manifests itself not merely against the hapten, but also against certain carrier-protein determinants that otherwise are not necessarily continuous with the implantation point of the hapten.

Feedback Control of Antibody Synthesis. As in numerous other biochemical processes, the synthesis of antibodies is inhibited by the products of its own reaction – the antibodies themselves. This phenomenon, called "feed-back inhibition," is absolutely specific and can be reproduced easily by passive immunization with the homologous antibody or its $F(ab)_2$ fragment (or Fab). Evidently, there is competition for the antigen between the combining site of the antibody and the specific receptor on the lymphocyte surface. The covering of the antigenic determinants by the homologous antibody prevents further recognition of the antigen as "non-self," a condition essential to the formation of antibodies.

IgM antibodies are capable only of inhibiting the synthesis of IgM, whereas IgG antibodies suppress the production of IgM as well as that of IgG. Antibodies of low affinity are incapable of inhibiting the synthesis of antibodies of high affinity because they do not compete efficiently with the lymphocyte receptors.

Theobald Smith demonstrated in 1909 in studies of the immunization of guinea pigs with mixtures of diphtheria toxin and antitoxin that antigen-antibody complexes with an excess of antibody have an inhibitory action; however, when there is an excess of antigen the immune response can even be enhanced by the adjuvant effect (phagocytosis of the complex and processing of the antigen). We shall see later that inhibition by feedback is utilized with success in the immunoprophylaxis of erythroblastosis fetalis (see Chap. 11).

Idiotypic Network Interaction. Feedback inhibition as just described is a major expression of a sophisticated active regulatory system of homeostasis involving many more elements. We are still at the beginning in our understanding of this regulatory system. Before we briefly outline the essentials of the current concepts of immune regulation, we shall introduce the necessary terminology and the already known elements.

An antigenic determinant is called *epitope*; this is a certain structural patch on an antigen molecule that can be recognized with various degree of precision by complementary patterns of antibody combining sites (*paratopes*). Antibody molecules themselves present epitopes to complementary paratopes. Epitopes of antibodies located at the constant parts of framework are called allotypes, those formed by the variable part are called idiotypes (see p. 97). Each single idiotypic epitope is called and *idiotope*. An idiotype then denotes a certain set of idiotopes representing the "internal image" of the antigen-binding site.

The demonstration that animals can be stimulated to make antibodies to the idiotopes of antibody molecules produced by other animals of the same species or strain indicates that a given animal possesses available paratopes that can recognize any idiotope occurring in the species, i.e., within the immune system of any given individual, any iditope can be recognized by a set of paratopes, and any paratope can recognize a set of idiotopes.

Thus, the immune system is an enormous and complex network of paratopes and idiotopes, and since antibody molecules occur both free and as receptor molecules on B and T lymphocytes, this network intertwines cells and molecules.

An important property of antigen-sensitive lymphocytes is their ability to respond either positively or negatively to a recognition signal, i.e., in this network, there are provisions for on/off switches; the suppression of an immune response by anti-idiotype antibodies has first been shown by Köhler and Cosenza, and Nisonoff.

Antibody Idiotopic Network. With these elements in hand, in 1974 K. N. Jerne proposed a network theory for the regulation of the immune response (Fig. 4.23). In this, a set of antibodies (Ab_1) [4] recognizes an epitope A of an antigen. The same set of antibodies Ab_1 will also recognize idiotopes present in paratopes of many antibodies Ab_2 within the immune system (internal image of epitope A). On the other hand, the paratopes of the antibodies Ab_1 consist of sets of idiotopes recognized by other sets of antibodies, Ab_3 (anti-idiotope antibodies). Since, for the sets of antibodies Ab_2 and Ab_3, and for all others, the same interconnections exist, this is an open-ended (infinite) network; however, as the effects of distal regulatory interactions will have to be transmitted along a chain, losses of definition can be expected at each step, resulting in a finite network. It is obvious that Ab_3 has suppressive, and that A and Ab_2 have stimulatory, properties with respect to Ab_1.

On the basis of these idiotopic interactions several properties of the immune response can be accounted for: Activation of specific antibody responses and their regulation; the elimination by the antigen of antibodies

---

4 Paratopes of antibodies recognizing a particular epitope need not be identical; also, idiotopes recognized by certain paratopes may belong to different paratopes

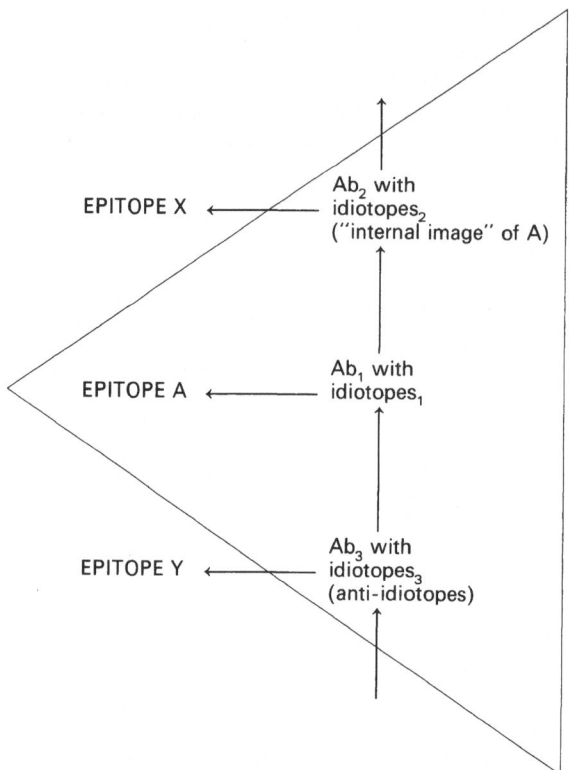

Fig. 4.23. Triad of epitopic and idiotopic antibodies forming an idiotopic network according to Jerne's theory. Ab_1 recognizes A, but also idiotopes on paratopes of a set of antibodies Ab_2 ("internal image" to A), which by themselves recognize epitope X, and idiotopes on still another set of antibodies. Idiotopes present in paratopes of the Ab_1 set are recognized, in turn, by paratopes of a set of antibodies Ab_3 (anti-idiotopic antibodies), themselves specific for epitopes Y unrelated to A. Again, idiotopes present in paratopes of these antibodies will serve as "internal image" for still other sets of antibodies, and so on. The triangle contains the elements of the basic triad

of set Ab_1 removes their inhibitory effect on the "internal image" (Ab_2) as well as their stimulatory effect on the anti-idiotopic set (Ab_3). Both effects favor an escape from suppression of cells of set Ab_1. On the other hand, the enhancement of set Ab_1 will tend to reverse these effects. The network attempts to restore its equilibrium.

Feedback inhibition of passively administered 7 S antibodies as described above removes the stimulatory effect of antigen A before antigen epitope A can activate the Ab_1 set, but beyond that may also suppress the set of internal-image antibodies, Ab_2, which diminishes the stimulatory effect for the Ab_1 set.

Low-zone tolerance (see Chap. 10) might be induced by an imbalance of activation: Low amounts of epitope A stimulate few Ab_1 producing cells; after proliferation the stimulation of the anti-idiotypic antibody set Ab_3 becomes dominant. In addition, unsaturated Ab-Ag complexes may provide a stronger stimulus to the Ab_3 set.

By now, the idiotypic network theory is widely accepted in its basic form. When Jerne proposed this theory, antibody molecules had been the best known part of the immune system; it laid, therefore, the groundwork for the theory. The firm existence and importance of various other parameters in this regulatory system such as helper and suppressor T cells have become clear only since then.

Control of Antibody Formation by Regulatory Cell Circuits. The development of T and B lymphocytes from precursors to effector cells follows similar differentiation patterns.

Initially, virgin precursor cells already committed with respect to effector function (see Chap. 2) and antigenic specificity (see p. 78) arise in the absence of antigen. Antigenic exposure triggers virgin precursors to differentiate to memory and effector cells. These antigen-dependent differentiation steps require help from (and are therefore regulated by) specific populations of T helper cells (THC$_1$). The recruitment of THC$_1$, in turn, is regulated by T suppressor cell populations (TSC$_1$) capable of specifically depleting individual THC$_1$. Recently, Cantor, Gershon and their colleagues demonstrated that the differentiation of TSC$_1$ from precursors to functionally active cells also requires help from T cells (THC$_2$), and these helper cells are distinct from the THC$_1$ which help precursor B cells to differentiate to antibody forming cells (feedback inhibition). It is not unreasonable to expect that the supply of the second population of THC$_2$ is specifically controlled by another suppressor cell population (TSC$_2$), and so on.

The regulation of these regulatory cells is thought to be realized via idiotope recognition whereby THC$_1$ possess paratopes (id$^-$)[5] complementary to be B cell receptor (id$^+$) and the TSC$_2$ paratopes (id$^+$); TSC$_2$ paratopes are, in turn, complementary to idiotopes of the THC$_2$ paratopes (id$^-$); the latter are again complementary to TSC$_1$

ent paratopes, see Chap. 6), whereby T and B cells recognize different epitopes.

On the basis of these data and other considerations, Herzenberg and colleagues extended Jerne's hypothesis and proposed a network of closed circles of regulatory interactions among cells and cell products which they termed circuits (in analogy to closed electronic circuits), capable of being switched between responsive (help), and nonresponsive (suppression) states. The basic or *Core Regulatory Circuits* (CRCs) are constructed by sets of overlapping TSC-THC triads in which TSC is flanked by two different THC's one which helps the TSC and the other which is its target; THC's will be similarly flanked by two different TSC's, one which is helped by the THC and the other which depletes it (for a given TSC, recognition restriction exists that prevents the depletion of its own THCs: a paratope X possessing an idiotope x recognized by a paratope Y$_x$ needs not to be complementary to any of the idiotopes y of paratope Y):

$$
\begin{array}{ccccccc}
\text{THC (2)} & \longrightarrow & \text{TSC (1)} & \dashrightarrow & \text{THC (1)} & \longrightarrow & \text{B} \\
\text{id}^- & & \text{id}^+ & & \text{id}^- & & \text{id}^+
\end{array}
$$

$$
\begin{array}{ccccc}
\text{TSC (2)} & \dashrightarrow & \text{THC (2)} & \longrightarrow & \text{TSC (1)} \\
\text{id}^+ & & \text{id}^- & & \text{id}^+
\end{array}
$$

$$
\begin{array}{ccccc}
\text{THC (3)} & \longrightarrow & \text{TSC (2)} & \dashrightarrow & \text{THC (2)} \\
\text{id}^- & & \text{id}^+ & & \text{id}^-
\end{array}
$$

$$
\begin{array}{ccccccccc}
\text{THC (3)} & \longrightarrow & \text{TSC (2)} & \dashrightarrow & \text{THC (2)} & \longrightarrow & \text{TSC (1)} & \dashrightarrow & \text{THC (1)} & \longrightarrow & \text{B} \\
\text{id}^- & & \text{id}^+ & & \text{id}^- & & \text{id}^+ & & \text{id}^- & & \text{id}^+
\end{array}
$$

CRC

paratopic idiotopes of THC$_1$. Each paratope corresponds to sets of idiotopes. The activation of these cells requires antigen as well (which, however, does not necessarily imply that a given T cell possess two *differ-*

5 Complementary *idiotypes* are referred to as id$^+$ and id$^-$; id should not be read as implying a single variable region structure but rather as a collective group of id$^-$ structures complementary to several id$^+$ V_H. The id structure produced by the B cell is assigned as id$^+$, the anti-id V_H structure of THC that helps the B cell is assigned id$^-$

A solid arrow in this diagram indicates help, a broken arrow suppression. This circuit configuration assumes that a THC that helps an id$^+$ B cell can also help an id$^-$ TSC. Depending upon which THC population is stimulated initially, the CRC tends to lock into either suppression or help configuration: if the THC(1) becomes activated first, it stimulates the TSC(2), which, in turn, suppresses the THC(2); therefore, the TSC(1) remains unactivated and the THC(1) can expand. On the other hand, if the THC(2) becomes activated first, the circuit will drive itself into the suppression configuration and lock there. The configuration of the CRC depends, therefore, ultimately on the regulatory interactions that control THC(1) or THC(2) stimulation. Such regulatory interactions can be constructed as *auxiliary Regulatory Circuits* (ARCs) by inclusion of antibodies and antigens in the circuit.

However, before we go on, three points should be emphysized and kept in mind: (1) None of the different lymphocytes (B, T helper, T suppressor lymphocytes) are stimulated without the help of macrophages which have to present the epitope to lymphocytes with appropriate receptors; when macrophages, epitope, id⁺Ig, and lymphocytes form a complex (bridge), macrophages release a stimulatory factor for the bridged lymphocyte. (2) The same receptor on lymphocytes recognizing id also recognizes an epitope on the antigen, and since THCid⁻ and Bid⁺ as well as TSCid⁺ have different receptors (although complementary), they probably recognize different antigenic epitopes; the epitope recognized by T cells is called "carrier," the epitope recognized by B cells is called hapten. And (3), for one epitope there is not only one but many CRCs; and further, for each antigen with numerous different epitopes, there will be even more CRCs involved in the overall reaction to them. In some of the CRCs, THC(1) will have an id⁻ fitting better to that id⁺ which has high affinity for the epitope than that of THC(2); in others, THC(2) will have the better fitting id⁻.

Under these provisions, ARCs may look as follows: At the beginning of an immune response, macrophages presenting the antigen-epitopes bound to any badly or well fitting id⁺Ig to THCs (and B cells") will stimulate those THCs (and B cells) that are bridged. Different B cells will secrete id⁺Ig with different affinity; soon, the poorly-fitting id⁺Ig will occur freely displaced from the epitope by the better-fitting id⁺Ig. The free id⁺Ig will bind to "its" THCid⁻ and will prevent its further stimu-

lation, i.e., will cause suppression of this THC. Those id⁺Ig fitting best an epitope will prevail and continue via macrophages to stimulate "their" THC; this process will go on, and more and more specific antibodies (with high affinity) will be stimulated until all the antigen is eliminated. Then, even the best-fitting id⁺Ig will occur freely, and stimulation of THCs (and B cells) possessing complementary (best-fitting) id⁻ will cease. Of the many CRCs involved in the response to one particular antigen, only a few may have the constellation THC(1)id⁻ high fit-THC(2)id⁻ low fit, but these will secure a positive immune response overall. In cases where antigens with few repetitive epitopes are used, such constellations may not arise, and the result might be one of no response. There are known parameters, influencing the availability of certain CRC combinations in respect to certain antigen-epitopes, which will be discussed in Chap. 6. There, we shall also discuss how the immune system may distinguish those epitopes against which a positive reaction is desired from those against which, if possible, no reaction should arise, namely the constituents of the individual's own organism.

References

Burnet FM (1959) The clonal selection theory of acquired immunity. Cambridge University Press, Cambridge, England

Cantor H, Gershon RK (1979) Immunological circuits: cellular compositon. Fed Proc 38:2058

Capra JD, Kehoe JM (1975) Hypervariable regions, idiotypy, and the antibody combining site. Adv Immunol 20:1

Cazernave PA (1974) Similar idiotypes in antibody-forming cells synthesizing immunoglobulins without detectable functions. Proc Natl Acad Sci (USA) 71:4500

Dunnick W et al. (1980) An immunoglobulin deletion mutant with implications for the heavy chain switch and RNA splicing. Nature 286:669

Grubb R (1970) The genetic markers of human immunoglobulins. Springer, Berlin, Heidelberg, New York

Herzenberg LA et al. (1980) Regulatory circuits and antibody responses. Eur J Immunol 10:1

Hilschmann N et al. (1978) Genetic determination of antibody specificity. Naturwissenschaften 65:616

Honjo T, Kataoka T (1978) Organization of immunoglobulin heavy chain genes and allelic deletion model. Proc Natl Acad Sci (USA) 75:2140

Hozumi N, Tonegawa S (1976) Evidence for somatic rearrangement of immunoglobulin genes coding for variable and constant regions. Proc Natl Soc Acad Sci (USA) 73:3628

Ishizaka K (1970) The identification and significance of gamma-E. In: Good RA, Fisher DW (eds) Immunobiology. Sinauer, Stanford, Conn.

Jerne NK (1974) Toward a network theory of the immune system. Ann Immunol (Institut Pasteur) 125C:373

Kabat EA (1976) Structural concepts in immunology and immunochemistry, 2nd ed. Holt, Rinehart & Winston, New York

Kabat EA (1978) Variable region genes for the immunoglobulin framework are assembled from small segments of DNA. A hypothesis. Proc Natl Acad Sci (USA) 75:2429

Köhler G, Milstein C (1975) Continuous cultures of fused cells secreting antibody of predefined specificity. Nature 256:495

Koshland ME (1975) Structure and function of the J chain. Adv Immunol 20:41

Low TLK (1975) Structure, function, and evolutionary relationship of Fc domains of human immunoglobulins A, G, M and E. Science 191:390

Maki R et al. (1980) Exon shuffling generates an immunoglobulin heavy chain gene. Proc Natl Acad Sci (USA) 77:2138

Melchers F et al. (eds) Lymphocyte hybridomas. Curr Topics Microbiol Immunol 81

Milstein C, Lennox ES (1980) The use of monoclonal antibody technique in the study of developing cell surfaces. Curr Topics Dev Biol 14:1

Molgaard HV (1980) Assembly of immunoglobulin heavy chain genes. Nature 286:657

Oudin J (1977) L'allotypie. Congr francophone int Immunol INSERM, Paris

Richards FF, Konigsberg WH (1973) Speculations how specific are antibodies. Immunochem 10:545

Sakano H et al. (1980) Two types of somatic recombination are necessary for the generation of complete immunoglobulin heavy chain genes. Nature 286:676

Shur PH (1972) Human gamma-G subclasses. Proc Clin Immunol 1:71

Singer PA et al. (1980) Different species of messenger RNA encode receptor and secretory IgM μ chains differing at their carboxy termini. Nature 285:294

Tonegawa S (1983) Somatic generation of antibody diversity. Nature 302:575–581

Tonegawa S et al. (1978) Sequence of a mouse germline gene for a variable region of an immunoglobulin light chain. Proc Natl Acad Sci (USA) 75:1485

Tonegawa S et al. (1981) Somatic reorganization of immunoglobulin genes during lymphocyte differentiation. Cold Spring Harbor Symp Quant Biol 45:839

Voisin GA (1980) Role of antibody classes in the regulatory facilitation reaction. Immunol Rev 49:3

Woodland R, Cantor H (1978) Idiotypic specific T helper cells are required to induce idiotype-positive B memory cells to secrete antibody. Eur J Immunol 8:600

Chapter 5   Complement

WILMAR DIAS DA SILVA

Contents

Complement 115
  Total Titration of Hemolytic Complement. . 116
  Complement as a Multifactorial System . . . 117
  Nomenclature 118
Sequential Reaction of Components
  in Immune Hemolysis 119
  First Step 119
  Second Step 120
  Third Step 122
  Fourth Step 123
  Fifth Step 123
  Sixth Step 124
  Seventh Step 124
Regulation of the Classical Pathway 126
Quantitative Determination of Components . . 126
Morphological Consequences of the
  Immunocytotoxic Reactions 127
Immunobiologic Activities of Complement . . 127
  Hemolysis 127
  Bacteriolysis 127
  Anaphylatoxins 128
  Chemotactic Factors 129
  Opsonization 130
  Complement-Dependent Liberation
   of Histamine 130
  Formation of Kinins 131
  Activation of Enzymes 131
  Immunological and Paraimmunological
   Tissue Injuries 131
  The Complement System as an Effector
   Mechanism in the Host Defense Against
   Infectious Agents 132
Activation Mechanisms of the Alternative
  Complement Pathways 133
  Alternative Pathway (Properdin System) . . 133
  Thrombin-Arachidonic Acid Pathway . . . 136
Effect of Complement on the Solubilization
  of Immune Complexes 137
Biosynthesis of Complement Components and
  Certain Hereditary Deficiencies 137
References 137

Complement

Pfeiffer and Issaeff observed in 1894 that cholera vibrios disintegrated when injected into the peritoneal cavities of previously immunized guinea pigs. Bordet demonstrated that the microorganisms also were lysed within minutes when placed in vitro in the presence of serum obtained from immunized animals; however, if the serum was heated to 56 °C for 30 min, or simply allowed to age for a few days, it lost its lytic activity even though the antibodies were preserved. The addition of fresh serum obtained from nonimmune animals restored the lytic activity of serum. This experiment demonstrated that the bacteriolytic action of serum of immunized animals depended upon two factors, one (the antibody) specific and thermostabile, and another that was thermolabile and nonspecific, existing in immune serum as well as in normal serum. The latter, initially termed alexin, is now called complement (C). Any immunologic reaction, as in the example cited above (Pfeiffer's phenomenon), is initiated by a specific combination of antigens and antibodies. From this point, a series of reactions is unleashed, humoral or cellular in nature, whose final expression is the production of tissue injury.

The union of the antigen and antibody in itself is an innocuous event, and antigen–antibody complexes resulting from this union are capable of producing cellular lesions only in collaboration with accessory systems. Complement is the effector system in reactions between antigens and humoral antibodies. This system may be defined as a group of factors (primarily enzymes) present in normal serum that do not increase with the immunization process and that are capable of interacting with different antigen–antibody complexes. If the antigens make up part of the structure of the cellular membrane, the participation of complement in the antigen–antibody reaction that occurs there causes an irreversible cellular lesion, terminating in lysis of that particular cell. As a result of the cytotoxic effects produced by complement during its activation, various orders of consequences can occur: lysis of bacteria (bacteriolysis); phagocytosis of certain particulate antigens that have been coated by antibodies (opsonization); alterations in the cellular membrane that lead to the lysis of erythrocytes (immune hemolysis) or of nucleated cells (cytolysis); production of substances capable of liberating histamine from mast cells or from smooth muscle cells (anaphylatoxins); formation of substances that attract leukocytes (chemotactic factors), etc. Finally, by the activation of the complement system, factors are formed that are necessary for the initiation of the inflammatory reaction that occurs in certain forms of immunologic tissue injury. Of the models of direct tissue injury mediated by complement, immune hemolysis has been investigated most thoroughly. The advantage of this model, which employs sheep erythrocytes sensitized with rabbit antibodies, and fresh guinea pig or human serum as a source of complement, lies in the precision of the information obtained.

Total Titration of Hemolytic Complement

Immune hemolysis was described by Bordet in 1909, but adequate methods for the rigorous quantitative determination of the hemolytic titer of complement in the serum have only been available since 1945, when advantage was taken of the role of the divalent cations Ca^{2+} and Mg^{2+} in the unleashing of the reaction. Much appreciation is owed to Manfred Mayer for the clarification of many aspects of the kinetics of immune hemolysis. Its general reaction can be represented as follows:

E + A → EA; EA + C → Stroma + Hemoglobin

where E represents sheep erythrocytes, A, antisheep erythrocyte antibodies produced

in rabbits, EA, sensitized erythrocytes; and C, complement.

For the titration of C, a standardized quantity of EA (5×10^8) is incubated with varying quantities of C, in a constant volume (usually 7.5 ml), with the pH of the medium maintained at 7.4–7.5 by an adequate isotonic buffer (saline veronal or triethanolamine buffer) containing Ca^{2+} (1.5×10^{-4} M). Incubation is performed for 90 min at 37 °C when guinea pig serum is used, or at 32 °C in the case of human serum. The degree of hemolysis is determined by measuring the quantity of hemoglobin liberated in each mixture. The mixtures are centrifuged, and the supernatants are examined spectrophotometrically at 540 nm. When the percentage of hemolyzed red cells is plotted against the quantity of C added, a sigmoidal dose-response curve is obtained (Fig. 5.1).

The graph shown in Fig. 5.1 verifies that the curve becomes asymptotic at the point where the hemolysis value approaches 100%. For this reason, it is best to titrate the complement at the linear part of the curve, with the unit of complement (CH_{50}) defined as the quantity that produces 50% hemolysis under the standardized conditions described previously. The relation between the percentage of hemolysis, y, and the quantity of complement, x, is given by the equation:

$$y = \frac{x^n}{x^n + K^n}$$

from which is derived the van Krogh equation:

$$x = K \left(\frac{y}{1-y}\right) 1/n,$$

in which x is the quantity of complement; y, the percentage of hemolysis; n, a constant whose reciprocal defines the inclination of the curve; and K, a constant expressing the 50% unit of complement. When there is 50% hemolysis, $y/(1-y-) = 1$ and x becomes equal to K (CH_{50} dose).

The curve described by van Krogh's equation is sigmoidal when $1/n > 1$ and, under

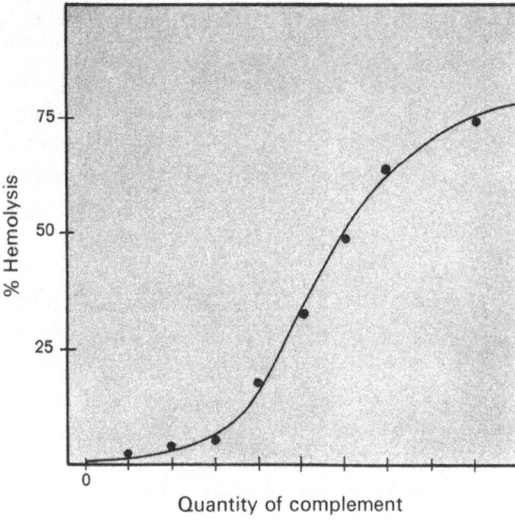

Fig. 5.1. Dose-response curve in the assay of complement (arithmetic scale)

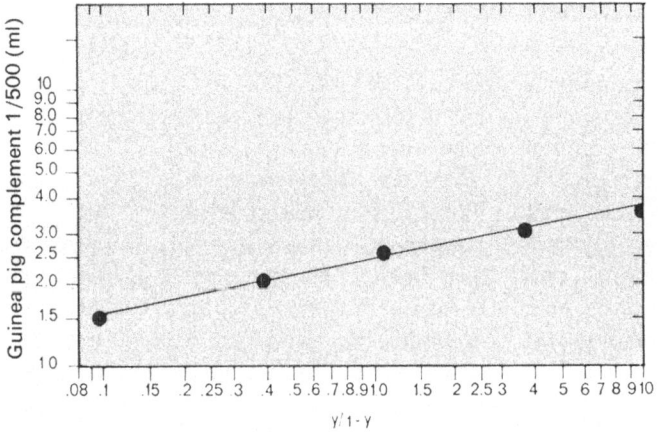

Fig. 5.2. Dose-response curve in determining the concentration of complement: log x versus log (y/1−y)

normal conditions, the value of $1/n$ should vary around 0.2 ($\pm 10\%$).

When a determination is made of the CH_{50} units in a serum, it is convenient to prepare a graph (Fig. 5.2) plotting $\log x$ along the ordinate against $\log [y/(1-y)]$ along the abscissa. With this formula, a straight line is obtained whose equation is

$$\log x = \log K + \frac{1}{n} \log \left(\frac{y}{1-y}\right).$$

The intersection of this line with the ordinate axis ($\log x = 0$) gives a quantity of serum that corresponds to one CH_{50} unit, for $\log (y/1-y) = 0$, $y = 0.5$. Guinea pig serum contains 200–300 CH_{50}/ml and human serum, 40–60 CH_{50}/ml.

Complement as a Multifactorial System

The liberation of hemoglobin in immune hemolysis, or the liberation of other cellular constituents in other forms of cellular injury mediated by complement, represents the final event in a sequential reaction. The multiplicity of components taking part in this reaction was verified in 1912, when Ferrata demonstrated that the serum fractions corresponding to the euglobulins and to the pseudoglobulins, obtained by dialysis of· fresh guinea pig serum against water, were hemolytically inactive by themselves, but regained their original hemolytic activity upon reassociation. Experiments in which first one fraction was added to the erythrocytes and then, after washing the cells, the other was added, revealed that the euglobulin fraction was fixed first, followed by the pseudoglobulin fraction. The former was thus termed the midpiece, or C1, and the second was called the end piece, or C2. Later, two other components were recognized – both thermostable – through the treatment of human serum with cobra venom or zymosan (C3) and with ammonia or hydrazine (C4).

The designations R1, R2, R3, and R4 are given to selectively deficient serums (called R-reactives), which serve, respectively, for the demonstration of C1, C2, C3, and C4 (Table 5.1).

The availability of the R-reactives also permits the titration of each of the components. For example, the titer of a serum in C1 is in-

dicated by the greatest dilution that produces 50% hemolysis of EA in the presence of a standardized concentration of R1.

Until 1958 only four complement components were known. The component that formerly was termed C3 ("classic" C3) is today recognized as a mixture of distinct proteins, with individual structures and functions, now called C3, C5, C6, C7, C8, and C9. Moreover, C1 can be divided into three subcomponents designated C1q, C1r, and C1s. These 11 proteins react sequentially in the fashion of a cascade. Some important properties of the components of complement are reproduced in Table 5.2.

Nomenclature

In accord with the nomenclature recommended by a group of experts convened by the World Health Organization, complement is designated by the symbol C, and the components are expressed by that symbol followed by a corresponding number (C1, C4, etc.).

The activated components are designated by a horizontal bar over the numeral of the respective symbol, e.g., $\overline{C1}$ = activated C1. The small letter "i" at the end of the symbol indicates a component that has lost its activity, e.g., C4i = inactivated C4. The products resulting from the cleavage of peptide linkages are represented by the general formulas Cna and Cnb, e.g., C3a and C3b or C5a and C5b.

Table 5.1. Separation of the classic components of complement

Treatment of the serum	R-Reactive	Components Present
Dialysis against		
pH 5.5 buffer, $\mu=0.02$		
Supernatant	R1	C2, C3, C4
Precipitate	R2	C1, C3, C4
Zymosan (2–3 mg/ml), 1 h at 37 °C	R3	C1, C2, C4
Hydrazine 0.02–0.03 M		
1 h at 37 °C	R4	C1, C2, C4
30 min at 56 °C	Inactivated serum	C3, C4

Table 5.2. Properties of the components of human complement

Components	C1q	C1r	C1s	C4	C2	C3	C5	C6	C7	C8	C9	C4bp	CIR
Synonyms	–	–	C1– esterase	$\beta_1 E$	–	$\beta_1 C$	$\beta_1 F$	–	–	–	–	–	–
Approx. mol. wt. ($\times 10^3$)	388	168	79	206	117	185	185	125	120	150	79	590	205
Sedimentation constant	11 S	7 S	4 S	10 S	6 S	9.5 S	8.7 S	6 S	7 S	8 S	4 S	7 S	–
Electrophoretic mobility	γ_2	β	α_2	β_1	β_2	β_1	β_1	β_2	β_2	γ_1	α_1	β	–
Concentration serum (μg/ml)	100–200	–	20	430	30	~1200	75	60	60	20	2–10	–	–
Congenital deficiency				Guinea pig	Man	Guinea pig	Mouse	Rabbit				–	–
Thermolability at 56 °C, 30 min	+	++	+	–	+	–	+	–	+	+	+	–	–

Sequential Reaction of Components in Immune Hemolysis

Figure 5.3 shows the reaction sequence of the complement components as established for immune hemolysis. This sequence is also valid for the lysis of other animal cells and for bacteria, and it is the same in cell-free systems with soluble preformed antigen–antibody complexes. The hemolysis of sheep erythrocytes (E) produced by rabbit anti-sheep red cell antibodies (A) and human or guinea pig complement, proceeds in eight steps:

(1) $E + A \longrightarrow EA$

(2) $EA + C1 \xrightarrow{Ca^{2+}} EAC\overline{1}$

(3) $EAC\overline{1} + C4 \longrightarrow EAC\overline{1, 4b}$

(4) $EAC\overline{1, 4b}, + C2 \xrightarrow{Mg^{2+}} EAC\overline{1, 4b, 2a}$

(5) $EAC\overline{1, 4b, 2a}, + C3 \longrightarrow EAC\overline{1, 4b, 2a, 3b}$

(6) $EAC\overline{1, 4b, 2a, 3b}, + C5 + C6 + C7 \longrightarrow$
$EAC\overline{1, 4b, 2a, 3b, 5b, 6, 7}$

(7) $EAC\overline{1, 4b, 2a, 3b, 5b, 6, 7} + C8 + C9 \longrightarrow E^*$

(8) $E^* \longrightarrow Stroma + Hemoglobin$

First Step

$E + A \rightarrow EA$.

In the first step, there is a specific union between antibodies (A) and antigens (E) localized on the surfaces of erythrocytes. There is indirect evidence that a single molecule of IgM or two molecules of IgG localized near one another on the cell surface are sufficient to sensitize it, making it capable of initiating the activation of complement. This idea agrees with the finding that, if an excess quantity of cells is mixed with a given quantity of IgM, the number of sensitized cells remains constant, whereas the same would not occur if IgG were used in place of IgM. Thus, antibodies of the IgM class tend to be much more efficient than those of the IgG class.

The necessity of having a pairing of the IgG molecules is implied in the fact that the corresponding groups with which they combine must be extremely close on the surface of the erythrocyte. Because the antigens of the Rh

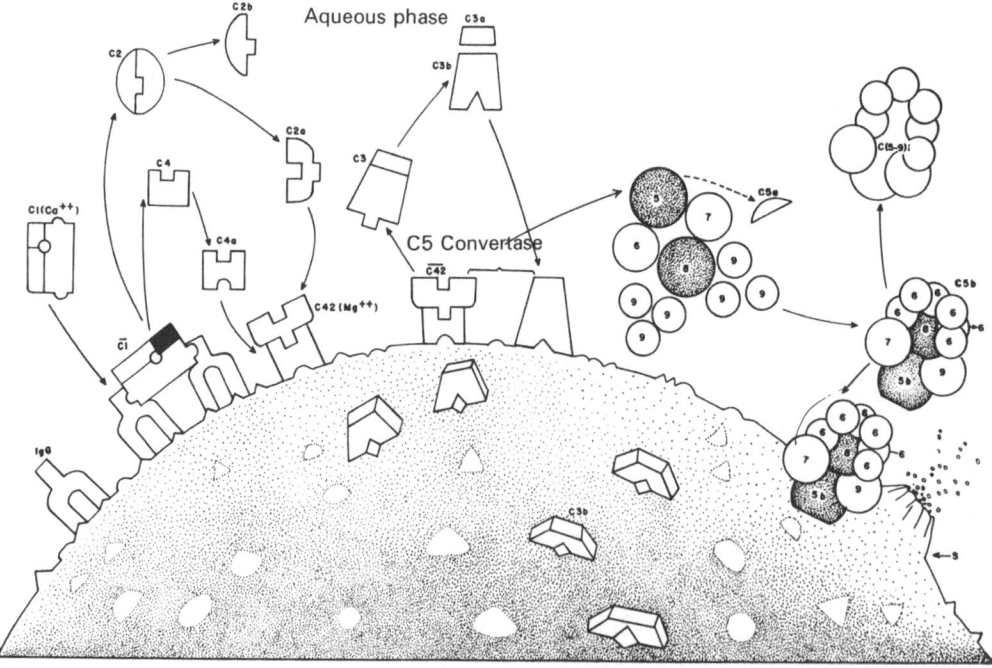

Fig. 5.3. Cascade reaction of the complement components in specific cytolysis

system, and some other isoantigens, are widely dispersed over the erythrocyte membrane, the foregoing considerations explain the inefficiency of antibodies to such antigens in sensitizing erythrocytes for immune hemolysis.

The antigenic determinants involved in immune hemolysis do not necessarily need to be natural constituents of the cellular membrane. Antigenic groups can be artificially linked to the membrane, and one can achieve hemolysis by the binding of antibodies specific for this group and the addition of complement. Immune complexes prepared in the zone of equivalence, or in slight antigen excess, activate complement more efficiently than do those found in regions with extreme antigen excess, where lattice-type structures do not form. Moreover, hybrid antibodies artificially prepared (antibodies synthesized from two half-molecules – one heavy and one light chain – from two antibodies with different specificities), having only one combining site, do not form lattices, nor do they activate complement.

The initial activation appears to depend at least upon a pair of heavy chains properly arranged and spaced with respect to one another for exposure of the Fc fragment sites responsible for aggregation with $C1q$. $F(ab')_2$ fragments, obtained by the cleavage of IgG with pepsin, form complexes with corresponding antigens that do not activate C. This last appears decisive for the localization of $C1q$ combining sites in the parts of the heavy chains that form the Fc fragment.

Not all antibodies that form complexes are capable of fixing guinea pig complement, which is usually used in routine tests. For example, the antibodies of birds do not activate mammalian complement. Moreover, in species whose antibodies are capable of fixing complement, only antibodies belonging to specific classes of immunoglobulins are really efficient. Thus, IgM and some subtypes of human IgG can fix complement, whereas IgA and IgE cannot.

Nonspecific aggregates of IgG, formed by warming at 63 °C for 10 min or by chemical aggregation with BDB (bis-diazobenzidine) also activate complement efficiently.

Second Step

$$EA + C1 \xrightarrow{Ca^{2+}} EA\overline{C1}.$$

The reaction between complement and red blood cells requires Ca^{2+} and Mg^{2+} ions, and the velocity of the reaction is greater at 37 °C than at 0 °C. These observations suggest that at least some of the complement components are enzymes that under normal conditions are encountered in serum in the form of proenzymes.

$C1$ forms a macromolecular complex composed of three subunits, designated $C1q$, $C1r$, and $C1s$, joined together by Ca^{2+} ions. Breaking this down with chelating agents such as EDTA (ethylenediaminetetraacetic acid), the complex dissociates into its subunits, which themselves can be separated by DEAE-cellulose (diethylaminoethyl-cellulose) column chromatography. In its macromolecular form, $C1$ combines, through domains localized in $C1q$, with special sites positioned on the Fc portion of the antibody molecule, which become accessible when the antibody molecules combine with the antigen $C1q$ is a macromolecule consisting of six triple-stranded subunits each composed of one A, one B and one C chain linked by S-S bond. For 78 residues near the N-amino acid the chains have a collagen-like sequence with a disaccharide gal-glu attached to many hydroxyllysine residues. Ultrastructural analysis indicates that each of six subunits has a globular domain at the end of its collagenlike strand. $C1q$ has stable combining sites and therefore requires no activation. On binding to immunoglobulin $C1q$ undergoes conformational changes that activate $C1r$ and $C1s$. Because $C1q$ possesses five or six valences per antibody molecule, each valence therefore could localize in the peripheral subunits. $C1q$ also is capable of interacting with IgG molecules and of precipitating preformed antigen-antibody complexes. Analysis through ultracentrifugation of the complexes formed by IgG and

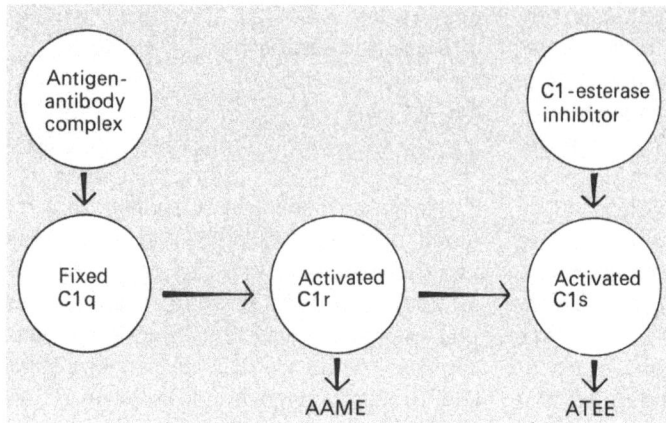

Fig. 5.4. Esterolytic activities of activated C 1

C1q molecules indicates that they have a 15 S sedimentation coefficient; apparently they are composed of six IgG molecules per single C1q molecule. Complexes of IgM and C1q are formed in an analogous manner.

Study of this stage of immune hemolysis has revealed that (1) after attachment to the EA membrane, C1 takes on the activated C$\overline{1}$ form, capable of hydrolyzing certain synthetic amino acid esters such as ATEE (N-acetyl-L-tyrosine-ethyl ester); and (2) the hemolytic activity as well as the esterolytic activity of C1 is blocked by DFP (diisopropyl fluorophosphate) and other inhibitors of esterase activity.

If EA or an adequate antigen-antibody complex interacts with C1, two esterase activities, distinct in terms of specificity, (Fig. 5.4) occur. The first, associated with C1r, hydrolyzes AAME (N-acetyl-arginine-methyl ester), whereas the other, associated with C1s, hydrolyzes ATEE (N-acetyl-L-tyrosine-ethyl ester) or TAME (N-p-toluenesulfonyl-methyl ester). The latter is commonly called C1-esterase and represents the hemolytically active form of C1. The component C1 treated with EDTA loses its macromolecular form by virtue of the removal of the Ca^{2+} ions. DEAE-cellulose column chromatography of C1 thus treated permits its resolution into three subcomponents C1q, C1r, and C1s (Fig. 5.5). Activation of C1s only occurs, however, when

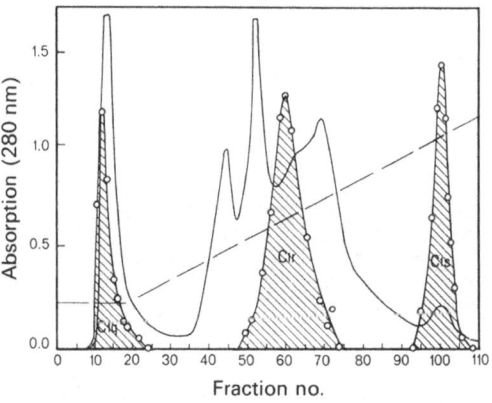

Fig. 5.5. Chromatographic resolution of C1 treated with EDTA. [Lepow IH, et al., (1962) J Exp Med 117:983]

the three subcomponents reassociate following the addition of Ca^{2+} ions. In these, the Ca^{2+} ions would be integrally part of the macromolecular C1 complex.

The normal serum of diverse species, including human and guinea pig, contains an inhibitor of C1-esterase (C1-E). The inhibitor is an acid-labile α$_2$ globulin with a 3 S sedimentation constant and a molecular weight of 90,000. It is destroyed by heating to 63 °C and by treatment with ether. Highly purified preparations of this inhibitor impede the activity of C1-esterase in the proportion of one unit of inhibitor for ten units of enzyme. Deficiency of C1 inhibitor see Table 12.7 (p. 380).

Third Step

$$EAC\overline{1} + C4 \rightarrow EAC\overline{1,4b}.$$

After the formation of $EAC\overline{1}$, the ensuing stage of immune hemolysis involves reaction with C4 to form the intermediate complex $EAC\overline{1,4}$ (see Fig. 5.3). The formation of this complex occurs efficiently only when C1 is present in its enzymatically active form on the surface of the sensitized erythrocyte. The inhibition of C1 with DFP, with anti-C1-esterase antibodies, or with purified preparations of C1-esterase inhibitor impedes the formation of the $EAC\overline{1,4}$ complex. Once this complex is formed, C1 can be inactivated by EDTA without affecting the activity of C4. Is not C44 itself linked to C1, but rather to binding sites located on the membrane of the red blood cell or on the antibody molecule.

Human C4 has been obtained in a highly purified form. It is composed of three disulfide-linked polypeptide chains of 93,000 (α), 75,000 (β), and 32,000 (δ) mol.wt. The α-chain contains an internal thiolester linkage which upon activation provides a site for attachment to the surface of the target cell through covalent attachment and by hydrophobic forces.

The treatment of a purified preparation of C4 with C1-esterase results in modifications of its electrophoretic mobility and in a small but detectable reduction in its sedimentation constant to 9.5 S (Fig. 5.6). These modifications result from the cleavage of the C4 molecule into a small fragment (C4a) with a molecular weight of approximately 15,000, and into a larger fragment that combines with the membranes of red blood cells (C4b), C4b activity is controlled by the plasma proteins C4bp and C3b/C4b inactivator (I). Cleavage of fluid-phase C4b by I requires the presence of C4bp. Surface-bound C4b is, however, split by I in the absence of C4bp, although the presence of this cofactor greatly accelerates the reaction. This larger fragment also contains the acceptor sites for C2 molecules. The availability of purified preparations of C4 has permitted a series of studies regarding the biochemistry of this stage of immune hemolysis. It has been ascertained, for example,

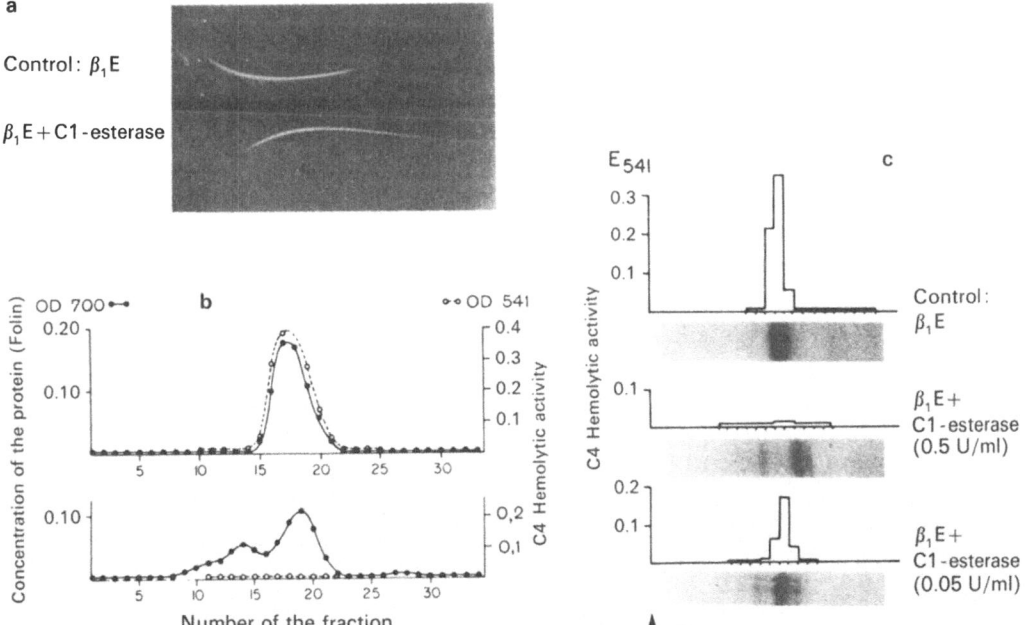

Fig. 5.6. The effect of purified C1-esterase on purified C4, demonstrable by **a** immunoelectrophoresis, **b** electrophoresis, and **c** through ultracentrifugation. [Müller-Eberhard JM, Lepow IH (1965) J Exp Med 121:819]

that C1-esterase probably acts upon the c4 molecules in two ways: first, in creating the conditions necessary for the linking of C4 molecules to the cellular membrane or to antigen-antibody complexes; later, in preparing them for combination with the C2 molecules (see Fig. 5.3). The sites of the C4 molecule responsible for its combination with C2 molecules are different from the sites responsible for its fixation to the cellular membrane. These last sites are unstable, and easily inactivated if the C4b molecules do not encounter their receptors on the cellular membrane. However, the sites for the fixation of C2 molecules are more stable, remaining active long after activation by C1-esterase.

Fourth Step

$$EAC\overline{1, 4b} + C2 \xrightarrow{Mg^{2+}} EAC\overline{1, 4b, 2a}$$

C2 is a β_2-globulin with a molecular weight of approximately 117,000 daltons. Treatment of C2 with iodoacetic acid or with p-chloromercuribenzoate destroys its hemolytic activity, whereas treatment with iodine increases this activity. This suggests that C2 molecules possess sulfhydryl groups essential for their activity. The reaction proceeds in two stages. In the first, in a reaction that requires Mg^{2+} ions, C2 molecules are linked, reversibly, to the EA C$\overline{1,4b}$ complex; in the second stage, depending upon temperature, C1 cleaves the C2 molecules that have just joined, producing two fragments: one active (C$\overline{2a}$) that binds firmly, but not irreversibly, to C4, the other inactive (C2b – mol. wt. 34,000 daltons), which dissociates in the liquid phase (see Fig. 5.3). The C$\overline{2a}$ fragment has a molecular weight of 83,000 daltons and contains the active sites for the C$\overline{4b}$–C$\overline{2a}$ complex, an enzyme provisionally termed C3-convertase because of its action in "converting" C3, in terms of electrophoretic mobility, from a protein that migrates to the β region into one that migrates to the α-protein region.

The complex EAC$\overline{1,4b,2a}$ is unstable, with a half-life of approximately 12 min at 32 °C. If C2 loses its activity, it is liberated in the aqueous phase, the complex thus reverting to the EAC$\overline{1,4b}$ stage. This last phenomenon is usually referred to as "decay".

The C$\overline{4b}$–C$\overline{2a}$ (C3-convertase) complex has a molecular weight of 305,000 daltons, which corresponds approximately to the sum of the values for C$\overline{4b}$ and C$\overline{2a}$. Its formation thus involves four distinct steps: (1) reversible interaction between the C4 and C1 molecules; (2) cleavage of C4 by C1-esterase into C$\overline{4a}$ and C4b, whereby the latter carries acceptor sites for activated C$\overline{2}$; (3) by action of C1-esterase, C2 is split into C$\overline{2a}$ and C2b; (4) finally C$\overline{2a}$ binds tightly to C$\overline{4b}$. Although Mg^{2+} is necessary for this reaction, EDTA causes neither dissociation nor inhibition of activity once the complex is formed. C3-convertase, formed from C2 oxidized with iodine (C2^{oxi}), is a considerably more active and more stable enzyme than that formed with native C2. This finding suggests that the transformation of S–H groups in S–S bridges is important for the enzymatic activity as well as for the stability of the bimolecular complex. It can also be assumed that the S–S bridges on the C2 molecule are close neighbors of the C4b combining region.

Fifth Step

$$EAC\overline{1, 4b, 2a} + C3 \rightarrow EAC\overline{1, 4b, 2a, 3b}.$$

C3 is a β-protein with a 9.5 S sedimentation constant and a molecular weight of approximately 185,000 daltons. It consists of two polypeptide chains (α and β) with molecular weights of 110,000 and 80,000 daltons, respectively, linked by disulfide bridges. The α-chain contains an intramolecular thiolester bond which becomes the reactive group of the metastable binding site of proteolytically produced C3b (Fig. 5.9, top). This internal thiolester linkage provides the covalent binding site of the C3b molecules for the surface of target cells. cDNA probes for mouse and human C3 have been made and were sequenced; the majority of the genomic DNA coding for C3 has now been identified. With the help of these clones (and by other means) it has been possible to show that the C3 gene in man is found on the 19th chromosome. Upon activation, the C3 molecules are split, giving rise to a large fragment, C3b, which is responsible for the hemolytic activity of C3, and a small fragment, C3a, with an approximate molecular weight of 9,000 daltons, which is liberated in the liquid phase and possesses pharmacologically important properties (see Fig. 5.3). This fragment (C3a) can be liberated by treatment of highly purified preparations of C3 with the C4b, 2a (C3-convertase) complex, as well as by the action of trypsin or corbra venom derived enzymes. During activation, C3a is separated from the N-terminal end of the C3α chain. The remaining part of the C3 molecule (C3b) is immediately bound to the membrane and forms an intermediate complex EAC1, 4b, 2a, 3b (C5-convertase). C1 does not take part in this reaction, because the reaction also occurs when C1-free EAC4b, 2a complex is used. If the C3b molecule does not attach quickly enough to the cell membrane, it loses its activity and is converted into the hemolytically inactive form, C3bi.

The influence of the C3b inactivator (conglutinin activating factor) together with the regulatory protein H on the bound C3b causes its decay into a fragment, C3d (mol.wt. ca. 25,000), which remains in the membrane, a small piece that represents the C3α chain, and the remaining part of the α chain with the entire β chain, which passes into the liquid phase. The binding of C3b apparently occurs via the C3d fragment. All available findings indicate that all physiologically active fragments of C3 are derived from cleavage of the α chain: C3a, C3b, C3c, and C3d.

Sixth Step

EAC$\overline{1, 4b, 2a, 3b}$ + C5 + C6 + C7 → EAC$\overline{1,}$ $\overline{4b, 2a, 3b}$, 5b, 6, 7.

Little is known about the mechanisms involved in the reaction of C5, C6, and C7. Analysis of the interactions of C6 and C7 with C5 through ultracentrifugation indicates that each of these can interact independently of the other; however, it is not clear

whether the two components compete for the same site on the C5 molecule. C5 is composed of two disulfide-linked polypeptide chains of 105,000 (α) and 75,000 (β) molecular weight and is apparently evolutionarily related to C4 and C3 components. It appears that the C5 convertase, comprising of C4b, C2a, C3b, contains the enzymatically active site for proteolysis of C5 on the C4b, C2a complex, C3b serving to present the substrate C5 in appropriated form to be cleaved. This was suggested by the observation that peptides containing residues of aromatic amino acids – e.g., glycyl-L-tyrosine – that are hydrolyzed by the intermediate complex EAC1, 4b, 2a, 3b, inhibit the conversion of this complex to the succeeding stage EAC1, 4b, 2a, 3b, 5b, 6, 7. The first phase of this reaction would therefore be the cleavage of the C5 molecule into C5a and C5b, followed by the aggregation of C5b with C$\overline{6}$ and C$\overline{7}$, to form the trimolecular complex C5b, C6, C7. It has been suggested that C6 is a serine-esterase enzyme but the role of this enzymatic site on the later sequence reaction has not yet envisioned. This aggregate attaches immediately to the cellular membrane, though there is some evidence that activated C$\overline{7}$ acts upon the membrane without linking to it permanently. Treatment of the EAC 1,4b,2a,3b,5b,6,7 complex with anti-C5 antibodies inhibits the combination of C8 with the cell membrane, suggesting that C6 and C7 are components responsible for the activation of C8 (see Fig. 5.3).

Seventh Step

EAC$\overline{1, 4b, 2a, 3b, 5b, 6, 7}$ + C8 + C9 → E* → Hemolysis.

Müller-Eberhard and co-workers suggested that the production of lesions by complement on the cell membrane was provoked by a decamolecular complex involving components C5–C9. After the cleavage of C5 into C$\overline{5a}$ and C$\overline{5b}$ by the C$\overline{4b, 2a, 3b}$ (C5-convertase) enzyme, C5b, C6, and C7 could link to the membrane in the form of a complex. The geometric form of this suggested complex is triangular, each component contributing a molecule in order to form a triangle. Because the molecular weight of C5b is 165,000 daltons and the molecular weights of C6 and C7 are 100,000 daltons each, the complex has a total weight of 365,000 daltons. The central region of the triangle accommodates a C8 molecule that is linked by simple adsorption to each of the components of the trimolecular complex. The complex, now tetramolecular, assumes the form of a tetrahedron. The connected C8 molecule is also capable of fixing six or more C9 molecules. Because the molecular weight of C8 is 150,000 and

that of C9 is 79,000, the decamolecular complex $C5b_1-C6_1-C7_1-C8_1-C9_6$ has a molecular weight of 995,000.

This molecular arrangement of the six last components was proposed based upon the following information: (1) $C\overline{5b}$, C6, and C7 are tied to the membrane of the target cell in intimate proximity with one another; (2) the $C\overline{5b}, \overline{C6}, \overline{C7}$ complex consitutes the combining site for C8; and (3) C8 possesses many combining sites for C9. This model is in accord with the possible allosteric effector functions of C9, suggested by earlier observations, in which C9 can be substituted by chelating compounds such as 1–10–phenanthrolene and 2,2′-bipyridine.

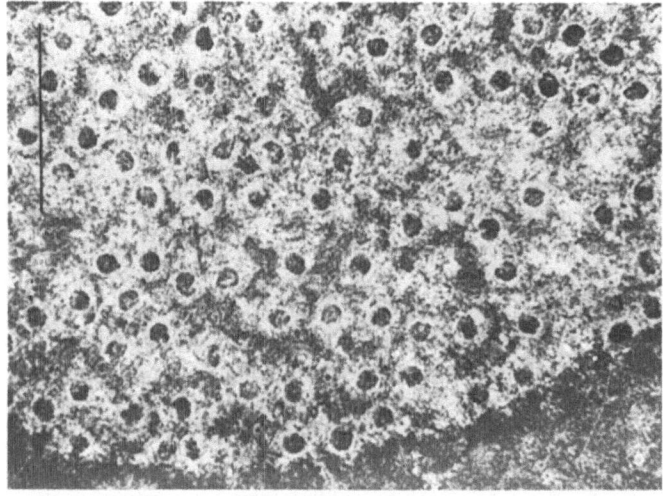

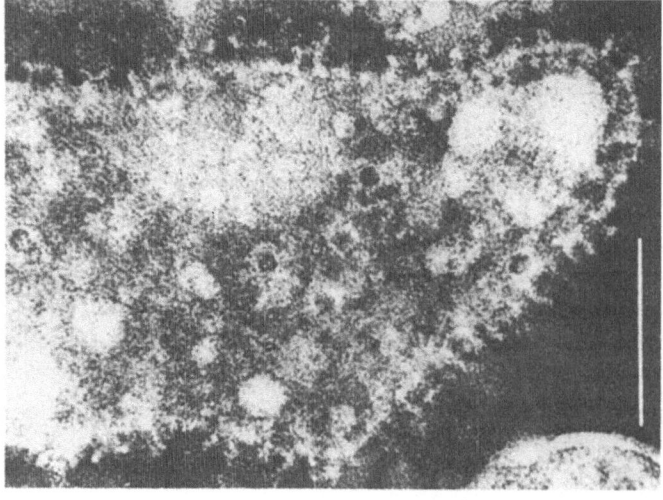

Fig. 5.7. Production of holes in the cell membrane (sheep and human erythrocytes) during cytolysis by complement

The mechanism by which this decamolecular complex injures the cellular membrane is unclear. The initial suggestion as to the activation of phospholipases was not confirmed in experiments using artificial membranes containing labeled phospholipids as substrates for the terminal components of complement. These experiments suggested that the lesion could occur by hydrophobic interactions between complement and the lipids of the cellular membrane.

The morphologic characteristics of the lesions on the surface of the cellular membrane (Fig. 5.7) become apparent immediately after fixation of C8. The subsequent interaction of the C5–C8 complex with C9 results in "functional lesions."

These "functional lesions" are in fact protein chanels, internally hydrophilic and externally hydrophobic, inserted into the bilayer cell membrane. The channels are lined by polymers of C9 the size of which being estimated as high as dodecamers.

Besides immune complexes two other kinds of molecular complexes may also activate the classical pathway. Cells infected with some virus (e.g. oncornaviruses, RNA tumor viruses) and expressing viral proteins on their surface or the viral particles by themself are able to interact with C1q, activate C1s, form C4b, C2a, cleave C3 and form C5b–C9 complex which promotes their lysis. On the other hand, C-reactive protein, a nonimmunoglobulin protein which sharply increases in the plasma during the onset of acute infections has also the capacity to activate the classical pathway. Although this protein forms calcium-dependent precipitating complexes with somatic C-polysaccharide of pneumococcus, and of several other bacteria and fungi, its mechanism of complement activation is poorly understood.

Regulation of the Classical Pathway

Mechanism of control of activation of this pathway have been localized in at least three points of the early sequence of the reactions: a) control of the activation of C1s and of its activity by the inhibitor of C1 esterase; b) self-control of the C4b, C2a convertase by the intrinsic decay of its enzymatic activity (half-life of 12 min at 32 °C); c) C4b- or C3b-mediated reactions, i.e. capability to bind membranes or immuneaggregates to assemble active C4b, C2a (C3 convertase) and C4b, C2a, C3b (C5 convertase) are controled by the serum proteins C4-binding protein (C4bp) and C3b, C4b inactivator (I) and the protein H. Cleavage of fluid-phase C4b by I requires the presence of C4bp whereas cell surface bond C4b is, although to a lesser extent split by I in absence ofC4bp. In addition, membrane-associated regulatory proteins seem to be of major imprtance under in vivo conditions.

Quantitative Determination of Components

A method for the quantitative determination of the individual components of complement based upon hemolytic activity was introduced by Meyer in 1961, following the formulation of his "one-hit theory" for immune hemolysis. This theory takes the position that a single molecule of any of the components of complement, at some stage in the sequence of reactions, is sufficient to produce a lesion on the surface of the erythrocyte that in turn is sufficient for lysis. The number of hemolytically active sites of each component could then be represented by $[Z = -\ln(1-y)]$, the negative natural logarithm of the number of cells not lysed. For 63% hemolysis, $Z = 1$, which corresponds to one hemolytically active site per cell. Because this method does not compute the unsuccessful reactions, the results represent the estimated minimum and thus are expressed in terms of "effective molecules." From an operational point of view, the method consists of making a graph in which the arithmetic values of Z are plotted against the dilutions of serum. To obtain the number of effective molecules of a specific complement component, it suffices to multiply the graphically obtained value corresponding to $Z = 1$ by the reciprocal of the dilution and by the number of erythrocytes in the mixture, and then to convert for 1 ml of serum.

Morphological Consequences of the Immunocytotoxic Reactions

Lesions produced in the cellular membrane by the action of antibody and complement have been visualized with the electron microscope using negative staining techniques. The lesions produced in the membranes of erythrocytes and in bacterial membranes are exhibited as relatively circular holes 80 Å–100 Å in diameter (Fig. 5.7). Studies of the effect of complement upon the lipopolysaccharide *Veillonella alcalescens* suggest that the lesions produced in the membrane are not actual orifices, but only the accumulation of micelles in the lipoprotein layer of the erythrocyte surface.

Nucleated cells, such as those of Kreb's ascites tumor, after interacting with antibodies reveal invaginations and interdigitations of the cellular membrane. The addition of complement to these cells produces swelling of the mitochondria and of the membranes of the endoplasmic reticulum; larger perinuclear pores are also noted. Dis-

turbances in control of cellular permeability are manifested initially by the loss of K^+, amino acids, and ribonucleotides. The cell swells and, as a consequence of osmotic lysis, macromolecules such as proteins and nucleic acids are liberated.

Immunobiologic Activities of Complement

During the sequential reaction of the complement system, various biologic activities emerge, associated alternatively with activated components or with products of cleavage. Table 5.3 shows these different activities and the component or components that participate in their production.

Hemolysis

Immune hemolysis utilizes the 11 complement components for its realization. Due to its great reproducibility and its considerable ease of execution, this reaction has been frequently used in studies of the biochemistry of the activation of complement.

Bacteriolysis

Gram-negative bacteria are susceptible to the action of antibody and complement; all

Table 5.3. Biologic activities associated with products resulting from the sequential reaction of complement

Biologic activity	Components involved in the process of production									Originating component (s)
	C1	C2	C4	C3	C5	C6	C7	C8	C9	
Hemolysis	+	+	+	+	+	+	+	+	+	C8, C9
Bacteriolysis	+	+	+	+	+	+	+	+	+	C8, C9
Anaphylatoxins	+	+	+	+	+	−	−	−	−	C4, C3 and C5
Chemotaxis	+	+	+	+	+	+	+	−	−	C5
Opsonization	+	+	+	+	+	−	−	−	−	C3
Immunoadherence	+	+	+	+	−	−	−	−	−	C3
Conglutination	+	+	+	+	−	−	−	−	−	C3
Immunoconglutination	+	+	+	+	−	−	−	−	−	C3
Activation of kinin	−	+	+?	−	−	−	−	−	−	C2
Enzymes	+	+	+	+	−	−	−	−	−	C1 r, C1 s, C4–C2, C3
Liberation of histamine	+	+	+	+	+?	+?	−	−	−	C4, C3, C5
Production of glomerulonephritis	+	+	+	+	?	?	?	?	?	?
Production of pulmonary edema	+	+	+	+	?	?	?	?		C3, C5

11 components, apparently, are also necessary. The final lesion involves the cell wall, leading to the formation of spheroplasts (cf. Chap. 7, p. 201).

Anaphylatoxins

The term "anaphylatoxin" was employed by Friedburger in 1910 to describe the property of inducing a syndrome similar to anaphylactic shock that some sera acquire when treated with preformed antigen–antibody aggregates. It was later verified that sera treated with polysaccharide complexes such as agar, zymosan, dextrans, etc, also acquire this property. Subsequent investigations demonstrated that the sera containing anaphylatoxin exhibited the following pharmacologic properties: (1) production of spasmodic contractions in smooth muscle (guinea pig ileum), followed by tachyphylaxis after administration of another dose; (2) capacity to liberate histamines from mastocytes and to produce degranulation (in guinea pigs) or extrusion (in rats and mice) of the metachromatic granulations encountered in the cytoplasm of these cells; (3) inability to contract the smooth musculature of the uterus of the rat in estrus; and (4) capacity to produce an increase in vascular permeability.

Based on the fact that sera previously heated to 56 °C did not form anaphylatoxin, Friedburger suggested in 1911 that complement could be involved in its formation. For nearly 50 years, this hypothesis remained unexplored, probably because of lack of greater knowledge of the biochemical events related to the activation of the complement system. This hypothesis was tested only after it became possible to obtain components of complement in a highly purified form. These investigations demonstrated that during the sequential reaction of complement, three products of cleavage were formed, derived from C4, C3 and the other from C5, representing the anaphylatoxins.

Anaphylatoxin Derived from C3. The biologically active fragment $C\overline{3a}$ originates from the cleavage of C3 by C3-convertase,

according to the following reaction:

$$C3 \xrightarrow{\overline{C4b-2a}} C\overline{3a} + C\overline{3b}$$

The fragment $C\overline{3a}$ represents approximately 4% of the original C3 molecule, has a molecular weight of around 9,000, and migrates during electrophoresis at pH 9 toward the cathode. The basic character of this fragment was confirmed by amino-acid analysis, which revealed a ratio of 1.65 between the basic and the acid residues. The $C\overline{3a}$ fragment is composed of a small carbohydrate portion bound to the peptide portion, which contains four residues of cysteine, serine as the N-terminal residue, and leucine as the C-terminal residue. This residue of leucine links $C\overline{3a}$ to the remaining portion of the original C3 molecule.

Aside from C3-convertase, other enzymes such as trypsin, plasmin, thrombin, and the CVF,Bb complex resulting from the combination between the 7S factor present in cobra venom (CVF) and the Bb fragment of factor B also break down C3 molecules, forming the same fragments.

Anaphylatoxin derived from C4, C4a, although less active, posses similar activities as C3a.

Anaphylatoxin Derived from C5. The biologically active fragment $C\overline{5a}$ originates from the cleavage of C5 by the activating enzyme $C\overline{4b,2a,3b}$ according to the reaction:

$$C5 \xrightarrow{\overline{C4b,2a,3b}} C\overline{5a} + C\overline{5b}$$

This $C\overline{5a}$ fragment has a molecular weight of 10,000–15,000. It can also be formed by treating purified preparations of C5 with trypsin.

The two fragments $C\overline{3a}$ and $C\overline{5a}$ possess all the properties attributed to anaphylatoxin. Table 5.4 shows the similarities as well as the differences in the pharmacologic behavior of these two products.

As Table 5.4 indicates, the anaphylatoxin derived from C3 ($C\overline{3a}$) degranulates and

Table 5.4. Biologic properties of the fragments C$\overline{3a}$ and C$\overline{5a}$ obtained by cleavage of components C3 and C5, respectively

Fragment	Enzymes responsible for cleavage	Contraction of guinea pig ileum	Morphologic alterations of mastocytes		Liberation of histamine by the tissues	
			Rat	Guinea pig	Rat	Guinea pig
C3a	C$\overline{4b-2a}$	+	+	+	+	+
C3a	Trypsin	+	+	+	+	+
C3a	Plasmin	+	+	+	+	+
C3a	CVF, Bb complex	+	+	+	+	+
C4a	C$\overline{1s}$	+	−	−	−	−
C5a	C$\overline{4b-2a-3b}$	+	−	+	−	+
C5a	Trypsin	+	−	+	−	+

liberates histamine from mastocytes in rats and guinea pigs, whereas the anaphylatoxin derived from C5 (C$\overline{5a}$) is active only for guinea pig mastocytes. These differences in biologic specificity suggest that the two anaphylatoxins act upon chemically distinct receptors. In these terms, guinea pig mastocytes would have receptors for both anaphylatoxins, whereas rat mastocytes would only have receptors for C$\overline{3a}$. It has been determined that preparations of guinea pig ileum desensitized to one of the anaphylatoxins, for example, by successive additions of C$\overline{3a}$, respond fully to the addition of the same dose of C$\overline{5a}$. These results also suggest that the two anaphylatoxins act upon different receptors.

In normal human serum there is an anaphylatoxin inhibitor. It is a β-globulin, thermolabile at 56 °C, which inactivates C$\overline{3a}$ as well as C$\overline{5a}$. It has a molecular weight of 300,000 and the activity of carboxypeptidase B, and probably is identical to carboxypeptidase N. The presence of this inhibitor in the serum could explain the absence of anaphylatoxic activity in samples of human serum treated with antigen–antibody complexes, agar, C1-esterase, or anaphylatoxinforming agents.

C$\overline{3a}$ and C$\overline{5a}$ seem to be involved in the pathogenesis of the acute respiratory distress syndrome (*ARDS*). This syndrom is initiated by massive complement activation, mainly through the alternative pathway, and thereby generation of C$\overline{3a}$ and C$\overline{5a}$. Complement activation can be induced through a variety of activators: In sepsis patients, gram-negative bacteria induce activation. Artificial membranes, tubings and other materials in machines used for hemodialysis or bypass-operations similarly activate complement. Proteolytic enzymes released from the tissue in polytrauma patients or in the course of pancreatitis directly cleave C3 and C5 and generate C$\overline{3a}$ and C$\overline{5a}$. In each case, the anaphylatoxins are able to bind to granulocytes and to induce their aggregation. The cells accumulate in the lung capillaries and adhere to the endothelium. The subsequent local release of lysosomal enzymes, prostaglandins and toxic oxygen derivatives induces tissue damage associated with an increased vasopermeability resulting in massive and frequently fatal edema.

Chemotactic Factors

Also called chemotaxins, these are substances that promote the migration of leukocytes from an area of lesser to an area of greater density in a concentration gradient of the chemotactic substance. Studies of chemotaxis originally were performed in vivo by local injections of the chemotactic factor, in order to follow histologically the

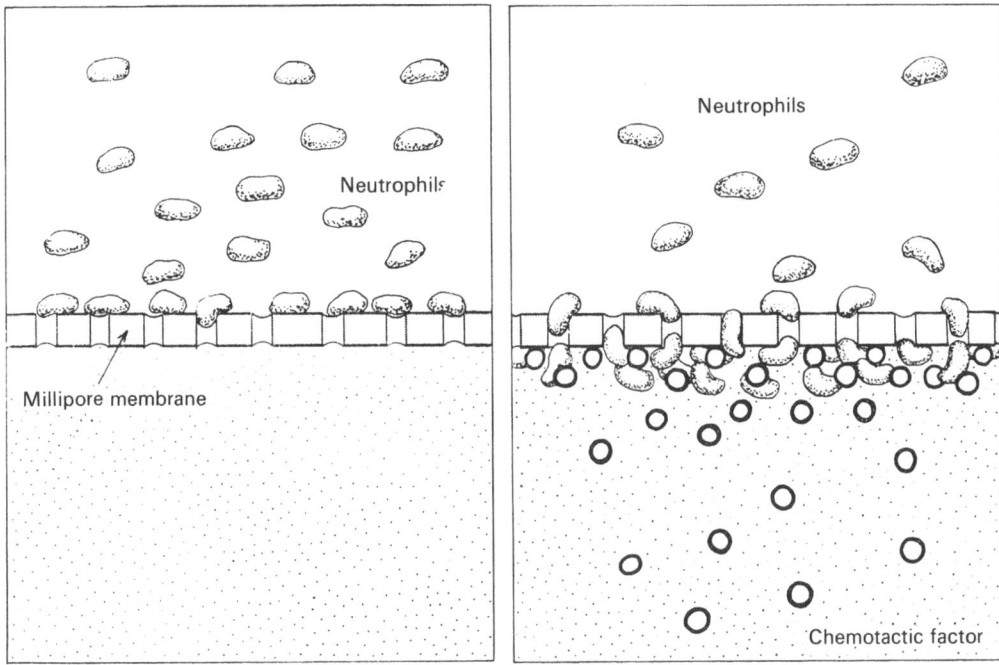

Fig. 5.8. Schema of the technique for demonstrating chemotactic factor

movement of leukocytes to the injected locale. Experiments of this type are now carried out in vitro, using appropriate chambers formed into two equal compartments of nonoxidizing metal separated by a microporous disk. The pores of this disk measure 650 nm and permit penetration of cells from the compartments. The chemotactic substance to be tested is placed in one compartment and the leukocytes in the other. Leukocytes migrating to the compartment that contains the chemotactic substance penetrate, by ameboid movements, into the membrane and are retained there (Fig. 5.8). Development of this in vitro method permitted the study of various chemotactic activities formed during the activation of the complement system. Chemotactic activity was shown for the fragment C 5 a, by proteolytic enzymes obtained from β-hemolytic streptococci of group A, and in the macromolecular complex formed by C 5–C 6–C 7.

The chemotaxis induced by any of these factors is related to the activation of an es-

terase linked to the leukocytes, from which the increased directional motility of these cells results.

Opsonization

Opsonins are substances that modify particles that are to be phagocytosed so as to cause them to be more easily ingested by phagocytic cells. Experiments designed to verify that complement components sensitize particulate substances by direct opsonization were conducted by inducing the adhesion of these substances to the surfaces of red blood cells. The results of these studies indicated that erythrophagocytosis could occur only after fixation by C 3 and was not augmented by the addition of the other complement components.

Complement-Dependent Liberation of Histamine

When rat mastocytes isolated from the peritoneal cavity are incubated at 37 °C with antimastocytic sera or with antigamma globulin inactivated at 50 °C, liberation of histamine occurs only with the addition of fresh serum. To verify that complement components were necessary, experiments were performed with purified preparations of complement. It was thereby possible to demonstrate that the liberation of histamine occurred only in the presence of C1, C4, C2, C3, and C5, with the necessity for C6 remaining in doubt. With the use of inhibitors whose spectrum of inhibition is well defined, the activation of an esterolytic enzyme in mastocytes was shown; it appears to be related to the process of liberation of histamine in anaphylaxis. The demonstration that C5 initiates the lesion in the erythrocyte membranes suggests that the factor responsible for the liberation of histamines is related to this component.

A similar phenomenon was observed when mastocytes isolated from the peritoneum of mice were treated in vitro with 19S fractions of rabbit anti-Forssman serum. The presence of heterophilic antigens on the surfaces of mastocytes was thus demonstrated.

Formation of Kinins

Numerous attempts to demonstrate the formation of kinins during the activation of complement have furnished inconclusive results. The first indirect evidence that this could occur was encountered in sera of patients with hereditary angioneurotic edema. In such sera, in addition to an accentuated increase of C1-esterase and a depression of the titers of C4 and C2, a peptide has been found that increases the vascular permeability of the rat uterus, but that differs, in certain respects, from bradykinin and from lysobradykinin. Subsequent experiments have shown that treatment of purified preparations of C4 and C2 with C1-esterase induces an activity similar to that of kinins, but in the conditions under which the experiments were performed, it was not possible to determine the nature of its relationship to C4 or to C2.

Activation of Enzymes

During the sequential activation of complement, four enzymes were activated, each with an already well-characterized spectrum of activity. These enzymatic activities are the esterases associated with C1r and C1s, the proteolytic activity associated with the bimolecular C4–C2 complex, and the dipeptidase associated with $C\overline{3b}$. Although the natural substances of these enzymes are encountered in the complement system itself, the possibility cannot be excluded that structural substrates also appear to be localized in plasma components not related to complement or making up a part of the composition of cellular membranes.

Immunological and Paraimmunological Tissue Injuries

There is an appreciable number of tissue damages in which the complement system undoubtedly plays an important role.
Glomerulonephritis produced by nephrotoxic sera or by deposit of circulating antigen-antibody complexes are mediated by the complement system. This syndrome is accompanied by fixation of immunoglobulins and complement components in various patterns on renal glomeruli.

Complement-dependent tissue injuries are the *pulmonary edema* produced experimentally by injecting nephrotoxic serum in rats or clinically observed in the human Goodpasture's syndrome, both lesions being initiated by the combination of specific antibodies with antigenic determinants of the basal membrane walls. In the first case, previous decomplementation of rats with CoF abrogate the establishment of the lesions. In the second case, the onset of the pulmonary crises coincides with a marked complement consumption.

The classical *Arthus reaction,* a cutaneous inflammation that could be elicited in rabbits undergoing sensitization to a foreign serum, was described by Arthus in 1903. Rabbits were injected into the skin each day with horse serum and the local response observed. During the first 4 days no response to the injections occured; after the fifth injection edematous and finally hemorrhagic and necrotic reactions appeared in the site several hours after the injection. Subsequently, it was demonstrated that the intensity of the reaction was dependent a) of the amount of circulating precipitating antibodies (0.12 mg N, 4.5 mg N and 0.22 mg N for active, direct passive and reversed passive Arthus reactions in rabbits, respectively); b) of the antibody class (guinea pig IgG2 e.g.), this later exigency lying in the immunoglobulin capacity to activate the complement system by the classical pathway; and c) of a normal serum complement level. The events leading to the establishment of the final lesion, an acute vasculitis i.e., deposition of immunocomplexes, activation of the complement system, chemotaxis of circulating cells and production and release of pharmacological mediators, are described in Chap. 10.

The Complement System as an Effector Mechanism in the Host Defense Against Infectious Agents

The complement system has been implicated as one of the first defense mechanisms in a nonimmune host. During its activation process which is initiated by the recruitment of $C3b$-like $C3$ molecules and by the surface of the invader pathogens, and leading to the creation of $C3b$, Bb, bearing sites on their surface follows: conversion of $C3$ into $C3b$ and $C3a$; deposition of $C3b$ molecules on the surface of the invader particles; formation of sites $C3b$, Bb, P, $C3b$ (n) containing $C5$ convertase activity and therefore capable to cleave $C5$ into $C5b$ and $C5a$; and, finally, culminating with the formation and insertion of the $C5b$–$C9$ complex into the particle membrane. Destruction of the pathogen can then be accomplished by the combined action of the inflammatory cells attracted to the invaded tissue and by the lytic effect of the $C5b$–$C9$ attack complex. In the first case, the inflam-

matory cells are attracted by chemotatic agents generated directly through the activation of the complement system. $C5a$ stimulated the locomotion of all leukocytes except lymphocytes. Removal of carboxy terminal Arginine from $C5a$ either by carboxy peptidase B or the anaphylatoxin inactivator serum produces $C5a$-des-Arg. Because the enzymatic transformation of $C5a$ to $C5a$-des-Arg by serum is so rapid, $C5a$-des-Arg has been suggested as the natural chemotactic factor derived from $C5$. $C3$ fragments have been reported to be chemotactic for neutrophils. However, purified $C3a$ is reported to lack chemotactic activity and it has been suggested that previous reports to the contrary arise from contamination of the $C3a$ with highly active $C5a$ or $C5a$-des-Arg. This observation is not however decisive in view of reports that tissue extracts and certain synovial fluids contain chemotactic activity that is inhibited by anti-$C3$ but not by anti-$C5$.

The $C\overline{5\ 67}$ complex stimulates neutrophil locomotion, the relative amount of $C5$ in the mixtures seems to determine whether the chemotactic activity will be in the form of the complex $C\overline{5\ 67}$ or $C5a$ fragments. Experiments have also demonstrated that both fragments derived by cleavage of B, Ba and Bb, are also able to stimulate neutrophil locomotion. Bb appears however to be active only when complexed with $C3b$.

In addition to the complement derived chemotactic factors other chemotactic agents are also formed in the local environment with the inflammation is ensuing. These include: fibrinopeptide B which stimulates the locomotion of neutrophils and monocytes; leukoaggressin, a proteolytically derived product of human IgG and IgG4, mouse IgG and rabbit fast IgG that stimulates neutrophil migration; a small glycoprotein of 8,500 mol.wt. chemotactic for neutrophils is produced by neutrophils when they ingest urate crystals; B and T lymphocytes, particularly T lymphocytes produce lymphokines that induce the locomotion of neutrophils, basophils, eosinophils, monocytes and lymphocytes; histamine, released from mast cells is specifically chemotactic, in a narrow dose range, for eosinophils, an effect which is not blocked neither by H_1 nor H_2 specific blockers. Besides histamine, a group of preformed tetrapeptides (Valyl-glycyl-seryl-glutamic acid and alanyl-glycyl-seryl-glutamic acid) with preferential attraction for eosinophils (ECF–H) and a 160,000 mol.wt. chemotactic factor for neutrophils are also released from mast cells; finally, an important group of metabolites of arachidonic acid and related unsaturated fatty acids which stimulate leukocyte migration are the HETE (12-L-hydrocy-5,8,10,14 eicosatetraenoic acid) and HHT (12-L-hydroxy-5,8,10 heptadecatrienoic acid), products of the lipoxygenase or cyclooxygenase arachidonic acid cascade, respectively. The release of these agents from the mast cells occurs in consequence of an anaphylactic reaction or by the action of the anaphylatoxins $C4a$, $C3a$ or $C5a$. Once accumulated in the tissues the leukocytes adhere to the $C4b$, $C3b$ or $C5b$ bearing pathogen particles and according with the type of cells or their state of activation, the pathogen particles can be either phagocytosed or killed. In the first case the particles are internalized and subsequently destroyed through the synchronized action of the O_2 metabolites and by enzymes present in the cell lysosomes (see Chap. 11). In the second case, the leukocytes adhere to the particle surface, for example of some larval worms, via the $C3b$ moiety of $C3$ and kill them through the release of some leukocyte components. The most important of which appears to be the MBP (major basic protein).

Although this overal picture is a simplification all these phenomena have been demonstrated to occur by both *in vitro* or *in vivo* experiments. It is also important to emphasize that in an immune host the onset of these phenomena is vertiginous and increasingly intensified.

The mechanisms described above have been implicated, at least in some way, in the destruction of a number of pathogenic agents. Thus, activation of the alternative complement pathway leads to the lysis of the cercariae and of the newly transformed schistosomula of *S. mansoni*. $C3$ fragments covering these larvae can also mediated both, the adherence of eosinophils to the parasite surface and the subsequent release of their cytoplasma components including MBP. This pathway has been also implicated in the lysis of the tripomastigote bloodstream forms of *T. cruzi*, the causative agent of the American trypanosomiasis. In this case, however, the activation of the pathway is initiated by the specific combining of antibodies with antigen parasite cell surface, activation of $C1$, formation of $C4b$, $C2a$, cleavage of $C3$ and deposition of $C3b$ molecules on some strategically disposed sites of the parasite cell surface. Elimination of some fungi or gram negative bacteria is also thought to be accomplished through the activation of the alternative complement pathway.

Activation Mechanisms of the Alternative Complement Pathways

Alternative Pathway (Properdin System)

The alternative pathway of complement activation (APC) serves as a primary recognition mechanism in the nonimmune host for a variety of pathogenic organisms which are rich on polysaccharides. Surface-associatd sialic acid moieties perform a critical role in determining the capacity of a particle to activate the APC. Particles such as sheep erythrocytes, which contain an abundance of terminal sialic acid residues, are nonactivating surfaces for the alternative pathway, while activating particles such as zymosan and rabbit erythrocytes are relatively deficient in surface-associated sialic acid.

Several virulent microorganisms have capsular polysaccharides that contain terminal sialic acid residues. For example, *E. coli* containing the K 1 antigen, a homopolymer of sialic acid, exhibit decreased alternative pathway-metiated opsonization and enhanced resistance to phagocytosis when compared with non-K 1 strains of *E. coli.* This cell surface modulatory component appears, however, to be not the sole mechanism governing the activation of the properdin alternative pathway. Recently, a glycoprotein of 205,000 mol.wt. has been isolated from the membrane of human erythrocytes and identified as the C 3 b receptor (CR-1). This protein was characterized as an inhibitor of the alternative pathway C 3-convertase (C 3 b, Bb) and is a cofactor for the cleavage of the α′-chain of C 3 b.

The two membrane components, the surface polysaccharides, sialic acid rich moieties (SR) and the CR-1 glycoprotein and probably other membrane factors are the modulatory components with determine whether or not a particle will be an activator or a nonactivator of the alternative pathway. Consistent with this is the observation that trypomastigote bloodstream forms of *T. cruzi,* which are nonactivator particles become activators of the complement alternative pathway upon previous treatment with trypsin. Similarly, young schistosomula of *S. mansoni* which are activators of the complement alternative pathway, lose this activity few days after *in*

vitro incubation or when recovered from the lungs of experimentally infected mice. This developmental change could not however be reversed by treating the old schistosomula larvae with neuraminidase, heparinase, chondroitinase ABC or trypsin, enzymes which are known to convert other particle substances into activators of the ACPP. Six plasma proteins and at least two cell surface components comprising this pathway have been identified (Table 5.5).

It has been proposed that an internal thiolester linkage is present in the α′-chain of native C 3 molecules, which can either react with water to form functionally C 3 b like C 3 (C 3*) or upon enzymatic conversion of C 3 to C 3 b, allows C 3 b to form a bond with hydroxyl- or amino groups on the target cell surface (Fig. 5.9). The initiating event of the activation of the alternative pathway has been envisioned by a "spontaneous" hydrolysis of the thiolester of a certain minor proportion of C 3 molecules, the Bb-like C 3 has the other to capacity to bind one molecule of B, resulting in the C 3*,B-complex.

The formation of an effective C 3*,Bb-convertase upon cleavage of the bound B by D̄ and the subsequent cleavage of C 3 depends on the presence or the absence on the cell

Table 5.5. Properties of components of the alternative properdin complement pathway

Protein	Synonym	Localization	Average plasma Conc. (μg/ml)	Isoelectric point	Polypeptide chains	Apparent mol wt of the chains	Cleavage fragments
C3	–	Plasma	1,250	6.1–6.8	Two	120,000 80,000	C3b, C3a C3bi, C3c, C3d
P	Properdin	Plasma	25	9.5	Four identical chains	54,000	None
B	Factor B; C3-proactivator	Plasma	250	6.6–6.8	Single	93,000	Bb, Ba
D̄	C3-proactivator convertase	Plasma	2	7.2–7.5	Single	23,500	None
I	C3b-Inactivator; KAF	Plasma	50	5.8–6.1		55,000 42,000	None
H	β1 H	Plasma	500	5.8–6.2	Single	150,000	None
Cl R	C3b receptor	Cell surface	?	?	Single	205,000	?
SA-P	Sialic acid rich polysaccharides	Cell surface	?	?	?	?	?

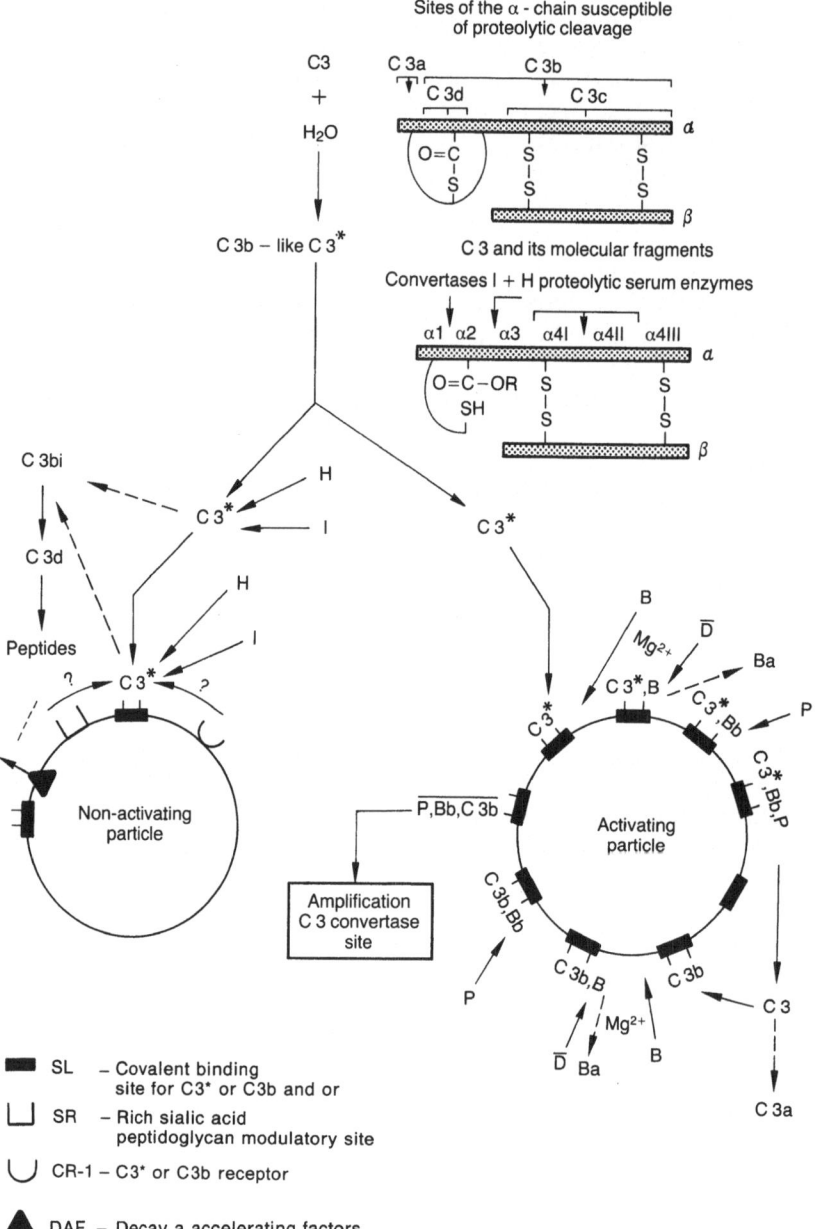

Fig. 5.9. Schematic representation of the alternative complement properdin pathway. *Top:* Formation of initial C3 convertase of the APC in plasma without proteolysis, by a low-rate direct hydrolysis of the thiolester bound present in native C3 molecules. This nucleophilic attack occurs at the asterisk(*) indicated in the residue of the peptide sequence Gly-Cys-Gly-Glu-Glu*-Asn-Met of the C3 α-chain. The steady hydrolysis of the thiolester would yield functionally active C3b-like C3 (C3*) without proteolytic release of C3a. Failure of C-g3b molecules to encounter an appropriate receptive surface results in their inactivation (Left). By contrary, the highly reactive form of the thiolester of the C3 molecules, once encountering activating particles, is capable to undergo transesterification with -OH groups on their carbohydrate-bearing surface components (Right). *Left:* Modulatory action of the cell surface associated components SR and CR-1 upon the attached C3* or C3b molecules on the SL sites leading to their cleavage into C3bi, C3d and small peptides by the regulatory proteins H and I. *Right:* In absence of the cell surface modulatory components SR and CR-1, the covalently bound C3* or C3b molecules are functionally able to form stable amplification C3 convertase sites, decay accelerating factors (DAF)

surface of the identified modulatory components SR or CR-1. The presence of one, bot or even unknown modulatory components increase the affinity constant of binding of H relative to B for C3b, thereby blocking formation of the alternative pathway C3b,Bb-convertase (Fig. 5.9, *left*). In contrast, the absence of these modulatory cell surface components on the activators particles or their artificial removal from the nonactivators particles increases the affinity constant of B to the bound C3* or C3b molecules, thus creating new cell surface sites containing C3b,Bb-convertase in an amplification molecular process (Fig. 5.9, *right*).

The lability of C3b,Bb (half-life of 4 min, at 30 °C), represents an intrinsic control that limits C3 cleavage by the amplification reaction of ACPP.

Two plasma proteins have been shown to stabilize the C3b, Bb-convertase prolonging its half-life at least tenfold. One of these proteins is P, a normal constituent of plasma first described by Pillemer and co-workers thirty years ago. The other is the C3 Nef, an ambigous name to design an IgG autoantibody directed to the C3b,Bb-complex which has been only detected in some patients with membranoproliferative glomerulonephrites or with partial lipodystrophy (Fig. 5.9, *right*).

The APC can also be activated in a fluid phase by the cobra venom factor (CVF), a glycoprotein isolated from the venom of cobra *Naja naja*. Addition of CVF to serum leads to the formation of a CVF,B-complex that enzymatically cleaves C3 into C3b and C3a. Factors $\bar{D}$ and Mg^{2+} are necessary for the formation of this complex. Because CVF appears to be functionally similar to C3b, but insensitive to the effect of I and H, the CVF,Bb-complex may function as an uncontrolled C3-convertase, thereby leading to be a complete exhaustion of C3 and the later reacting complement components.

The formation of a C-g5-convertase is essential for the generation of the C5b,C9 bivalent cytolytic membrane attack complex. Although the C5-cleaving enzyme of the classical pathway is comprised of C4tb, C2a, and C3b, the bimolecular complex carring the enzymatic site for proteolysis of C5 and C3b serving to present the substrate to permit its cleavage. Evidence has been accumulated that the alternative pathway C5-convertase is P,C3b,Bb with additional molecule(s) of C3b) which permits interaction of C5 with the stabilized P,C3b,B-complex in a manner analogous to the role of C3b in the classical pathway reaction of C4b, C2a, and C5.

Thrombin-Arachidonic Acid Pathway

Recent studies provide evidence that the thrombin-platelet aggregation and release of serotonin are significantly increased by the complement components C3, C5, C6, C7, C8, and C9. The process does not required any early reacting component either from the classical or the alternative pathway, but is initiated by the interaction of thrombin and C3 on the platelet surface and culminates in the formation of the membrane attack complex (C5b-9). Assembly of this macromolecular complex on the platelet surface initiates a transmembrane signal that modulates the arachidonic acid transformation pathway leading to the production of thromboxane A_2 as indicated by the inhibition of the whole process by aspirin and indometacin and by the formation of a significant amount of thromboxane B_2, the stable product of thromboxane A_2.

The sequence of reactions of this pathway could be schematically represented as following:

a) Thrombin (Th) + C3 + platelet → Th, C3b-like C3 complex-platelet surface component and formation of arachidonic acid from the platelet membrane phospholipids.

b) Th, C3b-like C3 + C5, C9 → C5b, C9 complex + arachidonic acid $\xrightarrow{\text{cyclo-oxygenase}}$ PG-endoperoxides $\xrightarrow{\text{thromboxanes synthetase}}$ thromboxane A_2 → thromboxane B_2.

Component	Species	Organ	Cell	
C1	Human, guinea pig	Intestine, GU[a]	Epithelial	**Table 5.6.** Cell and tissue synthesizing complement components
C1q	Human	Intestine, GU	Epithelial	
C1r	–	?	?	
C1s	Human	Intestine, GU	Epithelial	
C2	Human, guinea pig	Wide distribution	Macrophage	
C3	Human	Liver	Parenchymal cell	
C4	Human	Wide distribution	Macrophage	
C5	Human, mouse	Wide distribution	Macrophage	
C6	Rabbit	Liver	?	
C7	–	?	?	
C8	Pig	Wide distribution	?	
C9	Rat	Liver	Parenchymal cell	
C1-inhibitor	Human	Liver	Parenchymal	

[a] GU, genitourinary tract, excluding kidney. (According to Lachman, 1979)

Effect of Complement on the Solubilization of Immune Complexes

Studies show that immunocomplexes in the aqueous phase or bound to the cell membrane can be made soluble through the addition of complement. This reaction appears to be more effective when complement is activated via the ACP.

Defects in the homeostatic mechanism of circulating immunocomplexes through increased use, or because of a state of genetic deficiency of specific components of the complement or properdin system, are probably the basis for aggregation of immunocomplexes in tissue, leading to subsequent tissue damage.

Biosynthesis of Complement Components and Certain Hereditary Deficiencies

It is not known for all complement components which cell or tissue produces them. Recent studies suggest that C1 is synthesized in epithelial cells of the intestine and genitourinary tract (but not in the kidney); C2, C3, C4, and C5 are most probably synthesized in macrophages; C3, in addition, in parenchymal liver cells, as probably also C6, C9, and C1-inhibitor (Table 5.6).

The complement component C3 exists in different allotypic forms distinguishable by their electrophoretic mobility. C3 polymorphism has been verified in patients subjected to liver transplantation; after engraftment, the C3-allotype of the donor could be demonstrated. C4 also displays a polymorphism detected by electrophoretic mobility and serological markers, known in man as Chido and Rodgers.

The structural genes for the components C2, C4, and factor B are linked to the major histocompatibility complex.

Hereditary deficiencies of each complement component of the classical pathway have been studied in man; they are described in more detail in Chap. 12. Among inbred strains of laboratory animals, several deficiencies have been found: C5 in mice, C6 in rabbits, and C2, C4, and C3 in guinea pig.

References

Alper CH, Rosen FS (1971) Genetic aspects of the complement system. Adv Immunol 14:252

Bing DH (1979) The chemistry and physiology of the human plasma proteins. Pergamon Press, New York

Fearon DT (1979) Activation of the alternative pathway. Critical Reviews in Immunology 1(4):1–32

Gewurz H (1971) The immunologic role of complement. In: Good RA, Fisher DW (eds) Immunobiology. Sinauer, Stamford

Hugli TE (1981) The structural basis for anaphylatoxin and chemotactic functions of C3a, C4a and C5a. Critical Reviews in Immunology 1(4):324–336

Humphrey JH, Dourmashkin RR (1969) The lesions in cell membranes caused by complement. Adv Immunol 11:75

Lachman PL (1979) Complement. In: Sela E (ed) The antigen. Academic, New York

Lepow IH (1965) Serum complement and properdin. In: Santer M (ed) Immunological diseases. Little, Brown, Boston

Lepow IH et al. (1968) Nature and biological properties of human anaphylatoxin. In: Austen KF, Becker EL (eds) Biochemistry of acute allergic reactions. Blackwell, Oxford

Mayer MM (1961) Complement and complement fixation. In: Kabat EA, Mayer MM (eds) Experimental immunochemistry. Thomas, Springfield

Mayer MM (1973) The complement system. Sci Am 229:54

Medicus RG, Schreiber RD, Götze OJ, Müller-Eberhard HJ (1976) A molecular concept of the properdin pathway. Proc Natl Acad Sci 73:612

Müller-Eberhard H (1966) A molecular concept of immune cytolysis. Arch Path 82:205

Müller-Eberhard H (1969) Complement. Ann Rev Biochem 38:389

Müller-Eberhard H (1975) Complement. Ann Rev Biochem 44:697

Müller-Eberhard HJ, Schreiber RD (1980) Molecular biology and chemistry of the alternate pathway of complement. Adv Immunol 29:2

Müller-Eberhard HJ, Hoffmann LG, Mayer M (1977) Complement, Chap 17. In: Williams CA, Chase MW (eds) Methods in Immunology and Immunochemistry, vol IV. Academic Press

Spitzer RE (1977) The complement system. Pediatric Clinics of North America 24:341

Ward PA (1971) The role of complement in inflammation and hypersensitivity. In: Movat HZ (ed) Inflammation and hypersensitivity. Harper and Row, New York

Ward PA, Becker EL (1977) Biology of Leukotaxis. Rev Physiol Biochem Pharmacol 77:125–148

Chapter 6   The Major Histocompatibility Complex

DIETRICH GÖTZE and REINHARD BURGER

Contents

Histocompatibility Genes . . . . :. 139
Major Histocompatibility Complex
    (H–2) of the Mouse 141
    Congenic Strains 141
    Serology 143
The Major Histocompatibility Complex
    of Man (*HLA*) 148
    Serological Typing 148
    Cellular Typing 150
    Linkage Analysis of the HLA Complex . . . 154
Major Histocompatibility Complex
    of Other Species 154
Tissue Distribution of MHC Molecules 156
Biochemistry of MHC Molecules 158
    Class I Molecules: H–2K, D, L
    and HLA–A, B, C Molecules 159
Class II Molecules: *I* and *HLA-D*
    Region Molecules 161
    Class III Molecules: S-Protein 162
Function of *MHC* Molecules in the
    Immune Response 162
    Contribution to Antigen Recognition 162
    Genetic Restriction 164
    The T Cell Receptor: Antigen-Recognizing
    Element of T Cells 170
    Class III Molecules in the Immune Response . 174
MHC–Disease Association in Man 176
References 177

Histocompatibility Genes

At the beginning of this century, Tyzzer and Loeb showed that tumors of a strain of mice *(A/A)* grow normally if they are transplanted into mice of the same inbred strain (syngeneic, see Table 6.1); however, they are rejected by mice of another inbred strain (allogeneic, e.g., *B/B*). Mating experiments showed that susceptibility for tumor growth is genetically controlled: all F_1 animals of the cross $A/A \times B/B$ accepted tumors from both parental lines. Based on the percentage of accepted parental tumors in the F_2 generation, Little and Tyzzer calculated that in the mouse at least fifteen genes were responsible for the resistance to the parental tumor, because tumors grew in only 1.6% of the F_2 animals. According to the preceding example, if susceptibility were controlled by one gene, 75% of the F_2 animals would have been susceptible to the parental tumor tissue (50% A/B, 25% A/A, 25% B/B); if susceptibility were controlled by two genes, the number of susceptible animals would be reduced to 56% (9/16). In general, the percentage of F_2 animals in which a parental tumor grows is $(3/4)^n$, where n represents the number of different genes of both parental strains that control susceptibility. From these findings it was determined that susceptibility was controlled by several dominant genes.

In 1933, Haldane postulated that resistance (or susceptibility) is dependent on structures of the surface of the cell membrane which are different for each inbred strain and against which the recipient would react when its own differ from that of the donor. A few years later, Gorer (1936) demonstrated that there were indeed structures on the membranes of cells from inbred strains that could be revealed with antisera, and that were antigenically different for each inbred strain (alloantigen). He also showed that animals of an inbred strain that rejected a tumor from another inbred strain had antibodies in their serum reacting with cells of the inbred strain from which the tumor originated. Thus, Gorer demonstrated that genes responsible for susceptibility to tumor transplantation were identical to those that

Genetic relationship between donor and recipient	Noun (former term)	Adjective (former term)
Different species	Xenotransplant (heterotransplant)	Xenogenic (heterologous)
Same species, genetically different	Allotransplant (homotransplant)	Allogenic (homologous)
Same species, genetically identical (identical twins, animals of an inbred strain)	Isotransplant (isotransplant)	Syngenic, isogenic (isologous)
Donor = recipient	Autotransplant (autotransplant)	Autogenic (autologous)

Table 6.1. Terminology of histogenetic relationships

coded for alloantigenic structures, and that resistance to tumor transplantation was an immunologic phenomenon.

Shortly thereafter, Medawar showed that these observations were true not only for transplanted tumors but also for normal tissue grafts (e.g., skin); the rejection of normal tissue grafts was an immunological phenomenon. Structures on the cell surface, alloantigens, induced in a genetically different individual an immune reaction against the graft. Snell (1948) termed the antigens responsible for tissue compatibility *histocompatibility antigens* (H antigens) and the genes that control their expression, *histocompatibility genes* (H genes).

To study the effect and function of H genes and their products individually, Snell developed the concept of producing mouse strains that differ in only one H gene, the so-called congenic mouse strains. By developing such strains, the mouse became the experimental model par excellence in immunobiology.

In experiments with congenic mouse strains, Snell observed that not all the differences among H genes were equally strong in causing rejection: in some combinations transplanted tissue (e.g., skin) was rejected more quickly than in others. One gene in particular appeared to be responsible for acute rejection; this gene controlled the alloantigen designated by Gorer as antigen II, and that therefore was named the *H-2* gene. Allelic differences in this gene between recipient and donor of tissue grafts usually cause rejection within two weeks after engraftment,

whereas differences for other H genes led to delayed or chronic rejection. Tumor transplants were always rejected in cases of allelic differences at the *H-2* locus; however, this was not always true when there were differences in the alleles of other H genes. Thus, it appeared reasonable to distinguish two types of H genes: those that induce strong (major H gene), and those that induce weak (minor H genes) immune reaction. The major H gene was termed *major histocompatibility complex, MHC.* The minor H genes were summarized in general with a negative term, *non-MHC* genes. In the mouse, more than thirty *non-H-2* genes have been detected (*H-1, H-3, H-4, ...,* etc.). In most other species, including man, one may assume the existence of *non-MHC* genes, but they have not as yet been characterized.

Since the first description in the mouse, a major histocompatibility complex has been described for all better studied mammals, birds, and several lower vertebrates. Thus, the mouse *H-2* complex corresponds to the human *HLA* complex, to the *RhLA* complex in rhesus monkey, to the *DLA* complex in dog, to the *GPLA* complex in guinea pig, to the *RTl* complex in rat, and to the *B* complex in chicken. The genetic organization of these complexes appears to be extremely similar in all species thus far examined (with the possible exception of the mouse).

The elucidation of the *MHC* in terms of its phenotypic expression as well as function is based on the serological recognition and analysis of the cell surface molecules controlled by *MHC* genes. This serological and genetic analysis is performed in different ways depending upon the availability of inbred animals (for example, the mouse), or accessibility to outbred populations only (for example, man). The two different approaches will be discussed separately using the mouse as an example in which the analysis is based on inbred strains, and man in which the analysis is based upon population and family studies.

The Major Histocompatibility Complex (H-2) of the Mouse

Congenic Strains

Before we describe the mouse *MHC*, *H-2*, in terms of its serological properties, a brief summary on the laboratory mouse as used in these studies will follow.

Inbred strains are maintained by continuous brother–sister matings; after about twenty generations complete homozygosity for almost all alleles of the genome is achieved. In-

dividuals of an inbred strain are comparable to monozygous twins. An inbred strain differs in many alleles from other inbred strains or wild animals. If one of these alleles is a histocompatibility gene, one can determine the allogeneic difference by analysis of tumor or skin graft rejection and serological typing. If an allele donor strain (wild or inbred strain) A *(a/a)* is crossed with a background inbred strain B *(b/b)*, both genomes, *a* and *b*, will be "diluted" by half in the F_1 generation. Repeated crossing of the heterozygote *(a/b)* with the background strain B *(b/b)* and simultaneous selection for the allele H^a brings about in every subsequent generation a dilution of the A genome by half. In this way, after about 12 generations one has a mouse strain that has up to 99.999% the genome of the background strain B together with the H^a allele of the donor strain A (Fig. 6.1). Such a new inbred strain is now designated with the name of the background strain from which the genome originated (e.g., B 10) together with the symbol of the selected allele *(H-2ᵃ)*:

Production of H-2 complex congenic lines

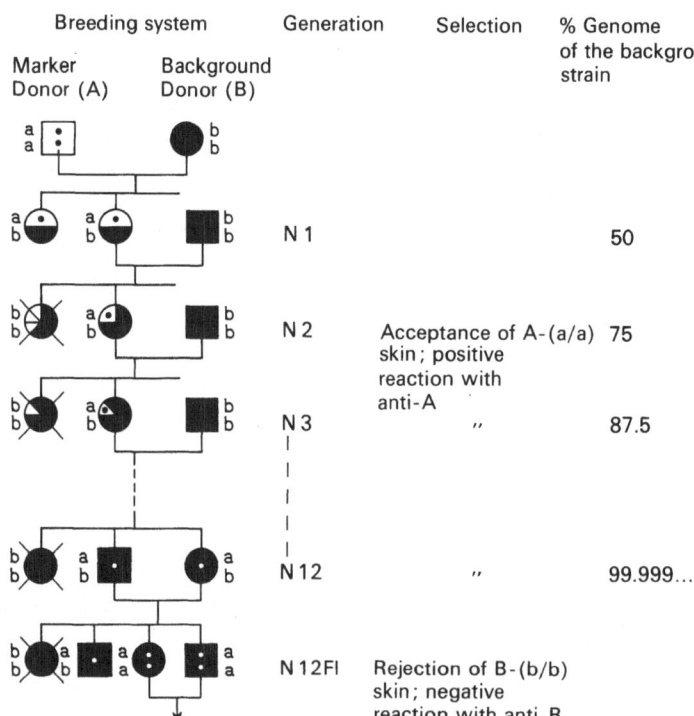

Fig. 6.1. Backcross system (NX) for the production of congenic strains of mice. Gen., backcross generation (N); A, donor strain; B, "background strain" (inbred); $a = H-2^a$; $b = H-2^b$, $H-2^a/H-2^b$ heterozygotes are selected through serotyping. [Modified from Klein J (1975) The biology of the mouse histocompatibility-2 complex. Springer, Berlin Heidelberg New York]

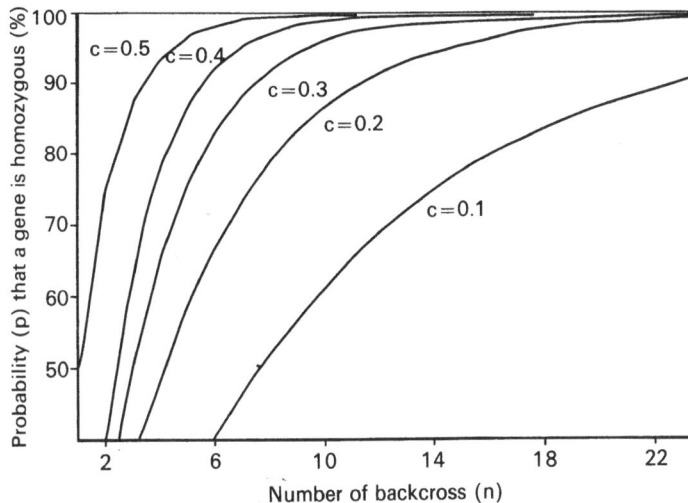

Fig. 6.2. Probability p (in percent) that any gene is homozygous if it is segregated from the selected gene ($c=0.5$) or is linked to the selected gene ($c=0.4$ to $c=0.1$), depending upon the number of backcrosses. Calculated according to the equation $p_n = 1 - (1-c)^{n-1}$, in which c is the recombination frequency and n, the number of backcrosses

B 10. $H\text{-}2^a$. This strain is $H\text{-}2$ congenic to B 10 (B 10. $H\text{-}2^b$); in a simpler form, only the allele symbol is written: B 10. A.

The degree of congeneity, i.e., the probability (p) that a desired gene will achieve homozygosity, can be calculated according to the equation,

$$p_n = 1 - (1-c)^{n-1}, \qquad (1)$$

where c is the recombination frequency between the H gene and any other gene and n, the number of backcrosses. To achieve homozygosity for all possible unlinked genes, 12 backcrosses are sufficient (Fig. 6.2.). However, to obtain homozygosity for all possible linked genes up to a distance of 10 recombination units, about 48 backcrosses are necessary (Fig. 6.2, curve $c=0.1$).

The most frequently used congenic inbred strains, together with their $H\text{-}2$ allele, donor strain, background strain, and inbred strains with the same $H\text{-}2$ type, are shown in Table 6.2.

Table 6.2. Some congenic inbred strains: H-2 haplotype, H-2 donor strain, background strain, and inbred strains with the same H-2 haplotype

Strain	H-2 type	H-2 donor	Background strain	Inbred strains with the same H-2 type
C57BL/10(B10)	b	C57BL/10(B10)	C57BL/10(B10)	129, C57BL/6 (B6), LP, A.BY, C3H.SW
B10.D2	d	DBA/2	B10	DBA/2, BALB/c
B10.A	a	A/WySn	B10	A/J
B10.M	f	Not inbred	B10	A.CA
B10.BR	k	C57BR	B10	C3H, CBA, AKR
B10.Q	q	DBA/1	B10	DBA/1, SWR
B10.RIII(71NS)	r	RIII	B10	RIII, LP.RIII
B10.S	s	A.SW	B10	A.SW, SJL
B10.PL	u	PL	B10	
A/WySn(A)	a	A/WySn	A/WySn(A)	A/J
A.BY	b	B10	A	C57BL/10, B6, 129, LP, C3H.SW
A.CA	f	Caracul	A	B10.M
A.SW	s	Swiss	A	B10.S, SJL

Serology

In the mouse, serology deals with planned immunizations using genetically uniform strains. The antisera obtained in such a reproducible way are then analyzed for their activity in such detail as to define as many antibodies as possible present in a given serum, and to establish all the determinants recognized by them. This is usually accomplished by testing the sera directly (hemagglutination, complement-dependent cytotoxicity test (see Chap. 7), after which absorption analysis with cells of all crossreacting strains is performed. This analysis is then followed by specifically designed mating experiments to establish linkage and, if possible allelism, of the genes coding for the detected determinants by segregation analysis.

Thus, let us consider an antiserum produced by immunization of an inbred strain B.B with tissue of another strain congenic to B (e.g., B.A). The B anti-A serum, which contains antibodies against alloantigens that are controlled by *H-2* genes, agglutinates or lyses (in the presence of complement) all cells that carry $H\text{-}2^a$ molecules. Using a large number of allogeneic strains, e.g., A, B, C, D, ..., etc., one will find that anti-A also reacts with cells from C, D, ..., etc. (crossreaction with determinants shared by molecules of different alleles). Selective absorption permits the detection of a complete spectrum of alloantigenic specificities (determinants) for the strains examined. For example, if the B anti-A serum reacts with cells of strains A, C, and D, one can assume the presence of at least one alloantigen, though more probably two or three. If after absorption with cells of C, the serum still reacts with A and D, it indicates that A and D cells possess a common alloantigen 1 which the cells of B animals (in which the serum was produced) and of C animals lack. If the serum still reacts with A and C cells after absorption with D cells, there is a second alloantigen 2 which is common to A and C cells but which the B and D cells lack; finally, if the reactivity against A cells re-

Table 6.3. Determination of antigenic determinants by cross-absorption

Reacting test cells	Reactivity of B anti-A serum after absorption with cells of				
	A	B	C	D	C+D
A (1, 2, 3)	–	+	+	+	+
B (0)	–	+	–	–	–
C (2)	–	+	–	+	–
D (1)	–	+	+	–	–

mains after the antiserum has been absorbed with C and D cells, it means that A cells have an alloantigen 3 that neither B, C, nor D cells carry. In the hypothetical example, B has none of the alloantigens, A has all three (1, 2, and 3), whereas C (antigen 2) and D (antigen 1) each have a different antigen in common with A (Table 6.3).

Using this scheme, one can choose all possible combinations to produce antisera and to analyze the sera by cross-absorption. Antigenic specificities (determinants) which can be detected on cells of the donor strain (against which the antiserum was produced) after the serum has been absorbed with cells of all cross-reacting strains, are called "private" antigens. These are characteristic for a specific *MHC (H-2)* allele when produced, analyzed, and applied within a limited test panel (here, A, B, C, and D). In our example, the private antigen for strain A is 3. Antigenic determinants found on cells of genetically different strains, i.e., cross-reacting antigens, are called "public" antigens (in our example, these are the antigens 1 and 2). The distinction between private and public determinants is only operational; in sufficiently large test panels, there is no difference in principle between these two types of determinants except that private determinants appear to occur less frequently than public determinants. In wild populations, private determinants are not characteristic of a specific allele; only sets of determinants define alleles.

***H-2 K,D* Genes: *Class I* Genes.** An accidental observation by Snell (1953) indicated that the *H-2* locus consisted not only of one gene. He observed that offspring of crosses between two strains of mice k/k and d/d accepted tumor grafts of a third inbred strain a/a, but that the parents of the k/d-F_1 hybrids did not. He explained this unexpected result with the hypothesis that the *H-2* locus consisted of two genes (*K* and *D*), and that the mice of strain a/a possessed one gene (*K*) from the k/k and the other (*D*) from the d/d parent, the combination being derived by recombination of the two chromosomes:

Mouse strain		
Phenotype	Genotype	
k/k	kk/kk	} Parents
d/d	dd/dd	
k/d	kk/dd	F_1 hybrid
a/a	kd/kd	recombinant

Since then, numerous additional recombinants for the *H-2* complex have been described. For historical reasons, one gene has kept the symbol *K*, and the other *D*. Different alleles are characterized by a small letter suffix with signifies the origin of the allele, e.g., the *K* allele of a b/b mouse is written K^b, the *D* allele D^b. The combination *K-D* is called a haplotype. Different haplotypes are indicated with small letters (e.g., $H-2^b$ represents the haplotype of a B10 mouse, $H-2^a$ the haplotype of an A or B10.A mouse, see Table 6.2. If such recombinant mouse strains are used to produce antisera, it can be shown that both genes control different alloantigens (K and D molecules, class I molecules, see p. 159), although both genes express a large number of shared determinants, e.g., each of the two genes controls one antigenic determinant that is typical for the specific *K* or *D* allele (private antigen), and several antigenic specificities that are shared by different *K* and/or *D* alleles (public specificities). The antigenic specificities are designated numerically in order of their detection, preceded by the designation of the encoding locus, for example K 33, D 2 (Table 6.4). Since the first description more

than 11 private K and 12 private D antigens have been found in standard inbred strains. When wild mice are typed with these reagents produced in inbred strain combinations, two remarkable results are obtained: first, the frequency of alleles encoding the different molecules is extremely low for all of them, in general below 2%; and second, the number of alleles which cannot be defined so far. is extremely high, i.e., more than 60% of the naturally occurring alleles are undetected by the available reagents. The number of alleles may turn out to be several hundred; we must keep in mind (see above) that the employed reagents do not truly characterize alleles. Thus, a molecule reacting with, say, anti-K 23, may not react with anti-K 25, a combination which defines the $H-2 K^k$ allele of the inbred strain against which the antisera had been produced. These numbers indicate a serological and molecular complexity and a genetic polymorphism unknown in any other genetic system (except antibody binding sites, see p. 91).

Immune Response Region Genes: *Class II Genes.* Specifically designed mating experiments between recombinants and inbred strains yielded new recombinants in which the new cross-over occurred between the *K* and *D* genes either extremely close to the *K* or near the *D* gene:

Mouse A.AL ($H-2^{al}$) × Mouse A.SW ($H-2^s$)

—K^k————D^d— =K^s====D^s=
—K^k————D^d— × =K^s====D^s=
                    ↓
        —K^k————D^d—
        =K^s====D^s=

—K^k— —D^d— | —K^k— —D^d—
=K^s= =D^s= | =K^s= =D^s=
      ↓ | ↓
=K^s——D^d— | =K^s——D^d—

Mouse A.TL ($H-2^{t1}$)   Mouse A.TH ($H-2^{t2}$)

When such recombinants having identical *K* and *D* alleles were reciprocally immunized, it was found, surprisingly, that the chromo-

Table 6.4. Antigen specificities of K and D molecules in inbred strains

Allele	Private	Public specificities																	
		3	5	8	11	25	34	35	36	37	38	39	42	45	46	47	52	53	54
H-2. K molecules																			
b	33	–	5	–	–	–	–	35	36	–	–	39	–	–	46	–	–	53	54
d	31	3	–	8	–	–	34	–	–	–	–	–	–	–	46	47	–	–	–
f	26	–	–	8	–	–	–	–	–	37	–	39	–	–	46	–	–	53	–
j	15	–	–	–	–	–	–	–	–	–	38	–	–	45	46	47	–	–	–
k	23	3	5	8	11	25	–	–	–	–	–	–	–	45	–	47	52	–	–
p	16	–	5	8	–	–	34	–	–	37	38	–	–	–	46	–	–	–	–
q	17	3	5	–	11	–	34	–	–	–	–	–	–	45	–	–	52	–	54
r	?	3	5	8	11	25	–	–	–	–	–	–	–	45	–	47	52	–	54
s	19	–	5	–	–	–	–	–	–	–	–	–	42	45	–	–	–	–	–
u	20	–	5	8	–	–	–	35	36	–	–	–	–	45	–	–	52	53	–
v	21	3	5	–	–	–	–	–	–	–	–	–	–	45	–	–	–	–	–

Allele	Private	Public specificities												
		3	6	13	35	36	41	42	43	44	49	50	51	55	56
H-2. D molecules														
b (j)	2	–	6	–	–	–	–	–	–	–	–	–	–	–	56
d (u)	4	3	6	13	35	36	41	42	43	44	49	50	–	–	–
f	9	–	6	–	–	–	–	–	–	–	–	–	–	–	56
k	32	3	–	–	–	–	–	–	–	–	49	–	–	–	–
p	22	3	6	–	35	–	41	–	–	–	49	–	–	–	–
q (v)	30	3	6	13	–	–	–	–	–	–	49	–	–	55	56
r	18	–	6	–	–	–	–	–	–	–	49	–	51	–	–
s	12	3	6	–	–	36	–	42	–	–	49	–	–	–	–

Table 6.5. Antigen chart of some specificities encoded at the $I-A$ locus (inbred strains)

H-2 Haplotype	Ia Antigens of the $I-A$ locus																						
	1	2	3	4	5	6	8	9	10	11	12	13	14	15	16	17	18	19	20	24	25	26	27
b	–	–	3	–	–	–	8	9	–	–	–	–	–	15	–	–	–	–	20	–	–	–	–
d	–	–	–	–	–	6	8	–	–	11	–	–	–	15	16	–	–	–	–	–	–	–	–
f	1	–	–	–	5	–	–	–	–	–	–	–	14	–	–	17	18	–	–	–	25	26	27
j	–	–	.	–	5	.	–	.	10	–	–	–	–	15	.	–	.	–	–	.	.	.	
k	1	2	3	–	–	–	–	–	–	–	–	–	–	15	–	17	18	19	–	–	25	26	–
p	–	–	–	–	5	6	–	–	–	–	–	13	–	–	–	–	–	–	–	.	.	.	.
q	–	–	3	–	5	–	–	9	10	–	–	13	–	–	16	–	–	–	–	–	–	–	–
r	1	–	3	–	5	–	–	–	–	–	12	–	–	–	–	17	–	19	–	24	25	26	–
s	–	–	–	4	5	–	–	9	–	–	12	–	–	–	–	17	18	–	–	24	–	–	27
u	1	–	.	–	5	.	–	.	–	–	–	–	–	–	.	17	.	–	–	24	.	.	.
v	–	–	.	–	5	.	8	.	–	–	–	–	–	15	.	–	.	–	–	.	.	.	.

somal section between the K and D genes also controlled alloantigens on the surface of cell membranes. Because genes of this region of the chromosome had already been characterized functionally, namely as genes that control the humoral immune response (*Im*mune *r*esponse genes, *Ir* genes), these genes were called *I* genes and the molecules that they control *I* region *a*ssociated (Ia) molecules (class II molecules, see p. 162). Thus far, two loci have been identified with serological methods: *I-A* which maps near the *K* locus, and *I-E* which is located to the right of *I-A*. Both loci are polymorphic with numerous antigen specificities designated by continuous numbers in order of their detection, preceded by the designation Ia (Table 6.5). Recent findings indicate that the *I-E* locus (and by analogy, the *I-A* locus) actually consists of two genes, E_α and E_β (and A_α and A_β), each encoding a polypeptide chain, which together form the membrane Ia molecule (see also p. 161). The E_α gene exists in two allelic forms, one expressing the E_α-polypeptide chain with the marker antigen Ia.7 (E_α^7), the other expressing no chain in the membrane (E_α^0). The E_β gene is highly polymorphic but is expressed only if combined with the E_α^7 allele, either in cis-position (linked on the same chromosome, recombinants) or in trans-position (located on the other chromosome, F_1 hybrids) (Table 6.6).

Ia molecules are characterized by two peculiarities that distinguish them both genetically and serologically from the K and D molecules: Ia molecules are found primarily on B lymphocytes and macrophages as well as stimulated T lymphocytes, but not in any other tissue.

Table 6.6. Ia determinants controlled by E_β and E_α loci

H-2 haplotype	E_β determinants[a]						E_α det.
	21	22	23	32	41	42	7
b	(–	22	–	32	.[b]	·)	0
d	–	–	23	–	–	–	7
j	.	.	.	32	–	–	7
k	–	22	–	32	–	42	7
p	21	–	–	32	–	–	7
q	(·	.	.	.	.	·)	0
r	–	–	–	32	–	–	7
s	(–	22	–	.	.	·)	0
u	.	.	.	32	–	–	7
v	.	.	.	32	41	42	7

[a] Determinants in parentheses are expressed on the cell surface only when the controlling E_β allele occurs in combination with the E_α^7 allele.
[b] Dot indicates unknown

The general terminology for the *I* region alleles corresponds to that of the *K* or *D* alleles, i.e., the *I* region of haplotype *H-2^a* is called *I^a*, that of the haplotype *H-2^b*, *I^b*. In recombinant haplotypes, the individual *MHC* loci are identified by the haplotype symbol of the parent strain from which they originate; e.g., for the previously described recombinant A.TL: *K^s-I^k-D^d* or *s k d = H-2^{t1}*, and A.TH: *K^s-I^s-D^d* or *s s d = H-2^{t2}*. The most common *H-2* recombinants, their origins, and the composition of their haplotypes are depicted in Table 6.7. The same numerical designation of alloantigens controlled by *K* and *D* genes indicates identical serological antigenic specificities; identical numerical designations for Ia antigens, however, characterize antigenic specificities that differ from those of the K and D antigens.

Linkage Analysis of the Mouse *H-2* Complex. On the basis of serologically determined phenotypes and corresponding breeding experiments, at least four genetic regions in the *MHC* of the mouse can be differentiated, linked in the following order: *K-I-S-D*. The *D* region consists of at least two loci, *D* and *L*, the order of which is unknown. The *L* gene product has been defined by capping (see p. 158) and a mutant *H-2^d* allele.

The *S* region also consists of at least two loci, the *Ss* (serum substance) gene, and the *Slp* (sex-limited protein) gene; the latter is expressed only in males within inbred strains – however, in wild mice it also occurs in females. The products of both genes are detectable in the serum and (passively?) attached to the membrane of erythrocytes. The *Ss* gene product has been shown to be the fourth complement component; the Slp substance has similar physicochemical properties, however, it is functionally not active as a complement component.

Within the *I* region, several loci can be identified: the *A*, the *A* locus (most probably three genes, A_{β_2}, A_{β_1} and A_α), the E_β locus, and the E_α locus.

Closely linked to the *H-2* complex are several genes which also control the expression of

Table 6.7. Examples of H-2 recombinant strains and their origin

F₁-hybrid origin	H-2 type	H-2 complex alleles K Aβ Aα Eβ Eα S D	New H-2 haplotype K Aβ Aα Eβ Eα S D	Strain	H-2 type
Xᵃ	k	k k k k 7 k k	k k k k|ᵇ 7 d d	B10.A	a
Y	d	d d d d 7 d d			
B10.A	a	k k k k 7 d d	b b b b | 7 d d	B10.A(5R)	i5
B10	b	b b b b 0 b b			
B10.A	a	k k k | k 7 d d	k k k | b 0 b b	B10.A(4R)	h4
B10	b	b b b | b 0 b b			
B10.A	a	k k k k 7 d | d	k k k k 7 d | b	B10.A(2R)	h2
B10	b	b b b b 0 b | b			
B10.A	a	k | k k k 7 d d	q | k k k 7 d d	B10.AQR	y1
T138	q	q | q q q 0 q q			
DBA/2	d	d d d d 7 d | d	k k k k 7 k | d	A.AL	a1
C3H	k	k k k k 7 k | k			
A.AL	a1	k | k k k 7 k d	s | k k k 7 k d	A.TL	t1
A.SW	s	s | s s s 0 s s			
A.AL	a1	k k k k 7 k | d	s s s s 0 s | d	A.TH	t2
A.SW	s	s s s s 0 s | s			
A.TL	t1	s k k k | 7 k d	s s s s | 7 k d	B10.HTT	t3
B10.S	s	s s s s | 0 s s			
B10.A	a	k k k k 7 d | d	s s s s 0 s | d	B10.S(7R)	t2
B10.S	s	s s s s 0 s | s			
A.TL	t1	s k k k 7 k | k	s k k k 7 k | f	A.TE	an1
A.CA	f	f f f f 0 f | f			
B10.AKR	k	k k k k 7 k | k	k k k k 7 k | q	B10.AKM	m
M	q	q q q q 0 q | q			
DBA/2	d	d d d d 7 d | d	d d d d 7 d | k	C3H.OH	02
C3H	k	k k k k 7 k | k			
DBA/2	d	d d d d 7 | d d	d d d d 7 | k k	C3H.OL	01
C3H	k	k k k k 7 | k k			

ᵃ The H-2 haplotype of B10.A was already existent before inbreeding; the parental strains of the F₁-hybrid are not known
ᵇ Bar designates position of cross-over

membrane components: the *Qa* loci and the *Tla* locus to the right of the *D* region. The former express molecules on subsets of B and T lymphocytes, the latter controls differentiation antigens on thymus cells. The relationship of these loci to the *H-2* complex proper is unclear.

To the left of the *K* locus is linked the *T/t*-complex, the genes of which control early ontogenic differentiation.

Several other genes syntenic to the *H-2* complex are also found in linkage with the *MHC*

in other species: *Glo* (glyoxalase), *Pgk* (phosphoglycerate kinase), *C3* (third complement component), *Pg-5* (urinary pepsinogen-5).

Cytogenetic studies of translocation indicated that the mouse *MHC* is localized on the seventeenth chromosome, and that the *K* locus lies nearer to the centromere than the *D* locus does (all chromosomes of the mouse inbred strains are acrocentric).

Figure 6.3 is a genetic map of the *H-2* complex. As will be evident, the gene structure of

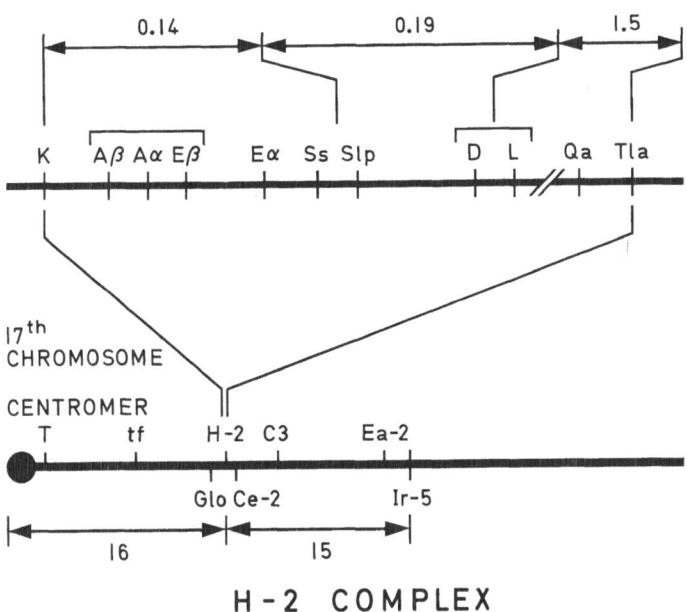

Fig. 6.3. Genetic map of the *H-2* complex and its vicinity. *T*, *T/t* complex (brachyury or short tail); *tf*, tufted; *Glo*, glyoxalase; *H-2*, major histocompatibility complex; *Ce-2*, kidney catalase; *C3*, complement component 3; *Ea-2*, erythrocyte antigen 2; *Ir-5*, immune response-5. The order of $A_\beta A_\alpha E_\beta$ and of *D, L* loci is not known. Also linked are: *Pgk-2*, phosphoglycerate kinase-2; *Apl*, acid phosphatase-liver; *Pg-5*, pepsinogen-5; *C3b*-receptor; *H-31; H-32; H-33;* and *H-39*

the *MHC* of the mouse differs from that of other species, including that of human: In the mouse, the *I* region is located between the two *H* loci, *K* and *D*; in all other species thus far examined, the genes that correspond to those included in the *I* region are found outside the *K* and *D* analogues. It is thought that the *K* and *D* genes originated by duplication of an ancestral gene during evolution and came to their present-day position by transposition.

The Major Histocompatibility Complex of Man (*HLA*)

Serological Typing

Leukocyte antigens (*HLA*), later defined as gene products of the human *MHC*, were first described by Dausset in 1956. Sera of patients who have had multiple transfusions and of multiparous women contain antibodies that agglutinate leukocytes and have specificity other than that exhibited by erythrocyte-agglutinating antibodies. It took almost ten years to discover that the leukocyte antigens were components of one

exceedingly complex genetic system: the human major histocompatibility complex.

Serological analysis of *HLA* molecules of a species consisting of outbred individuals only has to be performed differently from that of a species in which inbred strains are available, e.g., the mouse. In the outbred human population, no two unrelated individuals are genetically identical. Since genetic differences are also reflected in antigenic differences, antisera generated by immunization of an individual A by cells of an individual B will be unique. Although different antisera may contain antibodies to the same determinant(s), they will also contain antibodies to other determinants; and those other antibodies tend to obscure the determination of specificities. To analyze such antisera, it is necessary to apply a different approach from that used for the analysis described above of antisera produced in inbred mouse strains. Here, a large number of antisera has to be tested against a large panel of cells in order to find identical or antithetic reactivity patterns. The reactivity of each antiserum with each single cell of a large panel has to be compared with the reactivity of all other antisera individually. In order to find significant positive (identical reactivity) or negative (antithetical reactivity) associations of reactivity patterns, statistical methods are applied by first constructing a 2×2 contingency table, and then to determine the significance of the associations in this table by either the χ^2-test or the correlation coefficient test.

An example of such an analysis is given in Fig. 6.4. Here, van Rood and his colleagues analyzed the reactivity of 63 antisera with a panel of 40 individuals. The positive and negative reactions with each cell were compared with those of all others, i.e., that of lymphocyte 1 was compared with that of 39 others, that of lymphocyte 2 with the remaining 38, etc. In this way, 820 (20×41) independent comparisons had to be performed. Only for one pair were all reactions identical, and only four pairs showed 95% identical reactions.

Applying this approach and analyzing sera from multiparous women which contain antibodies against leukocyte antigens of the paternal haplotype transmitted to the children, it was possible to describe groups of antigens that acted as though they were controlled by alleles of the same gene (i.e., they never appeared together), and others that occurred together indicating that the products of at least two closely linked genes could be demonstrated. Family studies confirmed this contention of at least two genes: *HLA-A* and *HLA-B*. Studies in the past few years have shown that a third gene is located between *HLA-A* and *HLA-B* which controls membrane antigens, but which appears to be less polymorphic than the two others: *HLA-C*. With the help of monoclonal antibodies produced from hybridoma cells obtained by fusing spleen cells of mice immunized against human cells with myeloma cells, several additional antigens has been discovered of which the encoding genes are closely linked to *HLA-B*. At least four sets of genes has been defined with these reagents as well as biochemical and cellular analysis (see below): *HLA-DZ, HLA-DR, HLA-DQ* (formerly called *DC*), and *HLA-DP* (formerly called *SB*; these antigens has

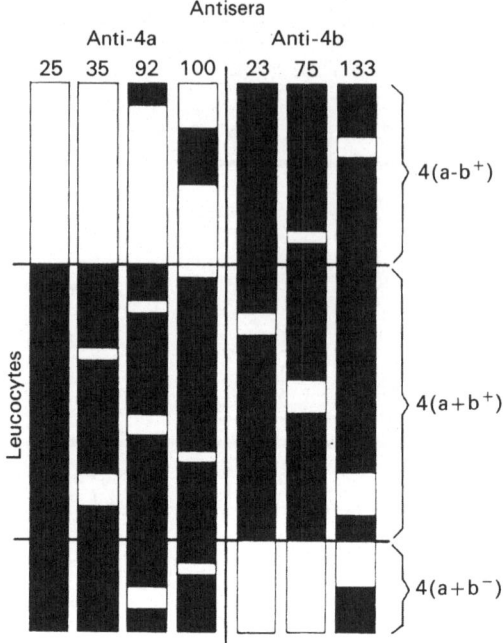

Fig. 6.4. Histogram of anti-4^a and anti-4^b reactions with leukocytes of a test panel (Van Rood)

been first detected by primary lymphocyte typing, see below). The whole region comprising these sets of genes is called *HLA-D*. It is the counterpart of the *I*-region of the mouse *H-2* system, whose determinants are called Ia (see p. 144) with *I-A* corresponding to *DQ* and *I-E* to *DR*, respectively.

To date, numerous HLA antigens have been identified on leukocytes; they represent the alleles of at least seven closely linked loci: *HLA-A* (formerly *first* or *LA* locus), *HLA-B* (formerly *second* or *FOUR* locus), *HLA-C* (formerly *third* or *Aj* locus), *HLA-DZ, HLA-DR, HLA-DQ* (formerly *DC*), and *HLA-DP* (formerly *SB*) (Table 66.8).

A part of the population that is not homozygous (which can be determined by family studies) cannot be characterized completely ("full house") for all alleles; this indicates that in addition to those already described, there are other alleles not yet identified by any antiserum ("blanks"). Furthermore, the more refined the serological analysis becomes, the more specificities are recognized

Table 6.8. Listing of recognized HLA specificities

A	B		C	D	DR	DQ	DPW1
A1	B5	BW48	CW1	DW1	DR1	DQW1	DPW1
A2	B7	B49	CW2	DW2	DR2	DQW2	DPW2
A3	B8	BW50	CW3	DW3	DR3	DQW3	DPW3
A9	B12	B51	CW4	DW4	DR4		DPW4
A10	B13	BW52	CW5	DW5	DR5		DPW5
A11	B14	BW53	CW6	DW6	DRW6		DPW6
AW19[a]	B15	BW54	CW7	DW7	DR7		
A23	B16	BW55	CW8	DW8	DRW8		
A24	B17	BW56		DW9	DRW9		
A25	B18	BW57		DW10	DRW10		
A26	B21	BW58		DW11	DRW11		
A28	BW22	BW59		DW12	DRW12		
A29	B27	BW60		DW13	DRW13		
A30	B35	BW61		DW14	DRW14		
A31	B37	BW62		DW15			
A32	B38	BW63		DW16	DEW52		
AW33	B39	BW64		DW17	DRW53		
AW34	B40	BW65		DW18			
AW36	BW41	BW67		DW19			
AW43	BW42	BW70					
AW66	B44	BW71					
AW68	B45	BW72					
AW69	BW46	BW73					
	BW47						
		BW4					
		BW6					

[a] w in front of the antigen notation indicates that the antigen was tested in a histocompatibility workshop but has not yet been recognized by the nomenclature committee of the World Health Organization (WHO)

as a group of specificities giving evidence for two or more antigens detected by a standard reagent (splitting). Thus, in the future, many more specificities will be added to the present chart.

Cellular Typing

Mixed Lymphocyte Culture Reaction. If lymphocytes of two unrelated individuals are cultivated together in vitro (mixed lymphocyte culture, MLC), after a few days (3–5) the culture contains lymphoblasts that are not observed when the cells of each person are cultivated individually for the same period of time. This transformation, from small lymphocytes to lymphoblasts, is called blast transformation. If ^{3}H-thymidine is added to the MLC after 3–4 days, it can be shown after an additional 16 h incubation

that the label has been incorporated into the DNA. These findings indicate not only that the lymphocytes are transformed but also that they synthesize new DNA, i.e., they proliferate. This entire process, transformation and proliferation, is called mixed lymphocyte reaction, MLR, and is, in the preceding example, a two-way reaction, because the lymphocytes of both individuals react.

This reaction occurs between lymphocytes only if they originate from histogenetically different individuals. It was thought originally that this reaction was caused by HLA-A and B antigens since there was a correlation of MLC reactivity and identity or disparity for HLA antigens in families. However, it was soon learned that A, B-identical lymphocytes of unrelated persons also exhibited strong MLC reactivity, i.e., they stimulated each other to transform and proliferate. Eventually, a family was found in which the lymphocytes of HLA-A and B-identical siblings exhibited MLC reactivity, indicating that the genes coding for HLA-A and -B molecules are different from those coding for lymphocyte-activating determinants (LAD) termed *HLA-D* gene(s).

If one of the reacting cell samples in the mixed lymphocyte culture is treated with mitomycin C or is irradiated with 2,500 R, these cells are no longer able to proliferate, but they are able to stimulate the untreated lymphocyte population to transform and proliferate. This set-up is called a "one-way reaction," and its use permits one to distinguish which of the two lymphocyte populations stimulates which. Applying this test, individual determinants can be defined.

Like the HLA-A, B, and C antigens, the membrane determinants responsible for the MLR are expressed codominantly, i.e., each individual has a maximum of two (if heterozygous) determinants on its lymphocytes. The testing of unrelated donors showed that there must be more than 20 allelic forms of this gene. Investigating selected families, one can in rare cases find persons who have inherited the same allele from both parents and are, therefore, *HLA-D* homozygous. Cells from this individual will stimulate all other cells that do not possess this allele; however, they will not stimulate those that carry the same allele in heterozygous or homozygous form (one-way stimulation) (Fig. 6.5). Using such homozygous typing cells (HTC), it is possible to characterize

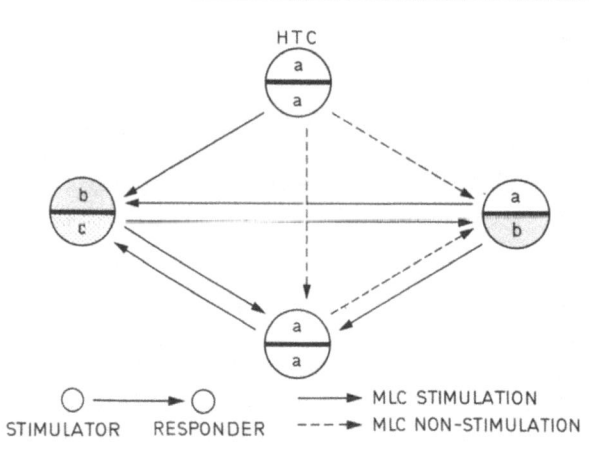

STIMULATOR RESPONDER

→ MLC STIMULATION

---→ MLC NON-STIMULATION

Fig. 6.5. Determination of HLA-D phenotype(s) with homozygous typing cells (HTC); a, b, and c represent *HLA-D* alleles

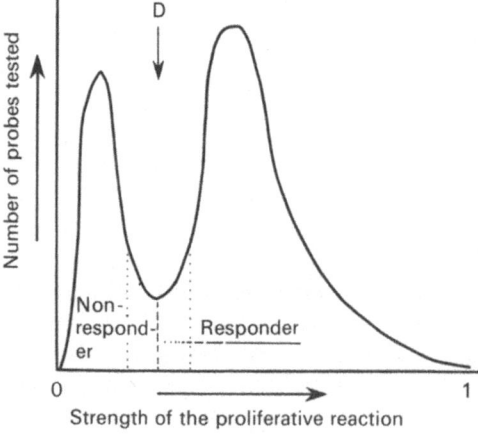

Fig. 6.6. MLR typing with homozygous reference cells as stimulator cells. D, discrimination value. Responder cells that exhibit a reaction <D are *nonresponders*, i.e., they have the *HLA-D* determinants of the reference cells; responder cells that exhibit a reaction >D are *responders*, i.e., they have *HLA-D* determinants that differ from those of the reference cells. D must be tested for each reference cell

other, unknown lymphocytes in terms of their HLA-D determinants by testing their ability to be stimulated by reference cells (Fig. 6.6). In this way, a number of homozygous reference cells with determinants HLA-Dw1 through Dw19 have been defined (Table 6.8).

The HLA-D phenotypic specificities defined by the mixed lymphocyte culture test with HTC's can not be clearly associated with one or the other of the *HLA-D* region subsets of products defined serologically or by PLT (see below). The HTCs are surely mixed reagents just like conventional alloantisera and the MLC responses are just like mixed serological reactions. They may detect mainly HLA-DR and HLA-DP determinants. For this reason, specificities defined by HTCs are designated HLA-Dw (w for workshop, i.e. the designation is provisional).

Primed Lymphocyte Typing. Fritz Bach first introduced primed lymphocyte typing (PLT) in 1975 as a means to accelerate cellular tissue typing for HLA-D. Responder cells were incubated with phenotypically HLA-A,B,C identical but HLA-D disparate stimulator cells treated with mitomycin or irradiation. After 10 days in culture, only stimulated responder cells survived. If these cells were incubated again with cells of unknown HLA-D type, only those which possessed an HLA-D type identical to the original stimulator cells provoked a secondary response; those which had an HLA-D antigen different from the original stimulator cell had no effect (no re-stimulation). Using a set of responder cells stimulated primarily by cells with different HLA-D type, HLA-D typing could be performed within 48 hours.

In 1980, S. Shaw could demonstrate, however, that this reaction was not exclusively related to HLA-D differences. Using HLA-A,B,C, *and* D identical responder-stimulator combinations, he found evidence for a new segregant series of B cell antigens (DP antigens, see p. 149) responsible for the stimulation.

Genetics

The genetic analysis of the HLA system is based on two factors: population and family studies.

In the genetic sense, a population is not only a group of individuals, but also a self-reproducing group whose gene constitution is described in terms of gene frequency. This frequency can be calculated from the corresponding phenotype frequency by direct counting of individuals that have a specific phenotype and division of the sum by the number of individuals in the population (in case of dominant genes). The frequency is expressed as a percentage. For example, we have two alleles, *A* and *B*, which present three phenotypes (genotypes): *AA*, *AB*, and *BB* (2%, 19%, and 79%, respectively). Because each individual has two genes, the percentages for *A* and *B* are: $2+9.5=11.5$ or $9.5+79=88.5$, i.e., the frequency of *A(p)* and *B(q)* is $p+q=0.115+0.885=1$.

In an ideal, large, panmictic population, in which the factors of migration, mutation, and selection play no role, there is a state of genetic equilibrium; i.e., genotype, as well as gene frequency, is constant from one generation to another. This characteristic is described by the Hardy-Weinberg theorem, expressed in the equation

$$(p+q)^2 = p^2 + 2\,pq + q^2 , \tag{2}$$

in which p and q are the gene frequencies of *A* and *B*. The gene frequency (p_A) can be calculated from the frequency of the phenotype frequency (f_A) with the help of equation (2), if $q=(1-p)$ is substituted (because $p+q=1$, see above):

$$f_A = p_A^2 + 2\,p_A(1-p_A) = 2\,p_A - p_A^2$$
$$1 - f_A = 1 - 2\,p_A + p_A^2 = (1-p_A)^2 \tag{3}$$
$$p_A = 1 - \sqrt{1-f_A}.$$

Linkage Equilibrium. According to the Hardy-Weinberg theorem, two conclusions can be drawn: (1) after one generation, the genotype of a gene with two alleles (A and B) will be present with a frequency of

p^2 AA:2 pq AB:$q^2 BB$, and (2) the frequency distribution will not change during the next generations, i.e., the population remains in equilibrium.

These conclusions apply to all autosomal gene loci, as long as they are considered individually. If two or more gene loci are considered at the same time , a state of equilibrium is not achieved after one generation. For example, in a population with the same number of $A_1 A_1 B_1 B_1$ and $A_2 A_2 B_2 B_2$ individuals (A and B are two loci each with alleles A_1 and A_2 or B_1 and B_2), the gene frequency for the two loci is then one-half, and from the nine possible genotypes, only one will appear after the first generation $(A_1 A_2 B_1 B_2)$. The others will appear in the subsequent generations, however, not exactly in equilibrium frequency. If one represents the frequency of each gene A_1, A_2, and B_1, B_2 with r, s, t, and u (r+s+t+u=1) and the frequency of the four gamete combinations: $A_1 B_1$, $A_1 B_2$, $A_2 B_1$, and $A_2 B_2$ with x_1, x_2, x_3, and x_4, whereby $x_1 + x_2 + x_3 + x_4 = 1$ and $r = x_1 + x_2$, $s = x_3 + x_4$, $t = x_1 + x_3$, and $u = x_2 + x_4$, then the population reaches equilibrium when $x_1 x_4 = x_2 x_3$. The difference, Δ,

$$\Delta = x_1 x_4 - x_2 x_3 \qquad (4)$$

describes the magnitude of the deviation from equilibrium, i.e., the magnitude of a linkage disequilibrium or a gametic association. The time necessary to achieve equilibrium is dependent upon the linkage relationship between the two genes and the initial value of Δ; if the two genes are not linked, Δ is halved with each generation. If both genes are linked, the value of Δ likewise decreases, but is dependent on the recombination frequency between A and B, according to the equation

$$\Delta_n = \Delta_0 (1 - rf)^n \rightarrow 0, \text{ if } n \rightarrow \infty, \qquad (5)$$

where Δ_0 is the initial value, Δ_n the Δ value after the nth generation, n the number of generations, and rf the recombination frequency in a generation. The smaller rf is,

the longer it will take until an equilibrium ($\Delta = 0$) is reached.

Linkage disequilibrium can occur in various ways: (1) migration, i.e., two populations with different gene frequencies, each of which is in equilibrium, mix; (2) selection, i.e., specific haplotypes (or alleles) have above all an advantage (disadvantage) for the survival of a population; and (3) gene drift, i.e., chance fluctuations of gene frequencies from one generation to another.

Haplotypes. If there is equilibrium, linked genes exhibit a basic difference in their behavior in families and populations. In a family, linked genes (haplotypes) show a "linkage association," whereas in the population no association is observed. If there is disequilibrium (which, with only a few exceptions, is the case in the human population), one can discover favored associations in population studies that would not be observed from family studies. Haplotype frequencies can be calculated using Δ according to the equation

$$x_{ij} = p_i P_j + D_{ij}, \qquad (6)$$

where p_i is the frequency of the allele i of the A locus, P_j the frequency of the allele j of the B locus, and D_{ij} the linkage association (see eq. 4 and Table 6.9) between the alleles. As shown in Table 6.9, there are several haplotypes in the North American population that do not occur in proportion to the fre-

Table 6.9. Significant associations of *HLA-A* and *-B* alleles in the North American population. Bodmer et al. 1977

Haplotype	Frequency	Δ value
A1 – B8	67.9	59.2
A3 – B7	38.0	27.6
A25 – B18	8.3	7.5
A26 – Bw38	10.0	9.2
A26 – Bw21[a]	11.4	10.3
A28 – B14	13.3	12.7
Aw30 – B18	7.2	7.2
Aw32 – Bw35[a]	13.5	13.0

[a] Significant among North American Blacks

quency of the alleles of both genes, but rather more frequently. Of these, the *HLA-A1-B8* haplotype occurs most frequently and is the characteristic haplotype for a Caucasian population.

Closely linked genes (with an rf between the loci of 0.001) are generally observed inherited as "one" gene in family studies, and different phenotypic characteristics of both genes can therefore be viewed incorrectly as being controlled by the same gene. Genetic studies of populations can uncover the difference between the gene and its linkage. Thus, family studies of the genetics of reactivity in a mixed lymphocyte culture clearly show that the genes responsible for the mixed lymphocyte culture are apparently identical to those that control the expression of the HLA-A and HLA-B antigens, because both characteristics are transfered together. Population studies, i.e., studies of the reactivity of lymphocytes of unrelated donors who were HLA-A and HLA-B identical, disclosed that *HLA-D* represents a different gene, which then could be proved by the finding of recombinant haplotypes in family studies.

Linkage Analysis of the HLA Complex

Until recently, linkage analyses in man were difficult, and with the exception of the sex chromosome-linked genes, few linkage groups were known. In the last few years, it has been possible, due to progress in somatic genetics and cell hybridization [1], to analyze linkage groups on autosomal chromosomes. The *HLA* complex forms a linkage group with phosphoglucomutase-3 (PGM-3), glyoxalase (GLO), and urine-pepsinogen-5 (Pg-5) on the short arm of the sixth chromosome. Analysis of recombinant haplotypes in families and gene cloning experiments

have shown that the loci of the *HLA* complex are linked in the order *HLA-DP—DQ—DR—DZ—C2—Bf—C4B—21OH—C4A—21OH'—B—C—Transferrin—A—* with the centromere at the left.

DP genes has been discovered by using primed lymphocytes as responding cells to HLA-A,B,C and D identical stimulator cells. *C2*, *C4B* and *C4A* control the expression of the respective complement components with the allotypes Chido and Rogers for C4. *Bf* controls the expression of factor B of the alternative pathways of complement. Also located within this chromosomal segment are the encoding genes for two adrenal 21-hydroxylase enzymes (*21OH* and *21OH'*) as well as the encoding gene for transferrin. Family studies also revealed that the loci controlling susceptibility for specific diseases are located between the *HLA-B* and *HLA-D* locus: *DS* genes (Disease Susceptibility) for the diseases multiple sclerosis (MS), Bechterew's disease (ankylosing spondylitis, AS), and celiac disease (CD), as well as others (see below, pp. 176). Another gene closely linked to *HLA* is that which regulates the immune response to pollen grain antigen (antigen E), and which is responsible for several asthmatic reactions. The data are summarized in Fig. 6.7.

Major Histocompatibility Complex of Other Species

The gene structure of MHC is similar for all species of animals examined thus far (Fig. 6.8). In addition to the two species already discussed at length, man and mouse, the following species have been studied in some detail: primates, particularly rhesus monkey and chimpanzee, cattle, horse, pig, dog, sheep, guinea pig, rabbit, rat, and among the birds, the chicken. Analysis of *MHC* in primates, dogs, and cattle were carried out by family and population studies, those in the other mentioned animals with the help of inbred strains. In primates

---

1 By this method, cells of different species are fused; after passage of such hybrid cells, chromosomes from one parent are usually lost. Parallel to the loss of certain chromosomes, certain phenotypic markers disappear. It is, therefore, possible to assign the genes of these markers to specific chromosomes which are, in turn, identified by banding patterns

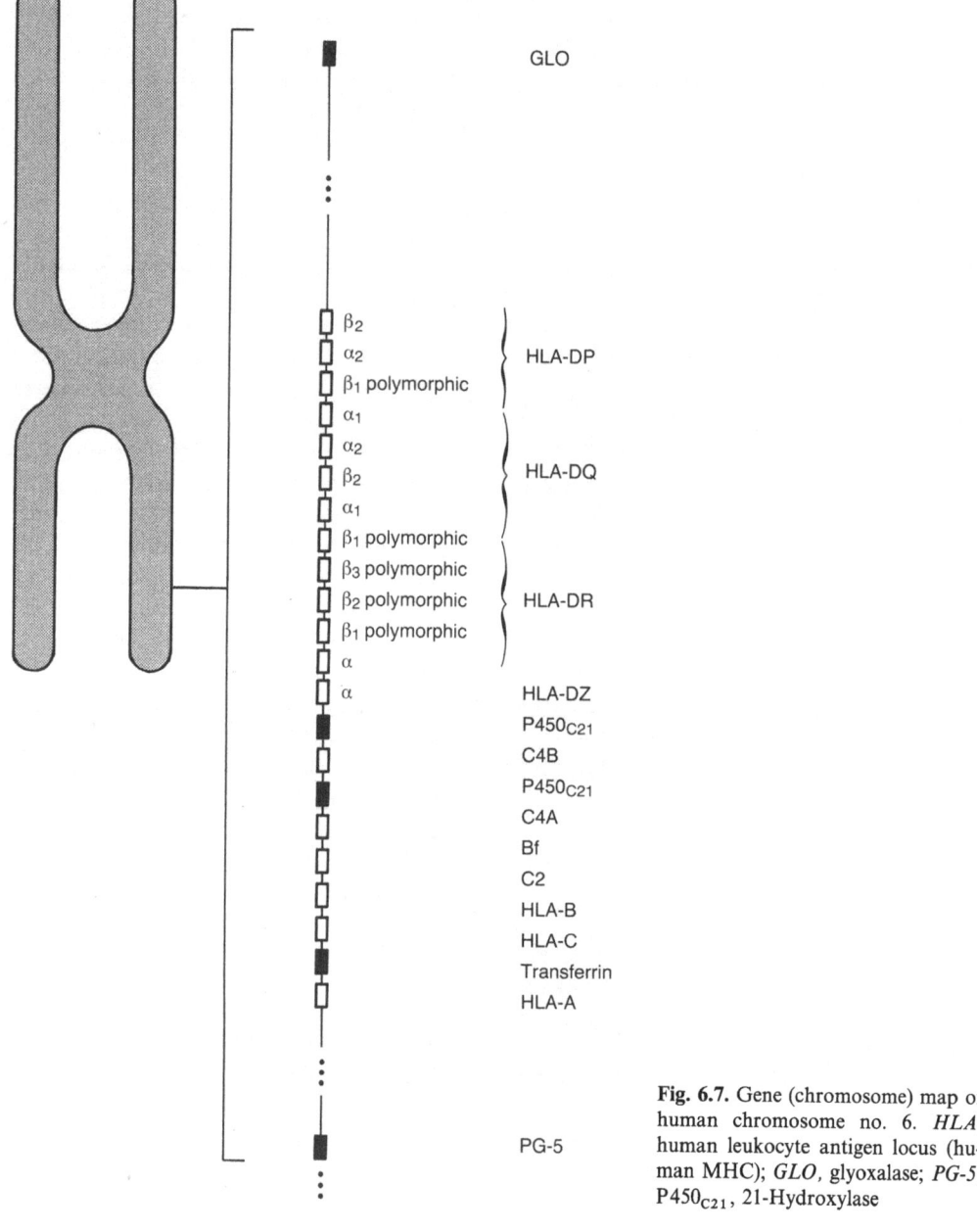

Fig. 6.7. Gene (chromosome) map of human chromosome no. 6. *HLA*, human leukocyte antigen locus (human MHC); *GLO*, glyoxalase; *PG-5*, $P450_{C21}$, 21-Hydroxylase

and dogs, two loci could be distinguished which control cell surface antigens like *HLA-A* and *B* or *H-2 K* and D, and one locus that controls reactivity in mixed lymphocyte culture like *HLA-D*. In the cattle, pig, and chicken, only two loci have thus far been found with certainty, one that controls reactivity in MLC, and one that codes for serologically detectable cell surface antigens like *HLA-A,B* or *H-2 K,D*. In the guinea pig and rat, it could be shown by biochemical methods that also here there are at least two genes controlling the expression of antigens analogous to the mouse K and D molecules. Furthermore, in the rat, two loci have been identified by their products which are analogous to the mouse *I-A* and *I-E* locus, respectively.

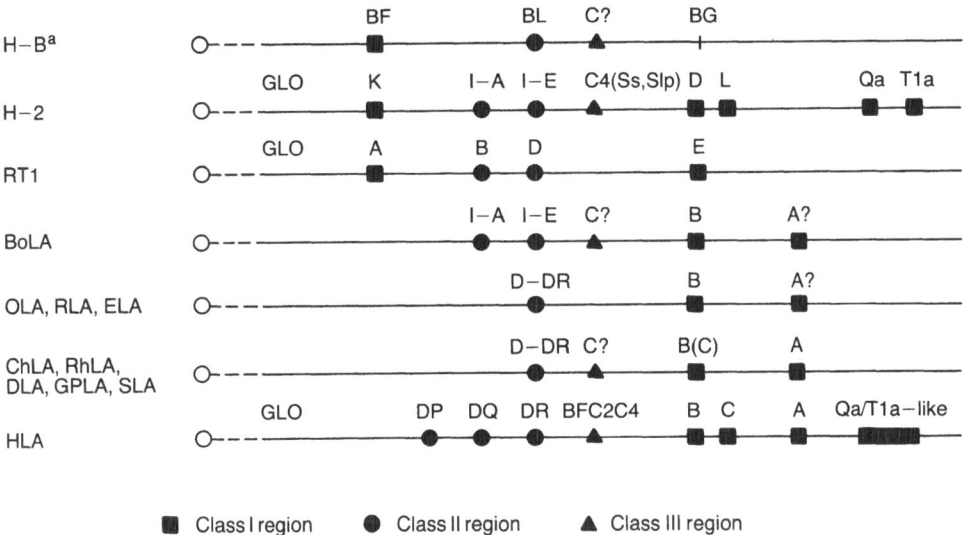

Fig. 6.8. Genetic organization of major histocompatibility complexes

[a] H-B, chicken; H-2, mouse; RT1, rat; BoLA, cattle; OLA, sheep; RLA, rabbit; ELA, horse; ChLA, chimpanzee; RhLA, rhesus monkey; DLA, dog; GPLA, guinea pig; SLA, swine; HLA, human.

In most of these species, genes were demonstrated which appear to be closely linked to the *MHC* and control the immune response (*Ir* genes) against certain antigens; in most cases in which a linkage order could be established, these genes are closely linked to or are identical to those controlling the mixed lymphocyte reactivity.

In the rhesus monkey and dog, the gene controlling the expression of the C3 proactivator (factor B) has been also shown to be linked to the *MHC*; the same has been found to be true for the gene controlling the expression of C4 in guinea pigs.

Tissue Distribution of MHC Molecules

Molecules whose phenotypic expression is controlled by *MHC* genes are demonstrable in different concentrations on different tissue cells. Detailed studies on this topic were carried out in the mouse. It is generally accepted that *K* and *D* molecules are present on all tissue cells with the exception of trophoblasts and the chorionic membrane. H-2 antigens were shown on embryos after the fourth day (late blastocyst); and HLA antigens were found also on human fetal tissue. The tissue distribution of MHC antigens is summarized in Table 6.10.

However, the concentration of MHC antigens varies noticeably for individual tissues: Liver cells exhibited only ca. 20%, kidney tissue ca. 5%, skeletal muscle tissue 0.5%, and brain cells only ca. 0.1% of the amount found on lymphatic cells. Erythrocytes also possess only a small amount of H antigen; mouse erythrocytes have about 10% in comparison to lymphatic cells, and human erythrocytes have considerably less.

I gene products (Ia antigen) exhibit restricted tissue distribution. They can best be demonstrated on lymphocytes, particularly on B lymphocytes; they are, however, also demonstrable on T lymphocytes (particularly on stimulated T lymphocytes), macrophages (and their tissue specific forms such as monocytes, Langerhans cells in the epidermis, Kupffer cells in the liver), and spermatozoa. They have not been found on thymus cells (provided they are unstimulated), nor on any other tissue studied thus far.

	H-2				HLA-			
	K	I	S	D	A	C	B	D
B lymphocytes	+	+	−	+	+	+	+	+
T lymphocytes	+	(+)ᵃ	−	+	+	+	+	(+)
Thymus cells	+	(+)ᵃ	−	+	+	+	+	·
Macrophages	+	+	+	+	+	·	+	+
Granulocytes	·	·	·	·	+	·	+	−
Reticulocytes	+	·	·	+	+	·	+	·
Erythrocytes	+	−	−	+	+	·	+	−
Thrombocytes	+	−	·	+	+	+	+	−
Fibroblasts	+	−	+	+	+	+	+	−
Endothelial cells	+	·	·	+	+	·	+	+
Epidermal cells	+	+	−	+	+	·	+	+
Liver	+	−	·	+	+	·	+	−
Kidney	+	−	·	+	+	·	+	−
Cardiac muscle	+	−	·	+	+	·	+	−
Skeletal muscle	+	−	·	+	+	·	+	−
Brain	+	−	·	+	(−)	·	(+)	·
Placenta	+	·	·	+	+	·	+	·
Spermatozoa	+	+	−	+	+	·	+	+
Ova	(+)	·	−	(+)	(+)	·	·	·
Trophoblasts	−	·	·	−	(+)	·	(+)	·
Blastocysts	+	·	·	+	·	·	·	·
Embryo	+	·	·	+	+	·	+	·

Table 6.10. Tissue distribution of antigens whose phenotypic expression is controlled by genes of the *H-2* or *HLA* complex

+ = present; − = absent; · = not tested; ( ) = demonstrable in extremely small amounts or only by absorption or conflicting results
ᵃ Clearly demonstrable on conA-stimulated (and allogen-stimulated) T (thymus) cells

The antigens are distributed evenly over the cell surface. By "capping" experiments (see below), it was shown that K, D, and Ia antigens are present on the membrane independently of each other (Fig. 6.9). In these experiments, the cells were first incubated with an antiserum that reacted specifically with the antigen of a locus, e.g., with the K antigen. After incubation at room temperature for 30 min, the serum was rinsed off and the cells were incubated with an antimouse Ig - serum to completely "cap" the K antigen. After an additional 30 min incubation (room temperature) the cells were washed and divided into several aliquots. The following steps were carried out at 0 °C: One aliquot was reincubated with the previously used antiserum; the other aliquots were incubated with an anti-H-2 D and an anti-Ia serum respectively. Finally, after washing

out the second antiserum, the cells were once again incubated with fluorescein-labeled antimouse-Ig (from goat or rabbit). After washing, the labeled cells were examined under a fluorescence microscope. Cells that were incubated twice with the same antiserum (anti-K) showed no label, whereas cells that in the second step were incubated with anti-H-2D or anti-Ia serum exhibited fluorescence, i.e., antigens that had bound antibodies of the first serum and were complexed by the anti-Ig serum on the membrane were pinocytosed and had not reappeared on the cell surface. On the other hand, antigens that were structurally independent of the K antigen were still demonstrable on the cell membrane. By the same method, public and private antigenic determinants have been shown to be on the same molecule.

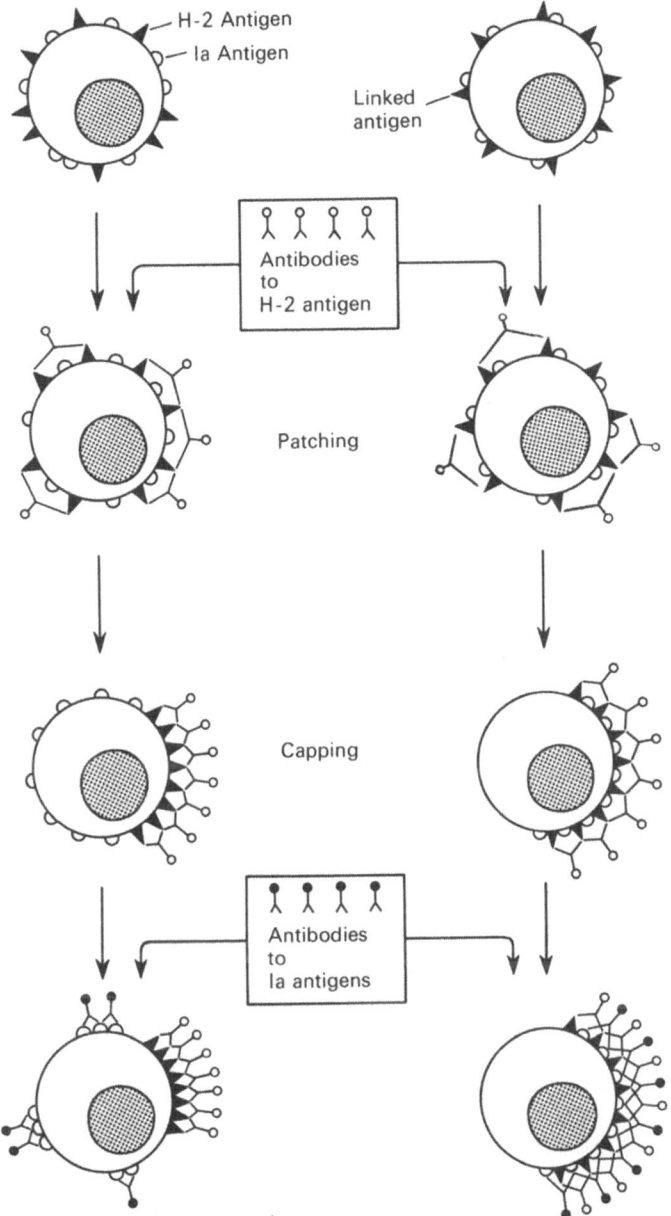

H-2 Antigen
Ia Antigen

Linked antigen

Antibodies to H-2 antigen

Patching

Capping

Antibodies to Ia antigens

Fig. 6.9. Schematic representation of capping

Biochemistry of MHC Molecules

Elucidation of the biochemical structure of molecules controlled by genes of the *MHC* was considerably impeded because they are integrated into the cell membrane and as such are not soluble in aqueous solutions. Cell membranes consist of a double layer of fatty acids and phospholipids whose polar groups are directed toward the inner and outer surfaces and whose nonpolar groups are pointed toward the interior of the membrane. The arrangement of the proteins on or in this layer can be imagined according to the model developed by Singer and Nicholson in 1972, in which the globular proteins "swim" in the double layer and have contact either with one surface or with both

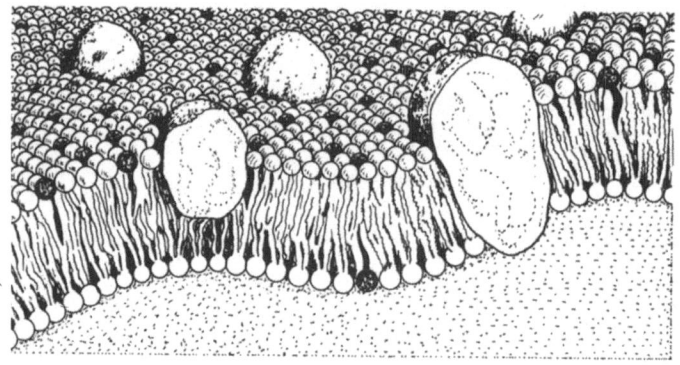

Fig. 6.10. "Fluid mosaic" membrane model according to Singer and Nicolson. Proteins swim like icebergs in the lipid-cholesterol double layer. [Singer SJ (1973) Architecture and topography of biological membranes. Hosp Prac 8:31–90]

(Fig. 6.10); they are kept stabilized in the membrane by hydrophobic sections in their structure immersed in the lipid phase.

The pioneering work on MHC biochemistry was done in the late 1960s by R.A. Reisfeld and his colleagues as well as S. Nathenson and his collaborators. Nathenson is credited with two methods that are in general use today: 1. Solubilization of membrane proteins by careful digestion of the cell membrane with papain, a proteolytic enzyme; and 2. Solubilization of membrane components, previously labeled with radioactive markers (either by external iodination with lactoperoxidase, or by internal labeling with ^{3}H- or ^{14}C-labeled amino acids) using a nonionic detergent, NP 40.

The detergent solubilized material is then ultracentrifuged. The MHC molecules are enriched by passing the preparation through a column of Sepharose B4 to which lentil lectin (a plant protein that binds sugars like glucose and mannose) is coupled. Since MHC molecules are glycoproteins they are retained on the lectin; after all not-bound proteins have been washed out, the MHC molecules are eluted with α-methyl mannoside. The MHC molecules in the partially purified fraction are then reacted with specific alloantisera. The complexes of MHC molecules with antibodies are precipitated with either a second antiserum (from rabbits or goats) specifically reacting with mouse immunoglobulins, or staphylococcus aureus–protein A which binds to the Fc portion of most mammalian IgG. The precipitate is then isolated by centrifugation,

and the MHC molecules are released from the complex by boiling in sodium dodecyl-sulfate (SDS) in the absence (non-reducing condition) or the presence (reducing condition) of 2-mercaptoethanol. The MHC molecules are separated from the immunoglobulins by SDS-polyacrylamide electrophoresis.

Class I Molecules:
H-2 K, D, L and HLA-A, B, C Molecules

With these two methods, the following results were obtained for the molecules K, D, and L, and HLA-A and B: After digestion with papain, a soluble component with a molecular weight of about 45,000 daltons or two components with molecular weights of about 34,000 and 12,000 daltons were obtained. If the purified molecules are dissolved in urea and analyzed either in this form or after reduction and alkylation by SDS-polyacrylamide electrophoresis, one finds two forms: a fraction with a molecular weight of 34,000 daltons and another with a molecular weight of 11,500 daltons. This finding leads to the conclusion that these molecules consist of two polypeptide chains held together by non-covalent bonds.

If H-molecules are isolated with detergent NP 40, different relationships are found. After being dissolved in urea, one finds, after SDS electrophoresis, two fractions with molecular weights of 45,000 and 11,500 daltons. If the larger protein is digested with papain, one obtains one piece of 34,000 daltons and one of ca. 12,000.

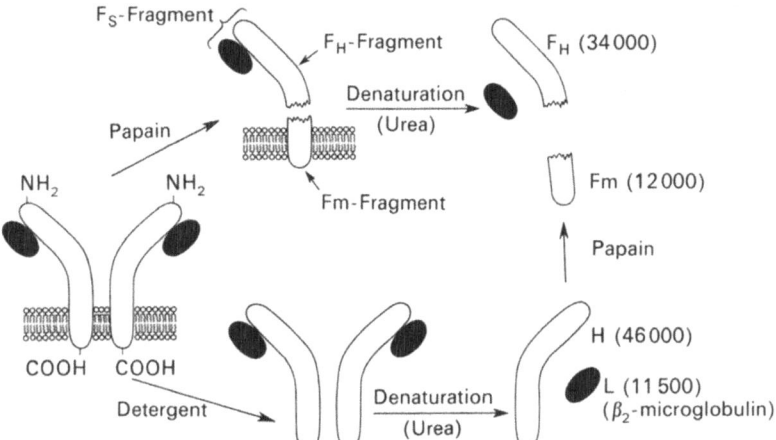

Fig. 6.11. Molecular structure of class I molecules (K,D or HLA-A,B): Solubilization with detergent (NP 40) yields a dimer composed of two heavy chains (H) and two light (β_2-microglobulin) chains. Solubilization through papain digestion yields a monomer (*Fs*, soluble fragment) of a shortened heavy chain and the light β_2-microglobulin chain (together their mol. wt. is 46,000 daltons). A polypeptide fragment of mol. wt. 10,000–12,000 daltons (*Fm*, membrane fragment) remains in the membrane

These findings yield the following picture of the structure of H molecules (Fig. 6.11): They are transmembrane glycoproteins with a molecular weight of 45,000 daltons (heavy chain), non-covalently associated with a large polypeptide (Fs = soluble fragment) of about 11,500 daltons (light chain). A polypeptide fragment of about 12,000 daltons can be cleaved from the heavy chain by papain. This fragments (Fm = membrane fragment) appears to remain in the membrane after isolation of the H molecule by papain digestion. The larger polypeptide, ca. 34,000 daltons, (F_H = heavy fragment) concists of a 30,000-dalton protein portion to which sugar is bound. According to Strominger, the polypeptide contains four half-cystines that form two intramolecular loops via S–S bridges. The light, 11,500-dalton chain can be characterized serologically as a protein that is also present in serum: β_2-microglobulin (β_2-MG). β_2-microglobulin has no H-antigen specificity; however, it appears to be important for the occurrence of the H molecule on the cell surface. In fact, it was discovered that tranformed cells that grow in suspension culture and exhibit no H molecule on their cell surface (Daudi cells) also have no β_2-MG. If

such cells are hybridized with other cells that normally have β_2-MG on their membranes, Daudi's own H-antigens whose specificity is known from the donor of the Daudi cells are expressed on the hybrids. A particularly exciting finding was the realization that β_2-MG had an unexpected high homology to certain C domains (see Chap. 4) of immunoglobulins; this homology concerns not only the amino-acid sequence, but also the number and position of two half-cysteines, both of which correspond exactly to the immunoglobulin domains. MHC molecules are cleaved with bromcyan or trypsin and the peptide mixture thus obtained is separated into two dimensions by thin-layer chromatography, the peptide divides in a characteristic manner. A comparison of MHC molecules of different serologic specificities indicates that they differ in up to 50% of their peptides. Using refined methods, primary structure (amino-acid sequence) analysis can be carried out on MHC molecules isolated by immunoprecipitation. It is evident from a comparison of the sequences of different K and D alleles of mouse-H, and human-H antigens, that there is considerable concordance in the primary structure; H-2K and H-2D molecules differ in approximately 35% to 45% of their amino acid residues, whereby neither K or D molecules exhibit a typical sequence; HLA molecules (A, B) differ in still fewer amino-acid residues: 5–10%. Even in a comparison of HLA-A, B and H-2K, D molelcules, about 40% of the amino-acid residues are identical; three positions appear particularly conservative. These findings clearly indicate a close relationship of the MHC products. Complete sequence data are only available for a few alleles of the H-2K and HLA-A and -B molecules. However, they indicate that there are three stretches of the primary structure that differ in 60% of more of their amino acids in different alleles, whereas the remainder part of the polypeptide chain shows only 10% or less variation. The highly variable areas are between the positions 65 and 80, and between 105 and 115. These areas are considered to be exposed to the outside and to represent the sites which are recognized by immune cells. On the other hand, the sequences within the disulfide loop including the residues 181–271 are totally conserved; this part of the sequence is homologous to Ig constant domains and β_2-MG.

HLA-C molecules are also studied using immunoprecipitation and they do not appear to differ from HLA-A, B molecules in their physico-chemical characteristics. Structural studies have not yet been carried out.

Class II Molecules:
I and *HLA-D* Region Molecules

Mouse I Region. Mouse Ia molecules (controlled by the *A* and *E* locus) are also glycoproteins and are composed of two polypeptide chains with molecular weights of about 32,000 and 28,000 daltons, termed α and β (i.e. $A_\alpha A_\beta$ and $E_\alpha E_\beta$). The molecules are not associated with β_2-microglobulin. Peptide mapping and N-terminal amino acid sequencing have provided the following information: The four murine chains A_α, A_β,

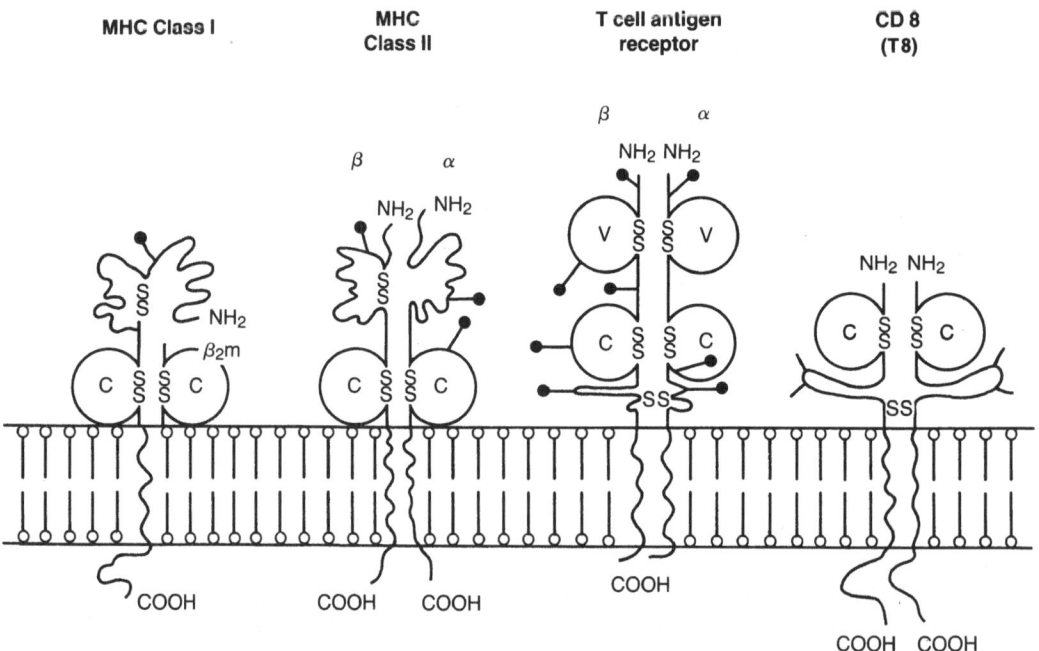

Fig. 6.12. Models for molecules found on T lymphocytes. Circles indicate segments related to domains with similarity to a *V* (variable) or *C* (constant) domain folding pattern. Double S symbols indicate possible positions of disulphide bounds but these are established only for MHC class I molecules. N-linked carbohydrate structures(●-) are determined by positions of AsnX Thr or Ser in the protein sequence. (Modified from Nature 314:579, 1985)

E_α, and E_β are not homologous to one another or to H molecules. Murine A_α and A_β are homologous to human DQ molecules; murine E_α and E_β are homologous to human DR (and rat Ia_α and Ia_β). The A and E α-chains of different alleles appear to differ only in a few amino acids or about 10% of their peptides. The A as well as E β-chains, however, show between 10% and 45% allelic variations.

Human *HLA-D* Region Molecules. There are at least three well defined subsets of products of the *HLA-D* region: HLA-DR, HLA-DQ (previously DC), and HLA-DP (previously SB).
Each product consists of a non-covalently associated combination of an α- and a β-chain. The α- and β-chains are substantially different from each other, and there is a evidence for at least five different α-gene products and seven different β-gene products in the *HLA-D* region. These genes appear to be arranged in subsets corresponding to the three subsets of products, where α- and β-chain products within a subset are significantly more similar to each other than they are to the products of one of the other subsets. The molecular weight of the α- and β-gene products is about 29,000 daltons for the protein part. The α-gene products possess additionally two N-linked carbohydrate moieties of about 3,000 dalton each, whereas the β-gene products possess only one N-linked moiety.
All the β-gene products are polymorphic, whereas of the α-gene products only $DQ_{\alpha 2}$ and $DQ_{\alpha 1}$ show some polymorphism. Different types of products have only about 30% of their sequences in common.
Points of contact between the α- and β-chains are different for DR and DQ to such an extent that is seems most unlikely that combinations of a DR α-chain and a DQ β-chain will form stable, fully functional products.
The membrane representation of the different class I and class II molecules is schematically shown in Fig. 6.12.

Class III Molecules:
S-Protein

The Ss protein has also been characterized: It represents the complement component C 4, and is a protein with a molecular weight of about 200,000 daltons, composed of three polypeptide chains with molecular weights of about 95,000, 70,000, and 33,000 daltons, respectively (see also Chap. 5).

Function of *MHC* Molecules
in the Immune Response

Contribution to Antigen Recognition

The two limbs of the immune system were originally regarded as more or less separate and independent mechanisms in the immune response: The B cell system providing the antibodies and the T cell system mediating the cellular immune reaction. However, after discovery of the T cell compartment it was recognized soon that there are intensive interactions between T and B cells and that in addition, a third cell population, the macrophage, is required for efficient activation of the immune system. These cellular interactions represent the major mechanism of regulation in immune recognition. Not until the seventies it was realized that the recognition process by T cells differs principally from B cells. T cells do not recognize foreign antigen per se but only upon "presentation" of the antigen in association with membrane proteins of the individual itself. This rule applies both for the recognition of antigen on the antigen presenting macrophage leading to activation of T-helper cells and for recognition of antigen by cytotoxic T cells. The membrane proteins of the individual contributing to these recognition process are encoded by a group of closely linked genes: the *MHC*. The products of this genetic region were initially detected by their interference with the transplantation of various organs and were therefore designated transplantation antigens.

Table 6.11. Synopsis of *MHC* gene classes

Characteristics	Class I	Class II	Class III
Designation	H molecules	Ia molecules	C3 convertase
Loci(mouse/man)	K,D,L/A,B,C	A, E/DR, DQ, DP	C4, C2, BF
No. of alleles	> 100	> 20	$\geqq 2$
No. of specificities	> 100	> 50	$\geqq 2$
Tissue distribution	All cells	Lymphocytes, macrophages	Serum
Biochemistry: chains	2	2	3 (C4); 1 (C2, B)
mo. wt.	45,000 D	α: 32,000 D	α: 95,000 D
	11.500 D(β_2-MG)	β: 28,000 D	β: 78,000 D
			γ: 33,000 D
Physiology	Target antigen for cytotoxic T cells (effector cells), self for cytotoxic T cells	Stimulation antigen for allogeneic immune reaction (MLR), self for helper/suppressor T cells (T-T, T-macrophage, T-B cell interaction)	Activation of lytic enzymes; opsonization; generation of anaphylatoxin, chemo-(leuko)-tactic substances

Transplantation and transplantation reactions obviously are unnatural situations and under the best of circumstances reveal only a special facet of the function of the *MHC* genes that is inherent in its cooperation in a specific immune response. The most attractive theory of the physiologic function of *MHC* genes has been presented by Burnet: *MHC* gene products signify SELF, i.e., indicate what the immune system should not react against unless this self is altered, for example by the occurrence of new antigenic determinants. Burnet's theory has become more plausible, particularly since the discovery that the MHC controls not only the humoral immune response but also the cellular immune response.

The most prominent feature of the *MHC* is the marked polymorphism of the *MHC* genes. There are many different alleles for each locus of the *MHC* resulting in homologous but distinct proteins. A combination of serological, biochemical and functional studies permitted a classification of the MHC into three groups (synopsis, see Table 6.11).

Class I Products of the MHC. The genes of *class I* code for membrane proteins present on all nucleated cells. Class I proteins represent a recognition element for cytotoxic T cells and are identical with the classical transplantation antigens. Biochemical analysis revealed the presence of two polypeptid chains. Only the heavy chain (molecular weight 45,000 dalton) is coded by the *MHC*. The smaller chain (molecular weight 12,000 dalton) is known as $\beta2$-microglobulin and is not coded by the *MHC* (see p. 159). The genetically controlled polymorphism affects only the heavy chain. The *class I* regions of the *MHC* are designated *HLA-A, -B* and *-C* in the human and *H-K, H2-D* and *H2-L* in the mouse.

Class II Products of the MHC. The genes of *class II* are encoding membrane proteins expressed predominantly on lymphoid cells and macrophages. The proteins consist of two polypeptide chains with a molecular weight of 33,000 dalton (α-chain) and 28,000 dalton (β-chain). The two chains are encoded by two different subregions of the *MHC* and are not associated with $\beta2$-microglobulin. These proteins are detactable serologically as Ia-antigens (I-region associated antigens). The corresponding analogous regions of the *MHC* are the *I-re-*

gion of the mouse or the *HLA-D*-region of the human. Both the *I*-region and the *HLA-D*-region can be subdivided into subregions (*I-A*, *I-E*, or *HLA-DP*, *-DQ* and *-DR*, respectively). The Ia-antigens represent the products of the functionally defined *Ir*-genes (*Immune response* genes, see below).

Class III Products of the MHC. The class III products differ principally from the class I and class II proteins. The class III proteins are soluble serum proteins instead of membrane proteins and are part of the complement system: C4 and C2 of the classical pathway and factor B of the alternative pathway of complement activation. Class III products were initially identified in the mouse as Ss-protein (serum substance); Ss-protein was subsequently recognized as murine C4. In the human there are two closely adjacent genes for C4 present on chromosome 6 and the corresponding proteins are structurally very similar. These genes arose probably by gene duplication. In the mouse there are also two genetic loci. The product of the first locus is the Ss protein (mouse-C4). Expression of the gene products of the second locus is under strict hormonal regulation and the protein is only expressed in the presence of male hormone. The protein was therefore designated Slp, six limited protein. Slp possesses no hemolytic activity. There are controversial opinions whether *class III* genes are just by chance located within the *MHC* or, alternatively whether these genes might contribute directly or indirectly to MHC-mediated function. The second hypothesis would provide an explanation for this unexpected genetic association between components of cell-mediated and humoral immune reaction.

There is one common feature of C4 and C2 and of factor B: All three components participate in the formation of C3-convertases,i.e. enzymes within the complement cascade with the capacity to cleave and thereby activate C3. The third component of complement, C3, has a central role in the complement system. C3 or its fragments generated upon C3 activation mediate a whole series biological functions contributing to host defense and to elicitation of inflammatory reaction (see Chap. 5). C3 fragments bind to defined receptors on the cell membrane (complement receptors) of various cell population and might subsequently modulate the regulatory functions of lymphoid cells. There are indications that C3-fragments affect processes in the induction phase of the immune response, i.e. those reaction steps governed by the MHC-class I and class II-products.

Genetic Restriction

The products of the *class I* and *class II* *MHC* genes have an essential role in both phases of an immune response: in the induction phase and in the effector phase. The induction phase includes all reactions triggered by encountering the foreign antigen and leading to the formation of T-helper cells with subsequent activation of B cells to antibody producing plasma cells or alternatively leading to specifically reactive cytolytic T cells in cases the antigen is cell-bound (transplantation, virus infection a.o.). Class I products are determining the recognition process of cytolytic T cells and control effector cell – target cell interaction. Class II products are involved in antigen recognition by T-helper cells and control T cell-macrophage and T cell – B cell interaction.

Functions of Class I-MHC Products. The role of class I MHC products in T-cell mediated cytolysis was recognized by Zinkernagel and Doherty in 1974. The following experimental system was used: For induction of specifically reactive inbred T cells, mice were infected with a virus, e.g. lymphochoriomeningitis (LCM)-virus. After an appropriate time interval T cells were obtained from the infected, i.e. immunized animals. In a second stage these T cells were incubated with various target cells in vitro. The target cells were obtained from mice of either identical or of distinct *MHC*-haplotype with regard to the original mouse strain used. The target cells were either infected with the same virus used initially for induction of the T cells or, alternatively, with an antigenically unrelated virus, e.g. Sendai- or Influenza-virus.

In controls, non-infected target cells were used. After labeling of the target cells with ^{51}Cr lysis of the target cells was detected by release of the incorporated ^{51}Cr from the cells (^{51}Cr-release assay). The following results were obtained in these studies.

Antigen (Virus)-Specific Immune Response. Lysis was only observed if the target cells were infected with the same virus as used for the initial sensitization: T cells from LCM-infected mice were only able to lyse LCM-virus bearing target cells but were unable to lyse e.g. influenza-virus infected target cells. This demonstrates the specificity of the immune response. Non-infected target cells remained unaffected revealing, as expected, the absence of reactivity to self antigens (self-tolerance).

MHC-Restricted Immune Response. The peculiar finding in these studies was that LCM-specific lysis was only observed if the LCM-infected target cells were obtained from the same mouse strain from which the cytolytic T cells originated. If the LCM-infected target cells were derived from mouse strains differing in their *MHC*-haplotype, no lysis was observed. This demonstrates that the appropriate antigen alone, in this case the LCM-virus, is required but not sufficient for lysis. In contrast, the constellation of the MHC products of the target cells determines also the capacity to induce lysis, i.e. about an efficient recognition by the T-lymphocyte (see Table 6.12). More detailed analysis revealed that effector cell and target cell had to share the *K*- or the *D*-alleles of the *MHC* for efficient lysis. Identity at the I region was, in general, not sufficient for cytolysis of the target cells.

These findings reveal a kind of dual specificity of T cells, namely 1. for the foreign antigen and concomitantly 2. for their own MHC antigen. In this sense the antigen-specific T cell response is narrowed or restricted to a genetically defined target cell and therefore the term "genetic restriction" was introduced. In a number of model systems these rules were confirmed using artificial antigens, e.g. antigens produced by modification of cells with trinitrophenol-(TNP) residues. The same results were obtained.

Functions of Class II Products. Since decades the association between the genetic constitution of an individual and its ability for the specific immune response is known. Clinical studies in 1887 indicate already a genetic element in susceptibility to diphtheria as shown by the increased frequency of this disease in some families. Major progress was obtained in model systems through the work of Benacerraf and McDevitt in the 1960s. These experiments revealed that there exists a genetically controlled ability (or inability) for an immune response to a given antigen. Different mouse strains were used which had a selective inability for antibody formation to certain synthetic poly-

Table 6.12. Specificity and H-2K, D restriction of virus-specific cytotoxic T effector cells

Target cell lysis (H-2 haplotype)		Effector cells stimulated with virus1	
		A($K^k D^k$)	B($K^d D^d$)
A	($K^k D^k$)	–	–
A$_{v1}$	($K^k D^k$)	+	–
A$_{v2}$	($K^k D^k$)	–	–
B	($K^d D^d$)	–	–
B$_{v1}$	($K^d D^d$)	–	+
B$_{v2}$	($K^d D^d$)	–	–
C	($K^k D^b$)	–	–
C$_{v1}$	($K^k D^b$)	+	–
D	($K^b D^k$)	–	–
D$_{v1}$	($K^b D^k$)	+	–
E	($K^d D^b$)	–	–
E$_{v1}$	($K^d D^b$)	–	+
F	($K^d D^b$)	–	–
F$_{v1}$	($K^d D^b$)	–	+

V1 = infected with virus 1
V2 = infected with virus 2

peptide antigens. This behaviour as "Non-responder" was restricted to some antigens, whereas the response of the same mouse strain to other antigens was absolutely normal. These synthetic polypeptides carry only a limited number of determinants because of their simple molecular structure. Therefore, the heterogeneity of the immune response, i.e. the number of responding lymphocyte-clones is relatively limited and

the failure to respond to these antigenic determinant(s) is easily detected.
The genes controlling this immune reactivity are designated "Ir-genes" (immune response-genes). Animals possessing the given allele ("Responder") are able to produce antibodies and to develop a T cell response (e.g. delayed type hypersensitivity reaction, T cell proliferation, lymphokine production etc.) whereas animals which do

Table 6.13. Mapping of *Ir-1A* (*I-A*) and *Ir-1C* (*I-E*) loci in the *H-2* complex

Strain	H-2 complex loci							Response
	K	A_β	A_α	E_β	E_α	S	D	
1. *Ir-1A* (*I-A*) locus controlled response to (H, G)-A-L[a]								
B10	b	**b**	**b**	b	0	b	b	Low
B10.D2	d	**d**	**d**	d	7	d	d	Low
B19.BR	k	**k**	**k**	k	7	k	k	High
B10.S	s	**s**	**s**	s	0	s	s	Low
B10.A(4R)	k	**k**	**k**	b	0	b	b	High
A.TL	s	**k**	**k**	k	7	k	d	High
B10.A(5R)	b	**b**	**b**	b	7	d	d	Low
2. *Ir-1C* (*I-E*) locus controlled response to GLT[b]								
B10	b	b	b	**b**	**0**	b	b	Low
B10.D2	d	d	d	**d**	7	d	d	High
D2.GD	d	d	d	**b**	**0**	b	b	Low
HTG	d	d	d	**d**	7	b	b	High
B10.A(5R)[c]	b	b	b	**b**	7	d	d	High

[a] (H, G)–A-L: synthetic polymer of alanin (A) and lysine (L) with histidin (H) and glutamine (G) as end groups
[b] GLT: linear terpolymer of $(Glu^{57}\text{-}Lys^{38}\text{-}Tyr^5)$
[c] E_β^b is a high-responder allele; it is, however, not expressed in B10 (*H–2ᵇ*) mice because of the E_α^o allele (see p. 146)

Table 6.14. Immune response to GKØ[a] by the *I-E* genes

Strain	H-2 complex loci							Response
	K	A_β	A_α	E_β	E_α	S	D	
B10	b	b	b	**b**	**0**	b	b	Low
B10.D2	d	d	d	**d**	7	d	d	High
B10.BR	k	k	k	**k**	7	k	k	Low
B10.S	s	s	s	**s**	**0**	s	s	Low
B10.A(5R)	b	b	b	**b**	7	d	d	High
B10.S(9R)	s	s	s	**s**	7	d	d	High
B10.S(7R)	s	s	s	**s**	**0**	s	d	Low
B19.A(2R)	k	k	k	**k**	7	d	b	Low
B10.A(4R)	k	k	k	**b**	**0**	b	b	Low
B10.HTT	s	s	s	**s**	7	k	d	High
D2.GD	d	d	d	**d**	**0**	b	b	Low

[a] GLØ: polymer of glutamin, lysine, and phenylalanin
Whenever the high-responder alleles E_β^b, E_β^d, E_β^s, are expressed, i.e., linked to the E_α^7, the high-response phenotype appears; E_β^k is a low responder allele

not possess the allele (Non-Responder) are unable to develop the specific immune response. The Ir-genes are localized in the I-region of the MHC (Table 6.13 and 6.14). The hitherto recognized loci *I-A* and *I-E* each control the expression of two polypeptide chains, A_α and A_β, and E_α and E_β. An additional immune response locus, *Ir-1 B* (formerly *Ir-IgG*) located between *I-A* and *I-E* has been proposed to explain the response pattern to an immunoglobulin allotype (IgG), lactate dehydrogenase-B (LDH_B), and ribonuclease (RNase). Extensive serological, biochemical, and cellular (MLC, CML) analysis failed to give proof for the existence of a product of such a proposed gene. Furthermore, the response to RNase can easily be explained as a result of control by the *I-E* genes after it has been found that the E_β-chain is not expressed in the sole presence of the E_a^0 allele (see p. 146). Therefore, it appears likely that the control of the immune response against IgG and LDH_B is controlled by both the *A* and the *E* genes, and in order to obtain high response both genes must be present as high-responder alleles. Actually, the response to LDH_B was thought to be controlled by two genes, the proposed *Ir-1 B* and E_α.

Regulation of the immune response by MHC-linked *Ir* genes occurs at the level of T-B cell and macrophage-T cell interaction; thymectomized mice that are high responders to a certain antigen form only minimal amounts of antibodies (IgM) comparable to that of low-responder animals. However, if mice that are low responders for a certain antigen are immunized with this antigen after it has been coupled to a carrier (e.g. BSA), these mice are capable of forming antibodies against the antigen (Fig. 6.13). (In addition to *Ir* genes mentioned so far, there are other genes influencing antibody formation. Some of these are closely linked to genes that control antibody allotypes, and it is thought that the failure to form antibodies in this case is due to the lack of a gene coding for the antigen-specific variable region (antigen binding site) of the immunoglobulin. Here, antibody formation cannot

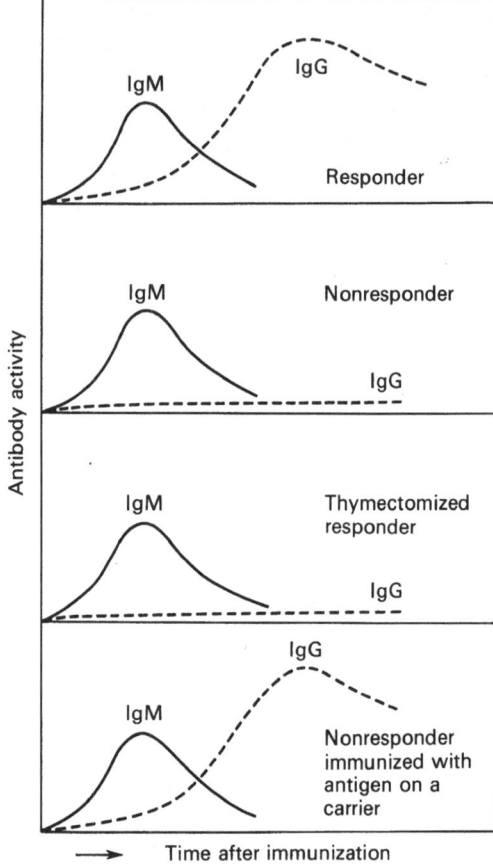

Fig. 6.13. Formation of antibodies against antigens for which the immune response is *Ir-1* controlled. Responders exhibit normal IgM and IgG responses, whereas nonresponders show only an IgM response. If the responder is thymectomized, it behaves like a nonresponder; on the other hand, if nonresponders are injected with antigen after it is linked to a carrier, normal IgM and IgG responses can also be shown

be restored by coupling the antigen on a carrier.)

Features of *Ir* Genes. In summary, *Ir* gene function exhibits the following characteristics:

a) *Ir*-genes are inherited as an autosomal, dominant fashion.

b) *Ir*-genes are localized in the *I*-region of the *MHC*.

c) *Ir*-genes influence the ability for an immune response in a selective fashion, depending on the structure of the given antigen. In fact, minor changes of single amino acids in side chains of the synthetic polypeptide antigen changes the responder/non-responder behaviour.

d) *Ir*-genes affect only the antibody response to T cell dependent antigens.

e) *Ir*-genes control the antigen-specific T cell response.

f) The presence of given *Ir*-genes is associated with the expression of certain serologically detectable determinants of Ia-antigens.

The contribution of *I*-region products in the induction of an immune response was shown in 1972 by Kindred and Shreffler and in 1973 by Shevach and Rosenthal. The interaction between T cells and macrophages or between T cells and B cells exhibited the same phenomenon of "genetic restriction" as described above for cytolytic T cells. For these studies, T cells were obtained from animals of a given strain, which were immunized previously with a given antigen. In parallel, macrophages of the same strain were pretreated ("pulsed") with the same antigen to permit antigen uptake and processing. These antigen-presenting macrophages were then cultured in vitro with the T cells. The specific T cells recognize the antigen and a marked T cell proliferative response is observed. There was no response if a different non-related antigen was used or if the macrophages were obtained from a *MHC*-distinct strain. Genetic analysis revealed that the restriction elements are localized in the *I* region. Efficient T cell-macrophage interaction, or similarly T cell–B cell cooperation, only occured if the partner cells exhibited compatibility in the *I*-region of the *MHC*.

The *I*-region exhibits therefore three major features: The *Ir*-genes are located in this region; restriction elements for cellular cooperation are associated with the *I*-region and finally Ia antigens on the cell surface are encoded also by the same region. A series of quite sophisticated experiments revealed that these three phenomena are different aspects of the same group of proteins namely the Ia-antigens. These proteins re-

present the products of the *Ir* genes and function at the same time as restriction elements. The fine structure of the Ia-antigens as it is detectable through their pattern of antigenic determinants determines obviously whether or not an immune response is induced by a certain foreign antigen.

The role of Ia-antigens as restriction elements can be explained by two, principally distinct hypotheses:

The first model emphasizes the role of T cell differentiation and development of the T cell repertoir for foreign antigens. The second model proposes a central role of the macrophage and a critical function of this cell in antigen-presentation. According to the first hypothesis I-region products might influence selection processes in the thymus and the diversification of T cells. MHC products present on thymus epithelium or on thymus macrophages are obviously of major importance in these selection processes. The nature of the MHC products (i.e. MHC-haplotype dependent) might determine the development of selective holes in the T cells repertoire leading to non-responsiveness against a given antigen. The particular configuration of the given self-MHC-molecule might resemble in its molecular shape a certain foreign antigen. The immunological tolerance to self-MHC products would then also extend to this antigen. In an individual of a different *MHC*-haplotype these holes in the repertoire would then affect the response to different antigens. The responder/non-responder status and the genetic restriction are according to this model the consequence of T cell selection processes and independend of exogenous foreign antigen. According to the second hypothesis, the specific *Ir*-gene function reflects the capacity of Ia-antigens on macrophages or B cells to form an effective association with fragments of the foreign antigen. These antigen fragments might bind to defined sites on the Ia-molecule thereby forming the immunogenic complex recognized by the T cell (Fig. 6.14). The nature of the Ia-antigen pattern in an individual controls the ex-

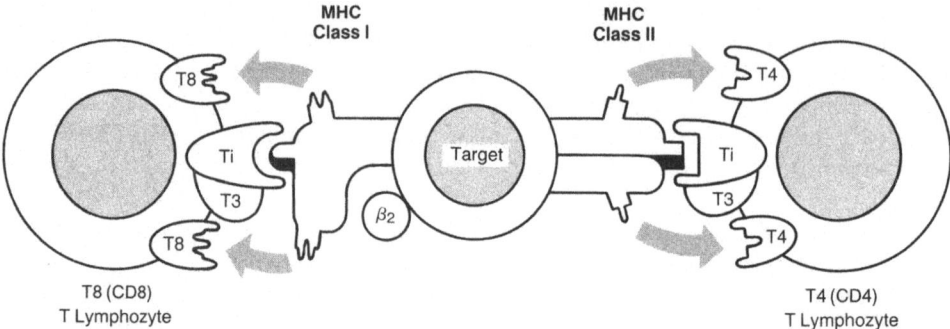

Fig. 6.14. Model for the interaction of T lymphocytes with antigen. Presented by macrophages (target) in association with MHC class I (left) or with MHC class II (right) molecules. Ti/T3, T cell antigen receptor; T8 (CD8), marker for cytotoxic/suppressor T lymphocytes, probably interacting with a constant part of MHC class I molecules; T4 (CD4), marker for helper T lymphocytes, probably interacting with a constant part of MHC class II molecules, β_2, beta-2-microglobulin. [From Reinherz et al. (1984) Immunol. Rev. 81:95–129]

pression of appropriate binding sites for a given antigen required for efficient presentation. The absence of appropriate binding sites might therefore result in non-responsiveness to this antigen. Genetic restriction is in this model the consequence of the priming event. Under in vivo condition, the first encounter of a T cell with foreign antigen would involve antigen presenting macrophages of its own *MHC*-haplotype. This process would subsequently lead to selective induction of T cells specific for the complex consisting of foreign antigen and self-MHC. In a secondary immune response the initially selected T cells would only recognize the same Ag-MHC complex effectively. Despite a large series of elaborate experiments no clear-cut decision is reached so far for one or the other hypothesis. There is convincing evidence for either one and further studies are required. Such studies involve for instance "chimera" experiments in which the selection processes of T cells are manipulated and the influence of MHC products born by thymus cells on the T cell selection process can be studied. The term "chimera" reflects the fact that in these experimental animals the immunocompetent cells or their precursors are of different origin (donor type) than the recipient's cells; these chimeras therefore represent a mixture of genetically heterogenous cell populations.

***MHC*-Restriction and Host Defense.** From a teleological point of view the phenomenon of genetic restriction must be of advantage for the species; otherwise it should not exist. The major role of the immune system under physiological conditions is obviously the defense against pathogenic microorganisms. The main function of cytotoxic T cells is the lysis of virus-infected cells. The fact that viral antigen alone is not sufficient to trigger T cell activation but additional (class I-MHC) membrane proteins are required might facilite a kind of focussing of the specific T cells to virus-infected cells. An inefficient triggering of the T cell's cytotoxic potential by e.g. circulating fragments of viral proteins is avoided through the requirement for dual recognition. On the other hand, lysis of the virus-infected cells leads of course to destruction of the host's cells which might be required for vital functions of the organism. There is a similar situation for the class II MHC restricted T cells. These cells are mainly T-helper cells known as the major source for lymphokines. Activation of macrophages by lymphokines results in an increased bactericidal acitivity of these phagocytic cells. The fact that T cells do not recognize bacterial antigen per se but only in the association with macrophage Ia-antigens again helps to focus the specific defense mechanism to those sites of the individual where elimina-

Table 6.15. Properties of interleukin-1 (IL-1) and interleukin-2 (IL-2)

Chemical and biological properties	Interleukin-1		Interleukin-2	
	Murine	Human	Murine	Human
Produced by	Macrophages		Ly-1$^+$ T cells	Lymphocytes
Size (gel filtration)	16,000		30,000	15,000
Elution from DEAE ion exchange	0.05–0.1 M		0.15 M	0.05 M
resin pH 7.5	NaCl		NaCl	NaCl
Isoelectric points	5.0–5.5	6.5–7.5	4.3, 4.9	6.0–6.5
Stable in pH range	2.0–9.0		2.0–9.0	
Absorbed on activated murine T cells	unknown		Yes	Yes
Stimulate growth of murine T-cell lines	No	No	Yes	Yes
Stimulate proliferation of murine thymocytes in presence of ConA or PHA under culture conditions where these mitogens alone are limiting	No	No	Yes	Yes
Generate CTL in murine thymocyte cultures and nude spleen cultures	No	No	Yes	Yes
Stimulate antibody response to heterologous erythrocyte antigens in nude spleen cultures	Yes	Yes	Yes	Yes
Activity MHC restricted	No	No	No	No
Activity antigen-specific	No	No	No	No

tion of bacteria is required. Thus, release of macrophage activating factor(s) occurs in the tissue only in the immediate vicinity of an infection. This prevents inefficient lymphokine release as it might be triggered otherwise by free, soluble bacterial fragments or products not associated with the macrophage.

The marked polymorphism of the MHC products has also to be considered under the aspect of host defense. Polymorphism of the two loci for class I antigens (e.g. *H2-K* and *H2-D* in the mouse) in combination with the normally heterozygous state of an individual drastically reduces the chance that a given pathogen might mimic in its antigenic structure the host MHC products. Due to the host's tolerance against its own MHC proteins, such mimicry would provide an efficient excape mechanism for the parasite.

The Nature of Allo-Reactivity. T lymphocytes from an individual respond vigorously against allogeneic MHC antigens, i.e. MHC of another genetically unrelated individual of the same species.

A very high proportion (1–3%) of all T cells is reactive for a given alloantigen. Therefore, by extrapolation the major part if not all of the T cell repertoire should be committed to recognition of the species alloantigens instead of foreign antigen. Recent studies of T cell populations and especially of T cell clones provided an explanation for this unexpected high frequency of alloreactive T cells. Convincing data revealed that T cells specific for a given antigen in the context with self MHC products are also able to recognize certain alloantigens. It seems that the antigenic structure present in certain sites of the alloantigen molecule resembles or mimics the complex of foreign antigen associated with self-MHC products. The apparent specificity of a T cell for alloantigen therefore represents actually a cross-reactivity in T cell recognition.

The T Cell Receptor:
Antigen-Recognizing Element of T Cells

T lymphocytes circulate in the body as small resting lymphocytes. Upon encounter with a foreign antigen, those T cells with ability to recognize this antigen are activated: Blast transformation occurs followed by proliferation and differentiation to functionally active effector T cells or regulatory T cells. A prerequisite for T cell activation is the specific recognition of the antigen by the individual, specifically reactive T cell. T cells aquire their specificity during differentiation and diversification processes under the influence of the thymus.

The repertoir of T lymphocytes to foreign antigens is probably of a comparable magnitude as the repertoir of B cells for antibody formation. The clonal selection theory obviously also applies for the T cell compartment of the immune response. A T lymphocyte with a specificity for a given foreign antigen 1 should possess a structural element on its surface mediating the specific recognition of this antigen. A second T lymphocyte of different antigen specificity should consequently bear a recognition element of different structure able to react selectively with the antigen 2. Therefore, the functional diversity of T cells in antigen recognition must reflect the presence of specific antigen recognizing elements on the cell surface complementary in their structure to the antigen. This cellular element on the T cell membrane for antigen recognition is called T cell receptor.

T Cell Clones as Homogenous Cell Populations. Identification of the T cell receptor became possible through advances mainly in two immunological techniques and their efficient application: Firstly, the establishment of the hybridoma-technique for the production of monoclonal antibodies and, secondly, the establishment of techniques for maintaining specific and functionally active T cell clones in vitro.

T cells originating from a single cell (i.e. a T cell clone) can be grown in semisolid media if the appropriate antigenic stimulus, growth factors (e.g. Interleukin 2) and nutrients are provided. The individual T cells specific for the antigen grow to colonies

similar to be bacterial colony. The T cells of a given colony can be expanded by repeated stimulation with the corresponding antigen. These cells are of monoclonal nature and all cells should therefore possess an identical antigen recognition structure which, in turn, should differ from another clone with a different antigen specificity.

An alternative for producing monoclonal T cells is T cell hybridization. This technique is similar to the hybridoma technique for production of monoclonal antibodies. T cells from an immunized animal (mouse) are hybridized to an appropriate T cell tumor and the resulting T cell lines growing from individual hybrid cells are screened for specific reactivity to the antigens (e.g. by lymphokine production upon response to the antigen). These antigen-specific and also *MHC*-restricted T cell clones or hybrids provide the ideal starting material for analyis of the T cell receptor at the clonal level. Monoclonal antibodies were raised after immunization with these monoclonal T cells. Antibodies were selected which reacted exclusively with the T cell clone used for immunization but not with other, closely related T cell clones. Such antibodies detect obviously a "clonotypic" determinant. The only candidate bearing such clonotypic (or idiotypic) determinants linked to the antigen-specificity of a given T cell clone is the T cell receptor of this particular clone. These antibodies interfere specifically with the antigen recognition of the corresponding T cell clone and are directed against a T cell specific membrane protein, the T cell receptor. It consists of two subunits with similar molecular weight (α-chain of 45,000 to 50,000 dalton; β-chain of 40,000 to 45,000 dalton). Both the α- and β-chain have, like the light and heavy chains of immunoglobulins, constant and variable regions recognizing the antigen in association with MHC products.

The genes of the α-chain are located on chromosome 14 in man and chromosome 14 in mice; the β-chain genes are located on chromosome 7 in man and chromosome 6 in mice. (In mice, genes of a third

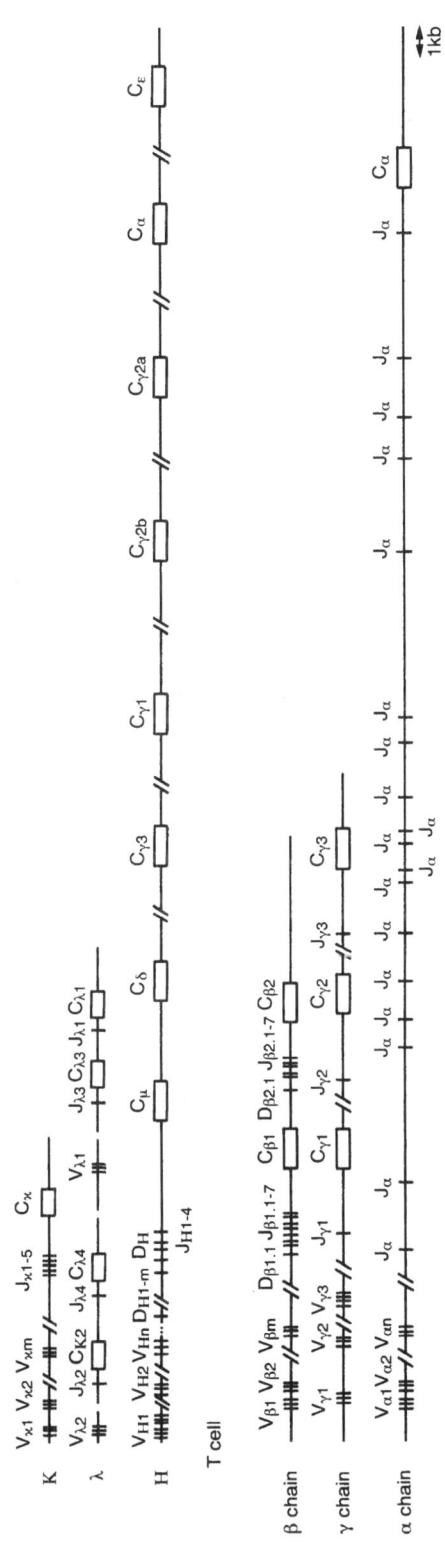

Fig. 6.15. Schematic diagram of the gene organization for the immunoglobulin and T cell receptor gene family. Boxes indicate the C genes, vertical lines the V, D or J gene segments. [Modifies from Winoto A, Mjolsness S, Hood L (1985) Nature 316:832–836]

chain, γ, has been described localized on chromosome 13.)

T Cell Receptor Genes. The organization of the genomic DNA encoding the α- and β-chain of the T cell receptor is similar to the heavy chain of Ig. The V region of the β-chain is encoded by V (variable), D (diversity) and J (joining) gene segments which rearrange with one of two C_β segments. The V region of the α-chain is encoded by V and J gene segments only; unusual is the apparently high number of J gene segments (Fig. 6.15). These gene segments rearrange in the course of T cell differentiation and diversification to give the final V region gene. The regulation of the rearrangement process remains to be clarified. The generation of diversity in the T cell receptor resembles principally the B cell. Multiple germline gene segments for the T cell receptor V region are present in the germline. Joining events in the combination of the different gene segments and somatic mutation contribute to the generation of diversity as well as the particular association in the combination of a certain α- and β-chain. There are no T cell receptor isotypes known comparable to the different Ig classes, i.e. the same T cell receptor gene segments are expressed in cytotoxic T cells as in T helper cells.

T Cell Receptor Associated Proteins. The T cell receptor is apparently associated in the membrane with another protein, the T3(CD3) antigen, to form a macromolecular complex. The T3(CD3) antigen consists of three polypeptides which are tightly bound to the T cell receptor heterodimer protein. In contrast to the α- and β-chain of the T cell receptor, the three chains of the T3(CD3) antigen are invariant in that they do not exhibit clonotypic variation and therefore do not contribute to antigen specificity of the T cell. Their function might be the formation of ion channels through the T cell membrane after previous antigen-binding to the α- and β subunits of the T cell receptor (Table 6.16).

Table 6.16. Cluster of differentiation (CD) antigens found on T cells/thymocytes

Antigen	Cell expression	Molecular weight
CD1	Thymocytes	45,000 d
(T6)		12,000 d
CD2	E-rosette forming	50,000 d
(T11)	T cells	
CD3	Mature T cells	19,000 d
(T3)		29,000 d
CD4	T helper cells	55,000 d
(T4)		
CD7	All T cells	41,000 d
CD8	Cytotoxic/	31,000 d
(T8)	suppressor T cells	32,000 d

In addition to the T3(CD3) antigen, two other T cell membrane proteins contribute indirectly to cell recognition: the T4(CD4) and T8(CD8) antigens. These proteins were – like many T cell markers - identified by monoclonal antibodies. The T4(CD4) antigen is mainly expressed on T cell recognizing antigen in association with MHC-class II antigen, i.e. the T helper cells. In contrast, the T8(CD8) antigen is predominantly expressed by cytotoxic T cells recognizing antigens in the context of MHC class I antigen. Therefore, the T4(CD4) and T8(CD8) antigens are obviously associated with the restriction specificity of T cells. These proteins might have a kind of accessory function in cellular interactions of T cells. The T4(CD4) or T8(CD8) proteins possibly facilitate the specific binding of the T cell to the MHC-complex. Loose binding of the T cell to its target cell might be mediated by the T4(CD4)- or T8(CD8)-proteins via interaction with MHC products (non-polymorphic regions of class II or class I, respectively) present on the target cells. This initial cellular contact might promote a more stable and specific interaction via the T cell receptor followed subsequently by T cell activation. The T4(CD4) and the T8(CD8) proteins exhibit, like T3(CD3), no structural heterogeneity and therefore do not contribute to T cell antigen specificity.

Comparison of Ig and T Cell Receptor. Ig and T cell receptor are encoded by clearly distinct genes. Nevertheless, the genomic organization for these proteins is similar. In addition, nucleotide sequence analysis revealed regions of partial homology between these genes implying common ancestry. The genes for Ig and the T cell receptor are also related in nucleotide sequence to other cell surface proteins involved in cellular interaction during various phases of the immune response. This group of proteins (the Ig-superfamily) might originate therefore from a primordial gene for a cell surface protein. Despite these similarities of Ig and T cell receptor there are the described principal differences in function. In summary:

Immunoglobulin
– binds foreign antigen per se
– binds soluble antigen
– does not require MHC products for antigen-binding
– is not associated with other proteins
– isotypes exist

T cell receptor
– does not bind antigen per se
– recognizes only antigen on the surface of other cells
– does not bind free soluble antigen

– requires MHC products for antigen-recognition
– is associated with T3(CD3) antigen to a macromolecular complex in the membrane
– isotypes unknown.

Class III Molecules in the Immune Response

A number of genes in this class that together control the expression or regulation of the level of serum proteins have recently been recognized as parts of the complement system. In several species, these are the components C2 and C4 of the classical complement pathway, and factor B of the alternative pathway.

The complement components C4 and C2 make up the C3-convertase of the classical pathway. This enzyme cleaves C3 to C3a and C3b, the active form of C3. The cleavage product Bb of factor B represents the enzymatically active moiety of the C3-convertase of the alternative pathway, also turning C3 into its active form C3b (Fig. 6.16).

The C4b,2a complex (C3-convertase) is formed when Ag–Ab complexes are present; particularly active Ab–Ag complexes

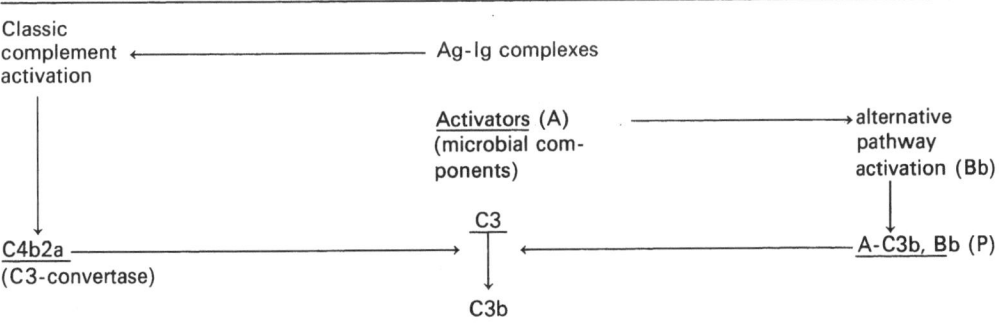

Classic complement activation ⟵————————— Ag-Ig complexes

Activators (A) —————————→ alternative
(microbial components) pathway activation (Bb)

C4b2a ————————————————→ C3 ⟵———————————— A-C3b, Bb (P)
(C3-convertase)   C3b

C3b:
Receptor on
Macrophages →· opsonization, phagocytosis

Convertase formation for
C5 → C5a and C5b → Anaphylatoxin; activator of lytic complement components C8 → C9

Underlined components are controlled genetically by MHC

Fig. 6.16. *MHC*-linked complement components that exhibit C3-convertase activity

are those formed with IgM as antibody, i.e., the kind of antibody that is already present in the serum and exhibits a high cross-reactivity (so-called preformed or natural antibodies), and is generated very early in the immune response, right after the first encounter of B cells with the antigen (and without the activating help of T cells). On the other hand, the alternative pathway is activated without antibodies by a variety of substances like zymosan present on or in microbial cell walls. In both instances, be it through the activated C 4 b, 2 a enzyme or the activated factor B, the complement component C 3 is converted into its active form C 3 b, which in 4 b, 2 a turn facilitates opsonization by macrophages through binding the antigen via C 3 b receptors. Possibly through activation of B lymphocytes, it effects liberation of chemo(leuko)tactic substances, and activates C 5 to C 5 b, the active component turning on the late complement chain enzymes, resulting in the lytic complex C $\overline{5 b, 6, 7, 8, 9}$ (see Chap. 5). The products of the *class III* genes fulfill a significant helper and enhancer function for the specific immune response, in particular for the digestion and elimination of infectious material such as bacteria, parasites, and particular antigens. The fact that the *MHC* has a significant regulative influence on an organism's defense against infections,

and that certain alleles of the *MHC* cause a low responder status in relation to certain infections, may explain the extreme polymorphism and genetic complexity of this genetic system. Homozygosity for a low-responder allele is considerably reduced by multiplication of a gene to several loci with similar functions, and the formation of multiple alleles for each of these loci. Furthermore, the observation that in populations certain alleles occur in association or linkage disequilibrium might be explained as minimizing unresponsiveness.

In summarizing the functions of the *MHC* (Table 6.17) one has the impression that it plays a significant role in the final differentiation of immunocompetent cells, particularly for the development of specificity of maturing T lymphocytes that come in contact with a substrate foreign to the organism (antigen), and a deciding role in the differentiation between *self* and *non-self* when the organism is infected by viruses, bacteria, parasites, or soluble antigens.

In this context – discrimination between *self* and *non-self* – can also be seen the phenomenon of linkage of specific *MHC* alleles with susceptibility to specific diseases, as is observed in the mouse and in man, particularly because most of these diseases involve a combination of infection and autoimmunity.

Table 6.17. Control of the immune system by the *H-2* complex

System	Expression	Effector	Interaction	Controlling H-2 locus
Humoral immunity	Antibody formation	B/plasma cells	T-helper cells, T-suppressor cells, macrophages	A, E
Cellular immunity	Cell-mediated cytotoxicity, graft rejection	T-killer cells	T-helper cells, macrophages	K, D
Auxiliary system	Phagocytosis, opsonization, chemotaxis	Complement factor B, C2, C4	Macrophages, monocytes, Ag-Ab complexes, B'-bacterium complex	S

Chromosome No. 17   C ————*K-A-E-S-D*————
                    H-2 complex

MHC–Disease Association in Man

The finding that inbred strains of mice exhibited different susceptibility to a tumor-inducing (oncogenic) virus (Gross virus), initiated the search for genes that play a specific role in viral oncogenesis. It was found that viral leukemogenesis is influenced by genes of the *H-2* complex. A similar relationship between susceptibility and the *H-2* haplotype could be determined for many other viruses: Tennant virus (RNA virus, lymphocytic leukemia); Friend virus (RNA, erythremia); Bittner virus (RNA, mammary carcinoma); lymphochoriomeningitis virus (RNA); vaccinia virus (DNA); and radiation-induced leukemia virus (RNA). In none of these cases, however, are genes of the *H-2* complex the only factors that control susceptibility.

These findings, and the fact that the immune response is controlled by genes of the *MHC*, induced investigators to search for associations between diseases and specific HLA antigens or haplotypes. An association of *HLA* alleles and tumor disease has not yet been convincingly presented, although in some neoplastic diseases certain

HLA antigens are increased in long-term survivors, which probably indicates an association between HLA and resistance. A number of diseases do exhibit a distinct association with certain *HLA* alleles or *HLA* haplotypes. Primarily these are autoimmune diseases, infectious diseases, and the sequelae (which may themselves be autoimmune diseases) of certain infectious diseases. A summary of the associations is given in Table 6.18.

The most significant association found is that between Bechterew's disease (ankylosing spondylitis) and HLA-B 27: 85% of patients with the disease are HLA-B 27-positive. The association is one-sided only: the presence of the antigen does not indicate that the person is susceptible to the disease. At present, there are only hypotheses concerning the underlying mechanisms of the association of *HLA* and disease. Several possibilities are discussed: Since the *MHC* is the major system regulating immune reactions (see p. 164), it is conceivable that under certain circumstances the normal immune response deviates, i.e., becomes suppressed or enhanced. That might be the case if the immunodominant epitope of a patho-

Table 6.18. Examples of HLA disease associations

Disease	Associated antigen	Relative risk	Disease	Associated antigen	Relative risk
Idiopathic hemochromatosis	A3, B7 B14	6.7	Multiple sclerosis	DR2	2.7
			Pernicious anemia	DR2	
Myasthema gravis	B8		Sicca syndrome	DR3	5.7
Graves' disease	B8, DR3	3.7	M. Addison	DR3	
Chronic acute Hepat.	B8, DR3		Myasthenia gravis	DR3	3.3
Psiorasis vulg.	B13, Bw57, Cw6	8.4	Celiac disease	DR3	11.6
			Juvenile diabetes	DR3, DR4	
Late onset AGS[a]	B14		Rheumatoid arthritis	Dr4	5.4
Ancylosing spondyltitis	B27	207.9			
			Pemphigus vulgaris	DR4	14.6
Reiter's disease	B27	37.1	Hashimoto thyreoiditis	DR5	
Subacute thyreoiditis quervain	B35		Kaposi sarkom	DR5	
M. Behçet	B51(5)	4.5	Dermatitis herpetiformis	DR7	17.3
Early onset AGS	Bw47				
Narcolepsy	DR2	358.1			
Goodpasture syndrome	DR2	13.8			

[a] Adrenogenital syndrome: 21-Hydroxylase deficiency

gen happens to be identical to an epitope of an *MHC* allele to which a complementary epitope (leading to anti-idiotypic reactions, see p. 162) is controlled by the same or the other allele class present in that individual. Indeed, in certain cases an association of susceptibility with *HLA* alleles was only apparent when certain *HLA* alleles occurred together in heterozygotes.

It has been shown that certain microorganisms possess epitopes similar or identical to epitopes of certain *MHC* alleles (i.e., streptococcal protein M and HLA); in these cases, an individual possessing such HLA alleles might be tolerant to those microorganisms (molecular mimicry).

On the other hand, genes that control the expression of complement components may explain the association if some alleles of this gene code for defective products. As discussed previously, the complement system plays a significant role in initiation or enhancement of the immune response. Preferential linkage of such alleles with certain *HLA* alleles could give the impression of an association with *HLA*. Clinically, complement-deficiencies can cause autoimmune disease-like syndromes (see Chap. 12).

Though there is as yet no explanation for the association, the clinical significance of these findings is obvious. HLA typing can be extremely important for diagnosis, particularly in the early phase of a disease. Furthermore, a known association can acquire prognostic and/or therapeutic value when more is known about the course of the disease in patients who either possess or do not possess the specific *HLA* allele. Thus, there is a correlation between the presence of HLA-D 2 allele and the progression of multiple sclerosis. On the other hand, HLA-A 9 and/or HLA-A 2 positive patients with acute lymphatic leukemia appear to have a better prognosis for survival than those who do not have these alleles.

It also appears possible to determine the risk for family members of persons who suffer from an *HLA*-associated disease, and on occasion to take prophylactic measures (e.g., vaccination for an infectious disease). Also,

HLA-disease associations should also be considered in genetic family counseling.

An association of MHC alleles with specific diseases in which not all diseased persons demonstrate such an association could lead to a new subdivision of certain diseases that today are viewed as units; without doubt, this would have repercussions on therapy and prognosis, and even on prevention.

Finally, an association between *HLA* and a specific disease also provides information about the etiology and pathogenesis of the disease, particularly concerning an infectious or immunologic (autoimmune) mechanism.

References

Albert E, Götze D (1977) The major histocompatibility system in man. In: Götze D (ed) The organisation of the major histocompatibility system in man and animals. Springer, New York, p 7

Albert ED, Baur MP, Mayr WR (eds) (1984) Histocompatibility Testing 1984. Springer, Heidelberg

Bernard A, Boumsell L, Dausset J, Milstein C, Schlossman SF (1984) Leucocyte Typing. Springer, Heidelberg

Bodmer WF, Batchelor JR, Bodmer JG, Festenstein H, Morris PJ (eds) (1978) Joint Report 1977. In: Histocompatibility testing 1977. Munksgaard, Copenhagen

Burnet FM (1970) Immunological surveillance. Pergamon, Sidney

Counce S, Smith P, Barth R, Snell GD (1956) Strong and weak histocompatibility gene differences in mice and their role in the rejection of homografts of tumors and skin. Ann Surg 144:198

Debré P, Kapp JA, Dorf ME, Benacerraf B (1975) Genetic control of specific immune suppression. II. H-2 linked dominant genetic control of immune suppression by the random copolymer L-gutamic acid[50]-L-tyrosine[50] (GT). J Exp Med 142:1447

Doherty P, Götze D, Trinchieri G, Zinkernagel RM (1976) Models for recognition of virally-modified cells by immune thymus-derived lymphocytes. Immunogenetics 3:517

Edidin M (1972) The tissue distribution and cellular localisation of transplantation antigens. In: Kahan BD, Reisfeld RA (eds) Transplantation antigens, markers of biological individuality. Academic, New York, p 125

Götze D, Reisfeld RA, Klein J (1973) Serologic evidence for antigens controlled by the Ir region in mice. J Exp Med 138:1003

Götze D (1976) Serologic characterization of Ia antigens and their relation to Ir genes. Immunogenetics 3:319

Götze D (ed) (1977) The major histocompatibility system in man and animals. Springer, Heidelberg

Hämmerling G, Mauve G, Goldberg E, McDevitt HO (1975) Tissue distribution of Ia antigens. Ia on spermatozoa, macrophages and epidermal cells. Immunogenetics 1:428

Jerne NK (1974) Toward a network theory of the immune system. Ann Immunol (Inst Pasteur) 125 C:373

Klein J (1975) The biology of the mouse histocompatibility-2 complex. Springer, New York

Meo T, Krasteff T, Shreffler DC (1975) Immunochemical characterization of murine H-2 controlled Ss (serum substance) protein through identification of its human homologue as the fourth component of complement. Proc Natl Acad Sci (Wash.) 72:4536

Möller G (ed) (1980) T cell stimulating growth factors. Immunol Rev 51

Reinherz EL, Haynes BF, Bernstein ID (1985) Leucocyte Typing II. Springer, New York

Revised nomenclature for antigen-nonspecific T cell proliferation and helper factors (1979) J Immunol 128:2928

Selwood N, Hedges A (1978) Transplantation antigens: A study in serological data analysis. Wiley, Chichester

Shaw S, Johnson SH, Shearer GM (1980) Evidence for a new segregant series of B cell antigens that are encoded in the HLA-D region and that stimulate secondary allogeneic proliferative and cytotoxic response. J Exp Med 152:565

Sheehy M, Sondel P, Bach M, Wank R, Bach F (1975) HLA typing: A rapid assay using primed lymphocytes. Science 188:1308

Shreffler DC, David CS (1975) The H-2 major histocompatibility complex and the I immune response region: Genetic variation, function and organization. Adv Immunol 20:125

Snell GD, Dausset J, Nathenson S (1976) Histocompatibility. Academic, New York

Solheim BG, Møller E, Ferrone S (1986) HLA class II antigens. Springer, Heidelberg

Svejgaard A, Platz P, Ryder LP, Staub-Nielsen L, Thomsen M (1975) HL-A and disease association – A survey. Transplant Rev 22:3

Thorsby E, Piazza A (1975) Joint report from the VI International Histocompatibility Workshop. II. Typing for HLA-D (LD-1 or MLC) determinants. In: Kissmeyer-Nielsen F (ed) Histocompatibility testing 1975. Munksgaard, Copenhagen, p 414

Tiwari JL, Terasaki PI (1985) HLA and disease associations. Springer, New York

Winoto A, Mjolsness S, Hood L (1985) Genomic organization of the genes encoding mouse T cell receptor α-chain. Nature 316:382

Chapter 7 Antigen–Antibody Interaction

Otto G. Bier

Contents

Serologic Reactions for Detection of Antibodies 179
In Vitro Serologic Reactions 180
   Precipitation 180
   Agglutination 187
   Immunofluorescence 194
   Complement Fixation 196
   Immunocytolysis 201
   Immunocytotoxicity 201
   Immunoadherence 202
   Conglutination and Immunoconglutination . 203
Serologic Reactions in Vivo 204
   Phagocytosis and Opsonization 204
   Neutralization of Toxins 209
   Protective Action of Antibacterial Sera . . . 212
Quantitative Study of the Antigen–Antibody
   Reaction 214
   Quantitative Precipitation 214
Applications of the Precipitation Reaction:
   Qualitative Precipitation 217
Quantitative Precipitation 217
Quantitative Inhibition of Specific
   Precipitation 219
Enzyme-linked Immunosorbent Assay
   (ELISA) 221
Quantitative Study of the Hapten–Antibody
   Reaction 221
Intermolecular Forces in the
   Antigen–Antibody Reaction 224
Comparative Sensitivities of Serologic
   Techniques 224
References 225

Serologic Reactions for Detection of Antibodies

The union of antibody and antigen gives rise to a series of reactions, the qualitative or semiquantitative study of which is the domain of serology.

The type of reaction observed depends upon the physical state of the antigen (soluble or particulate) and the experimental conditions of the test involved. If the antigen is a solu-ble protein, the reaction between the macro-molecules of the antigen and the antibody, in the proper proportions, results in the for-mation of an insoluble complex (precipi-tate). When the antigen is found on the sur-faces of particles (such as bacteria or ery-throcytes), the molecules of the divalent antibody form bridges with the particles and cause their agglutination (Fig. 7.1). In reactions with erythrocytes, when comple-ment as well as antibody is present, lesion sites form on the erythrocyte membrane through which hemoglobin is liberated. This is the phenomenon of specific hemolysis.

The intensity of a serologic reaction is gener-ally expressed in terms of "titer" – the dilu-tion of serum (or of antigen) in which a spe-cific effect is observed under certain ex-perimental conditions. Thus, for example, if a given serum prepared for experimentation in serial dilutions (1:10, 1:20, 1:40, etc.) produces agglutination at the 1:640 dilu-tion, but does not produce agglutination at 1:1280, it is said to have a titer of 1:640 or to contain 640 agglutinating units per unit of volume. In this type of test, the precision of the reading is obviously subjective and can vary by a factor of $\pm \log 2$ in repeated tests, so that only differences in the titers of two or more tubes of the reaction series are considered significant. In the case of specific hemolysis, however, one can, by using suc-cessive dilutions that vary by a factor of less than 2 and through spectrophotometric de-termination of the quantity of liberated he-moglobin, achieve a precision of $\pm 2\%$.

Although the verification of the intensity of serologic reactions is of inestimable practi-cal value in the diagnosis of infections, it is important to bear in mind that serologic

Reaction of the antibody with the
antigen in solution

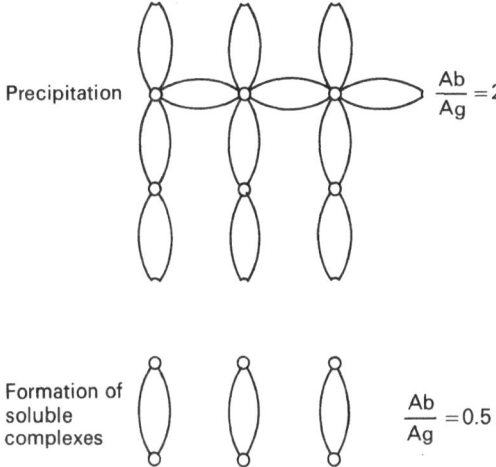

Precipitation $\dfrac{Ab}{Ag} = 2$

Formation of
soluble
complexes $\dfrac{Ab}{Ag} = 0.5$

Reaction of the antibody with the
particulate antigen

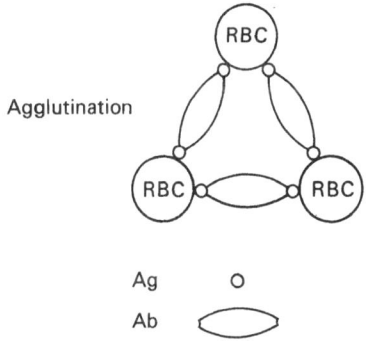

Agglutination

Ag   ○

Ab   ⬭

Fig. 7.1. Mechanisms of specific precipitation and agglutination

titer does not represent a measure of the
quantity of antibody, since it depends also
upon the quality of the antibody (as in
nonagglutinating or noncomplement-fixing
antibody) not to mention variations in function from antigen peculiarities and from
conditions inherent in the particular test.
In any case, when comparing the titers of
various antisera, one should use the same
dosage technique, including, whenever possible, previously standardized reference reagents (sera and antigens).

In Vitro Serologic Reactions

Precipitation

The easiest way of testing the reaction between an antibody and the corresponding
antigen in solution consists of layering the
two reagents and then observing, at the interface, the appearance of a disk or ring of
precipitation (ring test). This reaction, called
specific precipitation, occurs whenever the
antigenic macromolecule possesses two or
three or more combining sites for each of the
two combining sites of the bivalent antibody
molecule. If the antigen is univalent (hapten)
or just bivalent, soluble complexes are
formed and a precipitate is not observed
(Fig. 7.1). The same occurs when there is an
excess of antibody. There is no precipitation
when the multivalent antigen reacts with
univalent antibody fragments or with antibodies with weak affinity. In the latter case,
special methods must be used to detect the
presence of the antibody.
The quantitative reactions between antigen
and antibody in specific precipitates proceed
in variable proportions and are reversible.
Accordingly, the antibody (Ab)/antigen
(Ag) ratio in the precipitate decreases in proportion to the increase in the quantity of
antigen, until a molecular composition of
Ag_2Ab is attained, in which soluble complexes are formed:

$$Ag + Ab \longrightarrow AgAb + Ag \text{ Excess} \longrightarrow Ag_2Ab$$
$$\qquad\qquad\quad \text{(Precipitate)} \qquad\qquad \text{(Soluble complex)}$$

$$AgAb + H \text{ excess} \longrightarrow H_2Ab + Ag + H$$
$$\qquad\qquad \text{(Hapten)} \quad \text{(Soluble complex)}.$$

The latter reaction is the basis of the process
for purification of antibodies through the
elution of specific precipitates by the corresponding haptens.

Precipitation in Liquid Media. If, instead of
layering the antigen and the antibody as in
the ring test, aqueous solutions of the two
reagents are mixed, initially the mixture is
perfectly clear; after a while, there is a

progressively developing turbidity, or opalescence. After a certain period of time, a flocculate, or precipitate, forms that finally collects in the bottom of the tube. The quantity of precipitate is a function of the quantity of antibody present in the antiserum, as well as of the quantity of antigen added. Under these circumstances, if increasing quantities of antigen are added to a series of tubes containing a fixed quantity of antiserum (e.g., 1 ml), an increasing quantity of precipitate is formed, up to a maximum level. Beyond this level, the amount of precipitate diminishes because of the formation of soluble complexes by the antigen excess. By subtracting the quantity of antigen added from the quantity of precipitate formed at the level of maximum precipitation, one obtains the quantity of antibody present in the antiserum.

One can also measure the antibody (or the antigen) in precipitation reactions through determination of the time of the most rapid precipitation, which corresponds to the optimum proportion in which the two reagents combine (optimal proportions method). In the so-called alpha method (Dean and Webb), the concentration of the antiserum is maintained constant whereas that of the antigen is varied; in the beta method (Ramon), varying quantities of antiserum are added to a fixed quantity of antigen. In both methods, the optimum proportion corresponds to that in the tube in which precipitation first appears.

Titration of antibodies by this method is useful in the measurement of antitoxins produced in the horse (Ramon flocculation), whereby determination of the optimum relation is particularly clear because of the presence of precipitation inhibition (formation of soluble complexes) with excess antigen as well as with excess antibody.

The amount of toxin that yields optimal flocculation in the presence of one unit of antitoxin (AU) is called L_f and measures the combining power of the toxin. Vice-versa, the amount of antitoxin giving optimal flocculation with 1 L_f of toxin corresponds to one "Flocculating Unit of Antitoxin," which, in avid sera, is very close to *in vivo* AU (cf. p. 210).

Gel Precipitation. When an antigen mixture reacts with its antibodies (total antiserum) in a gel medium (agar, Agarose), multiple lines of precipitation are formed that correspond to the specific reactions of each component. It is thus possible by means of gel precipitation to analyse, using various techniques, the components of the antigen mixture (Fig. 7.2).

Simple Immunodiffusion. In this method, introduced by Oudin, the antigen, in aqueous solution, is layered in narrow-bore tubes above a column of 0.6% agar in which the antiserum has first been incorporated. As the solution diffuses through the gel, the antigenic components react with the antibodies to which they correspond. They thus form, in an excellent gradient, rings of precipitation. The position of these rings depends upon the concentration of the antigen and the time of diffusion. The greater the antigen concentration, the farther removed from the surface of the gel is the ring of precipitation. For a known concentration of antigen, the distance "h" from the ring to the gel–antigen interface is proportional to the square root of the diffusion time, according to Fick's law ($h = k\sqrt{t}$). The distance, therefore, increases after 1, 4, 9, and 16 days by a factor of 1, 2, 3, and 4 respectively; for example, if $k = 2$, the distance would be 2, 4, 6, and 8 mm after 1, 4, 9, and 16 days.

The specificity of the rings formed with the antigen mixture can be demonstrated clearly with absorption experiments, as exemplified in Fig. 7.3. With Oudin's test, the diffusion in the tube operates in only a single dimension. For the titration of immunoglobulins, however, Mancini introduced *simple radial diffusion*[1], in which different dilutions of a standard antigen and of an unknown prepa-

---

1 This is not to be confused with radioimmunodiffusion or radioimmunoelectrophoresis, in which radioactive antigens are used and the precipitation lines are revealed by autoradiography

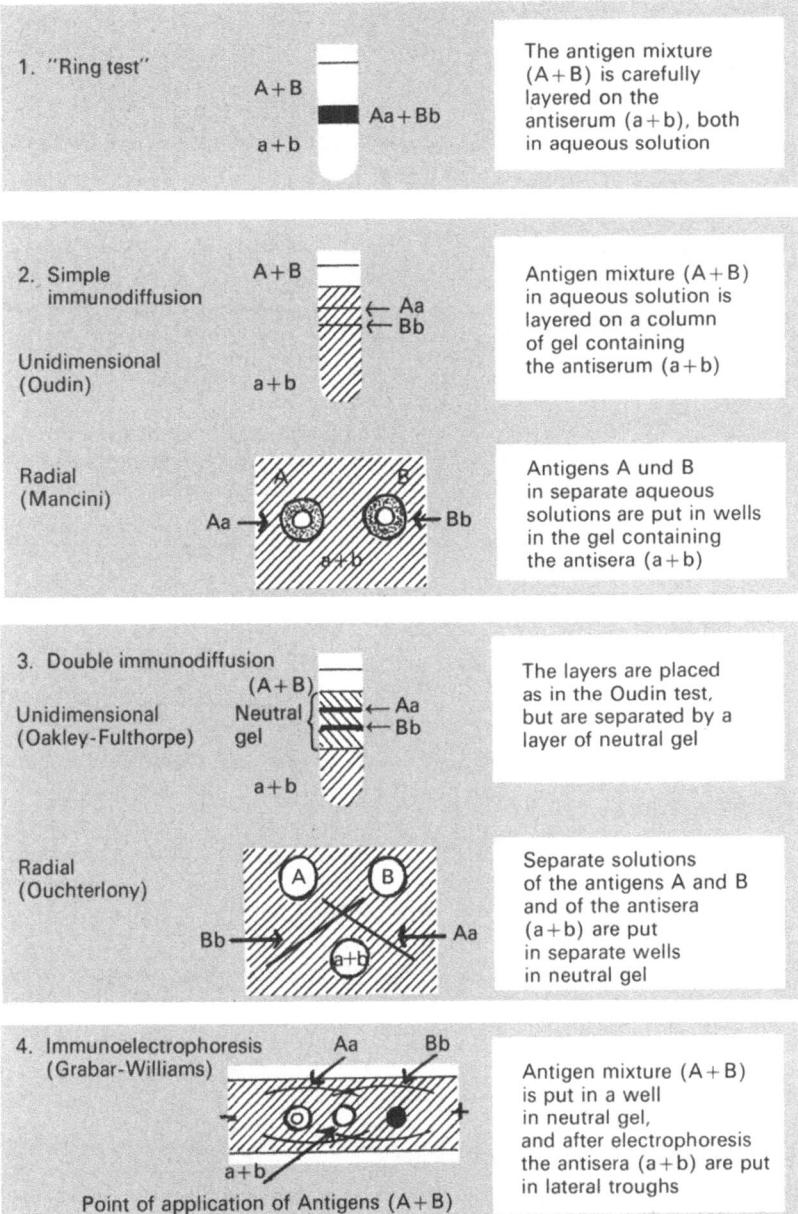

Fig. 7.2. Methods of immunochemical analysis by gel precipitation

ration are placed in separate wells made in a plate of gel in which specific antibody has been incorporated (immunoplate). The antigen diffuses radially, forming rings of precipitation whose diameters are proportional to the logarithm of the antigen concentration. The horizontal distance, m, between the parallel lines obtained with the standard

dilution (S) and unknown dilution (D) enables calculation of the relative potency of the latter (Fig. 7.4).

Double Immunodiffusion. Oakley and Fulthrope modified Oudin's technique, interposing a neutral layer of agar between the gel containing the antibody, located in the

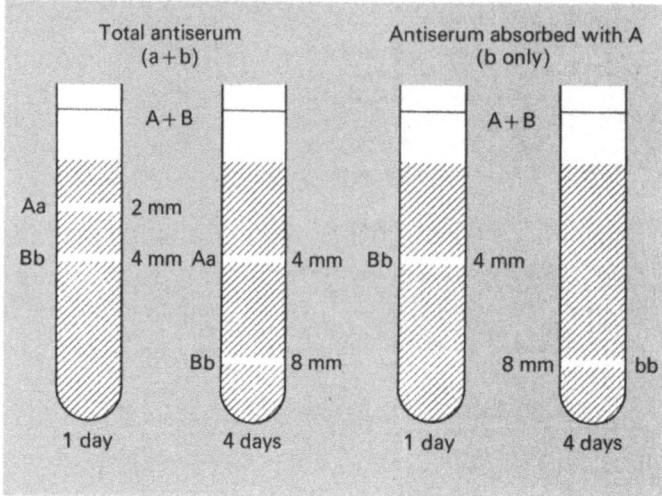

Fig. 7.3. Proof of specificities of the precipitation rings in Oudin's technique through absorption

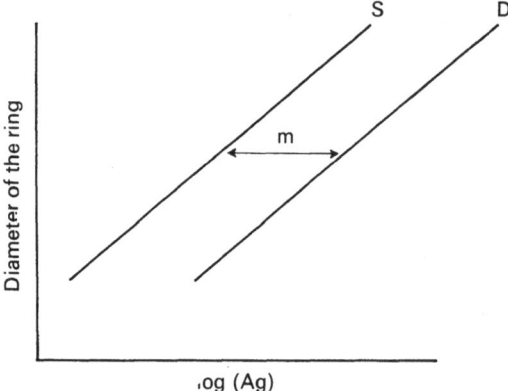

Fig. 7.4. Graph of relative antibody concentration in the Mancini test

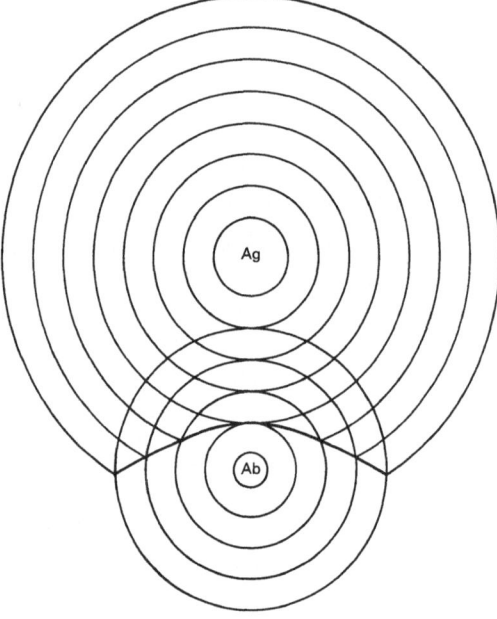

Fig. 7.5. Formation of precipitin line in the Ouchterlony plate

bottom of the tube, and the aqueous antigen solution, located on the surface. Under these conditions, the antigen diffuses from the bottom upward and the antibody diffuses from the top downward, forming a ring of precipitation in the neutral layer of gel. A variant of this technique (Preer) consists of placing a drop of antiserum in the bottom of the tube, covering it with a layer of neutral gel, and after solidification, adding the antigen solution.

In Oakley's technique, because the diffusion is double, it proceeds in a single dimension. However, in double radial diffusion, introduced by Ouchterlony, the antigen and the antibody – both in aqueous solutions – dif-

fuse into one another from proximate wells cut in a layer of neutral gel. Figure 7.5 illustrates the formation of the precipitin line in the Ouchterlony plate.

With the latter technique, numerous arrangements can be used, depending upon the experimental objectives. One of the most commonly used is that shown in Fig. 7.6. If the front wells contain the same (A 2) anti-

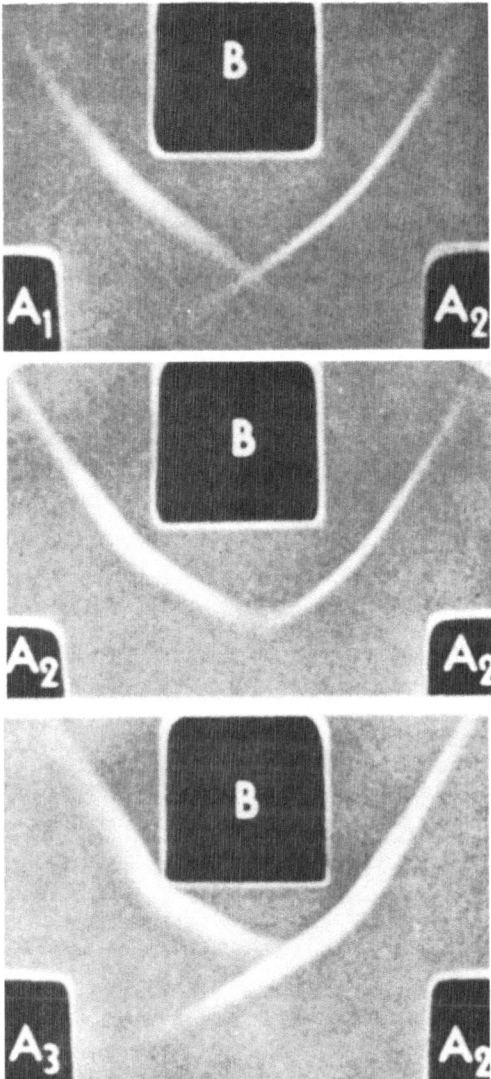

Fig. 7.6. Identical (complete or partial) and nonidentical reactions in double immunodiffusion

gen, a continuous line of precipitation (identity reaction) is formed. In the case of different antigens (A 1 and A 2) the lines intersect; when there is partial identity (e.g., A 2 and A 1, 2), a spur is formed in the direction of the monospecific antigen (here, A 2).

The use of immunodiffusion methods has permitted detailed analysis of the antigenic components of organic materials. For example, simple diffusion has shown that donkey's milk produces, with a homologous im-

mune serum, five rings of precipitation, three of which disappear when the immune serum is absorbed with horse milk. As many as ten antigenic components have been found in eggwhite, and even after three recrystallizations, chicken ovalbumin disclosed three antigenic impurities. Figure 7.7 illustrates, in diagrammatic form, some examples of antigen analysis with the Ouchterlony test.

Immunoelectrophoresis. Grabar and Williams combined electrophoresis with immunodiffusion and obtained a better separation of the lines of precipitation. In immunoelectrophoresis, an antigenic mixture is placed in a well in a plate of gel; after electrophoretic separation of the components, the antiserum (total) is added in a longitudinal trough (see Fig. 7.2, 4) along the path of electrophoretic migration.

In alkaline pH, the proteins, negatively charged, migrate toward the anode[2], and the components, separated along the axis of electrophoretic migration, diffuse radially to form a series of precipitation arcs with the specific antibodies diffusing from the lateral troughs in the gel.

Immunoelectrophoresis has a considerably greater power of resolution than that of immunodiffusion, making possible the separation of antigenically distinct components that have differing electrophoretic mobilities. For example, in normal human serum, immunoelectrophoretic analysis permits characterization of up to 30 components, instead of five (albumin, α_1, α_2, β, γ) as disclosed by simple paper electrophoresis or agar-gel electrophoresis. In ascending order of their electrophoretic mobilities, the

---

2 The electrophoretic mobilities are not determined from the point of application of the sample, but at a point situated to the left, in the direction of the cathode. This is because a current establishes itself in a direction opposite to that of electrophoretic migration. This current, called endosmosis, results from the fact that agar is not completely neutral and possesses an electronegative charge in relation to the buffer in which it is embedded. Under these conditions, since the support-gel is fixed, it is the buffer that moves in the direction of the cathode

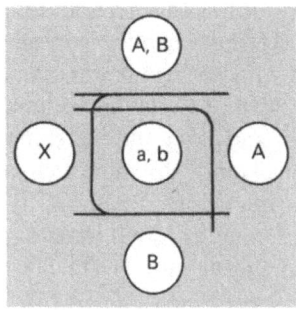

A and B are unrelated antigens;
X is partially identical to B,
but is not related to A

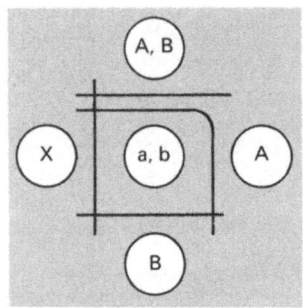

A, B, and X are unrelated

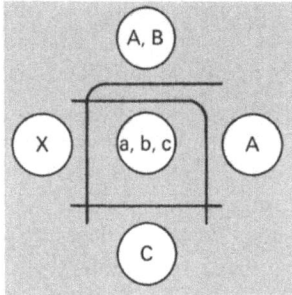

A, B, and C are unrelated
antigens; X is identical to B

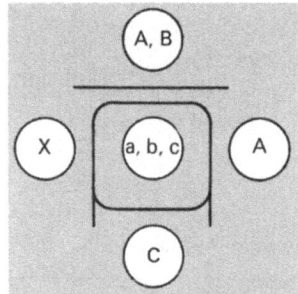

A and B are unrelated antigens;
A and C exhibit partial identity;
X is identical to A

Fig. 7.7. Example of antigenic
analysis in Ouchterlony plate

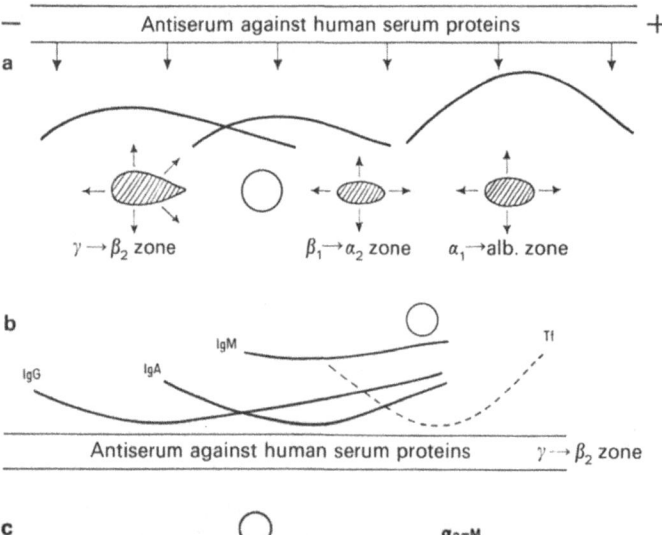

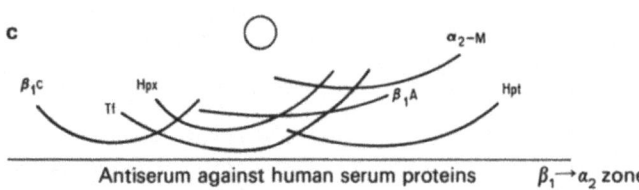

Fig. 7.8. Immunoelectrophoretic
separation of the principal protein
components of normal human
serum

components are differentiated as: γ and β_2 globulins (IgG, IgA, IgM); β_1 (siderophilin or transferrin); hemopexin (β_1B); β_1C–β_1A, β_1E, and β_F, corresponding to C3, C4, and C5; α_2 (haptoglobin, ceruloplasmin, α_2 macroglobulin), α_{1a} (antitrypsin), and albumin (Fig. 7.8).

Two-Dimensional Immunoelectrophoresis. Laurell has developed a new immunoelectrophoretic technique which, besides giving a marked increase in resolution, is especially valuable for quantitation. Electrophoresis of the antigen is carried out in one dimension, the gel is cut, unused gel is discarded and warm gel containing the antibody is poured onto the plate. A second electrophoresis is then carried out at a right angle to the initial direction of travel. After diffusion, distinct peaks are obtained whose areas are directly proportional to the concentration of antigen. In the Laurell technique, electrophoretic separation is achieved with a voltage of 10 V/m for at least 60 min (and not at 3–6 V/m as in the technique of Grabar and Williams), so that a cooling device is required.

For the titration of purified antigen the first electrophoretic separation is not necessary. Successive dilutions of the purified antigen are added to contiguous wells of the antibody containing gel, and electrophoresis is carried out at a right angle. As a consequence of the migration of antigen molecules precipitation cones are formed (rather like interplanetary rockets) and the procedure is therefore designated "rocket immunoelectrophoresis" (cf. Fig. 7.9).

Counterimmunoelectrophoresis. Another important technique is usually called "counterimmunoelectrophoresis" (a better designation is "immuno-osmophoresis") and consists of cutting wells about 8–10 mm apart in a gel plate. Antigen is added to one well, and antibody to the other. The antigen must migrate more quickly than the antibody at the pH used. After passage of the current, antigen migrates to the anode and antibody, because of endosmotic flow, travels in the opposite direction: $+\overrightarrow{Ab}\ \overleftarrow{Ag}-$. Consequently, the appearance of the precipitation line may occur within 20–30 min, instead of the 24–

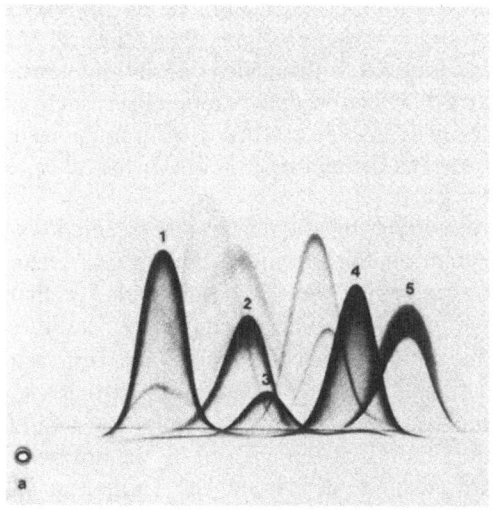 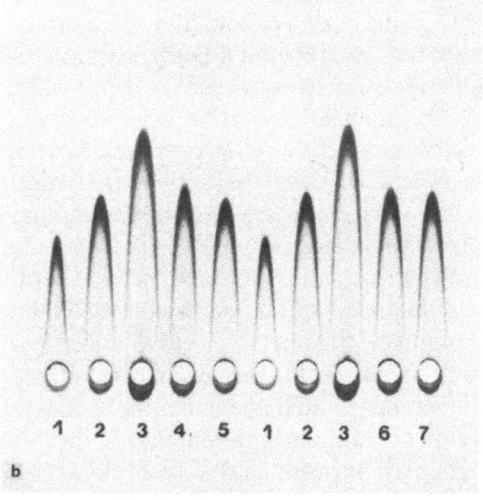

Fig. 7.9. a Two-dimensional immunoelectrophoresis (Laurell) Human serum samples were applied to well (*a*) of the first dimension and an oligospecific antiserum was mixed with the gel of the second dimension. Numbered precipitates correspond to following proteins: *1*) tranferrin; *2*) α_2-macroglobulin; *3*) ceruloplasmin; *4*) α_1-antitrypsin; *5*) α_1-glycoprotein. **b** Rocket immunoelectrophoresis. Anti-hemopexin was incorporated in the gel. Application wells 1–3: standard samples. Application wells 4–7: test samples

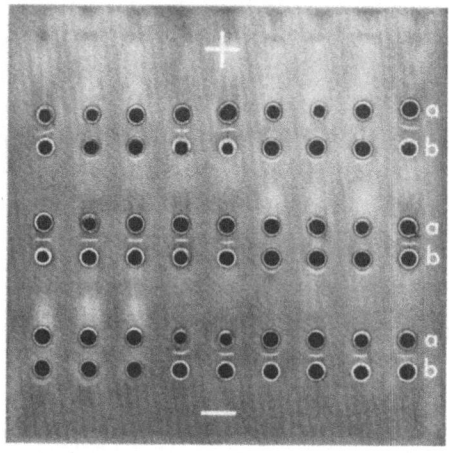

Fig. 7.10. Counterimmunoelectrophoresis. Application wells *a:* Rabbit serum ànti-HB$_s$ Application wells *b:* Human serum samples, HB$_s$-positive or negative

48 h required in the conventional Ouchterlony technique.

Counter-immunoelectrophoresis has proved to be extremely useful as a routine procedure to detect hepatitis HBs antigen (Australia antigen), in the rapid diagnosis of meningococcal meningitis (Fig. 7.10).

Agglutination

When a suspension of particles that bear antigenic determinants on their surfaces is mixed with the specific antiserum, large granules are formed that quickly sediment. This is the phenomenon of agglutination, described by Gruber and Durham at the beginning of the century.

The phenomenon may be observed with microbes or cells (erythrocytes, leukocytes, or other cells), in the activity of determinants naturally existing on the surface (direct agglutination), with cells (generally erythrocytes), or inert particles (latex, bentonite, etc.) artifically coated with a soluble antigen (indirect or passive agglutination). In any case, the mechanism of agglutination is fundamentally the same as that of specific precipitation, that is, the formation of bivalent antibody bridges that connect the antigenic determinants of adjacent particles (see Fig. 7.1).

As Bordet demonstrated, the presence of electrolytes constitutes a critical factor in agglutination: In the absence of salts, the particles fix the antibody, but are incapable of agglutinating. This fact caused the authors to espouse a two-stage theory, according to which the union of the antigen and the antibody (first stage) constituted the specific immunologic phenomenon, whereas agglutination represented only a secondary, nonspecific phenomenon (second stage) comparable to the flocculation of hydrophobic colloids by electrolytes. If this concept were accurate, mixing a suspension containing particles of two types, A and B, with an antiserum containing anti-A and anti-B antibodies would result in mixed granules of the two particles. However, in experiments with particles easily differentiated via microscopic examination, such as sheep or chicken erythrocytes, granules were observed containing only one or the other of the particles.

According to the currently accepted explanation, the relevance of salinity in its neutralization of the net negative charge that the particles exhibit in neutral pH, nullifies the repulsion between them and fosters a sufficient degree of attraction. In this way short-range noncovalent forces that assure the binding of the antigen by the antibody are able to determine the formation of bridges between adjacent particles.

Titration of Agglutinating Sera. The agglutinin titer of an antiserum is determined in a semiquantitative test in which decreasing quantities of serum (for example, 0.5-ml dilutions 1:10, 1:20, 1:40, etc) are reacted with a constant quantity of antigen (for example, 0.5 ml of a bacterial suspension containing $0.5–1.0 \times 10^9$ organisms per milliliter). After a period of incubation at the proper temperature, readings of the results are taken, noting the degree of agglutination $(++, +, -)$ by the nated eye, or with the aid of a magnifying lens. The agglutination titer is expressed in terms of the greatest dilution that gives rise to complete $(+++)$ or partial $(+)$ agglutination. As pointed out previously, the precision of this type of test is only $\pm 50\%$.

Various factors play an important role in the determination of agglutination titer:

1. The *presence of electrolytes* is essential to the phenomenon, and the pH of the diluent must not be excessively acidic or alkaline in order to avoid nonspecific results. Saline solution is generally utilized as diluent (1.9% NaCl solution), buffered to a pH of 7.2.

2. The *concentration of the antigenic suspension* also constitutes an important factor, for the greater the concentration of particles, the more rapid the agglutination. On the other hand, concentrated antigenic suspensions cause greater consumption of antibody and, consequently, lower agglutination titers.

3. The *temperature* at which the reaction occurs is important. The best temperature for the agglutination of microbes is 37 °C. In hemagglutination, e.g., in the study of the ABO or Rh blood groups, it is convenient to discriminate between the immune antibodies, which react better at 37 °C (warm agglutinins)[3] and the natural antibodies, which agglutinate better at 20 °C; there are also hemagglutinins, such as cryoagglutinins of atypical primary pneumonia or the anti-I agglutinins of acquired hemolytic anemias that react intensely only at 4 °C (cold agglutinins).

4. The *duration of incubation* is also important. One usually takes a first reading of the agglutination test after incubation for 1–2 h at 37 °C and then again after 24-h incubation at room temperature or under refrigeration at 4 °C. Agitation hastens considerably the results in tests performed on plates or on slides with concentrated antigenic suspensions (rapid agglutination). When the test is performed in tubes with diluted antigenic suspensions (slow agglutination), the results can be hastened through moderate centrifugation, followed by gradual resuspension of the sediment.

5. Certain antibodies called *incomplete antibodies* are incapable of agglutinating and, when coexisting with agglutinating antibodies, can block the fixation of the latter and produce a "prozone" of inhibition:

Dilution of the serum	1:10	1:20	1:40	1:80	1:160	1:320	1:640
Agglutination (Prozone)	−	−	+	+	+	+	−
						(Titer)	

Prozones are observed not uncommonly in certain antibacterial sera such as anti-*Brucella* sera. With anti-Rh antibodies, it is common to observe the exclusive occurrence of nonagglutinating antibodies, which may be disclosed for example through the utilization of diluents with high levels of albumin, the trypsinization of red blood cells, or the antiglobulin test.

It was thought at first that the incomplete antibodies were incapable of agglutinating because they were univalent. Today, however, we know that the lack of agglutiation of these antibodies is due to an inaccessible location of the antigenic determinants to which they correspond (Fig. 7.11), or to their weak avidity (low association constant).

It is obvious that an agglutination titer, even when determined under standardized conditions, does not denote the total level of antibodies in the serum, but only that of the predominant antibodies. Thus, for example, if A, B, and C antigens exist on the surface of a particle, the agglutination of these particles in the presence of a whole antiserum (antibodies a, b, and c) will be assured, in

---

3 Agglutinin is the term used for agglutinating antibodies

I

II

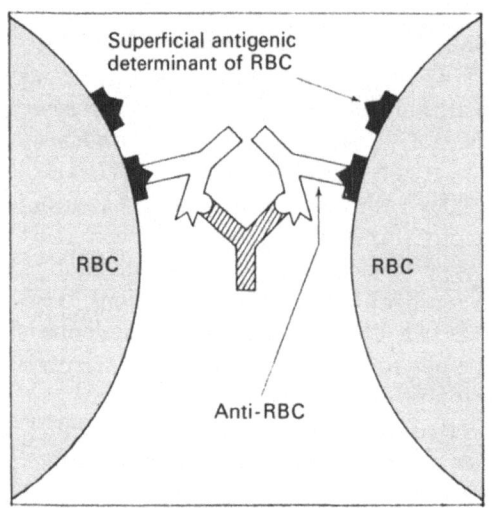
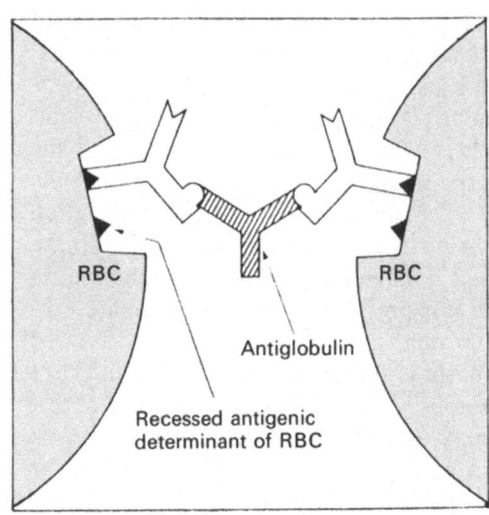

Fig. 7.11. Schematic representation of the absence of hemagglutination observed in certain systems, e.g., in the Rh system. According to interpretation I, the antibody, because it has combining sites that are too close together, cannot unite with two antigenic sites; whereas, according to interpretation II, the antibody is incapable of establishing linking bridges because of the deeply recessed location of the antigenic sites in crypts in the surface of the erythrocyte. In either case, the union can be assured by means of an antiglobulin serum (Coombs' test)

weak dilutions of antiserum, for any of the antibodies –

B-b-B-b-B-b-B
A-a-A-a-A-a-A
C-c-C-c-C-c-C

However, in an end-point dilution (titer), only the molecules of the antibody present in greatest quantity enter into play, e.g., for antibody a –

B   B   B   B
A-a-A-a-A-a-A
C   C   C   C

Somatic and Flagellar Agglutination. In motile bacteria such as *Salmonella*, agglutination can be of two types (Fig. 7.12):

1) *Flagellar* (H) *agglutination* occurs when microorganisms unite through their flagella, forming loose floccules that dissociate easily under agitation. This type of agglutination develops rapidly, enabling a reading of the H titer to be taken after 1–2 h of incubation[4].

2) *Somatic* (O) *agglutination* occurs when the union proceeds by way of antibody

bridges uniting the bacterial bodies so as to form compact granules, not easily dissociable. This type of agglutination develops slowly, in 24–48 h.

The agglutinogens (antigens that can be detected using agglutinating antibodies) responsible for these two types of reaction can be easily discriminated by heating the bacterial suspension at 100 °C: Such treatment destroys the H antigen without appreciably injuring the O antigen. On the other hand, the agglutinability of the O type is impeded in the presence of 0.5% formalin, which does not act upon H agglutination.

In *Salmonella*, the O antigen is represented by a polysaccharide composed of repeated units (galactose-mannose-ramnose) that – depending upon the mode of linkage among the sugars and/or upon the existence of lateral chains on the basic trisaccharide – ex-

---

4 The designations H and O are derived from German and were used primarily for the motile and nonmotile strains of *Proteus*: the former an invasive veil on the surface of the agar, which was compared to breath (Ger. *Hauch*) on a window pane; the other variant, O, grows in isolated colonies, without the invasive veil (Ger. *Ohne Hauch*)

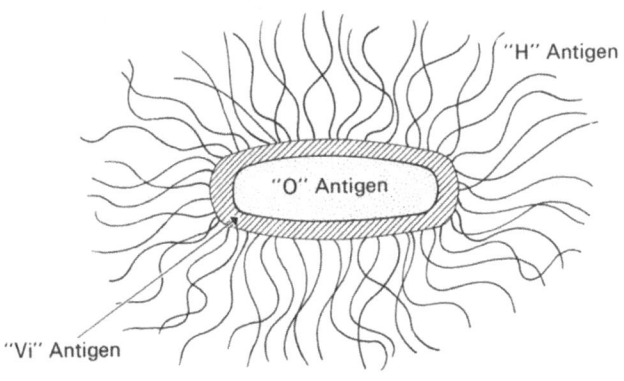

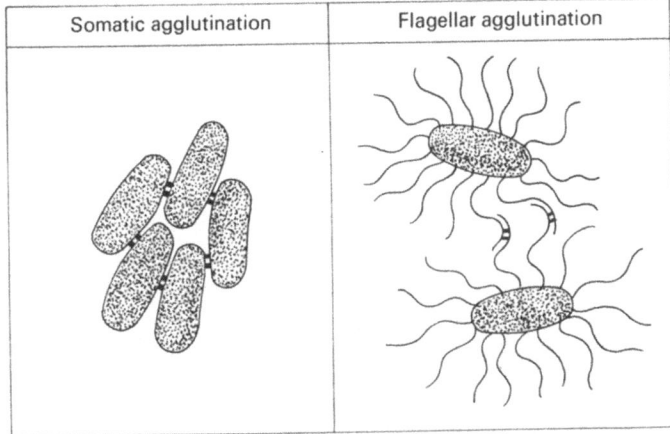

Fig. 7.12. Somatic and flagellar agglutination

hibit differing specificities (antigenic determinants). As for the flagellar antigens, we know that they are proteins, yet we know nothing about the chemical nature of their determinants.

Cross-Reactions in Microbial Agglutination. When two microbial species exhibit common antigens on their surfaces in addition to their specific antigens, or related antigens, cross-reactions occur among them; that is, the antiserum prepared with the homologous species is capable of agglutinating the heterologous species or vice versa.

We shall not occupy ourselves in this chapter with reactions due to related antigens, which can only be studied properly with the help of precipitation curves. Rather, we shall examine how cross-reactions due to group antigens can be distinguished utilizing the agglutinin absorption test.

Common antigens (group specific) and homologous antigens (type specific) can be represented by distinct molecules or by different regions of the same agglutinogen. In exemplifying this fact, the four species of *Salmonella* represented by the following abbreviated antigenic formulas are considered:

Salmonella paratyphi-B	4/b
Salmonella typhimurium	4/i
Salmonella anatum	3,10/e,h
Salmonella newington	3,15/e,h.

The first two are identical in respect of their somatic antigen (4) but differ in the flagellar antigens (b,i), whereas the last two possess identical flagellar antigens (e,h) but differ in one of the specificities of the O antigen (10 and 15).

If a rabbit is immunized with *S. paratyphi-B*, the total antiserum contains anti-4 + anti-b and, as such, agglutinates *S. paratyphi-B* (4/

b) as well as *S. typhimurium* (4/i). The same occurs with the anti-*typhimurium* (anti-4 + anti-i). However, by treating the anti-*paratyphi-B* serum with a thick suspension of *S. typhimurium*, we cause the absorption of the anti-4 agglutinin and thereby produce a monospecific anti-b antiserum.

Vice versa, the absorption of anti-*typhimurium* serum with *S. paratyphi-B* removes anti-4, leaving just anti-i. In this example, the common antigen and the specific antigens correspond to distinct molecules of the two agglutinogens.

The identical result is obtained, however, with the species *S. anatum* and *S. newington*, whose O specificities correspond to distinct regions of the respective agglutinogens:

$$\dfrac{(\text{Gal-}\alpha\,\overset{3}{\text{Man-Ra}})_n}{10} \qquad S.\ anatum$$

$$\dfrac{(\text{Gal-}\beta\,\overset{3}{\text{Man-Ra}})_n}{15} \qquad S.\ newington.$$

The 3,10 serum absorbed with 3,15 becomes monospecific anti-10 and, reciprocally, the anti-3,15 serum, absorbed with 3,10, becomes monospecific for 15.

The agglutinin absorption test has been widely utilized by bacteriologists for the differentiation of serologic types – in the enterobacteria group, for example. Utilizing monospecific sera obtained by absorption, more than 1,000 serotypes in the *Salmonella* genus can be distinguished (White-Kaufman table).

The determination of the agglutination titer of sera is important for the diagnosis of infections, as first demonstrated in typhoid fever (Widal's test). The agglutination absorption test permits differentiation of results due to a group reaction or to a mixed infection (Castellani's test). We might illustrate this by a case clinically characterized as typhoid fever, in which the serum of the patient exhibited an O agglutination titer of 1:640 for *S. typhosa* (9,12) and of 1:80 for *S. paratyphi-B* (4,12). Castellani's test (Table 7.1) may distinguish the group agglutination in a case of *S. typhosa* infection

Table 7.1. Model of Castellani's saturation of agglutinins test for the differentiation between group agglutination and mixed infection

Serum of the Patient	0 Agglutination with			
	T	B	T	B
Nonabsorbed	+	+	+	+
Absorbed with T	–	–	–	+
Absorbed with B	+	–	+	+
Interpretation:	Group agglutination		Mixed infection	

from that of a mixed infection of *S. typhosa* (T) and *S. paratyphi-B*.

Passive Hemagglutination. It is possible to fix antigens to the surfaces of erythrocytes or inert particles (colloid, latex, bentonite, etc.), making them agglutinable by the respective antibodies. With red blood cells (RBCs), this gives rise to passive or indirect hemagglutination, as opposed to natural or direct hemagglutination, which results from the interaction of antibodies with natural agglutinogens of the RBCs. Various antigens can be fixed simultaneously to the same RBC, which then becomes agglutinable by various antibodies. The same occurs in direct hemagglutination: the anti-RBC serum of sheep, for example, contains a mixture of antibodies with specificities directed against the various natural antigenic determinants of sheep RBCs.

Examples of natural hemagglutination include the agglutination of human erythrocytes by the serum of individuals with different blood groups; the agglutination of sheep erythrocytes by the serum of patients with infectious mononucleosis (Paul-Bunnell reaction); the cryohemagglutination of human O erythrocytes by the serum of patients with primary atypical pneumonia. Examples of passive agglutination include the agglutination of polystyrene (latex) or bentonite particles by the so-called rheumatoid factor; the agglutination of cholesterol crystals coated with cardiolipin by the serum of syphilis patients (Kline and VDRL tests); the passive hemagglutination tests with erythrocytes coated with specific agglutinogens, is utilized in the serodiagnosis of various infections because of their high sensitivity (detection of antibody quantities of the order of 0.003 µg).

Generally speaking, the polysaccharide antigens, when not highly purified [5], can attach directly to erythrocytes. Proteins, however, require prior treatment of the red blood cell with tannic acid (tanning – Boyden's technique), which makes it possible to obtain RBC suspensions specifically agglutinable in the presence of the respective antisera. It is not known for certain how tanning functions; it appears, however, that it not only causes a loose adsorption of the proteins to the red blood cell surfaces, but it also becomes easily agglutinable in the presence of small quantities of antibody. Occasionally, it causes nonspecific agglutination in the control tubes containing no antibody. This last inconvenience generally can be counterbalanced by the use of special diluents (e.g., saline solution with 1% normal rabbit serum).

In addition to tanning, other methods are also available for conjugating proteins to the red cell:

1) *Covalent bonding*. Covalent linkages are achieved by bifunctional molecules such as bidiazotized benzine (BDB), carbodiimide (CDI), glutaraldehyde (GA), and others.

2) *Metallic bridge*. Certain multivalent cations, Cr^+ in particular, modify the red blood cell surface, making it capable of adsorbing proteins.

3. *Immunologic bridge*. To avoid autoagglutinating suspensions because of the conjugation of erythrocytic proteins, one may resort to an interesting method that consists

of the following steps: (1) the protein antigen is conjugated by means of BDB with nonagglutinating anti-Rh antibodies; (2) the conjugate is then fixed to Rh-positive red cells (immunologic bridge).

Regardless of the method employed, the specificity of each amount of erythrocyte suspension must be controlled, for small variations in technique can noticeably affect the degree of autoagglutinability. Today there is a tendency to fix the erythrocytes before or after the fixation of the antigen to obtain suspensions that remain unchanged for months when maintained at 4 °C.

The erythrocytes most commonly used are human erythrocytes or sheep erythrocytes; in certain cases, however, there is an advantage in using erythrocytes from other species.

The quantity of antigen fixed to the erythrocytes is of major importance. It is advisable to determine the optimum quantity in preliminary experiments; that is, the quantity that produces the highest titer in comparison to a reference antiserum. The minimum number of molecules capable of "sensitizing" the erythrocytes can be determined by using antigens labeled with isotopes. The minimum number of molecules of O polysaccharide of *Salmonella* is of the order of 2,000 molecules per erythrocyte.

The hemagglutination reaction itself can be performed in tubes or, more conveniently, on plastic plates with wells in which different dilutions of serum to be tested are distributed along with a constant dose of the erythrocyte suspension. This latter technique is practical because it utilizes only 25 µl of serum. This assemblage, shown in Fig. 7.13, consists of a plastic plate with 75-µl wells and a metal loop titrator with a 25-µl capacity (Takatsy microtitrator). Into each well, 25 µl of diluent is pipetted; then 25 µl of the antiserum under study is deposited in the first well. The microtitrator is then dipped into the first well, and the solution is mixed well by rotating the stem of the microtitrator between the fingers. Then 25 µl of successive dilutions of serum at 1:2, 1:4, 1:8, etc. are passed successively from

---

5 Fixation of polysaccharides to red blood cells appears to depend upon the presence of ionized sugars (amino sugars, uronic acids). Thus, for example, the O polysaccharides of *Salmonella* obtained by alkaline hydrolysis, which possess the characteristics described previously, attach more easily to erythrocytes than do highly purified polysaccharides obtained through acid hydrolysis

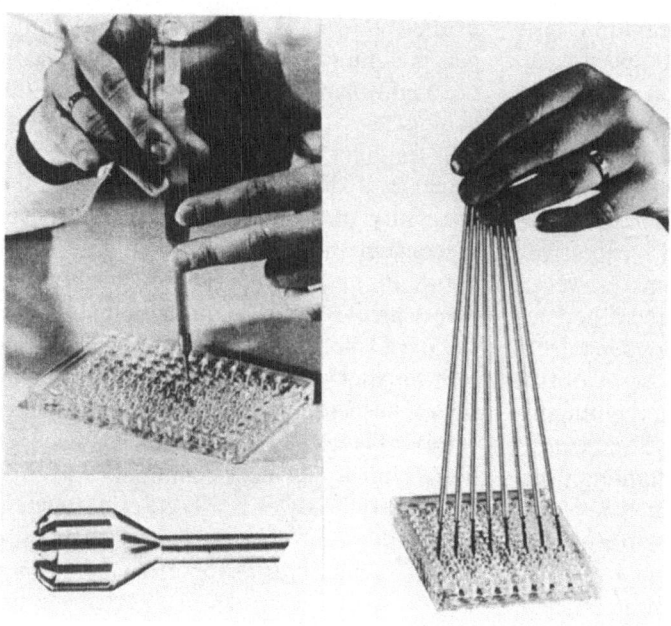

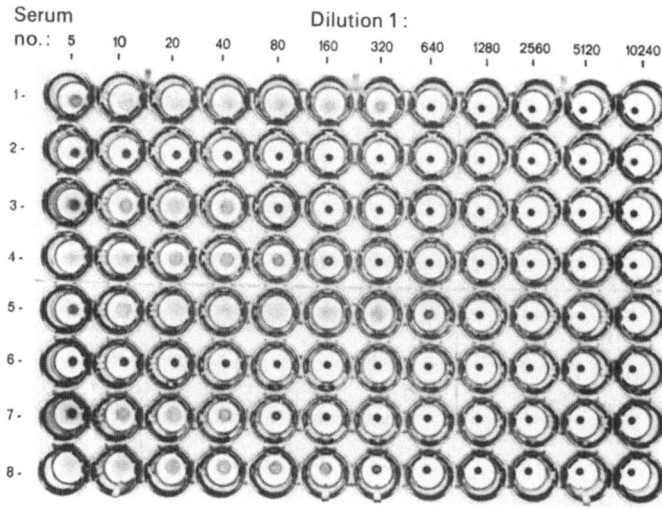

Fig. 7.13. Hemagglutination in the microtiter plate (Takatsy's microtitrator)

one well to another. Subsequently, 25 µl of 1% erythrocyte suspension is added, agitating carefully to mix the reagents. The plate is covered or placed in a humid chamber to prevent evaporation and incubated at the desired temperature. Results are generally read after 2 h at room temperature and after 12–24 h when refrigerated at 4 °C. In the tubes as well as in the plates, the results are in-

terpreted in conjunction with the pattern of the sediment, which exhibits the form of a button in negative reactions (−), that of a round plate with irregular borders in strongly positive reactions (4+), and with intermediate patterns in the +, 2+, and 3+ reactions (see Fig. 7.11, bottom). In case of doubt, the reading can be confirmed by gently resuspending the sediment and then observing with a lens the presence and size of the granules.

Immunofluorescence

It is possible to make the antigen–antibody reaction visible by labeling one of the reagents with substances called fluorochromes, which have the capacity to absorb luminous energy, to store it for short periods (10^{-9}–10^{-1} s), and then to emit it in the form of radiation of a greater wavelength. This mechanism of fluorescence is due essentially to the absorption of the energy of photons by electrons of peripheral orbits that move to occupy orbits more distant from the nucleus, inducing a state of excitability in the molecule. Such a state is, however, of extremely short duration, because the electrons quickly return to their former orbits, i.e., to a state of repose, due to the emission of luminous radiation. Because part of it is degraded into thermal or mechanical energy, the quanta of light emitted (fluorescence) have less energy, or greater wavelength, than that of the exciting radiation (Stokes law).

For this reason, anti-DNA antibodies labeled with fluorescein have an absorption maximum at approximately 490 nm [1 nm (nanometer) or millimicron (mµ) is equal to 10^{-9} m, or 10^{-6} mm], whereas its emission maximum takes place at around 530 nm. If a section or cellular smear is treated with labeled antibody, the cytoplasm appears blue, whereas the nucleus exhibits green-yellow fluorescence.

In addition to fluorescein, rhodamine B, which emits an orange-red fluorescence, is also frequently used. Both fluorochromes are used in the isothiocyanate form, which conjugates easily to proteins in alkaline pH (>9):

Fluorescein—N=C=S
  +Protein—NH$_2$ ⟶ Fl—N – C – N—Pr
                       | || |
                       H   S   H

(Isothiocyanate of fluorescein)

For microscopic observation of fluorescence, the following accessories are necessary: (1) a source of excitatory light; (2) a thermal filter; (3) an excitatory filter; (4) a dark-field (cardioid) condenser; and (5) a "barrier" or protector filter. The source of excitatory light is generally in the form of a quartz bulb with mercury vapor (Osram HB 200 lamp), which emits visible and ultraviolet radiation (below 400 nm).

The light proceeding from the excitatory source passes successively through the thermal filter and the excitatory filter – the latter permeable only to radiation of a wavelength around 435 nm, which is still situated in the band of absorption of the fluorescein. Next, the excitatory light is directed at the cardioid condenser, which projects it along the microscope's optical axis on to the preparation. The light transmitted by the preparation includes not only radiation of the same wavelength, but also radiation having a wavelength longer than that of the excitatory light (fluorescent). The barrier filter interposed between the preparation and the eyepiece protects the eye of the observer from short wavelength radiation that passes through the objective (Fig. 7.14).

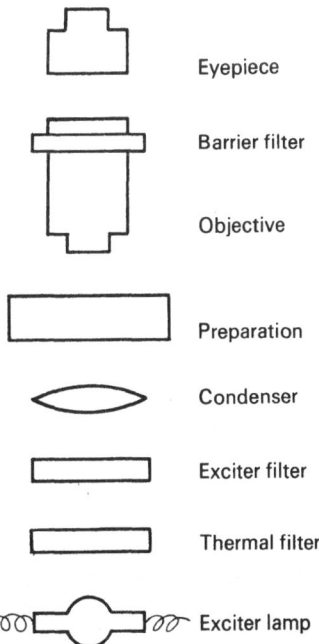

Eyepiece

Barrier filter

Objective

Preparation

Condenser

Exciter filter

Thermal filter

Exciter lamp

Fig. 7.14. The optical system in fluorescence microscopy

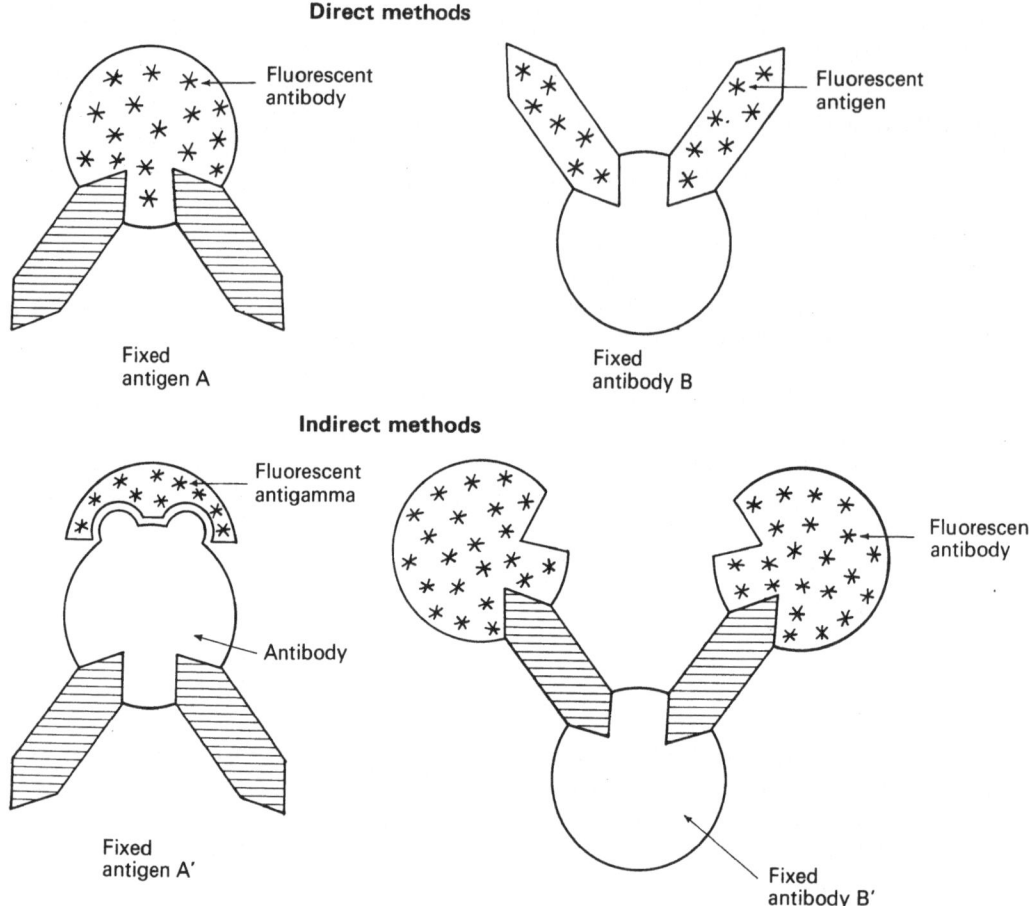

Fig. 7.15. Different methods of immunofluorescence

In principle, two techniques are utilized for the study of immunofluorescence (Fig. 7.15) 1) *Direct immunofluorescence*. This involves direct coloration of the antigen with labeled antibody. It is commonly used to identify microorganisms by immunofluorescence, e.g., *E.coli* (enteropathogenic serotypes), *Klebsiella* (serotypes), *Streptococcus* (Lancefield groups), *Gonococcus*, *B.pertussis*, *C.diphtheriae*, *Leptospira* (serotypes), and *Candida albicans*.
2) *Indirect immunofluorescence*. The specimen with attached antigen is treated with an unlabeled specific antibody and then, after washing, incubated with conjugated antigamma globulin produced against the immunoglobulin of the species from which the specific antibody originates.

The double-layer immunofluorescence just described is frequently utilized to demonstrate antimicrobial antibodies (serodiagnosis of syphilis, toxoplasmosis, leptospirosis, schistosomes, Chagas' disease, etc.), as well as to detect autoantibodies, e.g., antinuclear antibodies in lupus erythematosus or intercellular antibodies in pemphigus. There can also be formation of triple layers, as in the so-called sandwich technique. The first layer is an antigen–antibody complex, a second layer, unlabeled antibody against antibodies of the first layer, and the third, labeled antibody with a specificity directed against the second layer. This technique is used to demonstrate antibody on the surfaces of plasma cells, as performed by Coons and his associates.

The immunofluorescence reactions for the demonstration of complement fixation are similar to the sandwich technique. A first layer is composed of an antigen–antibody complex; a layer of complement is adsorbed to it; then a third level of labeled anticomplement is added. [Anticomplement is obtained by immunization with antigen-antibody complex or with zymosan-C3 (production of anti-β^1C serum).] The demonstration of complement fixation in vivo by immunofluorescence suggests that the lesions such as those that occur in the Arthus reaction (vasculitis), in certain forms of glomerulonephritis by the deposition of antigen–antibody complex or by cytotoxic antibodies, are produced by antigen–antibody complexes.

In any case, one must utilize reagents previously characterized as to their activity (titration of the conjugate to determine the optimum dose) and their specificity (absence of nonspecific fluorescence), which generally can be achieved by using conjugates obtained from potent antisera and with discrete labeling (low fluorochrome/protein ratio).

Complement Fixation

In combining with the antigen, certain antibodies affiliated with the IgG and IgM immunoglobulins form complexes capable of fixing complement. The phenomenon was discovered at the beginning of the century by Bordet and Gengou and quickly aroused great interest because of its application in the serodiagnosis of syphilis (Wassermann reaction). Today, numerous other infections are diagnosed by the complement fixation reaction (CF), e.g., Chagas' disease, South American blastomycosis, toxoplasmosis, echinococcosis, gonococcic infections, rickettsiosis, and numerous virus infections (psittacosis, lymphogranuloma, poliomyelitis, arbovirus infections, epidemic parotitis, influenza). Moreover, the CF test is also utilized, through the use of known antisera, to characterize the types and subtype of nu-

merous viruses, such as the aftosa viruses, the arboviruses, and the echoviruses.

The Qualitative Test. The complement fixation test can be summarized in the following manner:

I. Specific antigen (Ag)+C   Free C
 II. Anti-Ag antibody+C   Free C
  III. Anti-Ag+Ag+C

If EA (e.g., sheep erythrocytes sensitized by rabbit antisheep erythrocytes) is added to mixtures I and II, hemolysis occurs:

$$EA + free\ C = Hemolysis\,.$$

The addition of EA to mixture III, however, produces little or no hemolysis, for part or all of the complement mixed with the Ag-anti-Ag complex will have been consumed:

$$EA + fixed\ C \rightarrow Absence\ of\ hemolysis\,.$$

The qualitative test can be limited to the three tubes mentioned previously – I and II being antigen and serum controls, respectively, and III being the reaction tube. The mechanism of the test, in its two stages, is represented schematically in Fig. 7.16.

In the early days of serology, when the Wassermann reaction was introduced, the degree of fixation was evaluated by the percentage of hemolysis observed, expressing the results as $++++$ (absence of hemolysis), $+++$ (25% lysis), $++$ (50% lysis), and $+$ (75% lysis). Today, however, to evaluate the fixative potency of a serum, increasing dilutions of antiserum are mixed with adequate fixed amounts of antigen and complement, proceeding to a reading of the results in terms of the quantity of hemoglobin liberated in the supernatants, as previously described for the spectrophotometric measurement of complement-mediated hemoglobin release.

Quantitative Testing Methods. Two methods for quantitative testing should be mentioned here:

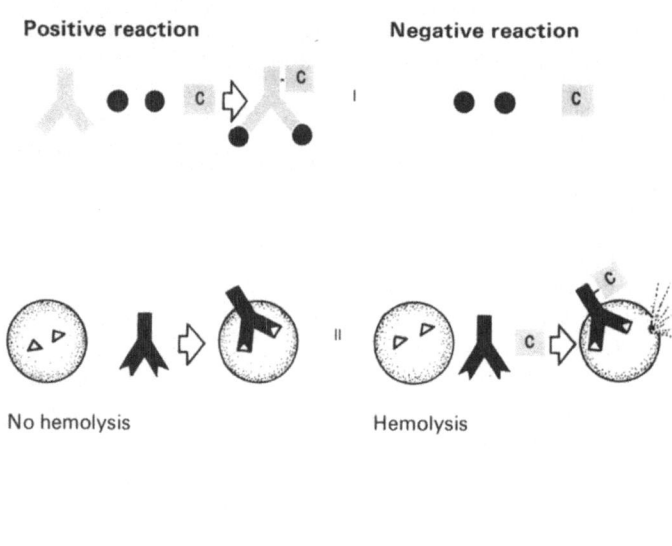

Positive reaction   **Negative reaction**

No hemolysis   Hemolysis

Wassermann antibody

Wassermann antigen
(cardiolipid)

C   Complement

Antisheep erythrocyte
antibody

Sheep erythrocytes (E)

Antigenic determinants
of E

Fig. 7.16. Mechanism of the Wassermann reaction for complement fixation

1) In the *macromethod of Mayer and associates,* dilutions of serum (or of antigen) are incubated for 20 h at 2°–4 °C with an optimum dose of antigen (or of serum) and an excess of complement, e.g., 100 CH_{50} units. Controls containing just serum $+C$ or antigen $+C$ are also included in the test, in order to detect any anticomplement activity in the reagents. After incubation the mixtures are diluted to measure the quantity of unfixed C and to determine the number of fixed CH_{50} units.

2) In *serodiagnostic tests* in which small quantities of complement (2–5 CH_{50} units) are used in such a way that the residual quantity of unfixed C is of the order of 0.8–1.2 CH_{50} units, the amount of complement fixation can be determined directly by addition of EA to the undiluted mixtures. Included in this category are the quantitative techniques (perhaps better described as semiquantitative) of Christiansen, of Maltaner and associates, of Stein and Van Ngu, and of others.

The introduction of Mayer's method permitted investigators to establish with precision the relations between antigen and antibody in the complement fixation reaction. By maintaining the antibody dose constant and varying the concentration of Ag, a CF curve is produced that notably resembles the curve of specific precipitation, clearly exhibiting a zone of inhibition by excess antigen (Fig. 7.17). However, when a fixed dose of Ag is added to a varying dose of immune serum, the curve changes and does not exhibit a zone of inhibition (Fig. 7.18). Still, in both cases the quantity of fixed C reaches a maximum that corresponds to the maximally reactive dose of antigen (in the tests with constant antiserum) or of serum (in the tests with constant antigen).

If we represent graphically the quantities of serum on the abscissa, and the number of units of complement fixed in the presence of maximally reactive doses of antigen on the ordinate, a sigmoid curve is obtained (Fig. 7.19). The fixation potency, expressed

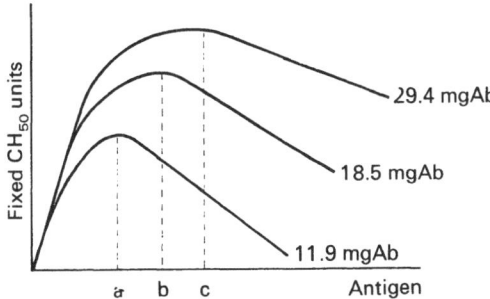

Fig. 7.17. Quantitative complement fixation studied by the macromethod of Mayer et al. in systems with constant levels of antibody (11.9 mg, 18.5 mg, and 29.4 mg) and variable amounts of antigen

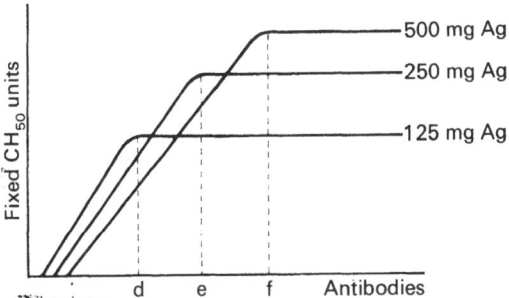

Fig. 7.18. Quantitative fixation of complement studied by the macromethod of Mayer et al. in systems with constant amounts of antigen (125 mg, 250 mg, and 500 mg) and variable amounts of antibody

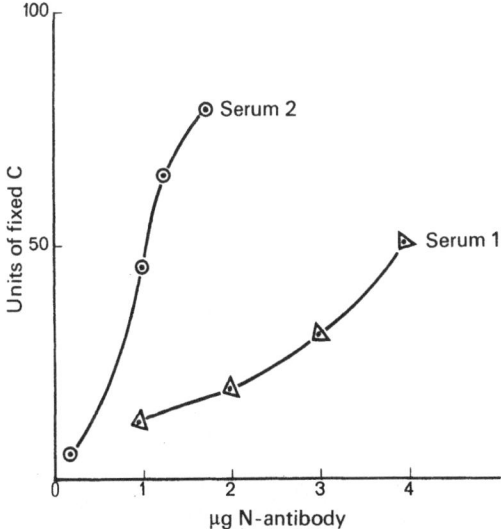

Fig. 7.19. Sigmoidal curve of the number of units of complement fixed by varying quantities of antibody, in the presence of optimum amounts of antigen. Determination of CH_{50}

in terms of CF_{50} (being the dose of serum at which 50% of the complement units involved are fixed) is found at the linear portion of the curve.

In the semiquantitative techniques, the maximally reactive dose of antigen is not established for each dilution of antiserum; rather, a dose capable of reacting optimally with a series of serum dilutions is utilized. To establish this dose, it is necessary to determine the curve of isofixation through experiments of the "checkerboard" type, in which the antigen and the serum are varied in perpendicular directions. The optimum doses are indicated by the minimum quantities of antibody (or antigen) and can be visualized easily by inspection of the isofixation curve (Table 7.2 and Fig. 7.20).

Under the conditions of the semiquantitative test, Maltaner and his associates verified the direct proportionality between $K'sa$, *the number of units of C required for 50% hemolysis in the presence of serum plus antigen*, and $1/D$, *the inverse of the serum dilution*, which permitted expression of the fixative titer in terms of the angular coefficient (slope) of the line $K'sa = b'(1/D)$. Since $K'sa$ is calculated by dividing n, the number of units of C used in the test, by the correlation factor (f) corresponding to the percentage of lysis, then

$$b' = D \times (n/f), \qquad (1)$$

in which $f = (y/1-y)h$ and h is the slope verified for the titration of the complement in the presence of serum or of antigen alone.

More precise experiments have shown, however, that the rigorously linear relation is that which is observed between $\log D$ and $\log(y/1-y)$, in accordance with the equation $\log D = \log T + h's \times \log y/1-$ in which $h's$ is the angular coefficient corresponding to the quantity of residual complement after the fixation reaction. From this equation, the following formula results for the calculation of fixative titer:

$$T = D \times (1/f). \qquad (2)$$

Antibody µg N/ml	Antigen µg N/ml							
	0.001	0.012	0.04	0.12	0.36	1.10	3.33	1.00
3.3	1ª	0	0	0	0	0	0	0
2.2	2	0	0	0	0	0	1	1
1.5	4	0	0	0	0	0	1	4
1.0	4	1	0	0	0	1	4	4
0.66	4	3	1	1	1	4	4	4
0.44	4	4	2	3	4	4	4	4
0.30	4	4	4	4	4	4	4	4

Table 7.2. Semiquantitative determination of the optimum antigen dose in the bovine serum albumin-rabbit antibovine serum albumin system in a test with five units of complement

ª 0, 1, 2, 3, and 4 represent, respectively, 0, 25%, 50%, 75%, and 100% hemolysis

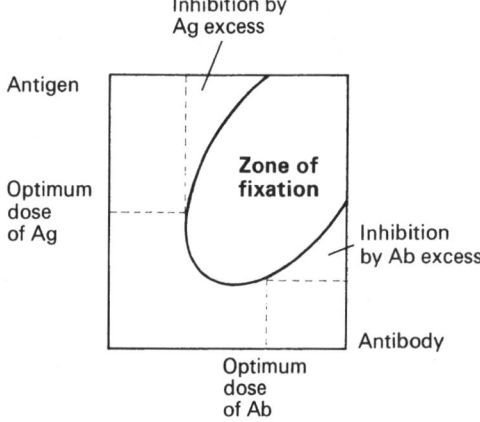

Fig. 7.20. Isofixation curve for the determination of the optimum concentration of antigen

Obviously, if $h=h's$, formula (1) gives a value equal to that of formula (2) or a multiple thereof. For example, if a serum at a dilution of 1/25 in the presence of the optimum antigen dose and in a test with 6 units of complement, produces 75.5% hemolysis where h is equal to $h's=0.2$, and $f'=f=1.25$, then the values of the titers calculated with the two formulas are:

$$b' = 25 \times 6/1.25 = 120,$$

$$T = 25 \times 1/1.25 = 20.$$

However, depending upon the number of units of C utilized in the test, the nature of the antigen or serum, and other factors, the value of $h's$ can differ considerably from that of h, imparting a corresponding differ-

ence to the calculation of fixative titer. In these cases, to avoid the calculation of new conversion factors, the titer can be determined graphically, as indicated in Fig. 7.21.

Mechanism of Complement Fixation. The mechanism of the fixation of complement is still obscure. Even the early immunologists sought to interpret it, with Ehrlich maintaining that complement fixation operates at the level of a special group (a complementophil group) of antibody binders (amboceptors), whereas Bordet attributed the phenomenon to the absorption properties of the antigen–antibody complex.

Modern immunologists, influenced by the works of Ishizaka and others, tend to favor the original point of view of Ehrlich, attributing primarily to the antibody the capacity to fix complement: (1) The immunoglobulins capable of fixing C in the presence of antigen also do so when aggregated by nonspecific means, such as by heat and by bisdiazobenzidine. (2) The binding property resides in the Fc fragment of the antibody molecule, because only this fragment becomes anticomplementary when aggregated, unlike the $F(ab')_2$ fragment. (3) When two immunoglobulins react, one an antigen and the other an antibody, C binding is observed only when the antibody immunoglobulin is capable of fixation – e.g., CF positive with rabbit anti-fowl gamma-globulin antibody, but not with bird anti-rabbit gamma-globulin, if rabbit or guinea pig serum is used as complement.

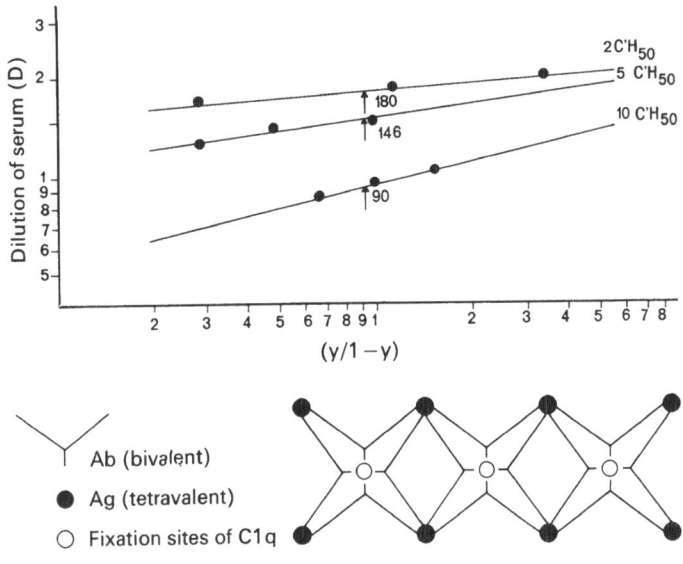

Fig. 7.21. Graphic determination of the fixation titer in the function of the curve log D versus log $(y/1-y)$

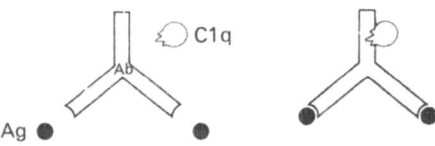

- ⊤ Ab (bivalent)
- ● Ag (tetravalent)
- ○ Fixation sites of C1q

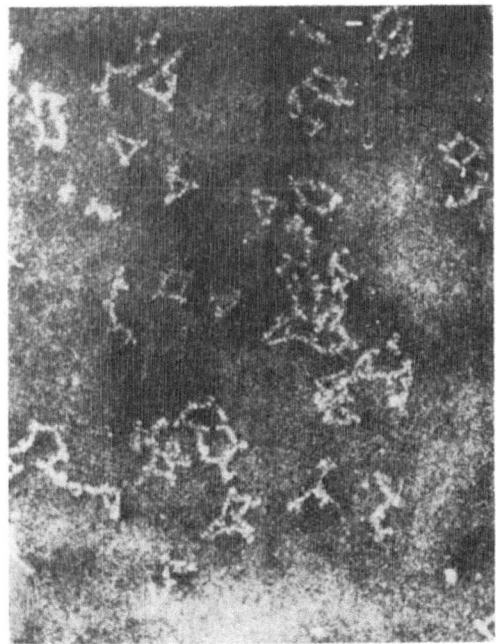

Fig. 7.23. Electron micrograph of antibody–hapten aggregates endowed with maximum capacity for complement fixation [Partial reproduction from Valentine RC, Green NN (1967) J Mol Biol 27:615

Relevant experimental data indicate, however, that simple aggregation is not sufficient to activate complement, and suggest that, in combining with the antigen, the antibody molecule exposes certain structures previously occluded in the C_H2 region of the Fc fragment, by a conformational mechanism comparable to the allosteric modification of enzyme molecules (Fig. 7.22).

In any case, electron microscopy shows that fixative capacity is associated with the formation of aggregates of four or more molecules of complete antibody, but not of Fab fragments (Fig. 7.23).

Effects of Complement Fixation on Cell Membranes. The fixation of components of complement to the surfaces of cells gives rise to a series of manifestations that can be catalogued as follows:

1. Effects arising from fixation of $C1 - C9$
   (a) Immunocytolysis
   (b) Immunocytotoxicity

Fig. 7.22. Mechanism of complement fixation by the antibody after its interaction with the specific antigen

2. Effects arising from fixation of C1 – C3
   (a) Immunoadherence
   (b) Immunoconglutination.

Immunocytolysis

Even in the early days of immunology, it was observed that bacteria or red blood cells, "sensitized" by the specific antibody, were lysed upon the addition of complement. We have already referred in detail to the mechanism of specific hemolysis, i.e., the sequential action of the C1–C9 components of complement. In this section, we deal only with the phenomenon of specific bacteriolysis, first observed in vitro after the inoculation of cholera vibrios into the peritonium of immunized rabbits. Under these conditions, whereas in the control animals examination of the peritoneal exudate revealed the presence of V. cholerae with its typical morphology and mobility, in immunized rabbits the vibrios quickly lost their mobility and disintegrated into granules (Pfeiffer's phenomenon). The phenomenon can be studied conveniently in vitro by mixing bacteria, immune serum, and complement, and determining the number of viable bacteria (bactericidal effect) by distributing the suspension on an agar plate and counting the colonies that are formed. Generally speaking, we can say that gram-negative bacteria (e.g., V. cholerae, S. typhosa, S. dysenteriae, E. coli, P. aeruginosa) are lysed and destroyed, whereas the gram-positive (e.g., gram-positive cocci, B. subtilis) are inhibited in their growth without concomitant lysis. In both cases, however, the cytocidal effect depends upon the sequential action of the nine components of complement: Serum of rabbits deficient in C6, for example, is incapable of exercising bactericidal action on S. typhosa.

With red blood cells, lysis appears to depend exclusively upon the initial formation of ultramicroscopic lesions on the cell membrane, with an initial increase in the permeability to substances of low molecular weight (entry of H_2O and Na, exit of K), followed by distention and rupture of the mem-

brane and by permeability to substances of high molecular weight (e.g., hemoglobin). In bacteria, however, this condition is not sufficient, because alteration of the cell wall is also necessary.

In gram-negative bacteria rich in phospholipids and with thin cell walls (10 mμ or less), the combining action of antibody and complement leads to the formation of damaged and defenseless spheroplasts, susceptible to lysis; in gram-positive bacteria, however, that have thick cell walls (15–50 mμ) and are poor in lipids, conditions are not favorable to the disintegration of the cell walls and lysis does not occur, although the lesion of the cytoplasmic membrane can have a bactericidal effect. Two experimental facts support this interpretation: (1) E. coli spheroplasts and B. subtilis protoplasts are lysed by the action of specific antibody plus complement; and (2) bacteria resistant to the action of antibody plus complement undergo lysis when lysozyme is added, which by destroying the cell wall exposes the damaged protoplasts.

Lysozyme is probably not the only non-specific adjuvant factor that operates in specific bacteriolysis. It is possible that the bactericidal action of normal serum, generally attributed to natural polyspecific antibodies, is enhanced by non-specific serum factors that may also, by themselves, activate the complement system.

In this connection, it is pertinent to mention the serum factor called properdin (from Latin, *perdere,* to destroy), a β-globulin not related to immunoglobulins, which is involved in the activation of complement by the alternative pathway (cf. p. 133).

Immunocytotoxicity

Immunocytoxicity describes antigen–antibody–complement interaction with the surface of a cell that does not result in cytolysis, but is accompanied by cytotoxicity activity, or structural alterations, and disturbances of cellular function (immobilization, increase in permeability, metabolic alterations).

The immobilization of *T. pallidum* (TPI test) by sera of patients with syphilis is an example of a reaction of this type. Mobile treponemas are mixed with the patient's serum and guinea pig complement. If the reaction is positive after incubation at 37 °C for 16–18 h, there is immobilization of the treponemas; there is no immobilization when normal serum is added or when complement is omitted. The long incubation time is necessary because the treponemas possess a coating of hyaluronic acid that impedes access of the antibody to the antigenic determinants (proteins) of the spirochete. The addition of lysozyme hastens the reaction.

An example of a cytotoxicity test that involves an increase in cellular permeability is the lymphocytotoxicity test, used currently to disclose histocompatibility antigens, with a view to selecting donors for tissue or organ grafts. A purified suspension of human lymphocytes is mixed with antiserum and complement (human, rabbit serum). After incubation at 37 °C, trypan blue (or eosin) is added. Under the microscope it can be seen that the injured cells have taken up the stain and appear blue (or dark red), whereas intact cell membranes do not allow the uptake of stain (microdye-exclusion test).

In the foregoing examples immunocytotoxicity was direct, i.e., resulted from the reaction of antibody with an antigen homologous to the target cell.

Immunocytotoxicity may, however, be indirect, in which case the reaction is with a heterologous antigen fixed to the target cell. An example of this kind is given by thrombocytopenic purpura developing in cases of allergy to allylisopropylacetylurea (Sedormid) or to quinidine. In this particular case, the secific antibody reacts with the drug bound to platelets, complement is activated and the result is thrombocytolysis and consequent thrombocytopenia.

Experimental glomerulonephritis provides examples of both direct and indirect immunocytotoxicity.

If rabbit anti-rat kidney is injected into the rat, massive and precocious proteinuria develops as a consequence of complement activation by immune complex(es) formed with antigen(s) of the basement membrane (BN) of rat glomeruli. If, however, like in the classical experiment of Masugi, a non-complement fixing antibody is used (goose anti-rabbit kidney serum into the rabbit), the proteinuria appears only after the formation of autoantibodies to the heterologous immunoglobulin fixed onto the BM, which then bind complement and are responsible for the delayed damage (indirect immunocytotoxicity).

Immunoadherence

Certain microorganisms, such as spirochetes and trypanosomes, when mixed with the specific antibody in a suspension of platelets and in the presence of complement, adhere to the platelets forming grains clearly evident by dark-field microscopic examination (Rieckenberg reaction). This phenomenon has been reinvestigated, and today it is called immunoadherence (IA) – the adhesion of antigen–antibody–complement complexes to the surfaces of the erythrocytes of primates[6] or to the platelets of other species, microscopically and macroscopically evidenced by the agglutination of the indicator particles.

Analysis of the role of complement in IA has shown that only the C1 and C3 components are involved, with the critical part being played by fixed C3; equal immunoadherence capacity is exhibited by the EAC $\overline{1,4,2,3}$; EAC $\overline{1,4,3}$; or EAC $\overline{4,3}$ complexes. Immunoadherence is an extremely sensitive serologic reaction that can be used for detecting minimal quantities of autoantibodies (e.g., in detecting levels of autoantibodies not disclosed by other reactions), or for the titration of C3. In addition to its serologic value for C3 titration and as an indicator for the complement binding reaction, an important role is attributed to immunoadherence in phagocytosis: Erythrocytes or bacteria, treated with specific anti-

---

6 In the case of human erythrocytes, the receptor is destroyed by neuraminidase

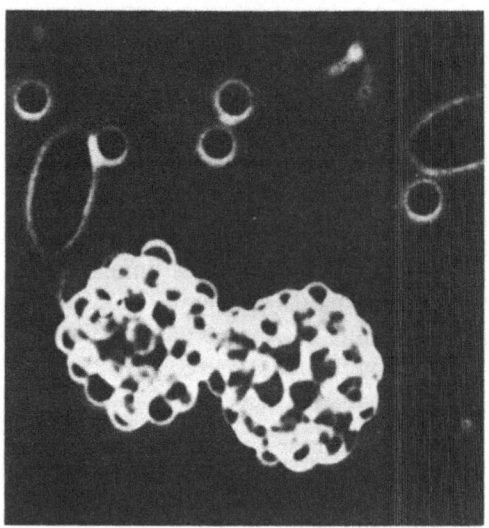

Fig. 7.24. Immunocytoadherence (Original Dr. G. Biozzi, Institut Curie, Paris)

bodies, can bind complement, and the coated C3b particles adhere not only to erythrocytes but also to the receptors of the macrophages.

Immunocytoadherence. Biozzi and associates used this term to describe rosettes formed by erythrocytes around the lymphocytes of immunized animals (Fig. 7.24). Thus, for example, the lymphocytes of the spleens of normal mice are capable only in small numbers of forming rosettes with sheep erythrocytes. If, however, mice are immunized with these erythrocytes, the number of rosettes increases gradually from the fourth day and in amounts paralleling the agglutination titer of the serum. The phenomenon is interpreted in terms of the formation of antibodies at the cellular level prior to their liberation by the lymphocytes that produced them. Interesting data have been obtained with this technique concerning the cytodynamics of the formation of antibodies.

Conglutination and Immunoconglutination

Conglutination is the active agglutination by a euglobulin[7] existing in bovine serum called conglutinin (K) of sensitized erythro-

cytes (E′A) that are coated with complement (C). Fresh horse serum is generally used in the conglutination reaction in a dose sufficient to provide an adequate quantity of C1, C4, C2, and C3, in the absence of hemolysis. The critical component is C3, which, when fixed (C3b), is under the influence of a serum β-globulin (mol. wt. 100,000), probably an enzyme: this is the conglutinogen-activating factor (KAF); which exposes the polysaccharide determinants, which in turn combine with K in the presence of Ca^{2+}, producing the conglutination phenomenon

$$EAC\,\overline{1,4,2,3b} + KAF + KCA^{2+} \rightarrow \text{Con-glutination.}$$

The conglutination reaction is important in serodiagnostics, since, like the specific hemolysis reaction, it serves as an indicator of free C in complement fixation tests (e.g., in the serodiagnosis of glanders).

Immunoconglutination is the agglutination of EAC$\overline{1,4,2,3b}$ by anti-non-gamma-autoantibodies of a specificity directed against determinants exposed on fixed C4 and C3. Such autoantibodies, called immunoconglutinins (IK), can be produced experimentally by the injection of bacteria that are sensitized (or else in vitro by a heteroantibody) and coated with complement (heterostimulated IK); they also are produced naturally, during infections, by microorganisms that coat the antibody and autologous complement (autostimulated IK).

A role in nonspecific resistance to infection has been attributed to the immunoconglutinins, which through an ŏpsonizing process promote phagocytosis and intracellular

---

7 The conglutinins can be purified through adsorption by zymosan in the presence of Ca^{2+} and subsequent elution by EDTA. The result is a highly asymmetric molecule, 7.8S, mol. wt. 750,000, not related to the gamma globulins, with an elevated level of glycine (18%). It is resistant to heating to 56 °C and to treatment with ammonium salts, mercaptoethanol, neuraminidase, and pepsin; however, it is easily destroyed by trypsin and by papain

digestion of bacteria by macrophages of the reticuloendothelial system.

Serologic Reactions in Vivo

Phagocytosis and Opsonization

Live cells have the capacity to engulf particles through an active process that involves the formation of hyaloplasmic membranes and bears the general term endocytosis: The term phagocytosis is used specifically for solid particles (from Greek *phag*, as in *phagein*, "to eat"), and pinocytosis is used with regard to the incorporation of liquids and the particles dissolved in them (from Greek *pin*, as in *pinein*, "to drink").

Whereas phagocytosis is characteristic of cells called phagocytes, pinocytosis is exhibited by all cells and probably constitutes a particular case of phagocytosis of inframicroscopic particles and macromolecules.

In both cases, the mechanism of engulfment is fundamentally identical. It is initiated by the adhesion of a particle to the cytoplasmic membrane, followed by invagination, which depends little and ends by sequestration of the particle in a cytoplasmic vacuole. At the same time, re-formation of the cytoplasmic membrane proceeds at the point of invagination (Fig. 7.25). It was formerly believed that phagocytosis depended upon a purely physical mechanism, i.e., the interplay of the forces of surface tension. However, today it is known that the reseal of the membrane after invagination is associated to an increased turnover of lysophospholipids. Phagocytosis, which in lower organisms represents the essential mechanism of nutrition (intracellular digestion), is also of fundamental importance for cleansing the organism (by scavenger cells)

through the removal of waste products of internal origin (e.g., dead cells or components of injured cells, denatured macromolecules), or through the elimination of foreign bodies, including microorganisms, regardless of their nature. As ingeniously recognized by Metchnikoff at the end of the last century, this latter process constitutes the basic defense mechanism against infections – in lower organisms as well as in the higher animals. In the latter, the digestive function becomes extracellular by means of enzymes situated in the gastrointestinal tract; however, some cells of mesenchymal origin still endure, scattered throughout the organism (fixed cells of the reticuloendothelial system) or accumulated at the sites of local inflammation, constituting an effective barrier to the penetration and dissemination of infectious agents, especially in immunized animals.

The Phagocytic Cells. In vertebrates, Metchnikoff distinguished two classes of phagocytes – microphages and macrophages.

Microphages correspond to polymorphonuclear leukocytes of the blood, capable of phagocytosis (neutrophils and eosinophils), whereas macrophages are cells found throughout the organism and include (1) the monocytes of the blood; (2) the endothelial cells of the hepatic (Kupfer cells), splenic (red pulp), and lymphatic sinusoids; and (3) free phagocytes encountered in the tissues (e.g., in the milky spots of the omentum) and in inflammatory exudates (e.g., in peritoneal exudate and in pulmonary alveoli).

As vital staining methods advanced, it became possible to characterize the macrophage system better on the basis of a common physiologic property. This property is

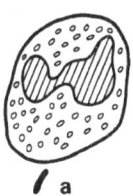 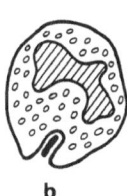 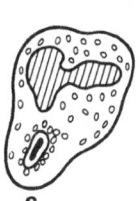 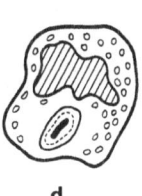

Fig. 7.25 a–d. Successive phases of phagocytosis. **a** Before engulfment, **b** cytoplasmic invagination, **c** formation of the phagocytic vacuole, **d** degranulation: evacuation of the enzymatic content of the lysozymes into the phagocytic vacuole

granulopexis, or the capacity of macrophages to capture electronegative-staining colloidal micelles (trypan blue, lithium-carmine, etc), or micelles of colloidal carbon, accumulating them in the form of granules in their cytoplasm.

For the group of cells endowed with the granulopexic function, Aschoff proposed the name reticuloendothelial system (RES). This system includes:

1) The monocytes of the blood
2) The histiocytes of the tissues
3) the microglia of the central nervous system
4) The reticular cells (weakly active) of the lymphatic tissues
5) The endothelial cells (very active) that coat the lymphatic and blood sinusoids (liver, spleen, bone marrow, adrenals, and anterior pituitary).

The macrophages encountered in the inflammatory exudates are thought to originate from monocytes in the blood or from tissue histiocytes.

Quantitative Study of Phagocytosis of Inert Particles by the RES. It is possible to study quantitatively the phagocytosis of inert particles by the RES by injecting into the vein of an animal a known quantity of a suspension of uniform-sized particles, sufficiently large that they cannot be eliminated by the blood. Under these conditions, study of the elimination of the inoculated colloid with time (elimination curve) permits evaluation of the intensity of the phagocytic function exercised by the reticuloendothelial cells that enter into contact with the blood. The quantitative relationship between the concentration C, at a particular time t, and the initial concentration C_0 is expressed by the equation

$$C = C_0 \times 10^{-kt}.$$

From the preceding equation, the value of k can easily be calculated (the phagocytic or granulopexic index) by

$$k = \frac{(\log C_0 - \log C)}{t}, \text{ or } \frac{(\log C_1 - \log C_2)}{(t_2 - t_1)},$$

which measures the phagocytic efficiency of reticuloendothelial cells that enter into contact with the injected colloid (Fig. 7.26). The value of k is inversely proportional to the quantity of colloid injected (d), so that

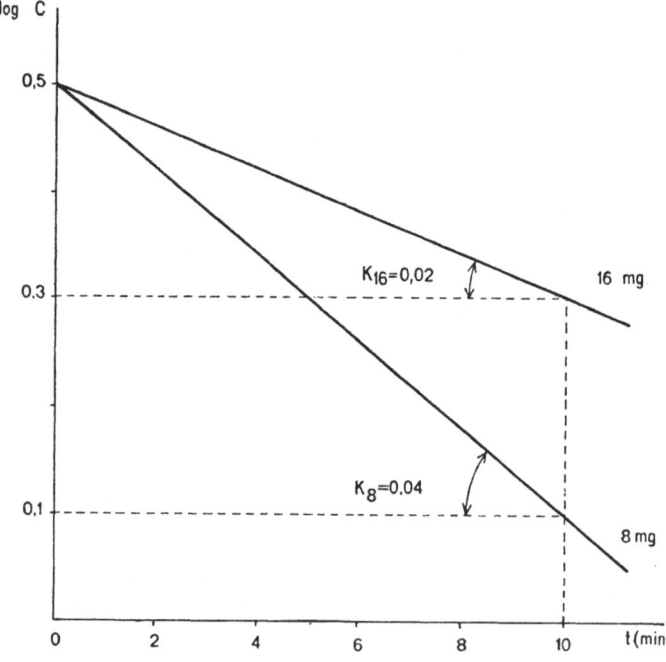

Fig. 7.26. Determination of the phagocytic index based upon the linear regression between the logarithm of the concentration of circulating carbon and the time elapsed

the product kd is essentially constant for each animal species. Thus, the kd product in the rat equals 0.208 in tests performed with colloidal carbon, which is to say that for a dose of carbon equaling 8 mg/100 g, the value of k equals 0.208/8 or 0.026, and that for a double dose, k is two times smaller (0.013).

In repeated tests, the values of k for constant doses of colloid in the same animal species vary considerably, e.g., in rats injected with 8 mg/100 g of colloidal carbon, $k = 0.026 \pm 0.015$. This variation is not due to a corresponding variation in phagocytic activity, but to a variation in the weight of the active tissue, i.e., the hepatosplenic tissue (W_{fb}), in relation to the total weight of the animal (W_t). In numerous determinations, it was verified that the k values were inversely proportional to the cube of the W_t/W_{fb} ratio; thus, multiplying the ratio by the cube root of k, a new constant is obtained – α (corrected phagocytic index), which expresses the phagocytic activity as a function of the relative weight of the active tissue:[8]

Unlike k, the α index is subject only to small variations ($\pm 10\%$), and it is effectively constant for any animal species, as illustrated by the 8 mg/100 g dose:

Index	Rat	Mouse	Rabbit
k	0.026	0.047	0.08
α	5.4	5.4	6.0

Quantitative Study of Phagocytosis of Bacteria by the RES. Applying the preceding method to the study of the elimination from the blood of bacteria labeled with radioactive isotopes, the identical quantitative relationship was confirmed. However, contrary to what occurred with the inert particles, the dose involved was not found to affect the value of the phagocytic index. This is easily

___

8 The active tissue is practically all represented by the hepatosplenic mass: After injection of colloidal carbon into mice, 90% can be recovered from the liver, 4% from the spleen

understood when one considers that the phagocytosis of bacteria (and not that of inert colloids) depends upon their interaction with serum components called opsonins, and therefore is subject to the influence of this limiting factor. Under these conditions, above a certain critical value of inoculum, the number of microorganisms phagocytosed corresponds to the maximum number that interacted with the limited level of opsonins available in the plasma of the animal involved.

Normal Opsonins and Immune Opsonins. It has long been known that the phagocytosis of microbes is facilitated by certain proteins existing in normal serum and, in a much more accentuated fashion, by specific antibodies against antigenic determinants of the microbial surfaces.

These substances are called opsonins (Greek *opsonein* "to soften food"), and the process is called opsonization; those in normal serum are called normal opsonins, whereas those in specific antisera are called immune opsonins.

Classically, immune opsonins (formerly called bacteriotropins) were distinguished from natural opsonins by their thermostability; the former remain active after being heated to 56 °C, whereas the latter are destroyed.

There is good evidence that immune opsonins are IgG antibodies which act directly as opsonins, because their Fc segments are able to combine with Fc-receptors on the surface of the phagocyte. Being able to fix complement, immune opsonins also generate C3B on the surface of the particle and may also utilize C3b-receptors on the phagocyte.

Normal opsonins are either thermolabile antibodies of the IgM type or serum factors of non-gamma globulin nature (heat labile serum factor or HLF) that are ineffective by themselves as opsonins, but being able to activate the complement system (the activation by HLF proceeds by the alternative pathway) may also promote the adhesion via C3b-receptors.

The adhesion via $C3b$ is called *opsonic adherence,* because of its analogy with *immunoadherence* (cf. p. 202).

Opsonic adherence is the sole element of opsonization in the case of normal opsonins, but is of secondary importance in the opsonization by immune opsonins of the IgG type.

The Role of Complement in Phagocytosis and the Mechanism of Ingestion. The action of complement in fostering phagocytosis can be evidenced clearly by in vitro and in vivo experiments. In the former, through study of the phagocytosis of sensitized erythrocytes (EA) treated with the various complement components, it has been verified that the phagocytosable complex corresponds to $EAC1,4,2,3$, in which the effect of $C5$ is minimal. Nevertheless, experiments with encapsulated pneumococci treated with fresh guinea pig serum evidenced participation, albeit to a lesser degree, of the $C5$ component. With in vivo experiments, the role of complement in phagocytosis is clearly indicated by the retarded elimination of labeled bacteria from the serum of animals lacking complement.

The relevant role of $C3$ can be interpreted as a function of the confirmed existence of receptors for $C\overline{3b}$ on the surfaces of polymorphonuclear cells and of monocytes, thereby assuring the initial stage of phagocytosis, i.e., the adhesion of the opsonized particle to the surface of the phagocyte.

The engulfment itself utilized high affinity receptors for Fc on phagocytes. Following opsonic adherence through $C3b$, the Fc portion of the opsonizing IgG antibody moves along the Fc receptors acting like a zipper to sequester the particle in a phagoxytic vacuole (phagosome), which in a later stage becomes a phagolysosome. The mechanism described above corresponds to the classical opsonization of humoral immunity and involves mainly polymorphonuclear leukocyts. Monocytes may also participate in this process, since they are equally provided with $C3b$ and Fc receptors. Macrophages may also be armed with

cytophilic antibodies or similar factors, e.g., the "specific macrophage arming factor" (SMAF) and thus be enabled to ingest the particle with or without previous opsonic adherence.

Determining Opsonin Concentrations. The classic methods for finding opsonin concentrations consist of comparing the average number (N') of bacteria phagocytized in a mixture of bacteria and leukocytes suspended in a medium containing the serum under study, with the value N, obtained with an identical mixture suspended in normal serum. The N'/N quotient represents the opsonization index of the serum in question. Thus, for instance, if in a counting of 50 leukocytes we encounter 120 phagocytized microorganisms in the suspension containing the patient's serum, and 200 in the suspension containing normal serum, we may conclude that the opsonization index of the patient's serum, and 200 in the suspension containing normal serum, we may conclude that the opsonization index of the patient's serum is 120/200 or 0.6, i.e., that the serum of the patient possesses 60% of normal opsonization power. A variant of this technique is the opsonocytophagic test, formerly used in the serodiagnosis of brucellosis. Today such tests have fallen into disuse, for they furnish no more diagnostic information than the simple direct or passive agglutination test.

For quantitative determination of the levels of opsonins in sera, the best method available is that based on the rapidity of elimination from the blood of bacteria labeled with radioactive isotopes. To avoid variations resulting from the level of natural opsonins in the experimental animals, a suspension of bacteria is injected and the initial k value is determined in the absence of the immune serum. Then the serum to be studied is injected and the new value of the phagocytic index, k', is determined. The difference, $k'-k$, permits calculation of the number of opsonizing units of the serum in question (Fig. 7.2.7) If we arbitrarily designate 0.01 as the value $k'-k$ for one opsonizing unit,

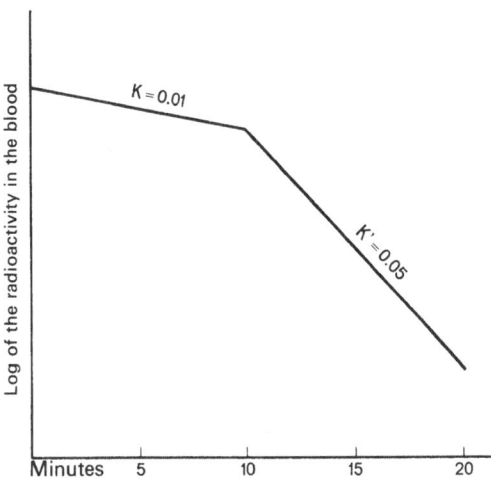

Fig. 7.27. Determination of immune opsonins by the velocity of elimination of *S. typhosa* labeled with [131]I. Biozzi et al., 1963

we can evaluate the number of opsonizing units (OU) of any serum using the formula

$$OU/ml = 1/V \times D \times 100 \; (k'-k),$$

in which V and D represent, respectively, the volume and the inverse of the dilution of the serum injected. Thus, for example, if in the testing of a mouse we obtain a k value of 0.01 and k' equals 0.05, for the injection of 0.1 ml of the 1:500 dilution of a determined antiserum, we can conclude that the level of opsonizing units is equal to

$$1/0.1 \times 500 \times 100 \; (k'-k), \quad \text{or} \quad 20,000 \; OU/ml.$$

The application of this method has indicated an impressive correlation between the specificity of the agglutination and that of the opsonizing activity in anti-salmonella sera. For example, different O variants of *S. typhimurium* (4,12; 1,4,12; 4,5,12; and 1,4,5,12) could be opsonized by the monospecific antiserum (anti-1,4,5 or 12) only if it possessed the respective antigenic determinants. The anti-H antibodies did not have any opsonizing power.

Postendocytic Phenomena: Intracellular Digestion. After the ingestion of opsonized

particles, due to increased anaerobic glycolysis, strong acidity (pH 3–pH 6) develops at the level of the phagocytic vacuoles. Moreover, phase microscopy discloses that degranulation of the polymorphonuclear vesicles takes place around the vacuoles – the granules being lysosomes containing numerous enzymes, in particular, acid and alkaline phospatases, ribonuclease, deoxyribonuclease, and β-glucuronidase. Electron microscopy reveals, in addition, that the membrane of the phagocytic vacuole (*phagosome*) fuses with the membranes of the lysosomes, forming *phagolysosomes*. The bactericidal contents of the lysosomes are thus discharged directly into the site in which the phagocytosed bacteria are encountered, without exposing the cytoplasm to the injurious effect of hydrolytic enzymes, as it occurs when granules are extruded outside the cell and provoke akute inflammation of surrounding tissues (cf. p. 324).

Aside from the lysosomic enzymes mentioned, two substances must be especially mentioned that are also liberated by lysosomes and probably constitute important agents in intracellular digestion: lysozyme and phagocytin.

Lysozyme is an acetylamino-polysaccharidase which exists in relatively high concentrations in the polymorphonuclear leukocytes and acts synergistically with antibody and complement in the lysis of gram-negative bacteria in vitro, possibly acting similarly in the phagocyte.

Phagocytin is a wide-spectrum, labile protein enzyme that acts upon gram-positive and gram-negative bacteria.

Many other bactericidal substances have been extracted from leukocytes (leukin, leukozymes, etc.), but their role in postendocytic digestion is doubtful. A synergistic and probably more effective mechanism of intracellular killing is provided in polymorphonuclear leukocytes by alterations in the oxidative metabolism (*respiratory burst*) that lead to intracellular formation of H_2O, hydrogenperoxide (HO_2^-) and superoxide (O_2^-) (cf. p. 324).

Immunophagocytes. Phagocytosed bacteria are not always destroyed by intracellular digestion. Microorganisms such as *D. pneumoniae*, *S. pyogenes*, and *K. pneumoniae* perish rapidly (in 15–30 min) after their ingestion by polymorphonuclear leukocytes; other bacteria, e.g., *M. tuberculosis*, *B. abortus*, *L. monocytogenes*, and *S. typhimurium*, are not destroyed following engulfment but remain alive in a state of latency in the interior of the phagocyte for long periods. The prolonged immunity that develops in response to infection by the bacteria mentioned previously or to immunization with the respective live vaccines (BCG vaccine against tuberculosis, live vaccines against bovine brucellosis) can be attributed to the persistence of such centers of latent or chronic infection. The mechanism by which this immunity develops is unknown. To explain the absence of multiplication of bacteria surviving in the interiors of the phagocytes, it was first thought that the macrophages of the immunized animal transformed into cells specifically capable of destroying the infectious agent (immunomacrophages).

Today it is known, however, that the resistance of the macrpohages is a cellular hypersensitiviy phenomenon induced by "activating" lymphokines liberated by the interaction of antigen with immune T cells.

The mechanism of the "activation" is still obscure, but it correlates with marked changes of the macrophage such as increased adhesion to plastic surfaces, more intense undulatory movements of the plasma membrane, and increased number of lysosomes. It should be noted, however, that although the activation results from a specific interaction, its expression is nonspecific: for example, macrophages of tuberculous animals, resistant to *M. tuberculosis*, also demonstrate resistance to unrelated bacteria such as *Brucella*, *Listeria monocytogenes*, and others.

It is also possible to produce in mice considerable resistance to infection by *S. typhimurium* by various treatments that substantially increase the value of the phagocytic index, k – such as via the injection of live BCG, of endotoxin, or of suspensions of killed *Corynebacterium parvum*.

Neutralization of Toxins

The bacterial exotoxins (diphteria, tetanus, *Cl. perfrigens*, botulin, and others) and the animal venoms (ophidic, arachnidic, scorpion, and others) are highly antigenic proteins that induce the formation of antibodies (antitoxins, antivenoms) capable of neutralizing the effects of the corresponding toxins. Discovered in 1890 by Behring and Kitasato, the antitoxins were the first known antibodies, for which relatively precise methods of titration have long been established.

Unit of toxin	Antitoxin added	Mode of administration	Reaction observed
MLD	–	Subcutaneous	Death in 4 days
MRD[a]	–	Intradermal	Minimum erythematous reaction
L_o[b]	1 AU	Subcutaneous	Minimum edematous reaction
L_T	1 AU	Intradermal	Minimum erythematous reaction
L_+	1 AU	Subcutaneous	Death in 4 days
L_f	1 AU	In vitro	Optimal flocculation

Table 7.3. Units of measurement for the diphtheria toxin

[a] The MRD, minimum reactive dose, is about 250–500 times less than the MLD

[b] Examples of experimental values for the doses above in a toxic filtrate: $L_o = 0.18$ ml, $L_t = 0.21$ ml, $L_f = 0.155$ ml

In Vivo Determination of Antitoxin Concentration. The fundamental research in this domain was performed by Ehrlich with the Diphteria toxin and antitoxin. To determine the neutralizing level of anti-diphteria serum, Ehrlich initially used as a base that dose of antiserum capable of neutralizing a test dose based upon 100 minimum lethal doses (MLD). This former unit is called antitoxic unit (abbreviated AU); the latter (MLD) he defined as the minimum 100%-lethal dose (death in 4 days) for guinea pigs weighting 250 g.

The instability of the diphteria toxin and its progressive transformation into atoxic

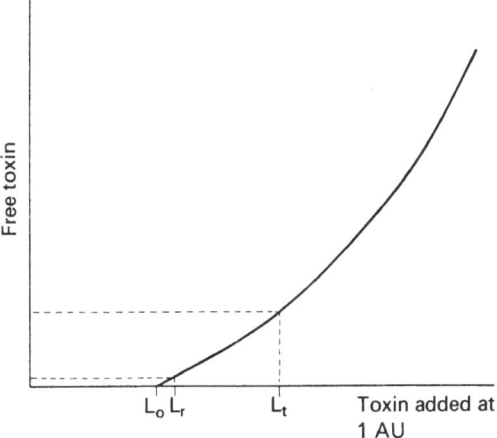

Fig. 7.28. Graphic presention of the relationship between L_0, L_r, L_+, and AE

(toxoid) molecules made it impossible to fix a test dose in terms of MLD. Consequently, Ehrlich had to define it in terms of combination units, through the use of a standard antitoxin, which today is obtained from international reference laboratories such as the National Institutes of Health in the United States.

Practically, it has proved more expedient to read a point from a dose greater than L_0, rather than the neutralization point (L_0). Ehrlich adapted as a point of reference the toxin mixture + 1 AU, which kills a guinea pig in 4 days; to the quantity of toxin contained in such a mixture, he gave the name "lethal limit" (L_+). Later, Römer adopted another reference point close to L_0, corresponding to the mixture that produces minimum local erythema when 0.2 ml of the mixture is injected intradermally. He called this new reference dose L_r (reaction limit). The different units of measure of diphteria toxin are described in Table 7.3; and Fig. 7.28 graphically presents the relationship of AU, L L_r, and L_+ to one another.

The assay of an unknown antitoxin involves two successive determinations: (1) standardization of the toxin, or determination of the test dose (L_r or L_+) in the presence of 1 AU furnished by the standard antitoxin; and (2) assay of the antitoxin by mixing successive dilutions of the antiserum containing the previously standardized toxin.

Neutralization of Toxins and Precipitation. When the antitoxins were discovered, precipitation of the toxin-antitoxin (TA) complex was not observed, and the effect of the antibody was characterized only by its vivo neutralizing power.

In 1922, it was recognized, however, that T and A, in optimum proportions, were capable of precipitation. This caused Ramon to develop an in vitro method for assaying antitoxins.

Quantitative studies of the reaction between T and A yielded curves similar to those obtained with other anti-protein pre-

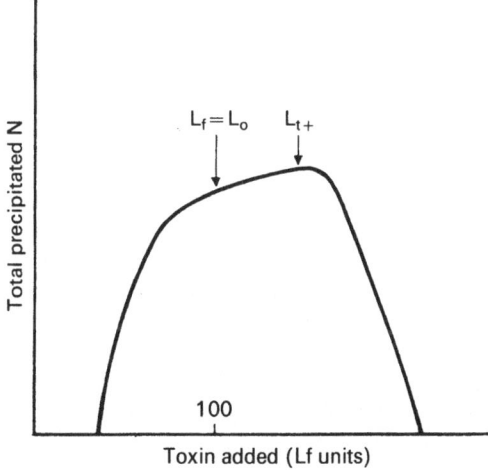

Fig. 7.29. Bell-shaped curve of the precipitation of diphtheria toxin by avid horse antitoxin, indicating the location of the points corresponding to L_f, L_0, and L_+

cipitating systems, making it possible to observe a curve of the "horse type" or of the "rabbit type," depending on the origin of the antitoxic immunoglobulin.

In the bell-shaped curve observed in the quantitative study of precipitation of diphteria toxin by horse antitoxin (Fig. 7.29), there is a maximum point corresponding to neutralization (L_0 and L_f in close proximity), and a second point remote from the first that corresponds to the L_+ dose.

Immunoglobulin Classes of Horse Antitoxin.
Equine antitoxins belong to two subclasses of IgG: 1) On initial immunization, to a fast component (γ_2 or γ_1 mobility) termed IgG(T); and 2) on continued immunization, to slow (γ_2) IgG.

The two antibodies can be separated by successive chromatography on DEAE- and CM-cellulose. The γ_2-antitoxin gives the "rabbit type" of precipitin curve (see Fig. 7.30), whereas IgG(T) gives the bell curve characteristic of Ramon flocculating antibodies (Fig. 7.27).

In other species (cattle, sheep, rabbit, monkey, and man) antitoxin is always associated with the slow, IgG fraction.

Avidity of Antitoxins. Certain antitoxins dissociate easily from the TA complex and are called non-avid, in contrast to those that form firm combinations and are thus called avid. This is an important characteristic to be checked for in antitoxic sera, because satisfactory therapeutic results cannot be expected with the use of non-avid antitoxins. Initially it was observed that certain TA mixtures were innocuous when injected subcutaneously, but demonstrated toxicity of an injected TA complex was dependent upon its concentration, this effect (no toxicity with subcutaneous, toxicity with intravenous injection) was found to result from the dilution of the TA complex.

Cinader proposed an index for measuring the avidity of antitoxins – the ratio

$$\frac{T/A}{T'/A'}$$

for the quantities of toxin and antitoxin required to constitute neutral mixtures with respect to two levels of toxin, T and T', with T' being less than T (for example ½T). If the Cinader index is greater than 1, the antitoxin is considered non-avid, revealing a capacity to dissociate from the TA complex upon dilution.

Another important value in determining the avidity of antitoxins is the ratio of the in vivo/in vitro concentrations, measured by the quotient

$$\frac{L_t}{L_f} \text{ or } \frac{L_r}{L_f}.$$

Non-avid antitoxin flocculates better than it neutralizes and consequently yields L_f values considerably lower than L_+, e.g.,

$$\frac{L_t}{L_f} = \frac{0.2}{0.1} = 2.$$

With avid antitoxins this ratio generally approaches a value of 1.

Flocculation. The minimal flocculation time, which corresponds to the complete neutralization of T by A, is called K_f and is inversely proportional to the concentrations of the participating reagents[9]. Thus, if T and A are in concentrated solutions, flocculation occurs rapidly. In fact, in adjacent tubes containing the optimal neutralizing mixture, flocculation occurs almost simultaneously. This prevents an exact determination of the tube corresponding to the flocculation optimum, which again indicates the value of K_f. On the other hand, if T and A are too dilute, only a light, late flocculation occurs, which cannot be clearly defined. Therefore it is necessary to use favorable concentrations, e.g., 2 ml of a 25 L_f/ml solution of toxin and variable amounts of antitoxin with about 50 flocculation units (Fig. 7.30).

---

9 The variation of K_f as a function of the concentrations of T and A is expressed as the empirical equation $\log K_f = a - b \log (A + T)$

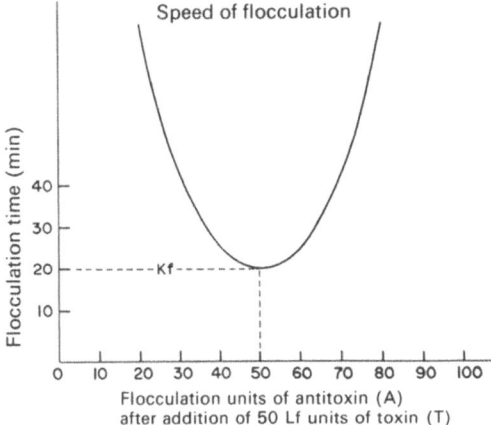

Fig. 7.30. Determination of K_f value

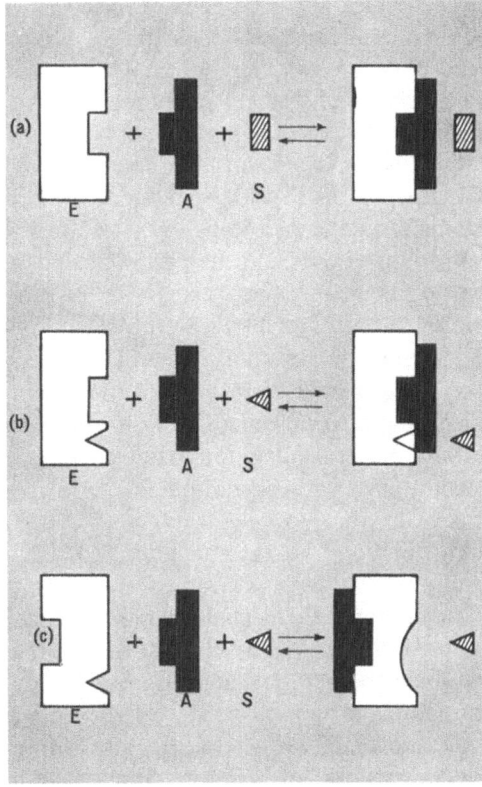

Fig. 7.31. Interpretation of the mechanism by which enzymes are neutralized by anti-enzymes (Original of O. G. Bier)

Determination of the K_f value is of great practical importance, because it depends not only on the optimal T/A ratio, but also on the inherent properties of the reagents: (1) If a known serum is used, an increased K_f value, i.e., a slow flocculation, suggest an alteration in T. (2) When the same toxin is used, slow flocculation signifies minimal avidity. Purified T and A result in rapid flocculation.

Mechanism of Neutralization. The mechanism for neutralization of toxins by antitoxins remains obscure but admits of three distinct possibilities (Fig. 7.29): (1) The antitoxin may bind, through competitive inhibition, at the level of the T site responsible for the toxicity. (2) The antitoxin may act at a site near the active T region and hinder the toxic effect by a steric hindrance mechanism. (3) The antitoxin may act upon a distant site and impede toxicity by an allosteric mechanism. With anti-enzymes, which can be considered in the case of antitoxins, possibility (1) can be excluded because for a fixed quantity of antibody, inhibition of enzymatic activity is not influenced by the increase in the concentration of the substrate. It is not possible, however, to decide between hypotheses (2) and (3).

Some experimental support for interpretation (2) is supplied by the fact that total in-

hibition occurs only when both enzyme and substrate are of low molecular weight, e.g., lecithinase from *Cl. perfringens* (30,000) and lecithin (1,200), with no inhibition occurring when the enzyme is of high molecular weight and the substrate is of low molecular weight, as occurs with the galactosidase (800,000)-lactose (350) system. When the enzyme is small and the substrate is large, e.g., with ribonuclease (14,000) and RNA ($n \times 10^6$), inhibition is partial.

Protective Action of Antibacterial Sera

The antibacterial sera are capable of passively protecting laboratory animals by the action of opsonizing bactericidal antibodies directed against surface antigens of the infecting microorganism. For example, anti-pneumococcus serum through its antibodies (carbohydrate S, type-specific) protects mice against pneumococcic infection by an alteration of the capsule, as evidenced by its swelling, which fosters the phagocytosis of virulent pneumococci.[10]

Examples of the same type are supplied by anti-*Hemophilus influenzae* serum, which also acts upon the capsular polysaccharide of the microorganism, and by anti-streptococcus serum, whose protective action is due to antibodies against the type-specific M protein of the beta-hemolytic streptococci.

In the case of intestinal bacteria (*V. cholerae*, *S. typhosa*, *S. dysenteriae*, and others), aside from their opsonizing action, antibodies with bactericidal action may play an important part, with or without bacteriolytic effect.

Early immunologists attributed to bacteriolysis (Pfeiffer's phenomenon) the role of the fundamental mechanism of immunity, but today it is generally considered that the cytotoxic and cytolytic actions mediated by antibody and complement (C1–C9) contribute, overall, as synergic factors within the framework of a more fundamental mechanism represented by phagocytosis followed by intracellular digestion. According to this interpretation, the action of the antibody–complement system resides essentially in a lesion of the cell wall, which conditions the transformation of the gram-negative bacteria into spheroplasts that are either lysed extracellularly, or more frequently, are destroyed in the interiors of macrophages that phagocytose them.[11]

Antibacterial antibodies can be either IgG or IgM, the latter appearing to be more active, whether as opsonizing agents or as bacteriocidins.

Viral neutralizing antibodies seem to act similarly to antitoxins by sterically hindering cellular adsorption and preventing the intimate adhesion that is required for the release of the viral nucleic acid into the host cell (cf. p. 336).

The mechanism for neutralization of viruses is exemplified by the much-studied model of the influenza virus (myxovirus), whose virion contains an internal group-specific S antigen associated with the nucleocapsid of the helical structure and an external V antigen, type-specific, associated with the coat or, more precisely, with the spicula that radiate from the surface of the viral particle. The V antigen is a glycoprotein and corresponds to hemagglutinin, being capable of establishing bridges between the virion and agglutinable erythrocytes. The formation of these bridges is assured by the presence, on the erythrocytic membrane, of a mucoprotein receptor with residual terminals of N-acetylneuraminic acid (sialic acid). Identical receptors are encountered on the surfaces of sensitized cells, and when free in the secretions they act as inhibitors.

In the presence of the anti-V antibody, the hemagglutinin is coated, and hemagglutination is inhibited. The hemagglutination-inhibition reaction can be considered the equivalent in vitro of the neutralization of the pathogenic effect in vivo, attributable to a blocking action of the antibody in relation to the fixation of the virus to the sensitized cells (target cells).

In practice, the in vivo neutralization test is performed by inoculation of a series of dilutions of serum with a constant number of viruses in tissue culture into a fertilized egg or into a sensitized animal, with 50% being adopted as a point of reference for the reading of the results. As with the T–A complex, the virus–antibody complex is reversible, dissociating upon dilution.

The anti-virus antibodies present in the immune sera can be either IgG or IgM immunoglobulins; in the secretions the predominant type is IgA, which is produced locally. Some authors contend that IgA antibodies play a part in immunization against influenza, which was practiced with success in the Soviet Union through nasal adminis-

---

10 The antibody against somatic carbohydrate C lacks protective action

11 The bactericidal action exhibited by immune sera against *S. typhosa* or *S. typhimurium* notwithstanding, there is evidence that the immunity against these microorganisms is fundamentally cellular and that it lies in their inability to multiply in the interior of the macrophages of an immunized animal (see Chap. 6)

tration of attenuated virus. It is also possible that the high degree of immunity obtained in the oral vaccination against poliomyelitis with attenuated virus may be attributed to local production of antibodies capable of neutralizing the virus in the intestines before it reaches the blood.

Quantitative Study of the Antigen-Antibody Reaction

Quantitative Precipitation

Precipitation Curve. Quantitative study of the specific precipitation reaction, initiated in 1929 with the introduction of a precise analytical method by Heidelberger and his associates in the United States, constituted the starting point of modern immuno-chemistry.

Increasing quantities of specific antigen[12] are added to a series of tubes containing a

---

12 Heidelberger and Kendall first used pneumococcal polysaccharide as antigen, which has the advantage that it does not interfere in the determination of the antibody protein as N. This problem has since been solved through the use of radioactively labeled antigens

constant quantity, say 1 ml, of rabbit anti-ovalbumin serum. After incubation at 0 °C and quantitatively transferred to micro-Kjedahl tubes to measure the content of protein nitrogen. Alternatively, any other method of measuring protein content can be used, such as colorimetric methods (biuret, Folin-Ciocalteu, and others) as well as ultraviolet absorption at 280 nm.

It has been verified under these conditions that the quantity of precipitate increases progressively with the quantity of antigen added until a maximum is reached, from which point the quantity begins to decline by virtue of the formation of soluble complexes due to antigen excess. Representative data from an experiment of this type are shown in Table 7.4 and in Fig. 7.32.

Figure 7.30 shows that the specific precipitation curve comprises three distinct segments: an initial ascending portion, a plateau corresponding to the precipitation maximum, and a descending terminal segment. These three segments are clearly delineated by examination of the supernatant from each reaction tube after centrifugation of the specific precipitates. Such tests can be performed either by means of the ring test

Table 7.4. Quantitative data of specific precipitation in the ovalbumin-rabbit anti-ovalbumin system[a]

Ag	Precipitate (Ag + Ab)	Ab	Weight ratio Ab/Ag	Molar ratio Ab/Ag	Test of the Supernatants
9	156	147	16.2	4	Antibody excess
40	526	486	12.2	3	Antibody excess
50	632	582	11.6	2.9	Antibody excess
74	794	720	9.7	2.4	Neither Ag nor Ab
82	830	748	9.1	2.3	Trace of Ag
90 (87)[b]	826	739	8.5	2.1	Antigen excess
98 (80)	820	731	8.2	2	Antigen excess
124 (87)	730	643	7.4	1.8	Antigen excess
307	106	–	–	–	Antigen excess
490	42	–	–	–	Antigen excess

[a] Addition of increasing amounts of ovalbumin to 1 ml of serum. Values expressed in μg N
[b] The values in parentheses correspond to the quantities of antigen in the precipitates, calculated by subtracting from the total Ag the quantity measured in the supernatant in the presence of a calibrated antiserum. The Ab/Ag molar ratio was obtained by dividing the weight ratio by the quotient of the molecular weights of the antibody and the antigen $(160,000/40,000 = 4)$

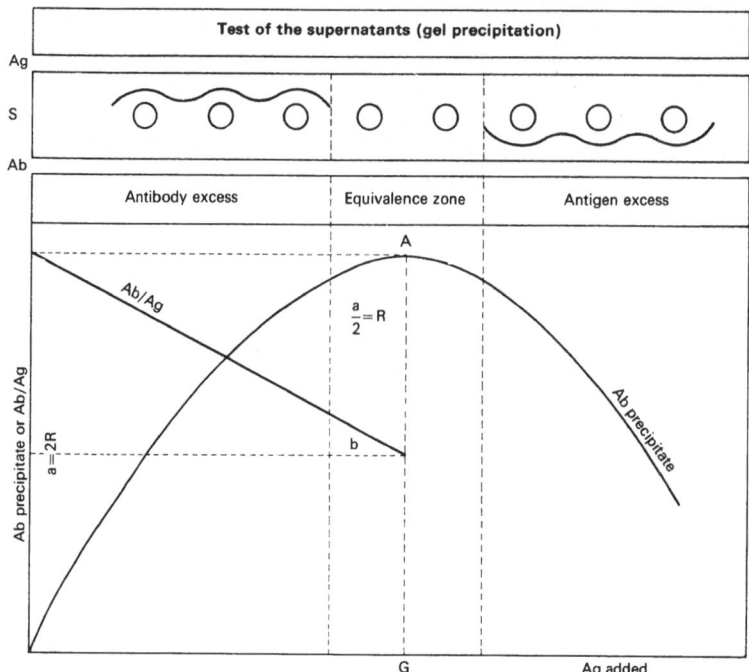

Fig. 7.32. Quantitative relationships in specific precipitation

in the proper capillary tubes, or by gel precipitation as indicated in the figure. Under these conditions, one can demonstrate that the initial (ascending) portion and the terminal (descending) portion correspond, respectively, to antibody-excess and antigen-excess zones, whereas the plateau region has an excess of neither. The plateau region thus depicts an equivalence zone in which the antigen and antibody are in optimum proportions and are incorporated into the precipitate.

The curve just described exhibits only the suggestion of an inhibition zone in the area of antigen excess; since this fact is commonly observed with rabbit antisera, this type of curve is called "rabbit type" or "precipitin type." With anti-protein horse sera (e.g. against diphteria toxin), the curve is different: it does not originate at 0 but rather from a positive abscissa value, and it has a characteristically bell-shaped form. Such antisera thus exhibit two inhibition zones, one for antibody excess and another for antigen excess. This type of curve is termed "horse type" or "flocculation type." In reality, horse antitoxin can exhibit both

types of curves, depending upon the nature of the immunoglobulin with which it is associated – IgG (precipitin type) or IgGT (flocculation type).

Quantitative Relationships in Specific Precipation. Figure 7.32 further shows that the antibody/antigen (Ab/Ag) weight ratio in the specific precipitates is a linear function of Ag, expressed by the equation

$$Ab/Ag = a - b(Ag) ,\qquad (1)$$

in which a (intersection with the ordinate axis) and b (slope of the line) are constants proper to each antiserum.
From eq. (1) we derive

$$Ab = a(Ag) - b(Ag^2) ,\qquad (2)$$

which permits calculation of the Ab value for each dose along the precipitation curve. In the example in Table 7.4, $a = 15.8$ and $b = 0.083$, so that the equation of the serum is

$$Ab = 15.8(Ag) - 0.083 \times Ag^2 ,$$

when Ag is expressed in µg N, or

$$Ab = 15.8(Ag) - 83 \times Ag^2$$

when Ag is expressed in mg N.
The absolute quantity of antibody in a serum corresponds to the value of Ab for the dose that maximally precipitates Ag. This dose can be calculated easily by the formula $A_{max} = a/2b$, which can be deduced from the relationship $b = R/Ag_{max}$ by taking into consideration the finding that a is approximately equal to 2 R (whereby $R = a/2$):

$$Ag_{max} = R/b = a/2 \, b \, .$$

Ab_{max} can be calculated from the equation

$$Ab_{max} = a(Ag_{max}) - b \times Ag_{max}{}^2;$$

then, substituting $a/2 \, b$ for Ag_{max},

$$Ab_{max} = a(a/2 \, b) \, -b(a^2/4 \, b^2) = a^2/4 \, b \, . \quad (3)$$

Applying eq. (3) to the antiserum in the example, we obtain

$$Ab_{max} = \frac{(15.8)^2}{4 \times 0.083} = 752 \, \mu gN \, ,$$

which is in close accord with the experimental value of 748 µg N (Table 8.4), corresponding to a slight antigen excess.
In Eq. (1), the constant a (which equals 2 R) denotes the degree of reactivity of the antibody, since evidently the greater the value of R, the greater is the quantity of Ag. The value of b depends not only on the quality, but also on the quantity of Ab, because b is

equal to R^2/Ab_{max} The latter ratio is calculated from $b = R/Ag_{max}$, substituting Ab_{max}/R for Ag_{max} (by definition, $R = Ab_{max}/Ag_{max}$, wehre $Ag_{max} = Ab_{max}/R$).
To compare the equations of various sera with respect to relative antibody qualities, it is necessary to eliminate the quantitative factor; this can be achieved by multiplying b by Ab_{max} to cancel out the denominator and make b equal to $R^2/1$.
Let us consider, for example, two antisera whose equations are

I) $Ab = 21.4 \, Ag - 101 \, Ag^2$,
II) $Ab = 21.4 \, Ag - 167 \, Ag^2$.

The two sera are seemingly different, because for one of them $b = 101$ whereas for the other $b = 167$. However, if we reduce eqs. I and II to the level of 1 mg of antibody by multiplying each b value by the respective Ab_{max} (1.136 for I, and 0.685 for II), a single equation results, denoting the identity of the two antisera:

$$Ab = 21.4 \, Ag - 114 \, Ag^2 \, .$$

The quantitive study of the specific precipitation reaction furthermore permits calculation of the molecular composition of the precipitates in the different zones of the precipitation curve. Thus, for example, in the ovalbumin-antiovalbumin system, the Ab/Ag ratio in the zone of extreme antigen excess is approximately equal to 5, whereas in the zone of extreme Ab excess, that figure is closer to 20. Since the molecular weights of the reagents involved are 40,000 and 160,000 daltons, the molar ratio of the com-

Table 7.5. Molecular composition of the precipitate for different immune systems (rabbit antibody)

Antigen	Molecular weight	A = 2R	Molar ratio	
			Equivalence	Extreme antigen excess
Ribonuclease	14,000	33	1,5	3
Ovalbumin	40,000	20	2,5	5
Serum albumin	60,000	15	3	6
Gamma globulin	160,000	7	3,7	7

plex in the extreme antibody-excess zone is

$$\frac{20/160,000}{1/40,000} = 5,$$

indicating an $AgAb_5$ complex. In the equivalence zone, the formula of the complex is $AgAb_{2.5}$, and in the antigen-excess zone it is $AgAb$ or Ag_2Ab.

The molecular weights of the antigens, the average a (or 2 R) values, and the respective molar ratios in the equivalence and extreme antigen-excess zones for different systems are shown in Table 7.5.

The molar Ab/Ag ratio in extreme Ag excess is frequently adopted as an estimate of the minimum number of determinants on the surface of the antigen molecule – as a measure of the valence of the Ag. However, this is a minimum estimate, for obviously there can be determinants incapable of uniting with the antibody because of steric hindrance; besides this, since the Ab is bivalent, a single antibody molecule can unite with two determinants of the same antigenic molecule.

Applications
of the Precipitation Reaction:
Qualitative Precipitation

The precipitation in liquid medium, in the form of the ring test, was introduced at the beginning of this century for the identification of blood stains in forensic investigations. Such identification was also useful for the discovery of hemophagocytic vectors.

The qualitative precipitation reaction is also used to diagnose infectious diseases, e.g., in the postmortem diagnosis of anthrax (Ascoli's reaction), and to identify bacteria, e.g., the Lancefield groups and the M-type streptococci. Today, precipitin reactions are used in the gel-precipitation form for antigenic analyses.

Quantitative Precipitation

Quantitative Assay of Antibodies. The absolute quantity of precipitins can be determined, in terms of milligrams of protein or of N per milliliter of antiserum, by means of the Heidelberger–Kendall method, or by analysis of the precipitate obtained through the addition, to a proper constant volume of antiserum, of a quantity of antigen slightly greater than the equivalence dose (see Table 7.4).

Even without analysis of the specific precipitates, it is possible to make an approximation of the level of precipitins by means of the so-called supernatants method, with its basis in the prior determination of the value of R, i.e., of the Ag/Ab ratio in the equivalence zone. Thus, for example, if to 1 ml of antiserum it is necessary to add 50 µg N ovalbumin so that a slight antigen excess remains in the supernatant – knowing that the value of R for the system involved is 10 – we could conclude that the antiserum contains approximately 500 µg of antibody (in N) per milliliter.

In the Heidelberger–Kendall method, the serum is maintained constant and the antigen is added in increasing quantitites to determine the maximum quantity of precipitate (slight Ag excess). However, one can determine comparatively the relative antibody content in different sera through the use of labeled antigens, (e.g., with ^{125}I or ^{131}I), thus determining the percentage of Ag incorporated into the specific precipitate. In the so-called P-80 method, the point of reference for the comparison is the dilution of serum corresponding to 80% incorporation (20% antigen excess in supernatant); this reference point generally is situated at the point of maximum precipitation.

In another method introduced by Farr for the assay of nonprecipitating antibodies,[13] the soluble complexes are precipitated by the addition to each tube of an equal volume

---

13 It was formerly thought that the non-precipitating antibodies were univalent, but equilibrium dialysis experiments have shown that such antibodies can be of low or high affinity. Possibly, the high affinity bivalent antibodies, when incapable of precipitation, possess an anomalous distribution of electric charges or other alterations that make a linkage with antigenic determinants impossible because of steric hindrance

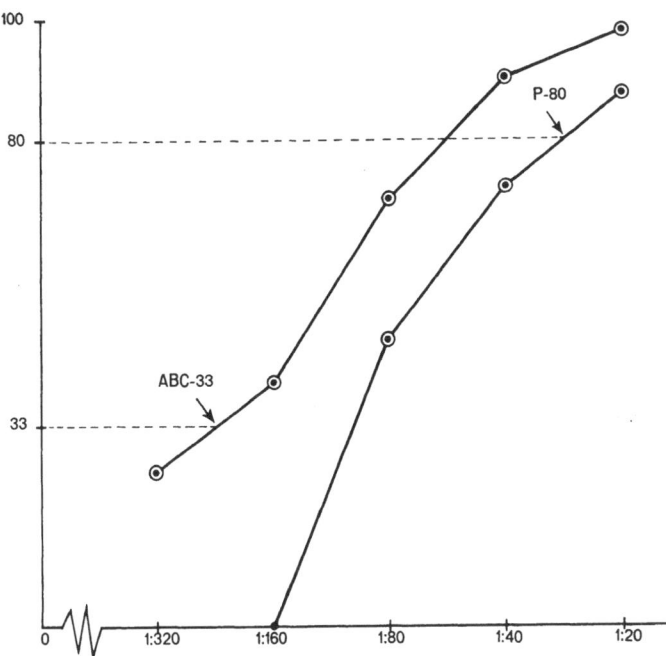

Fig. 7.33. Antibody concentrations measured by the ABC-33 and P-80 methods

of saturated ammonium sulfate solution, and the precipitates are analyzed after careful washing to determine the percentage of fixed antigen (ABC method, antigen-binding capacity). The point of reference in this method was arbitrarily fixed at one-third of incorporation (ABC-33), which represents a considerable excess of antigens in the supernatant (two-thirds of the antigen added). In Fig. 7.31, the parallel results are depicted for the assay of an antiserum by the P-80 and ABC-33 methods.

Farr's method incontestably is of great interest in the study of nonprecipitating systems, but it requires rigorous standardization of experimental conditions and is limited by the fact that it can be applied only to systems in which the antigen is not precipitated by semisaturated ammonium sulfate, as in the anti-ovalbumin or anti-albumin systems.

Assay of Antigens. Quantitative precipitation can be utilized for assaying antigens, provided that a monospecific antiserum calibrated for the antigen in question, is available. An important application of this tech-

nique is the assay of gamma globulins in cerebrospinal fluid, of great importance in neurologic diseases – particularly in multiple sclerosis and neurosyphilis, formerly diagnosed by a nonspecific test (benzoin colloidal reaction).

Study of Cross-Reactions. Quantitative precipitation is also of special interest in the study of cross-reactions; it permits differentiation of those that are due to the existence of common antigenic determinants from those that result from the interaction of similar (but not identical) determinants and fairly well adapted antibodies.

The former case is exemplified by the reactions between chicken and duck ovalbumin, or between the S 3 and S 8 pneumococcic polysaccharides and their respective antisera. In this last example, which has been particularly well studied by Heidelberger and his associates, the cross-reaction is due to the existence in both of the polysaccharides of repeated units of cellobiuronic acid (1,4-glucuronoglucose or GnGl), in which S 3 is a linear polymer of GnGl, whereas S 8 is composed of alternate units of

GnGl and of glucosyl-galactosyl (GlGa):

S 3 (GnGl)-(GnGl)-(GnGl)-(GnGl)-

S 8 (GnGl)-(GlGa)-(GnGl)-(GlGa)- .

Experimentation has confirmed what had been anticipated based upon the structure of the foregoing polysaccharides – that S 3, containing 100% GnGl residues per molecule, must precipitate better with anti-S 8 than does S 8 (only 50%) with anti-S 3.

The second type of cross-reaction embodies the reaction between similar antigenic determinants, e.g., m-azophenylsulfonate and m-azophenylarsonate, or 2,4-dinitrophenyl-lysyl and 2,4,6-trinitrobenzene.

In the case of common determinants, the heterologous reaction never reaches the maximum of the homologous reaction, with both curves exhibiting an equivalence zone clearly followed by an antigen-excess inhibition zone; however, if the cross-reaction occurs through similar determinants, the heterologous reaction curve can rise as high as that of the homologous reaction (when a sufficient quantity of antigen is added); however, it does not exhibit a distinct equivalence zone, and it forms soluble complexes only with difficulty because of the high degree of dissociation of the Ag-Ab complex.

Quantitative Inhibition of Specific Precipitation

Univalent antigens, incapable of precipitating, are nevertheless able to inhibit precipitation by the multivalent antigens. This inhibition can be studied quantitatively by mixing the antiserum first with an inhibitor and, second, with a multivalent antigen in a dose approximating equivalence. Thus, for example, if in the absence of inhibitor, the precipitation equaled 100 μg, whereas in the inhibitor's presence 80 μg was detected, we could say there was 20% inhibition. By comparing the inhibition percentages for different amounts of inhibitor, a dose corresponding to 50% inhibition can be determined and adopted for use in determining the relative potency of different inhibitors.

Three important applications are derived from quantitative inhibition of the Ag-Ab reaction.

1. *Determination of the size of the antibody-combining site.* From the pioneering work of Kabat with the human anti-dextran antibodies and dextran, it can be concluded that the "cavity," or combining site, of the antibody corresponds to a chain of six or seven glucose molecules. This conclusion resulted from inhibition experiments with different oligosaccharides of isomaltose (IM 2 to IM 7), in which it was verified that maximum inhibition was obtained with isomalto-hexose (IM 6) or with isomaltoheptose (IM 7). For different antisera, the relative inhibitive powers of the different oligosaccharides were variable, and this gave rise to an important additional conclusion, namely, that there was a heterogeneous population of antibodies with "cavities" of diverse sizes up to a maximum corresponding to IM 6 or IM 7. Experiments performed with other systems confirmed the data initially obtained with the dextran-antidextran reaction, that is, the antibody-combining site was capable of accommodating, at a maximum, six to seven glucose molecules or five to seven amino acids, with dimensions corresponding approximately to $34 \times 17 \times 7$ Å. The study of the dextran-antidextran system permitted further interesting inferences concerning the combining energies of the different groups of antigenic determinants. Based upon the proportionality existing between inhibitory potency and combining energy (ΔF^0), it was possible to evaluate the percentage contribution of each glucose to the total combining energy of IM 6. Although the first glucose (from the nonreductive end) contributed 40%, and the first three 90%, the increase from that point on was minimal (2%–5%). The group that contributed the greatest percentage of the total combining energy of the antigenic determinant was termed the "immunodominant group."

2. *Determination of the structure of the antigenic determinant.* Quantitative inhibition is also an important method for determining

the structure of the antigenic determinants. For example, the A, B, and H determinants of the substances of the AB0 blood-group system are inhibited, respectively, by N-acetyl-D-galactosamine (A), by D-galactose (B), and by D-fucose (H), indicating that these sugars are the immunodominant groups of the determinants in question. The structure of the A determinant was investigated further through quantitative inhibition with the following oligosaccharides obtained through acid or alkaline hydrolysis of the A substance:

α-D-GalNAc-(1- $\rightarrow$ 3)-β-D-Gal-(1- $\rightarrow$ 3)-D-GNAc

$$\alpha\text{-L-Fuc-(1-2)}$$
$$|$$
α-D-GalNAc-(1- $\rightarrow$ 3)-β-D-Gal-(1- $\rightarrow$ 4)-β-D-GNAc-R;

in which GalNac = N-acetyl-D-galactosamine; Gal = galactose, GNAc = N-acetyl-D-glucosamine, Fuc = fucose, and R is a radical resulting from the reduction of galactose. The reduced pentasaccharide was shown to be a more potent inhibitor than the trisaccharide, and the results of the quantitative inhibition taken together have permitted elucidation of the structure of the A determinants.

In addition to inhibition of specific precipitation, cross-reactions also can be used for the study of the structure of antigenic determinants. Using cross-reactions with antisera capable of reacting with antigens of known structure, Heidelberger studied the reactions of numerous polysaccharides with different type-specific horse sera. He was thus able to draw a conclusion concerning the unknown structures of those substances. For example, cross-reactions with anti-S2 could be due to residues of glucose, ramnose, or glucuronic acid; however, in the particular case of the reaction with acacia (gum arabic), it was possible to demonstrate that the reaction occurred with glucuronic acid, which otherwise constituted the immunodominant group of the S2-anti-S2 interaction. The anti-S14 serum reacts with polyglucoses as well as with terminal residues of galactose, which condition the cross-reaction with the

substances of the AB0 group system, as well as with certain gums and mucilages of vegetable origin.

3. *Radioimmunoassay*. This type of assay is extremely sensitive. It permits measurement of antigen quantities at the level of picograms, based upon the competitive action between an unlabeled antigen (Ag) and the same antigen (Ag^x) labeled with a radioactive isotope (usually ^{125}I) in the formation of immune complexes in the presence of a limited quantity of specific antibody (Ab), which is linked covalently to an insoluble matrix (e.g., particles of Sephadex), or in the form of an insoluble anti-Ab complex (co-precipitation double-antibody system).

In a hypothetical example, if to five molecules of bivalent antibody (10 combining sites) variable quantities of unlabeled antigen are first added, followed by a fixed dose of labeled antigen (10 molecules), the percentage of bound radioactivity (or the bound Ag^x/free Ag^x ratio) would decrease, as illustrated in Fig. 7.32 and in the graph of Fig. 7.33. Upon comparision with a reference curve obtained from an Ag solution of known concentration, one can determine, by the decrease in radio-

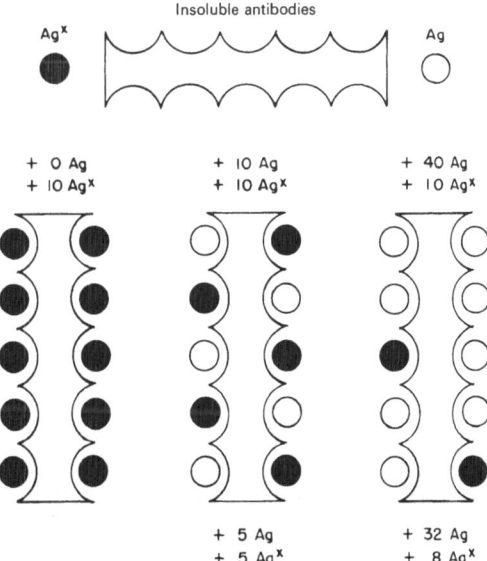

Fig. 7.34. Diagrammatic representation of the principle of the radioimmunoassay

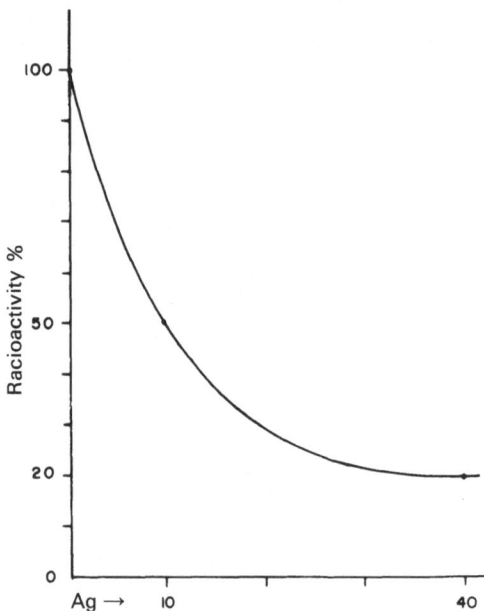

Fig. 7.35. Curve based upon the hypothetical example shown in Fig. 7.32: The drop in bound radioactivity due to the competitive action of Ag and Agˣ is approximately sigmoidal. When the antigen quantities are represented by logarithms along the abscissa, a straight line is obtained whose slope facilitates the calculation of the concentration of Ag in an unknown solution (once the standard curve is established)

activity, the quantity of antigen present in a solution of unknown concentration.

Radioimmunoassay has been used with excellent results in the detecting and assaying of peptides and hormones (steroids, insulin, growth hormone, ACTH, gonadotropin and chorionic gonadotropin, follicle-stimulating and luteinizing hormones, lactogenic, placental, and other hormones); of certain tumoral antigens (α-fetoprotein, carcinoembryonic antigen); of drugs (digoxin, morphine); of viral antigens (Hb); and of immunoglobulins (IgE).

Enzyme-linked Immunosorbent Assay (ELISA)

This method is in principle entirely analogous to direct or indirect immunofluorescence techniques. Instead of a fluorescent dye, an enzyme is conjugated to an antibody; horseradish peroxidase is most commonly used as enzyme, but virtually any enzyme can be employed as long as it is soluble, stable, and not present in biological fluids in quantities that would interfere with serum determinations. The test can be used to measure either antigen or antibody and is analogous to the radioallergosorbent test (RAST) (see p. 275). To measure antibody, antigen is fixed to a solid phase, incubated with test serum, and then reacted with enzyme-tagged anti-immunoglobulin. Enzyme activity adherent to the solid phase is measured spectrophotometrically, and then related to amount of antibody bound.

To measure antigen, antibody is bound to the solid phase, a test solution containing antigen is added, and then a second enzyme-labeled antibody is added. This test requires that at least two determinants are present on the antigen. Advantages of the enzyme immunoassay include sensitivity (ng/ml range), simplicity, stability of reagents, lack of radiation procedures, and that it is relatively inexpensive.

Quantitative Study of the Hapten-Antibody Reaction

The hapten–antibody reaction is a reversible reaction:

$$S + H \rightleftharpoons SH \, ,$$

in which S represents one reactive site on the antibody and H the hapten.

The total concentration of reactive sites, (SH) + (S), i.e., occupied plus vacant sites, is equal to the concentration of antibody molecules multiplied by their valence, n.

By subtracting (SH) = r, moles of hapten per mole of antibody at the concentration of free hapten (c), one obtains (S) = n − r.

The substitution of these values in equation (1) gives:

$$K = \frac{r}{(n-r)\,c} \, ,$$

from which $r/c = nK - rK$ (Scatchard's equation) by plotting r/c versus r, a straight line is obtained with slope K, intersecting

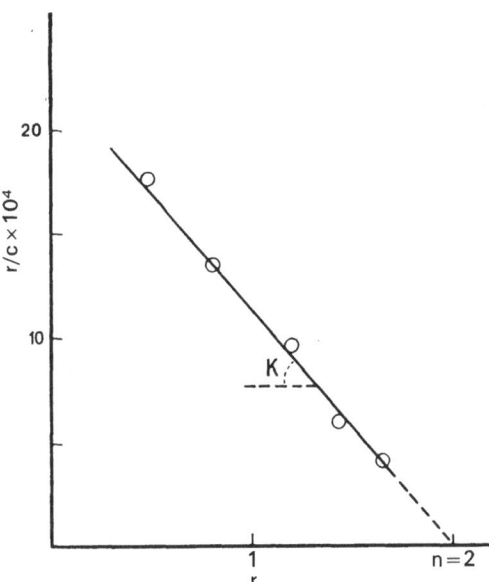

Fig. 7.36. Scatchard's equation (r/c vs. r)

Equilibrium Dialysis. Known amounts of purified antibody and hapten in a total volume of 1 ml are placed in a small cellophane tube, which is closed with a knot and put inside a glass flask with an equal volume of buffered saline. The mixture is agitated gently by rocking in a bath at constant temperature until the concentration of hapten in the exterior liquid reaches a constant value (equilibrium). The initial and final distribution of the molecules of hapten and antibody are illustrated in Fig. 7.37.

Where H is a colored compound, its concentration can be measured spectophotometrically. Otherwise, one should use a solution of labeled hapten. The experiment should include controls for the nonspecific adsorption of the hapten on the normal gamma globulins.

Knowing the value for the free concentration of H (c), one can determine by subtraction how many moles of H have combined with the antibody and, consequently, r can then be calculated, where r equals the number of moles of H fixed per mole of antibody. Table 7.6 illustrates the simplified protocol of an experiment of this type. If one supposes that the number of moles of H in the exterior phase of the tube in equilibrium is equal to 1.11×10^{-5}, then the quantity of free H in both sides is equal to 2.22×10^{-5} M. If tube 1 indicates nonspecific adsorption of 10% to the membrane, this value must be corrected by $(2.22 + 0.22) \times 10^{-5}$ or to 2.44×10^{-5}, and the quantity of H fixed by S can be estimated at $5 - 2.44$), i.e., at 2.56×10^{-5} M.

Since the total amount of antibody added is known (4×10^{-5} M), $r = 2.56/4 = 0.640$. $K^0(1/c)$ is equal to the reciprocal of 2.44×10^{-5}, or 0.41×10^5 M.

the abscissa at a value of $r = n$ (for $r/c = 0$, $rK = nK$) (cf. Fig. 7.36).

It thus becomes possible to calculate K and n if we know the values of r and c, which are obtained experimentally by special techniques (equilibrium dialysis, fluorescence quenching), described below.

Frequently, however, the variation r/c versus r is not linear in its full extension, so that the values for K are not uniform.[14]

It is convenient, therefore, to measure the affinity of antibodies by expressing them as a function of a median value K_0 (intrinsic association constant), which corresponds to the occupation of ½ the antibody sites, n. The substitution of $r = n/2$ in Eq. (1) leads to $K_0 = 1/c$.

The value of $((1/c)$ can also be estimated graphically as the middle of the K_n intersect, or the r/c value corresponding to $r = 1$.

14 To correct the effect of the heterogeneity of the antibodies in relation to the value of K, Sips' function (similar to Gauss's function) is used, which leads to the equation
$r/(n-r) = (K \times c)^a$,
in which a represents the index of heterogeneity. For $a = 1$ (absence of heterogeneity), the preceding equation is transformed into Scatchard's equation

Table 7.6. Simplified protocol of an equilibrium dialysis experiment

Tube no.	Interior	Exterior
1	0.15 M NaCl	5×10^{-5} M H
2	4×10^{-5} S	5×10^{-5} M H

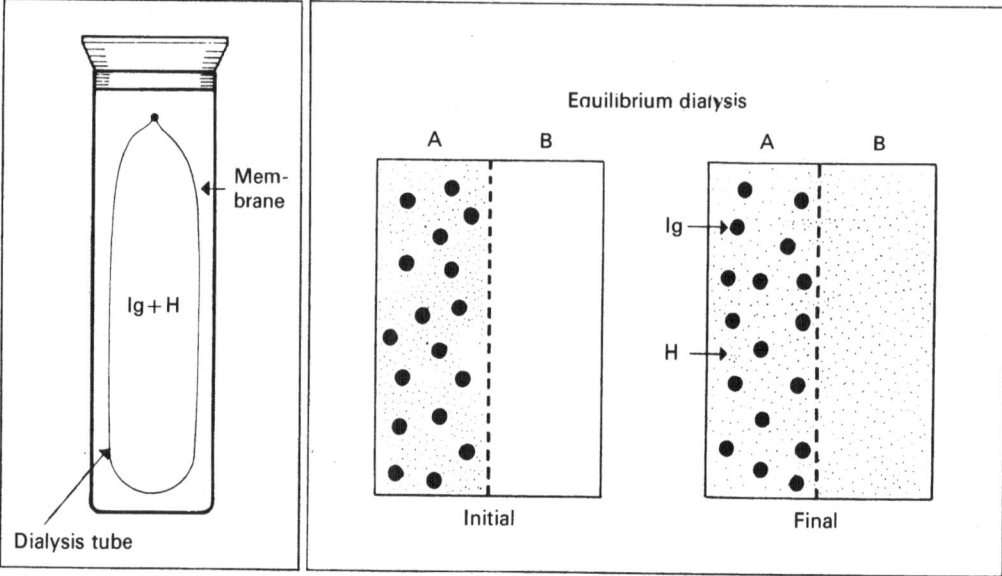

Fig. 7.37. Equilibrium dialysis

Fluorescence Quenching. The hapten-antibody reaction tends to extinguish part of the fluorescence that normally is exhibited by the immunoglobulin when irradiated with ultraviolet light (280 nm). This fluorescence quenching is due to residues tyrosine and of tryptophan found in the combining site of the antibody, which, when covered by the hapten, transmit to the latter the energy it has absorbed and that it should have emitted in the form of fluorescent light (330–350 nm).

The extent of quenching is proportional to the amount of hapten bound and can be used to derive the association constant of the antibody.

The technique of fluorescence quenching is advantageous in that it can be performed rapidly and requires only tiny quantities of antiserum; however, to be applied to unknown systems, it must always be run in parallel with an equilibrium dialysis, which is the standard method.

Thermodynamics of the Hapten–Antibody Reaction. Energy is the capacity to produce work, whereas so-called free energy (F) is that which produces maximum work. The value of F cannot be measured in absolute terms; however, it is possible to measure the positive or negative variations of F that occur when there are transformations in a system. In exothermic reactions – those that liberate energy – F has a positive value; in endothermic reactions – the inverse – energy must be furnished and F has a negative value.[15]

Free energy F is an exponential function of the association constant:

$$K° = e^{-\varDelta F/RT},$$

where

$$\varDelta F° = -RT \times \ln K° = -4.57 \times T \times \log K°.$$

For example, if the determination of $K°$, at the temperature of 25 °C (298 T) results in the value 1.57×10^5, the variation of free en-

---

15 Free energy (F) represents merely one part of the total energy (enthalpy or H); the other part includes a degraded form of energy associated with the disorder of the system, called entropy (S): $\varDelta H = \varDelta F + T\varDelta S$. To calculate the value of enthalpy (and, by subtraction, that of entropy), it is necessary to determine the association constants for two temperatures and to utilize Van t'Hoff's formula: $\varDelta H = R \times T_1 \times T_2 \times \ln(K_2/K_1)/(T_2 - T_1)$

ergy can be calculated as:

$$\Delta F^{\circ} = -4.57 \times 298 \times \log(1.57 \times 10^5) = -7.09 \text{ kcal/mol} .$$

For different Ag–Ab systems, different values for $-\Delta F^{\circ}$ are encountered from 6 to 11 kcal/mol, corresponding to values for K° between 1×10^4 and 1×10^9.

Intermolecular Forces in the Antigen–Antibody Reaction

The union of the antibody with the antigen, as with the union of an enzyme with the substrate, depends essentially upon the complementary adaptation of their tridimensional structures. This stereometric adaptation results in the mutual attraction of the opposed surfaces through short-reaching covalent forces that are inoperative between molecules not in sufficient proximity.

An analogous example is the glueing together of two fragments of a broken piece of china; after a layer of glue is brushed on the surface of each fragment, the two pieces must be held closely fitted together for a period of time. In the antigen–antibody reaction, the glue is represented by attractive forces which operate at the level of the combining sites of the reagents, subject to the complementary adaptation of their surfaces.

The following are the intermolecular forces that come together in the Ag–Ab union:

1. *Ionic or coulomb forces* result from the electrostatic attraction between ions of opposite charges, e.g., COO^- and NH_4^+.

2. *Polar attraction forces* occur between dipoles and between ions and dipoles. A particular case is represented by the hydrogen bond, in which H, linked covalently to an electronegative atom, is attracted by a pair of unshared electrons of another electronegative atom:

$$:\overset{..}{\underset{..}{F}}:H \longrightarrow :\overset{..}{\underset{..}{F}}: \quad \text{or} \quad F^-H^+ \longrightarrow F^- .$$

Though they are weak (3–7 kcal/mole), the numerous hydrogen bridges between the NH and CO groups of peptide bonds play

an important role in maintaining the secondary structure (alpha helix) of the proteins:

3. *Van der Waals forces* are the weakest forces (1–2 kcal/mol), operating only in a short radius of action, where the proximity of the molecules results in the induction of fluctuating charges originating from the attraction exercised by the nucleus of one of the atoms upon the electrons of the external orbit of the other atom and vice versa. Also called London forces, these intermolecular forces do not appear to play an important role in the Ag–Ab union.

4. *Apolar or hydrophobic bonds* occur in aqueous solution between apolar groupings. They work by virtue of their property of excluding the ordered network of H_2O molecules that are interposed between the dissolved molecules, furthering the approximation of these to the action radius of short-reaching forces – Van der Waals forces in particular. The hydrophobic residues of certain amino acids (alanine, phenylalanine, leucine, isoleucine, tyrosine, tryptophan, methionine) play a relevant role in the tertiary structure of the proteins.

Comparative Sensitivities of Serologic Techniques

The various methods for detecting antibodies exhibit greatly differing sensitivities, as indicated in Table 7.7, in terms of the concentration or of the absolute quantity of antibody that the respective reactions are capable of disclosing.

The determination of the minimum quantity of antibody evidenced by a reaction depends upon the underlying practical conditions, or more specifically, upon the volume of serum

| Method | Vol. of serum used in test (ml) | Sensitivity limit | | **Table 7.7.** Relative sensitivities of various immunologic techniques |
		µg N-Ab/ml	µg N-Ab	
Specific precipitation				
Qualitative:				
Ring test	0.1	2 – 5	0.2 – 0.5	
Gel diffusion				
Oudin	0.2	2 – 5	0.4 – 1.0	
Ouchterlony	0.1	5 – 10	0.5 – 1.0	
Preer	0.01	5 – 10	0.05 – 0.1	
Quantitative:				
Micro-Kjeldhal			20 (20 – 100)	
Mod. Markham			10 (10 – 100)	
Biuret (550 nm)			20 (20 – 100)	
Folin-Ciocalteu (750 nm)			2 (2 – 30)	
UV absorption (277 or 287 nm)			5 (5 – 100)	
Passive hemagglutination	0.1	0.03 – 0.06	0.003 – 0.006	
Complement fixation	0.1	0.5 – 1.0	0.05 – 0.01	
Diptheria toxin neutralization (Römer-Frazer test)	0.1	0.001-0.04	0.001 – 0.004	
Passive cutaneous anaphylaxis (rabbit-antibody, guinea pig skin)	0.1		0.003 – 0.006	
Radioimmunoassay; ELISA		µg-ng range	ng-pg range	

utilized and the inherent peculiarities of the individual test. Thus, for example, passive hemagglutination is capable of detecting 0.003–0.006 µg N of antibody in tests that utilize 0.1 ml of serum.

In cutaneous anaphylaxis (PCA) however, in which 0.03 µg of Ab-N can be detected, a serum that contains 0.3 µg Ab-N does not exhibit the PCA reaction because of the blocking action of normal immunoglobulins.

With the radioimmunoassay, serum at a dilution up to 10^{-6} can be used, and antigens such as corticosterone can be measured with precision in amounts as small as 5 pg $(1.5 \times 10^{-14} M)$.

References

Ackroyd FF, Turk JL (eds) (1970) Immunological methods. Blackwell, Oxford

Arquembourg PC, et al. (1970) Primer of immunoelectrophoresis. Ann Arbor Humphrey, Ann Arbor/ Mich.

Barret JT (1970) Textbook of immunology. An introduction to immunochemistry and immunobiology. CV Mosby, St. Louis

Berson SA, Yalov R (1968) General principles of radioimmunoassay. Clin Chim Acta 22:51

Burrows W (1951) Endotoxin. Ann Rev Microbiol 5:181

Campbell DH et al. (1970) Methods in immunology (2nd ed). WA Benjamin, New York

Chase MW, Williams CA, jr (1971) Methods in immunology and immunochemistry, vols I and II. Academic Press, New York

Coombs RRA, et al. (1961) The serology of conglutination and its relation to disease. Blackwell, Oxford

Coons AH (1958) Fluorescent antibody methods. In: Danielli JF (ed) General cytochemical methods. Academic Press, New York

Crowle AJ (1961) Immunodiffusion. Academic Press, New York

Davis BD, et al. (1967) Microbiology (2nd ed) Chaps 12–18. Harper & Row (Hoeber), New York

Dubos RJ, Hirsch JG (eds) (1965) Bacterial and myotic infections of man, 4th ed. Lippincott, Philadelphia

Eisen HN (1964) Equilibrium dialysis for measurement of antibody-hapten affinities. Methods in Med Res Yearbook 10:16

Fahey JL, McKelvey EM (1965) Quantitative determination of serum immunoglobin in antibody agar plate. J Immunol 94:84

Furth R van, et al. (1972) The mononuclear phagocytic system, monocytes and their precursor cells. Bull WHO 46:845

Givol D (1970) Procedures for sensitive radioimmunoassay. Int Atom Energy Agency 1245:15/72

Grabar P, Burtin P (1960) L'analyse immunoeléctrophorétique. Masson, Paris

Heidelberger M (1947) Immunochemistry of antigens and antibodies. In: Cooke (ed) Allergy in theory and practice. Saunders, Philadelphia

Heidelberger M (1969) Quantitative absolute methods in the study of antigen-antibody reactions. Bact Rev 3:49

Holborrow EJ (ed) (1970) Standardization in immunofluorescence (2nd ed). Blackwell, Oxford

Kabat EA (1961) Kabat and Mayer's Exp Immunochemistry, 2nd ed, Chaps 1–12. CC Thomas, Springield/III.

Kabat EA (1971) Einführung in die Immunchemie und Immunbiologie. Springer, Berlin Heidelberg New York

Kabat EA (1976) Structural concepts in immunology and immunochemistry, 2nd ed. Holt, Rinehart & Winston, New York

Karush F (1962) Immunological specificity and molecular structure. Adv Immunol 2:1

Kwapinski JBG (1972) Methodology of immunochemical and immunological research. Wiley, Chochester

Nairn RC (1969) Fluorescent protein tracing. Livingstone, Edinburgh

Oakley CL (1954) Bacterial toxins. Ann Rev Microbiol 8:411

Osler AG (1968) Quantitative study of complement fixation. Bact Rev 20:166

Ouchterlony O (1958/1962) Diffusion-in-gel methods for immunological analysis. Progr Allergy 5:1/6:30

Oudin J (1952) Specific precipitation in gels and its application to immunochemical analysis. In: Methods in Med Res Yearbook 5:335

Pappenheimer A, Jr (1948) Proteins of pathogenic bacteria. Adv Protein Chem 1:69

Pinckard RN, Weir DM (1973) In: Weir DM (ed) Handbook of exp immunology, 2nd ed. Blackwell, Oxford

Prevot AR (1950) Hemolysines et antihemolysines bactériennes. Le Sang 21:565

Raynaud M (1959) Heterogeneity of diphtheria antitoxin. In: Mechanisms of hypersensitivity. Little, Brown and Co, Boston

Relyveld EH (1959) Toxine et antitoxine diphtériques. Etude immunologique. Harmann, Paris

Schmidt H (1931) Die Praxis der Auswertung von Toxinen und Antitoxinen. Gustav Fischer, Jena

Staub AM, Raynaud M (1971) Cours d'Immunologie générale et de Sérologie de l'Institut Pasteur. CDU, Paris

Thomas L (1954) The physiological disturbances produced by endotoxins. An Rev Physiol 16:467

Van Heyningen WE (1954) Toxic Proteins. In: Neurath, Bailey (eds) The Proteins, vol II. Academic Press, New York

Westphal O (1957) Pyrogens. In: Second Macy Conf on Polysaccharides in Biology. Macy Foundation, New York

Zwilling R (1977) Immunologisches Praktikum. Gustav Fischer, Stuttgart

Chapter 8   Blood Groups

OTTO G. BIER

Contents

Erythrocytic Systems 227
  ABO System: Differentiation of Groups
    and Subgroups 227
  Lewis, Lutheran, and Secretory Systems:
    Differentiation and Genetic
    Interrelationships 230
  Chemistry and Biosynthesis
    of Group Substances 231
  MNSs and P Systems 232
  Rh System 234
  Other Erythrocytic Systems 236
Practical Applications of Immunohematology . 237
  Blood Groups and Transfusion 237
  Blood Groups and Maternal-Fetal
    Incompatibility 238
  Blood Groups and Autoimmune Hemolytic
    Anemia. 239
  Blood Groups and Forensic Medicine . . . 239
Anthropologic Applications
  of Immunohematology 241
References 241

The blood has always been regarded by man as an object of mystery and fascination – a vitalizing and rejuvenating element. Even ancient authors reported transferring the blood of animals, usually of sheep and dogs, to man. They noted that such transfusions invariably resulted in fever and hemoglobinuria, and terminated not infrequently in the death of the patient. Blundell (1818), who can be considered the father of the modern blood transfusion, recognized that when the recipient and the donor were of the same species, e.g., dog-to-dog or human-to-human transfusions, the tolerance was greater, although even then there were numerous accidents. The problem was not resolved until 1900, when Landsteiner, having discovered the blood groups of the ABO system, interpreted the post-transfusion reactions in terms of an interaction between the red cells of the donor and isoantibodies (or more properly, alloantibodies) existing in the serum of the recipient. About 40 years later, with the discovery of the Rh system by Levine, it was demonstrated that even the transfusion of blood compatible for the ABO system could give rise to transfusion reactions: These were attributable to anti-Rh alloantibodies contained in the serum of the recipient that had been induced by previous transfusions with Rh^+ red blood cells or by antigenic stimulation from fetal red blood cells during gestation. In addition to its importance in blood transfusions, we have already observed the practical importance of alloimmunization in the genesis of hemolytic disease in the newborn (erythroblastosis fetalis).

More recently, attention has been focused on the leukocyte groups, whose delineation is particularly important in connection with histocompatibility tests in organ transplantation and susceptibility for specific diseases (they are described in detail in Chaps. 6 and 9).

Erythrocytic Systems

ABO System: Differentiation of Groups and Subgroups

By allowing the red blood cells of six individuals (himself and five colleagues) to react with each other, Landsteiner characterized at the outset three blood types – today called O, A, and B. Less than one year later, a fourth group, AB, was discovered. The reactions exhibited by these four blood groups are shown in Table 8.1.

Table 8.1. Reactions of erythrocytes with antisera against the ABO blood group

Erythrocytes	Serum			
	O	A	B	AB
O	−	−	−	−
A	+	−	+	−
B	+	+	−	−
AB	+	+	+	−

Table 8.2. Differentiation of the subgroups A_1 and A_2

Test cells	B Serum (Anti-A + A_1)		
	Not absorbed	Absorbed with A_1	Absorbed with A_2
A_1 (A + A_1)	+	−	+
A_2 (A + H)	+	−	−

These reactions are easily interpreted in light of Landsteiner's rule, i.e., antibodies never occur in an individual against red blood cells of his own blood group; they appear only in response to erythrocyte antigens from a different individual (alloimmunization). Thus, for example, O erythrocytes are nonagglutinable in any serum, yet the serum of O individuals agglutinates all erythrocytes with the exception of O red cells. In contrast, AB red cells are agglutinated by any serum except that of AB individuals, and sera from AB individuals are incapable of agglutinating red cells of any of the ABO types. A red cells agglutinate in B serum, which is anti-A; similarly, B red cells agglutinate in A serum, which is anti-B.

In addition to the four classic groups of Landsteiner, subgroups of group A and group B are recognized – in particular the subgroups A_1 and A_2 which are differentiable by absorption tests. A_1 cells possess agglutinogens A and A_1, A_2 have A and H. Therefore, by absorbing a B serum with A erythrocytes, nothing is left, but if absorption is carried out with A_2 cells anti-A_1 remains in the serum (Table 8.2).

It was thought in the beginning that O red cells did not contain agglutinogen (*Ohne* or without antigen), but later it was recognized that they contain an agglutinogen now designated as H agglutinogen, which also occurs in A, B, and AB red cells, albeit in lesser quantities (it is almost abundant in A_2 or A_2B red cells). Only rare individuals of the Bombay type do not possess H and consequently are able to form anti-H.

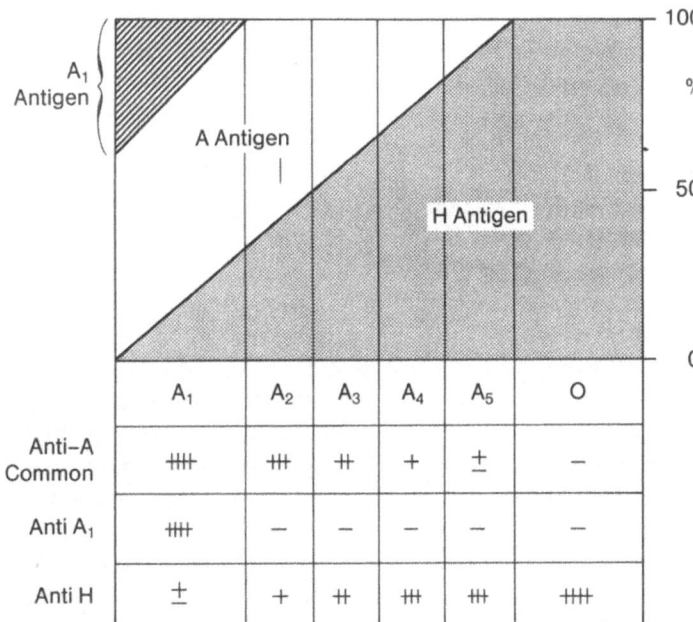

Fig. 8.1. Hypothetical distribution of A and H antigens in A subgroups. Levels of anti-A, anti-A_1, and anti-H are also indicated. (Reproduced from Zmijewski, CM, 1968, Immunohematology, Appleton-Century-Crofts, New York)

Test Cells	Serum O (anti-A+A$_1$+B)	Serum B (anti-A+A$_1$)	Serum A (anti-B)	Anti-A$_1$	Anti-H	
						Table 8.3. Typing of the ABO system
A$_1$(A+A$_1$)	+	+	−	−	±	
A$_2$(A)	+	+	−	−	+	
B	+	−	+	−	±	
A$_1$B	+	+	+	+	±	
A$_2$B	+	+	+	−	+	
O	−	−	−	−	++	
Bombay	−	−	−	−	−	

Besides A$_2$, other "weak" A phenotypes were described, such as A$_3$, A$_4$, A$_5$, Ax, Am etc, whose cells have an amount of agglutinogen A which is inversely proportional to that of H antigen, as illustrated in Fig. 8.1. Reproduced in Table 8.3 are the reactions necessary for the typing of the AB0 system, including subgroups A$_1$ and A$_2$ and the Bombay type.

The following serve as anti-A$_1$ reagents: (1) about 80% of B sera, which contain anti-A+A$_1$, when absorbed with A$_2$ red cells (A antigen only); (2) plant hemagglutinin (lectin) extracted from *Dolichos bifloris* seeds.

For anti-H reagents, the following can be used: (1) certain bovine sera (weak); (2) eel serum *(Anguilla anguilla)*, which is capable of reacting in high dilutions (1:100–1:500); (3) serum of Bombay individuals (extremely rare); and (4) lectins of *Ulex europeus* and *Lotus tetragonolobus*.

Genetics. The groups and subgroups of the ABO system are hereditary characteristics that are determined, according to Bernstein's theory, by a combination of three alleles – O, A, and B – with O being an amorphous recessive gene and the A and B genes being codominant. In accord with this scheme, the four classic groups (phenotypes) correspond to six genotypes: OO, AO, AA, BO, BB, and AB. With the further inclusion of subgroups A$_1$ and A$_2$, we must recognize ten genotypes corresponding to six phenotypes (Table 8.4).

The H antigen, present in all red cells (except the Bombay type), is not modified by

Table 8.4. Genotypes of the ABO system

Phenotype	Genotype	
	Homozygote	Heterozygote
O	OO	
A$_1$	A$_1$A$_1$	A$_1$A$_2$, A$_1$O
A$_2$	A$_2$A$_2$	A$_2$0
B	BB	B0
A$_1$B		A$_1$B
A$_2$B		A$_2$B

the amorphous O gene; hence the phenotype O results. The structural genes A and B act upon H (more intensely in A$_1$ individuals than in A$_2$ agglutinogens and yet leaving a certain quantity of H (incomplete conversion). Further details relating to the genetic control of the biosynthesis of these group substances are discussed below, in the treatment of the interrelations of the ABO and Lewis systems.

Alloantibodies of the ABO System. The alloantibodies of the ABO system can be either natural or immune antibodies. The former occur in normal serum, usually in low titers; they probably appear in response to natural stimuli resulting from the ubiquity of the blood group substances, especially in the bacteria of the intestinal tract. For example, chicks born and maintained in germ-free environments do not form hemagglutinins; yet they readily produce anti-B when E. coli, a carrier of B substance, is added to their diet. In man, agglutinogens exist on the red cells even at birth, but the natural hemagglutinins

Table 8.5. Characteristics differentiating natural and immune alloantibodies

Properties	Natural antibodies	Immune antibodies
Ig class	IgM or IgG	IgG
Heating at 70 °C	Labile	Stable
Optimum temperature	4–20 °C	37 °C
Agglutination in saline	+	+ or −
Agglutination in colloid medium	+	+
Hemolysis with complement	−	+

only begin to appear around the third month of life. Natural antibodies are usually of the IgM type (previously existing maternal agglutinins are of the IgG type, which are capable of crossing the placental barrier) and in contrast to he immune alloantibodies are destroyed by heating at 70 °C 10 min and act better at 4–20 °C ("cold antibodies") than at 37 °C ("warm antibodies"). Individuals exposed to natural antigenic stimuli evidently form antibodies only against antigens that do not exist on their own red cells (Landsteiner's rule) – in other words, against antigens for which tolerance has not developed during prenatal life.

Immune antibodies, particularly the anti-A_1 antibodies, develop in elevated titers in response to transfusion of incompatible blood (e.g., B into A, or A into O); through heterospecific pregnancy (e.g., a B fetus in an A or O mother): through exposure to biologic products containing group substances (e.g., tetanus or diphteria toxoids derived from cultures in peptonized mediums, or antitoxins purified through digestion with pepsin); and by the infection of purified group substances (Witebsky substances).

Table 8.5 summarizes the most important characteristics in the differentiation of natural and immune alloantibodies.

Lewis, Lutheran, and Secretory Systems: Differentiation and Genetic Interrelationships

In about 80% of all individuals, the substances A, B, and H are encountered only in red cells, whereas in the remaining 20%, blood group substances occur in mucous secretions (nonsecretor and secretor types). H-like substances have been demonstrated in secretions and in erythrocytes. These substances, termed Lewis (Le) substances, have two specificities, Le^a and Le^b. The former is encountered in secretions, as well as in the erythrocytes of nonsecretors, whereas Le^b is found in secretions and in the erythrocytes of secretors (Table 8.6).

Also associated with secretions is the Lutheran system, which contains two antigenic specificities: Lu^a in nonsecretors, and Lu^b in secretors.

The genetics of the Lutheran system remains obscure, although the genetic interrelationships between the Lewis system and the se-

Table 8.6. Genetic interaction between the AB0, Lewis, and secretory systems

Secretion genes	Other genes	Erythrocytes				Secretion			
		A or B	H	Le^a	Le^b	A or B	H	Le^a	Le^b
Se	A or B H Le	+	+	−	+	+	+	+	+ +
sese		+	+	+	−	−	−	+	−
Se	OO H Le	−	+	−	+	−	+	+	+ +
sese		+	+	+	−	−	−	+	−
Se	A or B H lele	+	+	−	−	+	+	−	−
sese		+	+	−	−	−	−	−	−
Se or	A,B,O hh Le	−	−	−	−	−	−	−	−
sese (Bombay)	A,B,O hh lele	−	−	−	−	−	−	−	−

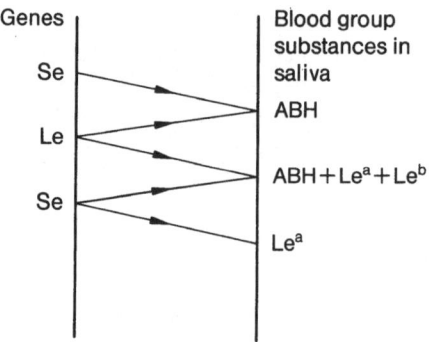

Fig. 8.2. Lewis-Secretor interaction in the formation of Le^b

cretory system have been clarified, largely due to the efforts of Ceppellini. The appearance of A, B, H, Le^a, and Le^b appear to result from the combined effect of four gene groups, which may act sequentially in the following order: Le-le (alleles for Lewis), Se-se (alleles for secretion), H-h, and O-A-B. The data summarized in Table 8.6 can be correctly interpreted only after a study of the chemistry of the group substances and of the genetic control of their biosynthesis. One can quickly infer, however, that the Le^b specificity results from interaction between the H and Le genes in individuals of the secretor type and that a double dose of the "se" gene can inhibit this interaction. When the Le, Se, and H genes are present, the Le^b substance appears in elevated concentrations in the secretions and part is absorbed onto the red cells; Le^a also is formed, but only in quantities insufficient to absorb onto the red cells (Fig. 8.2).

Chemistry and Biosynthesis of Group Substances

The substances responsible for the A, B, H, and Lewis specificities cannot easily be extracted from the red cells, because they occur in relatively small quantities and probably in association with lipids and proteins. For this reason, the chemical study of such substances has been conducted with materials isolated from body fluids: A, B, and H from secretors and Le^a from nonsecretors (see Table 8.6).

In human material, the level of group substances is particularly elevated in meconium, in amniotic fluid, and in the fluid of ovarian cysts. Appreciable quantities are also encountered in the saliva,[1] gastric juice, seminal fluid, urine, and blood serum. The animal sources that furnish the highest yields of A, B, and H substances are the gastric mucosa of the horse and the pig.

Among the methods available for the isolation and purification of group substances, that of Morgan and King is most widely used. It consists essentially of extraction with 90% phenol followed by precipitation with ethanol. Under these conditions, products can be obtained that satisfy the chemical and immunologic criteria for purity, such as constant solubility, homogeneity under ultracentrifugation and electrophoresis, and total precipitation by the specific immune serum.

Chemical analysis shows that the group substances are glycoproteins formed by a peptide skeleton, rich in serine and threonine, to which a polysaccharide chain is attached. This chain is composed of two amino sugars (D-N-acetylglycosamine and D-N-acetylgalactosamine) and two sugars (D-galactose and L-fucose).

The manner in which the units of the polysaccharide chain are associated was investigated particularly by Morgan and by Kabat and his colleagues. Following diverse approaches, they concluded that the immunodominant groups in question were D-N-acetylgalactosamine (GaN) for substance A, D-galactose (Ga) for substance B, and L-fucose (Fu) for substances H and Le^a, depending upon the position of linkage (Fig. 8.3).

Little is known concerning the biosynthesis of the polysaccharide precursor – which among other properties exhibits cross-reactivity with type XIV pneumococcic polysaccharide – except for the verification

---

1 Saliva from the A or B secretors inhibits the agglutination of the respective red cells by the corresponding antibodies: H saliva from H secretion inhibits the agglutination of 0 red cells by Ulex anti-H or eel serum

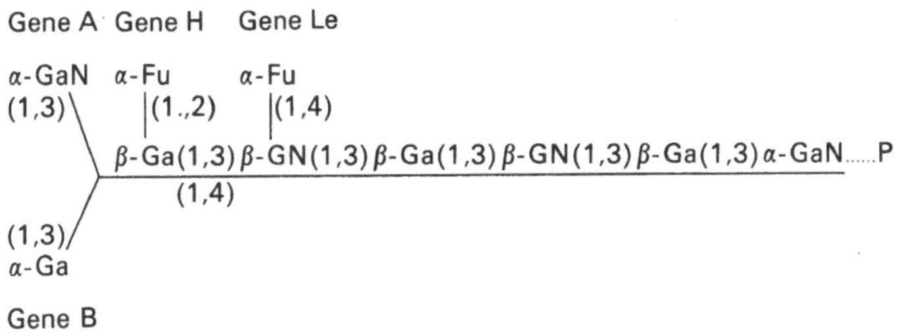

Gene A Gene H   Gene Le

α-GaN α-Fu   α-Fu
(1,3)\ |(1.,2) |(1,4)
       | β-Ga(1,3) β-GN(1,3) β-Ga(1,3) β-GN(1,3) β-Ga(1,3) α-GaN.....P
      /   (1,4)
(1,3)/
α-Ga

Gene B

Fig. 8.3. Structure of the blood-group substances, including the genes that participate in the biosynthesis

of a close relationship to the antigen I, present in virtually all adult red cells and responsible for acquired hemolytic anemias, due to production of cryoagglutinins. In fact, the degradation of substances A, B, and H by combined treatment with periodate and borohydrate (Smith's degradation) exposes determinants capable of reacting with anti-I.

The H substance is synthesized under the influence of the H gene through the addition of α-L-fucose in a (1,2) bond, from the acetylgalactose terminal of the precursor. In individuals deprived of the H allele, i.e., those that are "h" homozygotes, no formation of H occurs. These are the extremely rare Bombay individuals.

In the biosynthesis of the group substances, the precursor is first subjected to the action of the glucosyltransferase controlled by the Le gene, which promotes the addition of α-L-fucose to the subterminal acetylglucosamine in a (1,4) linkage. In this way, the Le^a substance results. Next, the H substance is formed. In secretors, there is an additional interaction between Le and H, from which the Le^b specificity results. Ultimately, the O-A-B genes come into play: O, being an amorphous gene, does not modify the H substance; however, the glucosyltransferases, controlled by the A and B genes cause binding of a (1,3) α-D-acetylgalactosamine (specificity A) and a (1,3) α-D-galactose (specificity B) to the D-galactose terminal.

Figure 8.3 shows that two precursors are possible: In the I chains, the linkage of the terminal galactose to the acetylglucosamine is (1,3); in the II chains, it is (1,4). The Lewis substances, which originate by the addition of L-fucose to the subterminal acetylglu-

cosamine through a (1,4) linkage can apparently only be formed from the I chains, because in the II chains, position 4 is occupied.

MNSs and P Systems

Two factors, M and N, were found on the red cells of each ABO group. No alloagglutinins exist in the serum for these factors, and it is necessary for their identification to utilize properly absorbed rabbit antisera (e.g., to immunize with OM red cells and absorb with ON red cells to obtain a specific anti-M serum). To identify the N factor, one can also use the lectins extracted from the seeds of *Vicia graminea*.

For the MN system, one can differentiate three groups: M, N, and MN. Because the antigens are controlled by codominant genes, the absence of both factors is never observed.

Initially, the MN system appeared to be the simplest blood-group system, but later it was recognized that it is genetically associated with another system (Ss) and that there are numerous antigenic variants of M and N, in addition to other antigens linked to the system that are nonallelic to Ss. Among these antigens, we might cite the Hu (Hunter) and He (Henshaw) factors, relatively frequent in blacks; and the Gr (Graydon), Vw (Verweyst), Mi^a (Miltenberger), and U factors.

Considering, however, only the alleles N,M and Ss, and assuming that such genes form four gene complexes – MS, NS, Ms, and Ns – in the MNSs system, then nine phenotypes corresponding to ten genotypes are differentiated.

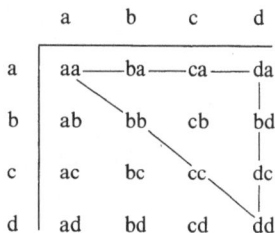

	a	b	c	d
a	aa——ba——ca——da			
b	ab	bb	cb	bd
c	ac	bc	cc	dc
d	ad	bd	cd	dd

In the foregoing diagram, the genes MS, NS, Ms, and Ns are represented, respectively, by a, b, c, and d. Of the ten genotypes included in the triangle on the right (the rest are duplicates), the genotype (encircled) will have an expression identical to that of the genotype ad (NSMs and MSNs), which reduces the number of phenotypes to nine:

MS, Ms, MSs, NS, Ns, NSs, MNS, Ms, and MNSs.

The P system was discovered by a method similar to that utilized in the study of the MN system, which ultimately was characterized as analogous to A_1–A_2, with three principal types, P_1, P_2, and p – this last being incapable of reacting with the antisera that identify the first two. Such p individuals are extremely rare. Their sera contain anti-P + P_1 (anti-Tj[a] or Jay) alloantibodies, which agglutinate the red cells of almost all individuals. Given the extreme rarity of p individuals, scattered all over the world, if one of these should require a transfusion, compatible blood might be obtained only through an international organization.

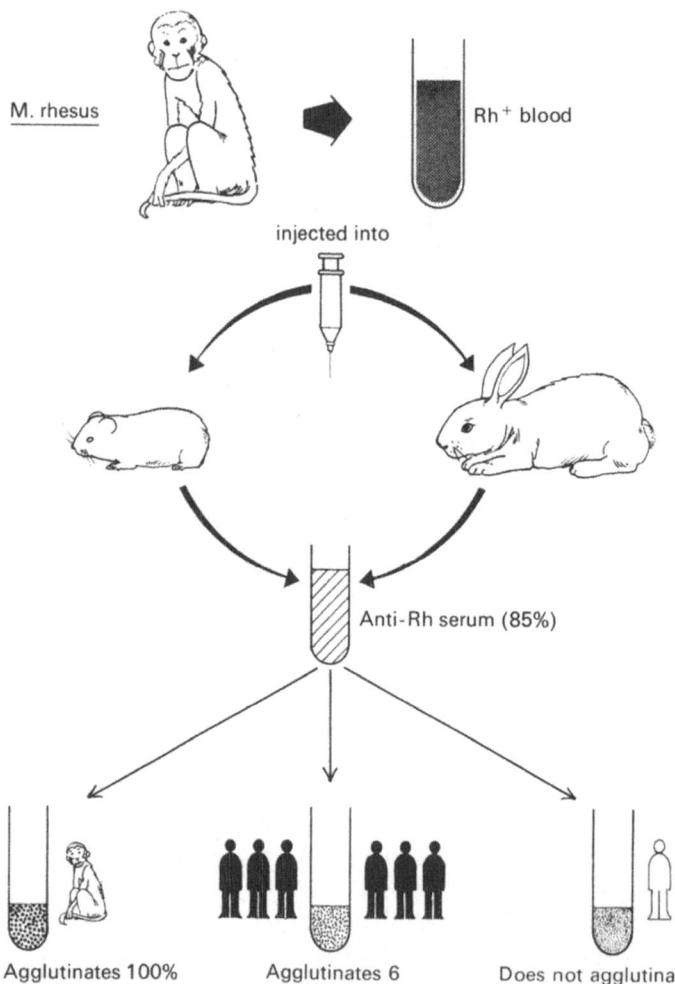

M. rhesus

Rh⁺ blood

injected into

Anti-Rh serum (85%)

Agglutinates 100% of erythrocytes of M. rhesus

Agglutinates 6 out of 7 human erythrocytes (Rh⁺)

Does not agglutinate 1 out of 7 human erythrocytes (Rh⁻)

Fig. 8.4. Protocol of experiments leading to the discovery of the Rh factor

Rh System

In 1939 Levine encountered in the body of a mother who had delivered a stillborn child an irregular agglutinin capable of agglutinating the blood of about 85% of white donors in the United States. Shortly thereafter, Landsteiner and Wiener reported that a similar serum could be produced in rabbits by the injection of red cells from the *Macacus rhesus*. The relationship between the two observations was evident, and the new agglutinogen, for which Levine had encountered an alloantibody, came to be called Rh (from rhesus), because of its occurrence on the red cells of this primate species (Fig. 8.4).

Factors and Agglutinogens. The Rh system which at first appeared simple (85% Rh^+ individuals and 15% Rh^- individuals), was later revealed to be highly complex because of the multiplicity of antigenic determinants and of their variants involved in the composition of the different types of agglutinogens.

Table 8.7. Nomenclature of the factors and agglutinogens of the Rh system

	Wiener	Fisher-Race
Factors	Rh_0	D
	rh'	C
	rh''	E
	hr'	c
	hr''	e
Agglutinogens	Rh_0	Dce
	Rh_1	DCe
	Rh_2	DcE
	Rh_z	DCE
	rh	−ce
	rh'	−Ce
	rh''	−cE
	rh^y	−CE

In addition to the original serum, two more alloantisera were soon encountered: one from patients subjected to multiple transfusions, which agglutinated 70% of human red blood cells; and another from the mother of an infant with fetal erythroblastosis, which agglutinated the blood cells of 30% of all individuals. The three antisera represented distinct antigenic determinants, which Wiener designated, respectively, Rh_0, rh', and rh''. Later, two antisera were encountered that exhibited reactions opposite to those of anti-rh' and anti-rh'' sera and thus were designated anti-hr' and anti-hr''. A third, postulated, antiserum, i.e., one that would react against anti-Rh_0, has not been discovered even though it is theoretically possible.

Thus, there are five antisera available for the determination of the principal factors of the Rh system; and with these, 32 (2^5) phenotypes can be identified. The determinants corresponding to these antisera, designated Rh_0, rh', hr'' by Wiener, are associated in groups of two or three to constitute the agglutinogens Rh_0, Rh_1, Rh_2, rh', and rh''.

Differing interpretations of the hereditary mechanism of the Rh system induced Wiener in the United States, and Fisher and Race in England to adopt a different nomenclature for the factors, whereby Wiener's nomenclature has the disadvantage of using identical symbols for certain factors and agglutinogens (e.g., Rh_0, rh', and rh''), but the advantage of being easier to pronounce when dealing with the type designations (e.g., Rh_1, Rh_2, instead of DCe/DcE) (Table 8.7).

Differentiation of Types. If we consider only the three anti-Rh sera first discovered, i.e.,

Table 8.8. Typing of erythrocytes for the Rh antigen with anti-C, D, and E Sera

Serum	Rh-negative types				Rh-positive types			
Anti-D	−	−	−	−	+	+	+	+
Anti-C	−	+	−	+	−	+	−	+
Anti-E	−	−	+	+	−	−	+	+
Phenotypes	rh	rh'	rh''	rh'rh''	Rh_0	Rh_1	Rh_2	Rh_1Rh_2
Per Wiener	cde	Cde	cdE	CdE	cDe	CDe	cDE	CDE
Per Fisher-Race	13	1.5	0.5	−	2	54	14	15
Percentages								

the anti-D (85%), anti-C (70%), and anti-E (30%), we can differentiate 8 (2^3) types, as indicated in Table 8.8 – in which the reactivity percentages for each type encountered among white populations are also listed.

The data in Table 8.8 enable us to calculate the percentages corresponding to the reaction incidence of each of the antisera. Thus, the anti-D serum (anti-Rh$_o$), which reacts only with red cells of the group to the right, i.e., Rh$^+$, corresponds to a reactivity frequency of $2+54+14+15=85\%$. The anti-C serum (anti-Rh') corresponds to a reactivity frequency of $1.5+54+15=70.5\%$, and the anti-E serum to one of $0.5+14+15=29.5\%$.

Clinically, interest is limited merely to differentiation of the Rh$^+$ group through the use of anti-D serum. However, in anthropologic or forensic studies, differentiation of the different genotypes as well as that of the different phenotypes becomes relevant. Of particular importance in this respect is the differentiation of the homozygous and heterozygous types, achieved through the use of anti-hr (anti-c, anti-e) sera.

Antigenic Variants. The Rh factors exhibit numerous antigenic variants (D^u, D^w, C^u, E^u, E^w, E^t, e^s, etc.) as well as compound antigens [G(CD), f(ce), V(ce^s), and others], which greatly increase the complexity of the system.

The D^u variant merits special mention. There is no specific antiserum at our disposal for this variant, but D^u erythrocytes react, albeit weakly, with anti-D, these reactions varying in intensity (strong D^u and weak D^u). Weak reactions require the antiglobulin test for their demonstration; in routine tests they can be falsely identified as Rh$^-$. Clinically, D^u-positive donors should be considered as Rh-positives, since they are able to immunize Rh-negative receptors and to produce harmful antibodies. The immunization of D^u-positive individuals by D-positive donors is, however, exceptional and controversial.

Genetics. Two genetic theories have been proposed for the Rh system. According to

Wiener, there is a single locus with six codominant alleles, whereas Fisher theorizes three closely linked loci, each of them with a pair of codominant alleles: D-d, C-c, E-e. The Fisher genes codify the appearance of the respective antigenic determinants, whereas the Wiener genes, termed r, r', r", R$_o$, R$_1$, and R$_2$, would represent genetic complexes capable of codifying three factors. Wiener originally postulated six genes; however, the possible existence of eight genes came to be recognized; two more were discovered and termed R$_z$ and R$_y$ (agglutinogens Rh$_z$ or CDE, and rh$_y$ or CdE):

$$
\begin{array}{l}
\text{E DCE or R}_0 \\
\text{e DCe or R}_1 \\
\text{E DcE or R}_2 \\
\text{e Dce or R}_y
\end{array}
\qquad
\begin{array}{l}
\text{E dCE or r}^y \\
\text{e dCe or r'} \\
\text{E dcE or r"} \\
\text{e dce or r .}
\end{array}
$$

Leaving aside the R$_z$ and r$_y$ genes, the eight Rh phenotypes mentioned in Table 8.8 correspond to 21 genotypes ($6 \times 7/2$) formed by six alleles:

Phenotype	Genotype
rh	rr
rh'	rr', r'r'
rh"	rr", r"r"
rh' rh"	r' r"
Rh$_0$	R$_0$r, R$_0$R$_0$
Rh$_1$	R$_0$r, R$_0$R$_1$, R$_1$R$_1$, R$_1$r', R$_1$r
Rh$_2$	R$_0$r", R$_0$R$_2$, R$_2$R$_2$, R$_2$r", R$_2$r
Rh$_1$ Rh$_2$	R$_1$R$_2$, R$_1$r", R$_2$r'

With the Fisher-Race nomenclature, the designation of the genotypes becomes more complicated: dce/dce instead of rr; DCe/DcE instead of R$_1$R$_2$, etc.

We might mention, finally, that the divergencies between the theories of Wiener and of Fisher lack practical importance.

It is really irrelevant to decide whether D, C, and E are separate molecules or different epitopes on a single molecule. The important point is that D, C, and E are inherited in bloc, as a haplotype (cf. p. 153), i.e., as half of the Rh genotype. As a matter of fact, and in favor of the theory of Fisher and Race, crossing over between frequent Rh chromosomes are observed and account for the appearance of rare Rh phenotypes, e.g., between r' (Cde) and $R_2(\bar{c}DE)$, originating the rare chromosome ry (CdE).

The existence of allelomorphs of C, D, and E has further complicated the genetics of the Rh system. The three allelic pairs postulated by Fisher have been contested by Wiener, who prefers to consider all genes codifying the Rh antigens as alleles of a single locus, each allele commanding a distinct large antigenic structure with multiple epitopes. It is also possible, however, to visualize the inheritance of Rh types in terms of a system of multiple alleles of three closely contigous loci.

Rh Alloantibodies. Unlike the ABO system, the Rh system does not produce natural antibodies; anti-Rh is encountered only in the sera of Rh$^-$ individuals immunized with Rh$^+$ red cells.

There are two anti-Rh varieties: (1) antibodies agglutinating in saline medium; and (2) antibodies capable of agglutinating only in colloidal medium, e.g., in diluents with high protein concentrations (compatible serum, bovine serum albumin).

It was thought originally that the nonagglutinating antibodies were incomplete antibodies, carrying only one combining site. However, this hypothesis was abandoned when it was recognized that such antibodies agglutinated erythrocytes in colloidal medium and that even in saline solution they were capable of agglutinating red cells previously treated with proteolytic enzymes (papain, bromelain, ficin). This gave rise to the suggestion that the incapacity for agglutination in saline medium could be attributed to the improper bridging of divalent antibodies with antigenic determinants unfavorably localized on the erythrocyte surface (cf. Fig. 7.11) or because the electric charge of the red cells did not permit sufficient approximation of their surfaces. According to the first hypothesis, the enzymatic treatment would have the effect of exposing the inaccessible or recessed sites: in the second case, the colloidal diluent causes a reduction of the zetapotential of the erythrocytes, thus making agglutination possible. Zeta potential refers to the difference of electrostatic potential between the net charges of the erythrocytic membrane and of the surface of the ionic cloud that envelops the particle, separating it from the suspension medium. For agglutination to occur, it is necessary that the zeta potential falls to a critical level that permits sufficient approximation for the establishment of bridges between particles by the divalent antibody.

Nonagglutinating antibodies can be demonstrated with the highly sensitive Coombs antiglobulin test. The test consists of adding an appropriate dilution of specific anti-human gamma-globulin serum to red cells previously incubated with the antiserum to be tested and then washed. The antiglobulin reacts with antigenic determinants of the Fc part of the fixed antibody, thus establishing the connecting bridges required for agglutination. In certain systems, such as Lewis, Kell, Kidd, and Xg^a, by virtue of the fixation of complement on the surface of the red cell, better results are obtained using anticomplement (anti-β 1 C)-disclosing serum. The Rh antibodies further differ from normal ABO agglutinins in that they are more active at 37 °C than at 4–20 °C. In fact, the Rh-anti-Rh interaction proceeds in vitro under conditions similar to those in which they exert their pathogenicity in vivo, i.e., in the presence of a high level of proteins and at 37 °C (warm agglutinins).

Other Erythrocytic Systems

Other erythrocytic systems should also be mentioned:

(1) Systems Revealed by the Coombs Test (with anti-nongamma or anticomplement). These include the Kell-Cellano (K-k), Duffy (Fy^a, Fy^b), Kidd (Jk^a, Jk^b), and Diego (Di^a, Di^b) systems.

(2) System I. Antigen I exists on almost all adult human red cells. It can be demonstrated with anti-I produced by the rare I-nega-

Table 8.9. Differentiation of systems other than ABO and Rh

System	Specific Antiserum			Phenotype	Genotype	%
MN	Anti-M	Anti-N				
	+	+		MN	MN	50.0
	+	−		MM	MM	25.0
	−	+		NN	NN	25.0
P	Anti-Tj^a (P, P$_1$)	Anti-P$_1$				
	+	+		P$_1$		75.0
	+	−		P$_2$		25.0
Lewis	Anti-Le^a	Anti-Le^b	Secretion			
	−	+	+	Le(a−b−)		70.0
	+	−	−	Le(a+b−)		25.0
	−	−	+ or −	Le(a−b−)		5.0
Lutheran	Anti-Lu^a	Anti-Lu^b				
	−	+		Lu(a−b+)	Lu^b Lu^b	92.0
	+	+		Lu(a+b−)	Lu^a Lu^a	7.9
	+	−		Lu(a+b−)	Lu^a Lu^b	0.1
Kell-Cellano	Anti-K	Anti-k				
	−	+		k	kk	90.0
	+	+		Kk	Kk	9.8
	+	−		K	KK	0.2
Duffy	Anti-Fy^a	Anti-Fy^b				
	+	−		Fy(a+b−)	Fy^a Fy^a	15.0
	−	+		Fy(a−b+)	Fy^b Fy^b	50.0
	+	+		Fy(a+b+)	Fy^a Fy^b	35.0
Kidd	Anti-Jk^a	Anti-Jk^b				
	+	+		Jk(a+b−)	Jk^a Jk^b	50.0
	+	−		Jk(a+b−)	Jk^a Jk^a	25.0
	−	+		Jk(a−b+)	Jk^b Jk^b	25.0
Xg	Anti-Xg^a					
	+			Xg(a−)		85(1) 65(2)
	−			Xg(a+)		15 35
Diego	Anti-Di^a					
	+			Di(a+)		36(3)
						8 − 12(4)

(1) Women. (2) Men. (3) South-American Indians. (4) Japanese

tive individuals (about 1 in 5,000). In the newborn, the reaction with anti-I is weak or absent, since the antigen develops during the first 2 years of life.

(3) System Xg. This system carries only one Xg^a antigen, which occurs more frequently in women (about 35%) than in men (about 15%) and appears to depend upon a gene linked to the X chromosome. The two phenotypes are Xg(a+) and Xg(a−).

(4) Public and Private Groups. These designations include certain extremely frequent antigens (Vel, Yt^a, Go^b, Gy^a) and some ex-

tremely rare antigens (Levay, Becker, Ven, Yt$_b$, and many others).

Data relating to systems other than ABO and Rh are summarized in Table 8.9.

Practical Applications of Immunohematology

Blood Groups and Transfusion

Transfusions without prior determination of the blood type may not be performed: Incompatibility between the sera of the donor and that of the recipient could result in severe shock. In addition to the benign reactions due to pyrogen release, the immediate and grave consequences of the transfusion of incompatible blood consist essentially of chills, precordial oppression, lumbar and abdominal pains, prickling sensations in the limbs, dyspnea, intravascular cyanosis of the face, hemoglobinuria, and renal complications sometimes resulting in fatal anuria. This incompatibility is caused principally by the transferred red cells, since the natural agglutinins in the plasma of the donor are diluted in the blood volume of the recipient. Furthermore, the anti-A and anti-B agglutinins involved bind in large part to the blood group substances existing in the fluids and tissues of the recipient. In light of this concept, O individuals were long considered universal donors, in contrast to AB types, who were thought incapable of donating blood to any other group, yet able to receive from all (universal recipients). A and B individuals can receive from their own types, but are able to donate only to their own types, but are able to donate only to their respective types or to AB types.

It is known today, however, that type O blood is not universally compatible and can be dangerous: it can exhibit elevated titers of anti-A and anti-B, even though these can be neutralized by the addition of group substances; furthermore, danger arises by virtue of potential incompatibility with respect to other systems – above all, the Rh system. Rh^- individuals repeatedly subjected to transfusions of Rh^+ blood or Rh^- women who have borne Rh^+ fetuses can acquire high titers of Rh antibodies, generally of the incomplete type, and thus can acquire high titers of Rh antibodies, generally of the incomplete type, and thus can exhibit grave reactions to the transfusion of Rh^+ blood. Even if type O Rh^- blood is used, or Rh^- blood of the same ABO group, a reaction can occur resulting from incompatibility relating to other systems. For this reason, in addition to determining the blood types of the recipient and the donor, it is advisable to perform cross-matching tests for compatibility – i.e., between the red cells of the donor and the serum of the recipient. The test should be carried out in colloidal medium and, if possible, a Coombs test also should be done to detect rare sensitivities to the Kell, Kidd, Duffy, and MNSs factors, among others.

Blood Groups and Maternal–Fetal Incompatibility

Antibodies from the maternal serum can cross the placenta and lyse the red cells of the fetus. This is observed principally when there is maternal–fetal incompatibility in relation to the Rh system, i.e., when the mother is Rh^- and the fetus (father) is Rh^+. The limiting factors involved are primarily the following: (1) the genotype of the father (if homozygous Rh^+, RR, the fetus is Rh^+ in 100% of cases; if heterozygous Rh^+, Rr, only in 50%); (2) the quantity of fetal red cells that manage to enter the maternal organism; and (3) the capacity of the mother to form the harmful alloantibody. In successive pregnancies, a booster (secondary stimulus) effect evidently occurs, which leads to more rapid and intense production of the alloantibody, thus increasing the possibility of injury to the fetus (Fig. 8.5). Of great value in diagnosing hemolytic disease of the newborn is the direct Coombs test, which consists of adding antiglobulin to red cells washed from the blood of the umbilical cord to detect sensitization in vivo of the fetal red cells. The test is also run during the pregnancy to determine the presence of maternal anti-Rh, with an eye toward taking measures designed to mitigate or to impede the appearance of fetal disease, either in the first parturition or in subsequent pregnancies.

Such measures include (1) exchange transfusion, or substitution of compatible serum for the bulk of the newborn's blood, laden as it is with harmful antibodies and toxic products resulting from red-cell destruction; and (2) prophylaxis for subsequent pregnancies with anti-D gamma globulin, administered within 24–48 h post partum.

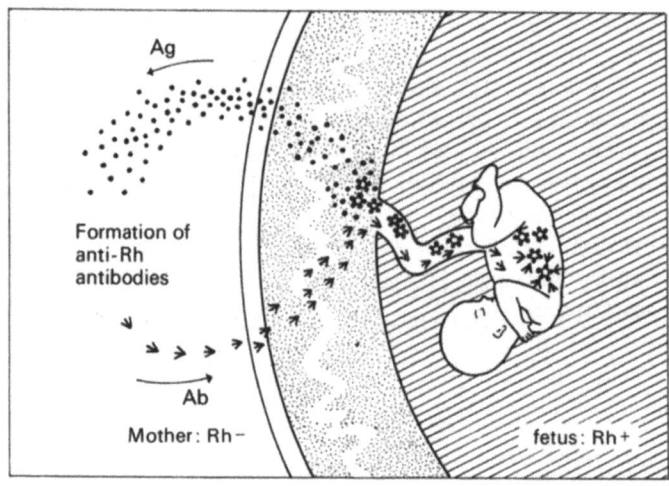

Ag

Formation of
anti-Rh
antibodies

Ab

Mother: Rh−

fetus: Rh+

Fig. 8.5. Pathogenesis of fetal erythroblastosis due to Rh incompatibility

Prophylaxis with anti-D gamma globulin has yielded excellent practical results, e.g., 0.17% anti-Rh production in treated mothers as against 12.7% in the control group – nearly 75 times less.

The small quantity of antibody required (about 300 µg) suggests that what occurs is not a total masking of the antigenic determinants of the fetal red cells, but rather a suppression of antibody synthesis by inhibition of the proliferation of the lymphoid cells involved in the formation of anti-D (feedback inhibition).

Blood Groups and Autoimmune Hemolytic Anemia

Autoimmune hemolytic anemias can be classified into two groups: (1) "cold" anemias, associated with antibodies that act at 4 °C, and (2) "warm" anemias, due to antibodies reacting at 37 °C.

The first group includes the following diseases: (a) the classic paroxysmal cold anemia of Donath and Landsteiner[2], formerly common, associated with syphilitic infection and characterized by a diphasic reac-

---

2 This is not to be confused with paroxysmal nocturnal hemoglobinuria, apparently associated with a defect of the erythrocytic membrane, which becomes particularly vulnerable to complement, without sensitization by antibodies (reactive hemolysis by C 567)

tion: fixation of the autohemolysin at 4 °C and lysis by complement at 37 °C; (b) the rapidly reversible hemolytic anemia observed in a certain percentage of primary atypical pneumonia cases caused by *Mycoplasma pneumoniae*; and (c) hemolytic anemia related to the Ii system.

The antibody involved in these anemias is of the IgM type and binds complement; red cells from patients generally are positive in the direct antiglobulin test using either anti-gamma or anti-nongamma (anti-C).

In the group of "warm" autoimmune hemolytic anemias, we mention only those produced by anti-e of the IgG type.

Blood Groups and Forensic Medicine

The individuality of the blood as revealed by determination of the blood groups is considerable; as such, numerous forensic applications are possible. Considering just 6 ABO groups, 9 MNS groups, 2 P groups, and the 18 Rh types differentiated by the anti-D, -C, -E, -c, and -e, we already have $6 \times 9 \times 2 \times 18$, or 1,944 different types. By computing further the remaining factors and variants of the erythrocytic groups, the serum allotypes, and the leukocytic groups, serologic individualization increases to millions of types, approximating the diversity of fingerprints. However, the methodologic

Table 8.10. Exclusion of paternity by the ABO system

Child	Mother	Excluded father
O	O	AB
	A	AB
	B	AB
A	O	O, B
	B	O, B
AB	A	O, A
	B	O, B
	AB	O

complexity inherent in differentiation militates against a use as widespread as that of fingerprints.

Aside from being utilized in the identification of blood stains, saliva, or sperm, and in investigations relating to the possibility of exchanged newborns, the determination of blood groups has been particularly useful for the exclusion of paternity (Table 8.10). Exclusion rests on the following principles: (1) A factor or agglutinogen not present in at least one of the parents is never encountered in their child. (2) The child can, however, lack a factor or agglutinogen present in one or both of the parents. (3) A type O man cannot father AB children or vice versa. (4) An N father cannot produce an M child or vice versa.

The following examples illustrate the importance of determining the erythrocytic groups in the exclusion of paternity, using only the ABO system.

1) *A Man of Group A_1 is Alleged to be the Father of Two Children, Types O and A_2; the Mother Belongs to Group O.*
Result: The possible genotypes of the father are A_{11}, A_1A_2, and A_1O. In the first possibility, he could not be the father of either of the two children; in the second, he could be the father of only one child O and not child A_2. The only possible conclusion, therefore, is that the accused man is conclusively not the father of one of the children; the test does not allow determination as to which one.

2) *Man of Group O is Alleged to be the Father of Two Children, Types O and A_2; the Mother Belongs to Group A_1.*
Results: The only possible genotype for the A_1 mother of an O child is A_1O; the genotype of the A_2 child must therefore be A_2O. Since the father does not have the A_2 gene that appears in the child, the child can only have been fathered by another man. The paternity of the man accused in relation to child A_2 therefore can be excluded.

3) *The Rh System is of Service in Solving Cases that Cannot be Resolved Relying Solely on the ABO and MN Systems. For Example:* $A_1/MN/Rh_1$ is alleged to have fathered a child $A_1/M/Rh_2$ with woman $A_1/MN/rh$. Exclusion, impossible by ABO and MN analysis, can be found in the fact that the man possesses factor C, absent in both mother and child; and also lacks factor E, absent in the mother but present in the child.

Besides ABO, MNSs, and Rh, other systems can and should be employed in disputed paternity, such as P, Lutheran, Kell, Duffy, Kidd, and Xg. Most people's erythrocytes have at least one antigen in each of these systems and its exclusion in the child is evidence of non-paternity.

Anti-Xg^a can only exclude men from the paternity of female children: an Xg(a+) man cannot have an Xg(a−) daughter and an Xg(a−) man cannot have a Xg(a+) daughter if the mother is Xg(a−).

The probability of exclusion is calculated by taking into account the frequency of the blood group in the population. For example, a man AB cannot be the father of a child O and since the frequency of this blood group in the population is around 40%, the man will have a chance of 40% to disprove the paternity before the ABO group of the child is known. Data of this kind indicate that for both ABO and MNSs, the chances of exclusion are approximately $1/6$, therefore $1/3$ for both systems. By adding Rh, the probability of exclusion rises to about 50% and by associating the other systems listed above it reaches 78%. By combining erythrocyte and leukocyte (HLA) antigens, the cumulative probability is around 95%.

The association of rare factors in the man and in the child but not in the mother strongyl suggest paternity.

Anthropologic Applications of Immunohematology

Considerable differences have been found in relation to the incidence of blood groups in different populations. For example, the Basques are characterized by a high percentage of Rh$^+$ (30%) and a low incidence of groups B, C^w, and Fy^a. Blacks exhibit high percentages of B (20%–25%), unlike the Eskimos and Australian aborigines who exhibit an increased frequency of A ($>50\%$). These differences admit of interesting speculations, although most are disputable. It was imagined, for example, that the ancestral human race was of type O and that the A and B genes emerged later, by mutation, first in Australia and Greenland and later in Central Asia and in Africa. Migrations would subsequently have determined the degree of intermixture of genes and the phenotype percentages observed in different countries. However, this theory encountered a serious drawback because A and B specificities appear in the anthropoid monkeys. Another interesting example is provided by the Diego factor (Di^a), encountered exclusively in Mongoloids and Brazilian Indians, appearing frequently in the latter.

Table 8.11 summarizes the approximate percentages represented by the different groups among six erythrocytic systems in white, black, and Brazilian Indian populations.

Analysis of Table 8.11 reveals that the percentages of the different blood groups in white Brazilian populations does not differ significantly from those continents (Europe, North America), and that the blacks exhibit figures resembling those of African blacks, yet with evidence of intermixture. In addition to the high incidence of B and the

Table 8.11. Approximate percentage incidence of the groups of six erythrocytic systems in different ethnical groups

Groups	Whites	Blacks	Indians
O	45	49	100
A	41	25	0
B	10	22	0
AB	4	4	0
M	30		49–80
N	20		1–9
MN	50		19–42
P$_+$	75	97	89
P$_-$	25	3	11
Rh$_+$	85	90	100
Rh$_-$	15	10	0
Di (a$_+$)	0		30–45
Di (a$_-$)	100		55–70
Fy (a$_+$)	65	35	40–75
Fy (a$_-$)	35	65	26–60

low incidence of Fy^a, the prominent feature is the frequency of sutter and V factors in blacks and their near nonexistence in other races. Additional characteristics of blacks are elevated frequencies of R$_0$ and D^u, as well as of rare factors of the MNSs system, such as Hunter and Henshaw.

The Indians exhibit genetic markers that surely indicate racial purity, such as the absence of the following antigens that have been sought but never encountered in them: A$_2$, Kell, Lewis (a), Berrian (Be), Henshaw (He), Lutheran (Lu^b), Sutter (Js^a), V of the Rh system. Verweyst (V^w) of the MN system, and Wright (Wr). Pure Indians are almost always O and Rh$^+$ (100% in the case of Brazilian Indians) and exhibit elevated frequencies of R^2 (DcE), Se, M, and Diego.

References

Amos DB, Ward FE (1975) Immunogenetics of the HL-A system. Physiol Rev 5:271

Boyd WC (1963) The lectins: Their present status. Vox Sang (Basel) 8:1

Fisher RA (1947) The rhesus factor. Am Sci 35:95

Goudemand M, Delmas-Marsalet Y (1967) Eléments de Immunohématologie. Flammarion, Paris

Kabat EA (1956) Blood group substances, their chemistry and immunochemistry. Academic, New York

Kabat EA (1976) Structural concepts in immunology and immunochemistry. Holt, Rinehart & Winston, New York

Levine P (1951) A brief review of the newer blood factors. Trans NY Acad Sci Sect II 13:205

Marcus DM (1969) The ABO and Lewis blood group system. Immunochemistry, genetics, and relation to disease. N Engl J Med 280:994

Mollison PL (1967) Blood transfusion in clinical medicine. Blackwell, Oxford

Morgan WTJ (1960) Croonian lecture: A contribution to human biochemical genetics. Proc Roy Soc B 151:308

Post RH, et al. (1968) Tabulations of phenotype and gene frequencies for 11 different genetic systems studied in the American Indian. In: Biomedical challenges presented by the Indian. PAHO/WHO, Washington

Prokop O, Uhlenbruck G (1969) Human blood and serum groups. McLauren, London

Race R R, Sanger R (1968) Blood groups in man, 5th edn. Blackwell, Oxford

Schiff F, Boyd WC (1942) Blood grouping technic. Interscience, New York

Schwartz LM, Miles W (1972) Blood Bank Technology, 2nd Ed. Williams & Wilkins, Baltimore

Springer GF (1971) Blood-group and Forrsman-antigenic-determinants shared between microbes and mammalian cells. Prog Allergy 15:19

Watkins W (1966) Blood group substances. Science 152:172

Wiener AS (1946) Blood groups and blood transfusion. C C Thomas, Springfield, Ill.

Wiener AS, Wexler IB (1958) Heredity of the blood groups. Grune & Strattan, New York

Zmijewski CM (1968) Immunohematology. Appleton-Century-Crofts, New York

Chapter 9   Hypersensitivity

Ivan Mota

Contents

Hypersensitivity 243
Classification 244
Anaphylaxis (Type I) 244
   Anaphylaxis in the Guinea Pig 245
   Mechanisms of Anaphylaxis 252
   Cells Involved in Anaphylaxis 255
   Antibodies Involved in Anaphylaxis 261
   Anaphylactic Phenomena in Man 267
   Tests for Detecting and Measuring IgE . . . 268
Cytotoxic Reaction (Type II) 278
Reaction by Antigen-Antibody Complexes
   (Type III) 279
   Methods for Detection of Immune Complexes 282
   Arthus Reaction 283
   Serum Sickness 284
Cell-Mediated Reactions 284
   Delayed Type Hypersensitivity, Type IV . . 284
   Reaction to Tuberculin 286
   Systemic Reaction to Tuberculin 287
   Delayed Reaction to Proteins 287
   Contact Sensitivity 287
   Transfer of Delayed Hypersensitivity 288
   The Effector Cell in Delayed
   Hypersensitivity 289
   Cellular Interaction in the Development
   of Delayed Hypersensitivity T Cell 290
   Mechanism of Target-Cell Destruction . . . 292
   Antigen Recognition by Cytotoxic T Cells . . 294
References 294

Hypersensitivity

Since it was established that an initial contact of the organism with certain infectious-toxic or noxious agents may result in the production of antibodies which protect the individual by lysing, neutralizing, or eliminating the foreign substance, numerous observations have indicated that the immunologic reaction does not always benefit the organism, and the organism is often damaged as a result. This type of harmful reaction is called an allergic or hypersensitivity reaction. The organism, tissue, or cell capable of exhibiting a hypersensitivity reaction is said to be sensitized. The allergic reactions, being immunologic reactions, are extremely specific, with the sensitized organism reacting exclusively with the antigenic determinant used for immunization or a similar structure. Hypersensitivity reactions are separated into two different types according to the time that elapses between the contact of the sensitized organism with the antigen and the macroscopic observation of the allergic phenomenon. Thus, whereas the so-called immediate hypersensitivity reactions require only minutes or a few hours to appear, delayed hypersensitivity reactions develop only after many hours. Today, although this criterion of the reaction time remains valid for classification of hypersensitivity reactions, it is understood that more important differences separate the two types. Thus, whereas reactions of the immediate type include all the reactions reproducible by various types of antibodies present in the serum – and which consequently can be transferred from one individual to another by antiserum – reactions of the delayed type depend upon sensitized cells and, therefore, are not transferable by antisera, but only by cells. The transfer of an immune state by cells is called adoptive immunization because the recipient organism adopts the cells of the donor that confer upon it the immunity acquired in another organism. The phenomenon of transferring a hypersensitivity state by cells is termed adoptive sensitization. Adoptive immunity as well as adoptive sensitization are possible only between isogenic individuals. Notably, whereas delayed hypersensitivity is transferable only by cells, immediate hypersensitivity is transferable either by antibodies or by cells.

Classification

The following scheme summarizes the classification of various types of hypersensitivity. Immediate hypersensitivity reactions include anaphylaxis, cytotoxic reactions, and the reactions due to antigen-antibody complexes. In all types of immediate hypersensitivity, an antigen-antibody reaction occurs, resulting in alterations in the tissues. In anaphylaxis, cells with membrane fixed antibodies are activated by the specific antigen and secretes biologically active substances (mediators) that cause tissue alterations; in cytotoxic reactions, it is the antigen that is associated with the cells. In reactions due to antigen-antibody complexes, neither the antigen nor the antibody is associated with the cells; the reaction ocurs in the extracellular fluid. In addition, whereas the last two reactions depend upon the presence of complement, the anaphylactic reactions proceed without activation of this system. Evidence indicates that in almost all these reactions, the response of the organism is due to the action of substances formed or liberated by the tissues through the antigen-antibody reaction. These substances, which usually possess intense pharmacologic activity, are called pharmacologic mediators. Diverse active substances are also produced in the delayed hypersensitivity reaction.

Hypersensitivity reactions	Immediate or Humoral	Anaphylaxis (type I)
		Cytotoxic reactions (type II)
		Reactions by antigen-antibody complexes (type III)
	Delayed or Cellular	Due to tuberculin or other proteins, infectious germs. Due to purified proteins. Due to simple chemical substances (contact dermatitis, type IV)

Anaphylaxis (Type I)

In an animal, the first injection of a nontoxic antigen (sensitizing dose) does not cause any reaction; however, after an interval of 2–3 weeks (sensitizing period), a second dose of the same antigen produces a violent reaction (symptomatically diverse depending upon the animal involved), which frequently is fatal. This phenomenon was observed for the first time by Portier and Richet (1902), who were investigating the toxic effect of extracts from the *Actiniaria* (sea anemone). Portier and Richet named this phenomenon anaphylaxis to indicate a status contrary to that of immunity (*ana*, against; and *phylaxis*, protection). Anaphylaxis later was observed in many laboratories where horse serum and other antigenic mixtures were injected into guinea pigs for experimental pur-

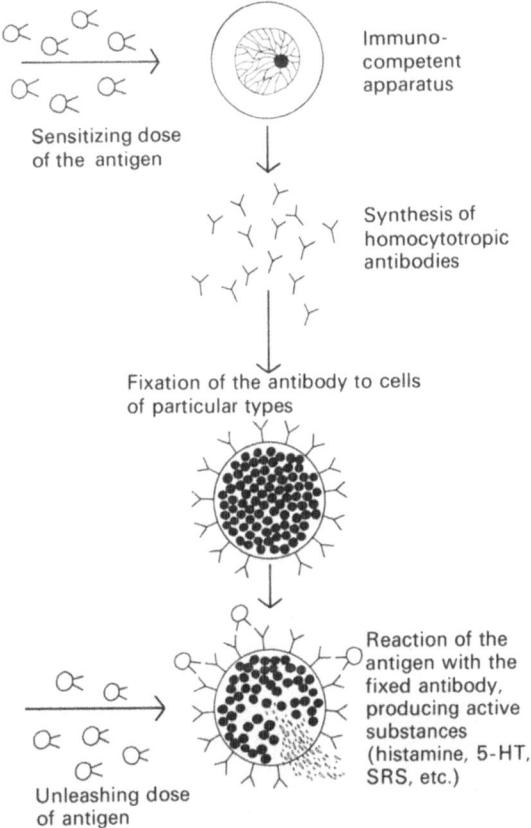

Fig. 9.1. Mechanism of the anaphylactic reaction

Table 9.1. Characteristics of anaphylaxis in different species

Species	Shock organ	Active substances liberated	Principal symptoms
Man	Lung + larynx	Histamine, kinins, SRS	Edema of the bronchia and larynx; emphysema
Dog	Hepatic veins	Histamine, kinins, SRS	Hepatic congestion; hemorrhage of intestinal mucosa
Guinea pig	Lung	Histamine, kinins, SRS	Emphysema
Rabbit	Pulmonary, circulation	Histamine, serotonin, SRS	Obstruction of the pulmonary capillaries by microthrombi of platelets and leukocytes. Failure of the right ventricle. Congestion of the abdominal organs
Rat	Intestines	Histamine, serotonin, SRS	Circulatory collapse, intestinal hemorrhage
Mouse	Intestines	Histamine, serotonin, SRS	Circulatory collapse, Intestinal hemorrhage

poses, and in human beings injected with antisera for treatment of infectious diseases. Anaphylaxis can appear either as a general phenomenon, affecting the entire organism, as always occurs when the antigen is injected intravenously, or as a localized phenomenon such as occurs when the antigen is injected extravascularly – e.g., intradermally or subcutaneously. The former is called systemic anaphylaxis, whereas the latter is termed local anaphylaxis. In either of these situations, the presence of the antigen, the specific antibody, and the cellular element to which the antibody is fixed are indispensable. The reaction between the antigen and the antibody results in a response of the target cell, i.e., the cell to which the antibody is fixed, which gives rise to the formation and liberation of mediators (Fig. 9.1). A summary of the symptomatology of systemic anaphylaxis, or anaphylactic shock, in different animal species is found in Table 9.1. The symptomatology of anaphylactic shock, although different for each species, results from a spasm of the smooth musculature, from an increase in capillary permeability, from an alteration in the distribution of the circulatory volume of the blood, and usually from a combination of these factors.

In this chapter, we first examine anaphylaxis in the guinea pig and then in man. In the interpretation of the latter is included a summation of thoughts obtained from clinical and experimental observations.

Anaphylaxis in the Guinea Pig

The guinea pig has been the species of choice for the study of anaphylactic phenomena due to the facility with which it becomes sensitized and the intensity with which it reacts to a second contact with the antigen. This species can be sensitized by any means of administration of the sensitizing dose, even by inhalation of an aerosol containing the antigen. A few weeks later, further contact with the same antigen, particularly intravenously, provokes intense symptomatology, characterized by severe puritis in the muzzle, contractions in the masticatory muscles, sneezing, spasmodic coughing, intense dyspnea, relaxation of sphincters with elimination of feces and urine, and in the final phase prostration with violent contractions of the respiratory muscles. The violence of the shock produces the death of the animal within a matter of minutes as a consequence of asphyxia resulting from constriction of the smooth musculature of the bronchia and bronchioli. Postmortem examination discloses lung emphysema due to retention of air in the alveoli from expiratory difficulties. The predominance of pulmonary alterations and of death by respiratory insufficiency characterizes the lung as the "shock organ" in the guinea pig. At an early date Dale (1920) attributed to histamine the anaphylactic phenomena in the guinea pig. He noted the essential similarity between anaphylactic shock in this species and the shock produced by the injection of histamine. Histamine liberated from sensitized tissues by the antigen was later obtained from the livers of dogs and the isolated lung of the guinea pig. These were the first demonstrations of the existence of a mediator in anaphylactic reactions. Acute anaphylaxis in the guinea pig appears to be due exclusively to the action of histamine, to which the smooth musculature of this species is extremely sensitive. However, today we know that many other mediadors are involved in anaphylaxis, as we will see later.

Protracted Shock. In contrast to the efficiency of the intravenous mode, sensitized animals in which the antigen is injected subcutaneously or intraperitoneally frequently do not exhibit acute respiratory symptoms, but present a different clinical picture. Protracted shock, as this manifestation is called, is characterized by prostration, hypothermia, and hypotension, with death occurring many hours after the animal is subjected to the second dose of the antigen. Upon postmortem examination, the emphysema characteristic of acute anaphylaxis is not observed, but hemorrhagic lesions are visible on the intestines. The nature and mechanism of this type of shock are unknown.

Passive Anaphylaxis. Shortly after recognition of anaphylaxis as an immunologic phenomenon, its transmission to an unsensitized animal by antisera obtained from actively sensitized animals was observed, thus demonstrating the dependence of this phenomenon upon the antibodies existing in the serum. Passive sensitization was extremely useful in the study of anaphylactic phenomena, for it permitted their study with known quantities of antibodies or with different classes, subclasses, and fragments of antibodies. On this matter, Zoltan Ovary gave very interesting and very important contributions using the passive cutaneous anaphylactic reaction (PCA). All anaphylactic phenomena obtained in the actively sensitized animal are also reproducible after passive sensitization. A primary insight resulting from the study of passive anaphylaxis was recognition of the existence of the so-called latent or sensitization period.

Sensitization Period. After the injection of the sensitizing dose of antibody, it is usually necessary that a given period of time elapses before administration of a second antigen dose produces an anaphylactic reaction. The interval between the application of the antibody and that of the antigen is called the latent or sensitization period. What happens during this period? This question remains without a definitive answer despite numerous attempts to provide one. This necessary interval suggests the existence of a process of fixation of the antibody to special receptors existing in certain types of cells of the tissues. Supportive of this idea is the fact that certain types of antibodies require a long sensitization period for the antigen to provoke an anaphylactic reaction of maximum intensity.

The necessity for fixation of the antibody to obtain an anaphylactic reaction is a possible explanation for the observation that antibodies of a certain animal species are not always capable of transmitting sensitivity to another species. For example, the guinea pig can be passively sensitized by rabbit, monkey, and human antibodies, but not by horse, goat, cattle, chicken, or rat antibodies.

Experiments in which the quantity of antiserum was varied and the sensitization period was kept constant have demonstrated a direct relationship between the quantity of antibody used for the sensitization and production of an anaphylactic reaction of maximum intensity, thus demonstrating the existence of an optimum antibody dose above which the effecfts are not modified. These experiments have also shown that, by increasing the quantity of antibody, one can reduce the sensitization period practically to zero when the quantity of antibody injected reaches levels far above the optimum dose for a sensitization period of 48 h. The anaphylaxis obtained under these conditions, i.e., with a large quantity of antibody and without a sensitization period, exhibits a clinical picture simular to the anaphylaxis obtained with small amounts of antibody after the sensitization period. It is called anaphylaxis by aggregation. In this situation anaphylaxis is triggered by antigen-antibody complexes formed extravascularly and it does not require a latent period. Some types of antigen-antibody complexes are able to cause anaphylaxis without previous antibody fixation leading to anaphylactic symptoms indistinguishable from those induced by anaphylaxis caused by combination of antigen with previously fixed antibody (see antigen-antibody reactions). It has been verified that preformed heat aggregates and immune complexes are able to bind to target cell surface through the Fc fragment but it is not known whether their binding site differs from that of IgE.

Passive Cutaneous Anaphylaxis. One of the simplest and most elegant techniques for the study of anaphylaxis is passive cutaneous anaphylaxis (PCA), which consists of sensitizing a small area of skin by intradermal injection of antiserum and, after an adequate sensitization period, injecting the antigen intravenously together with a dye such as Evans blue to facilitate reading of the reaction. The antigen rapidly reaches the sensitized site, reacts with the antibody and, by a mechanism to be discussed subsequently, produces an increase in local capillary permeability evidenced by the blue stain taken on by the area (Fig. 9.2). Passive cutaneous anaphylaxis also can be obtained by injecting the antibody into the blood, consequently, all of the animal's skin is sensitized. In this case, after an appropriate period of sensitization, the antigen is injected into the skin at any location. The human counterpart to passive cutaneous anaphylaxis is the Prausnitz-Küstner reaction (P.K. reaction) that was for many years used to study anaphylaxis in man.

Inverse Passive Cutaneous Anaphylaxis. Inverse passive cutaneous anaphylaxis (IPCA)

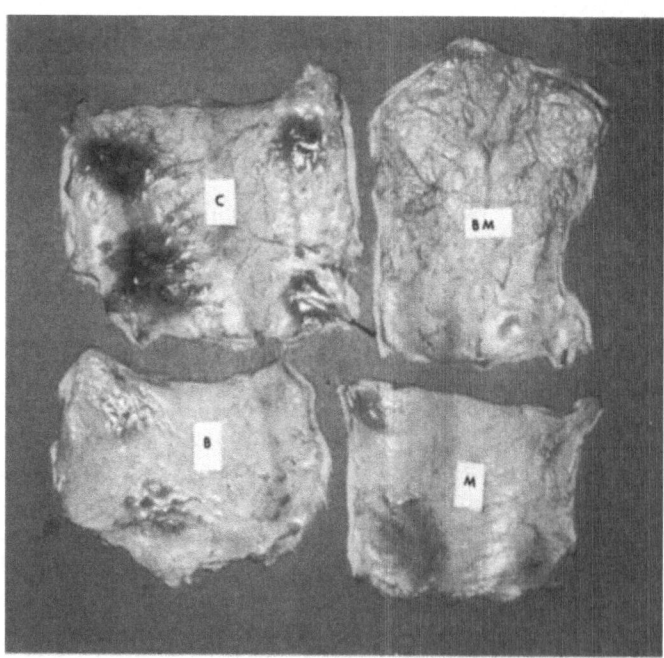

Fig. 9.2. Passive cutaneous anaphylaxis (*PCA*) in rats induced with reaginic antibody (IgE): *C* PCA in untreated control animal; *B* PCA in animal previously treated with serotonin inhibitor (diethylamide of D-bromolysergic acid (BOL-148): *M* PCA in animal treated with antihistamine (mepyramine): *MB* PCA in animal treated with BOL-148 in animal treated with BOL-148 and mepyramine. The necessity for the simultaneous presence of histamine and serotonin inhibitors to completely abolish the reaction indicates that these two mediators are responsible for the increase in capillary permeability that occurs in PCA of the rat induced with reaginic antibody. Mota I (1963) Life Sci 12:917

is produced when, instead of the antibody, the antigen is first injected into the skin and, after a sensitization period, the antibody is injected into the blood. The reaction is called inverse because of the inversion of the order of injection. It should be noted that IPCA is possible only when the antigen is a gamma globulin of a species whose antibody is capable of sensitizing the recipient species by direct PCA. Thus the guinea pig can be prepared for IPCA by using as antigen rabbit gamma globulin that is injected into the skin; there it is fixed to the cellular receptors as if it were an antibody. Later, upon reacting with the anti-rabbit gamma-globulin antibody injected intravenously, it produces a local anaphylactic reaction. However, if horse gamma globulin is used as antigen (which does not sensitize the guinea pig when used as antibody), subsequent injection of anti-equine gamma globulin does not produce anaphylaxis. This is explained by the apparent incapacity of the equine gamma globulin to attach to the cellular receptors of the guinea pig.

Homocytotropic and Heterocytotropic Antibodies. Antibodies able to sensitize cells so

that later contact with antigen induces anaphylactic reactions are called cytotropic antibodies. There are two types of cytotropic antibodies: homocytotropic and heterocytotropic.

Homocytotropic antibodies are capable of sensitizing the same species that produced them (they may or may not be capable of sensitizing another species), whereas heterocytotropic antibodies are incapable of sensitizing the same species that produced them, but are capable of sensitizing another species. The term anaphylactic antibodies includes both homocytotropic and heterocytotropic antibodies. Studies with anti-DNP and anti-picryl antibodies produced by hyperimmunized guinea pigs demonstrated the existence in this species of two populations of IgG possessing the same specificity, but differing in electrophoretic mobility. The population of antibodies migrating more rapidly was designated IgG_1 and the slower one IgG_2. When the biologic activity of these subclasses was analyzed, it was shown that whereas the IgG_1 antibodies were capable of passively sensitizing the guinea pig, the IgG_2 were incapable of doing so, but were capable of sensitizing an-

Table 9.2. Characteristics of the homocytoztopic antibodies

	Human[a] Type		Guinea pig[b] Type		Rat Type		Mouse Type		Dog Type	Rabbit Type	
	I	II	I	II	I	II	I	II	I	I	II
Immunoglobulin	IgG	IgE	IgG.	IgE	IgG_2	IgE	IgG	IgE	IgE	IgG	IgE
Electrophoretic mobility		$\gamma_{1/2}$	$\gamma_{1/2}$	?	$\gamma_{1/2}$	$\gamma_{1/2}$	$\gamma_{1/2}$	$\gamma_{1/2}$	$\gamma_{1/2}$	$\gamma_{1/2}$	$\gamma_{1/2}$
Sedimentation coefficient		7S	7S	?	7S	7S	7S	?	7S		
Complement fixation		0	0	?	+	0	0	?	?	+	0
Thermolability		+	0	+	0	+	0	+	+	0	0
Persistence in the skin		28 d	2–4 d	45 d	24 h	31 d	24 h	15 d	15 d	?	17 d
Optimum sensitization period		48 h	4–6 h	48 h	2–4 h	48–72 h	1–3 h	72 h	24–48 h	48 h	72 h
Transfer across placental barrier		0	+	?	?	0	?	?	?	?	?
Quantity present in the serum		Traces	+ + + +	Traces	+ + + +	Traces	+ + + +	Traces	Traces	+ + + +	Traces

[a] The existence of a type I homocytotropic antibody is probable, although not definite. Various works indicate the existence of a homocytotropic antibody belonging to IgG. In the dog, a type I homocytotropic antibody has not yet been identified
[b] Apparently, more than one type I homocytotropic antibody exists in the guinea pig

other species such as the mouse. IgG_1 and IgG_2 of the guinea pig are typical examples of homocytotropic and heterocytotropic antibodies, respectively. The homocytotropic antibodies appear capable of attaching only to homologous cellular receptors (or those of a closely related species), whereas the heterocytotropic antibodies do not have this capacity. The activity of the heterocytotropic antibodies is not clearly understood, but it is attributed hypothetically to the fact that these antibodies have molecular configurations capable of adapting to the cellular receptors of other species.

Among the homocytotropic antibodies, two types are distinguished (type I and type II) which are present in almost all species studied and are easily differentiable by their physicochemical and biologic properties (Table 9.2). Type I homocytotropic antibodies are characterized by high serum levels; by being resistant to heat (56 °C) and to treatment with mercaptoethanol followed by alkylation; by crossing the placental barrier; by exhibiting a short optimum sensitization period (2–4 h); and by persisting in the skin after passive sensitization for a maximum period of 24–72 h. The known type I antibodies are subclasses of IgG. The 7S IgG_1 immunoglobulin of the guinea pig is a typical example of this group. Type II homocytotropic antibodies are characterized by appearing in unusually low serum levels; by being destroyed by heat treatment and mercaptoethanol followed by alkylation; by not crossing the placental barrier; by possessing an optimum sensitization period of 48–72 h; and by persisting in the skin for many days after sensitization (> 30). Type II antibodies, such as the reaginic antibodies in man, rabbit, guinea pig, rat, and mouse (and perhaps also in other species) belong to a distinct class of antibodies, IgE. One peculiarity of IgE antibodies is the fact that they appear in elevated levels in the sera of individuals who are carriers of parasitic infection, particularly helminths (see p. 342). This contrasts with the modest levels obtained when the dead parasites or antigens extracted from them are injected into the organism – even when reinforced with an adjuvant. For example, high levels of reaginic antibodies directed against antigenic components of S. mansoni are encountered in individuals with schistosomiasis, as well as in monkeys and rabbits experimentally infected with this helminth. In contrast, single or repeated injections of extracts of the adult worm or of cercariae induce them only in modest levels. The reason for this difference is not known.

IgE Receptors and Antibody Fixation. The existence of a sensitization period in anaphylaxis suggests the necessity for the occurence of a union or fixation between the antibody molecule and cellular receptors. In man and higher primates, the fixation of IgE molecules on basophilic leukocytes and mastocytes is practically specific, because other classes of antibodies such as IgG are bound to these same cells by a factor of 100 less than the number of IgE molecules fixed. With the use of ^{125}I-labeled IgE, the number of receptors for IgE on the surface of basophils has been calculated to be 30,000–90,000. Rat mast cells have as many as 10^6 IgE receptors. The observation that the IgE molecules fixed to the cell can be dissociated from the receptors (at pH 4) without injuring them indicates that the union between the IgE molecules and the receptors is reversible and not covalent.

Mast cells and basophils have cell surface receptors highly specific for IgE. After being synthesized and secreted by plasma cells IgE molecules becomes fixed through its Fc to mast cells and basophils. Subsequent reaction with antigen activates the cell to secrete, probably by cross-linking of adjacent receptors. The characterization of the cell receptor for IgE has been facilitated by the use of rat basophils obtained from myeloid leukemia and mast cells isolated from rat peritoneal cavity. It was possible to label with radioactive iodine the cell membrane components of mast cells, saturate these cells with IgE, solubilize the cell membrane with nonionic detergent and co-precipitate

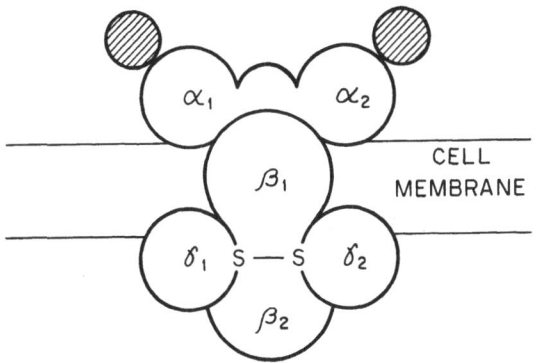

CELL
MEMBRANE

Fig. 9.3. Proposed structure of IgE receptor (modified from Metzger, 1984). Each receptor is made up of three polypeptide chains, designed α, β, and γ, each having two domains. α and β domains are held together by a less compact structure very susceptible to proteolysis; γ domains are joined by an S–S bridge. The site of insertion of IgE molecule is located in $\alpha 1$ domain. Shaded areas represent carbohydrates

the soluble radioactive IgE-receptor complex with antibody. The precipitated complex is then solubilized in sodium dodecyl sulfate and analyzed by polyacrylamide gel electrophoresis and gel filtration.

The IgE receptor seems to be made up of three polypeptide chains, α, β, and δ, each having two domains. The α_1 and α_2 and the β_1 and β_2 domains are joined by a less compact structure which is very susceptible to proteases whereas the δ_1 and δ_2 domains are joined by an S–S bridge. The α chain is partially exposed on the cell membrane and possess the site of insertion for the IgE molecule. The β and γ chains are intramembranous but cross the cytoplasmic side of the cell membrane and are exposed to the interior of the cell (see fig. 9.3).

Present understanding of the antibody structure responsible for fixation to the cell receptor is incomplete. However, some information on this was obtained from PCA experiments using antibody fragments by enzymatic digestion.

It appears that the capacity of the guinea pig IgG_1 antibody to attach to tissues and the inability of the IgG_2 of the same species to do the same depends upon differences in the structure of these molecules. Guinea pig IgG_1 and IgG_2 antibodies possess identical Fab and Fd fragments, yet differ in the antigenic properties of the Fc fragment. It is possible, therefore, that the Fc-fragment of the IgG_1 possesses a molecular configuration that permits its fixation to the cellular receptors – a configuration lacking in the

IgG_2. The importance of the Fc fragment in the fixation of antibody to the tissues was demonstrated using the PCA and IPCA techniques. In experiments in which guinea pigs were sensitized with whole (control) antibodies or with Fab and univalent 5S fragments obtained from the same antibody through papain digestion, the injection of antigen produced PCA only in the locations sensitized with the whole molecule or with the fragment containing the Fc part. The same results were obtained with IPCA (Fig. 9.4). In these experiments, guinea pigs were first injected intradermally with the Fab and Fc fragments obtained from rabbit antibodies and subsequently were given an intravenous injection of anti-rabbit gamma globulin. The antigen-antibody reaction produced an anaphylactic reaction only at the site injected with the Fc fragment capable of binding to the cellular receptors. The experiments pointed definitively to the Fc fragment as being responsible for this fixation.

The Fc fragments of IgG and IgE include $C_\gamma 2$, $C_\gamma 3$, and $C_\varepsilon 2$, and $C_\varepsilon 3$, and $C_\varepsilon 4$ domains, respectively. When subjected to different processes of enzymatic digestion, the Fc fragment can be cleaved into smaller fragments composed of either the C-terminal portion, corresponding roughly to $C_\varepsilon 3$ (in the case of IgG) and to $C_\varepsilon 3$ and $C_\varepsilon 4$ (in the case of IgE), or corresponding to the N-terminal portion of $C_\gamma 2$ and $C_\varepsilon 2$. Subsequent experiments investigating the function of the subfragments of immunoglobu-

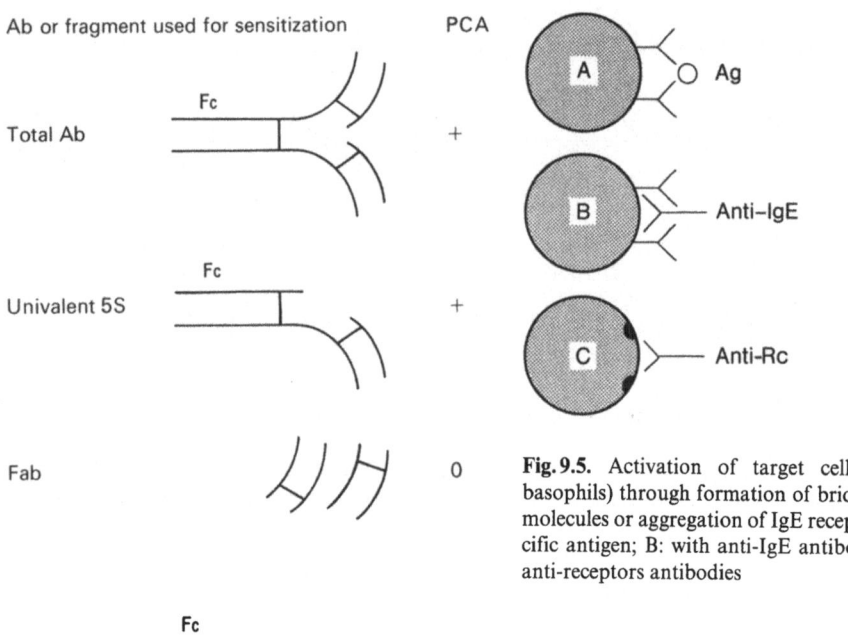

Fig. 9.4. Efficiency of the univalent 5S, Fab, and Fc fragments in inducing direct or inverse passive cutaneous anaphylaxis

Fig. 9.5. Activation of target cell (mastocytes or basophils) through formation of bridge between 2 IgE molecules or aggregation of IgE receptors. A: with specific antigen; B: with anti-IgE antibodies and C: with anti-receptors antibodies

lin produced from Fc pieces suggest that the entire Fc region is necessary for antibody fixation. It should be remembered that the anaphylactic reaction is a complex phenomenon, and even when it appears that the entire Fc region is necessary for antibody fixation, it does not prelude that the domains cannot contribute for the binding with separate and distinct steps. It is possible that there are specific quaternary interactions among the Fc domains and that the binding may be formed jointly by both $C_\varepsilon 3$ and $C_\varepsilon 4$ domains. It has been suggested that disulfide bonds in the $C_\varepsilon 1$ and $C_\varepsilon 2$ are essential for the orientation of the $C_\varepsilon 3$ and $C_\varepsilon 4$ domains and the spacial relationship of the two former domains may also be implicated in the ability of IgE to bind to its receptor.

Valence of the Antigen and Antibody in Anaphylactic Reactions. The use of antibodies and antigens of known valence in PCA experiments led to the conclusion that whereas the antigen must be at least bivalent, the antibody can be monovalent, although two molecules of antibody must be involved in the reaction. This conclusion is based on experiments in which the efficiency of monovalent, divalent, or multivalent haptens in producing anaphylaxis was studied, verifying that the univalent haptens were incapable of producing PCA whereas equimolar solutions of divalent or multivalent haptens demonstrated equal efficiency for production of PCA. In experiments with this system, Levine studied the capacity of a monovalent hybrid hapten containing one BPO grouping (Benzylpenicilloil) and one DNP grouping to produce PCA reactions in guinea pigs sensitized with anti-BPO or anti-DNP or with anti-BPO and anti-DNP simultaneously. Challenge of the sensitized animals with the monovalent hapten induced a PCA reaction only in the animals simultaneously sensitized with anti-BPO and anti-DNP. It was also shown that monovalent fragments such as the 5S fragment or artificially prepared monovalent antibodies are capable of producing anaphylaxis when bound to the target cell. It is accepted, then, that at least two conditions need to be satified for an anaphylactic reaction to occur: (1) fixation of the antibody by the Fc piece to the cellular receptors; (2) reaction of the fixed antibody with bi- or multivalent antigens to form a complex involving two or more antibody molecules. Apparently, it is sufficient that the antigen molecule forms a bridge to unite two active sites of two antibody molecules bound to the tissues (Fig. 9.5).

Mechanism of Anaphylaxis

Pharmacologic Mediators. The term mediator is applied to substances liberated directly or indirectly as a consequence of antigen–antibody combination that are responsible for the various manifestations of immediate hypersensitivity. Some of the mediators exist preformed in the cells; some are formed in the cells during the hypersensitivity reaction, whereas others are formed by the activation of humoral enzymatic systems. Mediators can be liberated from the cells by cytotoxic mechanisms and by noncytotoxic mechanisms. In cytotoxic liberation, irreversible lesions of the cellular membrane occur along with loss of control of cellular permeability, which leads to the loss to the external medium of the mediator and other cell constituents. Cytotoxic liberation results generally from the lytic action of the terminal components of the complement system activated in the classic or the alternate manner (see Chap. 5). With anaphylactic (nontoxic) liberation, selective passage of the mediator(s) to the exterior occurs without either irreversible lesions in the cellular membrane or

Table 9.3. Mediators for anaphylactic reactions

Mediators	Origin	Identifying properties
Histamine	Mastocytes	Contracts guinea pig ileum
	Basophils	Does not contract rat uterus
	Platelets	Inhibited by the antihistamines
Serotonin	Enterochromaffin cells	Contracts guinea pig ileum and rat uterus
	Mastocytes	
		Inhibited by lysergic acid
	Platelets	
Lys-Arg-Pro-Pro-Gly-Phe-Ser-Pro-Phe-Arg Bradykinin	Plasma α-globulin	Contracts guinea pig ileum and rat uterus Inhibited neither by lysergic acid nor by antihistamines
Slow-reacting substance (SRS)	Mastocytes Polymorphonuclear cells?	Contracts guinea pig ilusm Does *not* contract rat uterus
(Unknown structure)	Others?	Not inhibited by antihistamines
Prostaglandins	?	Contracts rat stomach and colon; Contracts chicken rectum
ECF–A	Mastocytes	Chemotactic for eosinophils
PAF (phospholipids)	Mastocytes Basophils	Activation of platelets

the death of the cell. Noncytotoxic liberation probably involves a mechanism equal or similar to that of secretion (see Table 9.3).

Histamine. Histamine, a product of the decarboxylation of histidine, which is widely distributed in nature, is located in mammalian tissue primarily in the granules of the mastocytes. In the blood of some species such as man, histamine is localized in the leukocytes, particularly in basophils, whereas in rabbit blood it is also found in the platelets. Histamine causes contraction of the smooth muscle of the intestine and uterus of the guinea pig, dog, and cat; and of the smooth muscle of the veins and arterioles of various species; in addition, it causes vasodilation and increasing permeability of the capillaries. Histamine activity is mediated by two receptors defined pharmacologically by the antagonistic effect of specific antihistamines. The contraction of smooth muscle induced by histamine is blocked by the classical antihistamines like mepyramine and diphenhydramine. However, the stimulation of gastric acid secretion inducec by histamine is not blocked by these antihistamines. This led Schild to suggest the existence of two histamine receptors, H_1 and H_2 of which only the first is blocked by classical antihistamines. The existence of two receptors was confirmed by Black et al., who synthesize a new antihistamine, burimamide, and verified that this drug although not inhibiting the histamine induced smooth muscle contraction, did inhibit the histamine-induced gastric acid secretion. In anaphylactic reactions, histamine is liberated from the tissues of numerous species and, in some of them such as the guinea pig, the intravenous injection of histamine reproduce a clinical picture similar to that of anaphylactic shock. The histamine liberated from the tissues of various species for the most part originates from the mastocytes, the basophilic leukocytes, and/or the platelets. The importance of histamine as a mediator of anaphylaxis depends upon the species considered and particularly upon the sensitivity of its smooth muscle to this substance. Thus, histamine is the most important mediator in anaphylactic shock of the guinea pig, contributes considerably to hypotension in anaphylactic shock of the dog, and appears to be responsible for certain phenomena of anaphylaxis in man, such as edema of the glottis and urticaria. In other species such as the rat and mouse, its role in anaphylaxis appears minor.

Serotonin. Serotonin (5-hydroxytryptamine) results from the decarboxylation of tryptophan after introduction of an –OH group in the indole ring. In most species, it is encountered principally in the intestinal mucosa, in the brain, and in the platelets. In the rat and mouse, it also is localized in mastocyte granules. This substance is liberated, during anaphylaxis, by the platelets of rabbit blood and by the mastocytes of rat and mouse tissue. In the mouse, it also appears to originate from the argentaffin cells of the intestinal tract: Serotonin produces contraction of smooth muscle and augments capillary permeability in many species. There is no evidence indicating its participation in the anaphylactic phenomena in man and in the guinea pig. It appears to play a more important role in the rat and mouse, due to the greater sensitivity of their tissues to this substance. It has been suggested that the simultaneous action of serotonin and histamine is of fundamental importance in the anaphylactic shock of the mouse.

Bradykinin. The kinins or kallidins, of which the better known is bradykinin or kalidin II, originate from precursors or kininogens (α-globulins) existing in the plasma, under the influence of enzymes called kallikreins:

(1) Bradykininogen + kallikrein → lysyl-bradykinin
(decapeptide) or kallidin I
(2) Lysylbradykinin + aminopeptidase → bradykinin
(nonapeptide) or kallidin II.

Bradykinin produces contraction of the smooth musculature, increases capillary permeability, and has a greater vasodilatory action than any other known substance. It also stimulates pain fibres. Experimental data suggest its participation in anaphylactic phenomena. It has been detected during anaphylactic shock in the blood of various species, and a diminution of bradykinogen occurs in the plasma of the rabbit and dog during anaphylaxis.

Slow-Reacting Substance. This substance, usually called SRS, is characterized by the ability to cause gradual contraction of the smooth musculature of various species. SRS has been chemically characterized as a mixture of linear compounds derived from arachidonic acid through the action of lipoxygenases. The first component of SRS to have its completed structure known was leukotriene, LTC4, which was later synthesized. This and similar compounds (see Fig. 9.6) are termed leukotrienes because they are made by leukocytes and have three conjugated double bonds. Studies with the synthetic compounds have shown that these substances are extremely potent, being 100 to 1,000 times more potent than histamine or prostaglandins in their effect on the bronchial tissues (see also p. 347). Unlike histamine and serotonin, it does not preexist in the tissues, but is formed during anaphylaxis. It was detected initially in the perfusion fluid of the isolated lungs of sensitized guinea pigs – and later in the lungs of man, rabbit, and monkey. Human bronchi are extremely sensitive to the action of

SRS, unlike guinea pig bronchi. SRS has been detected together with histamine in the perfusion fluid from lungs of asthmatic patients after the addition of antigen to which the patients have been sensitized. It is possible that SRS plays an important role in human asthma, contributing to the contraction of the bronchi.

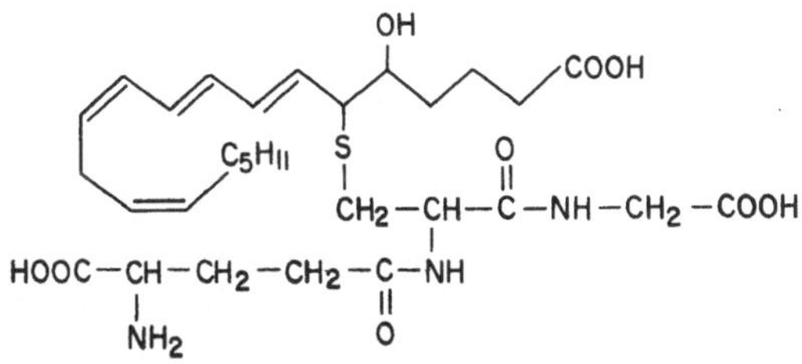

Eosinophil Chemotactic Factor (ECF). It has been observed that several factors capable of specifically attracting eosinophils appear in the tissues of humans and other species in anaphylactic reactions. One of these named eosinophil chemotactic factor of anaphylaxis (ECF-A) is constituted by two tetrapeptides VAL-GLY-SER-GLU and ALA-GLY-SER-GLU. They exist preformed in mast cells and basophils and, besides their chemotactic effect on eosinophils, they increase (or reveal) the $C3b$ receptors of these cells. There are indications that larger eosinophil chemotactic polypeptides are also secreted by mast cells in anaphylaxis. It is probable that the old observation of an eosinophil infiltrate in the tissues after an anaphylactic reaction may be in part explained by the release of these factors.

Neutrophil Chemotactic Factor (NCF). A chemotactic factor for neutrophils was found in extracts of basophils and mast cells and in the venous effluent collected from the arm of a patient sensitized to cold. This mediator may play an important role in the anaphylactic inflammatory process.

Prostaglandins. Prostaglandins are cyclic fatty acids containing 20 carbon atoms derived from unsaturated fatty acids such as arachidonic acid. Release of arachidonic acid, by the effect of phospholipase A_2 on phosphatidylcholine on mast cell membrane is very fast occurring within 30 s of anaphylactic cell activation. Other membrane phospholipids are also affected by phospholipase C and diglyceride with release of more arachidonic acid. Oxydative metabolism of arachidonic acid via the

Fig. 9.6. Leukotriene LTC4. Note the three conjugated double-bonds. Other SRS components like LTD4 and LTE4 possess slightly different structure

cyclooxygenase pathway originates two cyclic endoperoxydes, PGD2 and PGH2. In human and rat mast cells, PGH2 is converted to PGD2 by action of PGD2 synthetase. Rat mast cells activated by reversed anaphylaxis produce about 8.0 ng of PGD2 per 10^6 cells and human lung mast cells activated by antigen-human IgE produce as much as 97 ng of PGD2 per 10^6 cells. 9 α-hydroxy,11,15-dioxo-2,3,4,5-tetranorprostane-1,20dioic acid, a major metabolite of PDG2, has been found in urine of patients with mastocytosis (there are only traces of this metabolite in normal human urine) suggesting that synthesis of PGD2 occurs *in vivo* by human mast cells. Since human lung fragments activated by an IgE-dependent stimulus, produce PGD2, PGE2, PGF1, PGF2, and thromboxane A2, whereas activated human mast cells produce only PGD2, it is probable that the other mediators are produced by other cells.

Prostaglandins are involved in many physiological and pathological conditions including anaphylactic inflammatory reactions. They are generated in human and guinea pig lung after *in vitro* anaphylaxis and the plasma level of their metabolites is increased in asthma patients immediately after an attack. Among other effects, prostaglandins increase venous permeability, relax bronchial smooth muscles and have anti-inflammatory acitivity. Depending on the dose, prostaglandins affect other mediators inhibiting or potentiating their secretion (usually potentiation occurs with very low doses). In anaphylaxis, prostaglandins are generated from mast cells, basophils, eosinophils and probably other cells.

Platelet Activator Factor (PAF). PAF's are lipids secreted by activated mast cells and basophils in anaphylactic reactions that are able to induce release of histamine and serotonin from platelets. PAF induces secretion of platelet granules in a non-cytotoxic way that is dependent on calcium ions and energy. *In vivo,* PAF increased vascular permeability, favors intravascular coagulation and induces platelet accumulation.

PAF has been obtained from human and rabbit leucocytes (probably due to their content in basophils) and its structure was reported as 2-acylglyceryl-phosphorylcholine (see Fig. 9.9, p. 260). It is inactivated by phospholipases A2, C, and D.

Heparin. To these mediators one might add heparin, a proteoglycan responsible for the metachromatic coloration of the mastocyte and basophil granules. Recently, ^{35}S-labeled heparin was extracted from human lung cells enriched for mast cells. The calculated human lung mast cell heparin content is between 2.4 to 7.8 µg per 10^6 cells which gives a ratio of histamine to heparin on a weight basis of about 1:2.4 which is similar to that of intact lung fragments, implying that heparin in human lung is largely confined to mast cells. Heparin is liberated during anaphylactic shock in the dog, coming particularly from liver mast cells. Its only known effect in this species is to prevent blood coagulation. It does not seem to play any role in the pathogenesis of anaphylaxis in other species.

Cells Involved in Anaphylaxis

The target cells of anaphylaxis are those cells which have anaphylactic antibodies fixed to their membrane receptors and are activated in presence of the specific antigen (allergen). This definition includes mastocytes and basophils which are primary target cells but other secondary target cells are also involved in anaphylaxis.

Mastocytes. The mastocytes are cells of the connective tissue characterized by an extreme abundance of granules that totally fill the cytoplasm, frequently to the point of impeding the visibility of the nucleus. These granules are composed principally of glycoproteins; they stain metachromatically due to their mucopolysaccharide sulfate content. In the majority of species, the mastocytes are extremely rich in histamine and heparine and, in the rat and mouse, are also rich in serotonin. The histamine present in the mas-

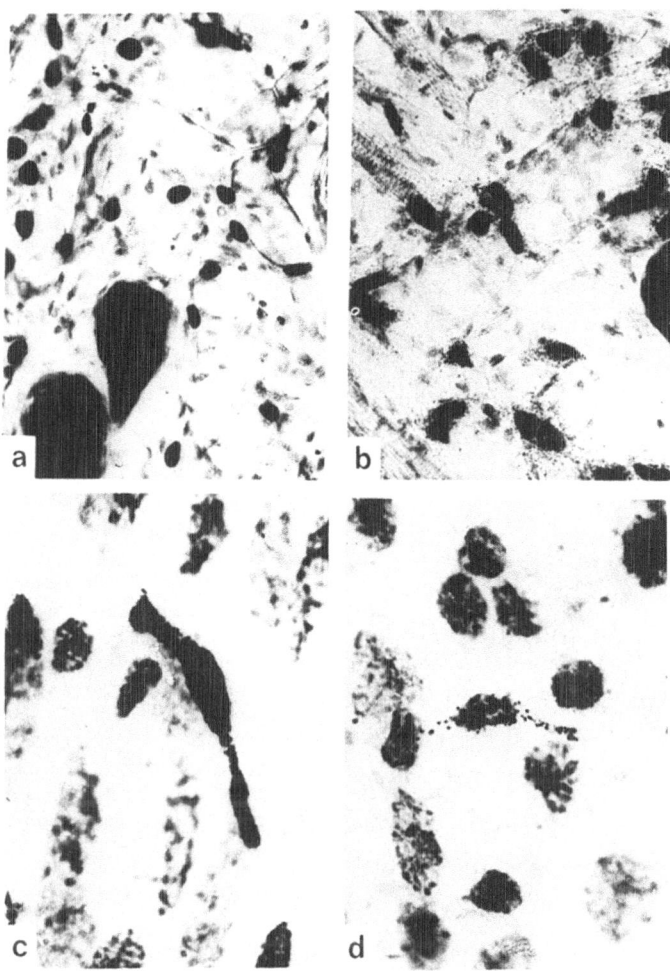

Fig. 9.7 a–d. Morphologic alterations of the mastocytes in anaphylaxis. **a** Mastocytes in the skin of unsensitized rats injected with ovalbumin. Note the distinct outlines of these cells and the absence of extracellular granules. **b** Mastocytes in the skin of rats injected to ovalbumin after intravenous injection of the antigen. Note the considerable extrusion of the granules and the imprecise outline of the cells. **c** Normal appearance of the mastocytes in the guinea pig mesentery. Note the cytoplasm totally filled with granules that conceal the nucleus. **d** Mastocytes of the mesentery of a sensitized guinea pig after contact with the antigen. Note the disappearance of most of the granules, leaving the nucleus visible. There is no extrusion of the granules as occurs in the rat. Mota I (1953) Tese de Livre Docencia, Universidade de Sao Paulo; Mota I, Vugman I (1956) Nature 177:427; Mota I (1959) J Physiol 147:425

tocytes is synthesized from histidine through an enzyme, histidinodecarboxylase, whereas serotonin is synthesized from tryptophan through the activity of 5-hydroxytryptophanodecarboxylase. All of these substances are found in the cytoplasmic granules of the mastocytes (see also pp. 8 and 344). Although Ehrlich described the mast cells as early as in 1877 only in the past 28 years has its physiological role begun to be understood. There are three important landmarks in the recent history of mast cells: the demonstration by Wilander (1937) that these cells contain heparin, the demonstration by Riley and West (1953) that tissue histamine is also located in these cells and the demonstration by Mota (1963) that the mast cell plays an essential role in anaphylaxis.

Morphologic alterations of the mastocytes have been described in active anaphylaxis in man, monkey, dog, guinea pig, pig, rat, and mouse (Fig. 9.7). In the guinea pig and rat, the agents that inhibit the liberation of histamine simultaneously inhibit the morphologic alterations of the mastocytes. When first observed these alterations were attributed to the presence of certain types of hypothetical antibodies bound to the cellular membrane of the mastocytes, which, upon reacting with the specific antigen, caused the cellular reaction, together with activation and liberation of substances of intense pharmacologic activity. Experiments with

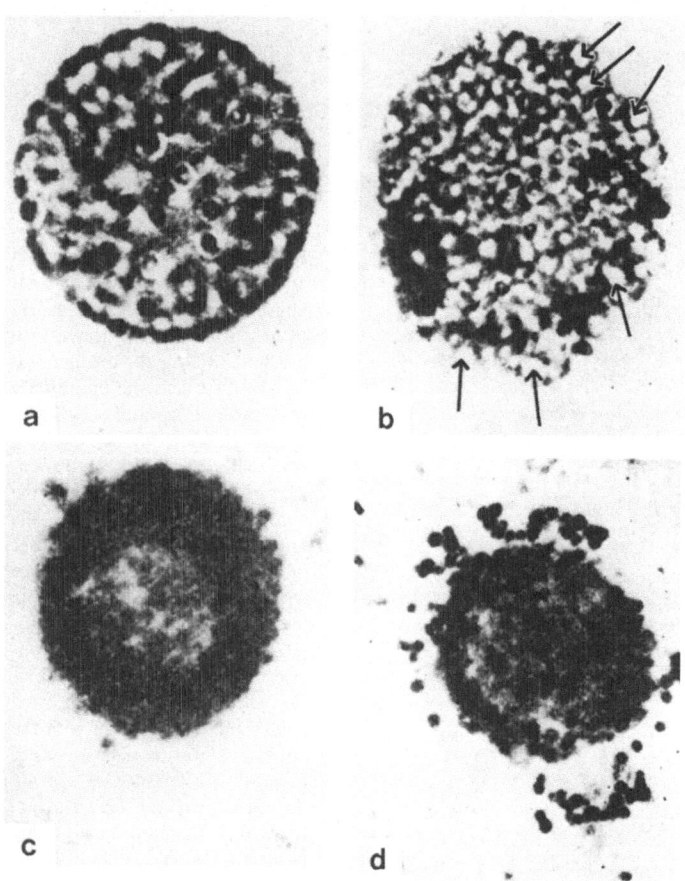

a   b

c   d

Fig. 9.8 a–d. Response to antigen by mastocytes isolated from the abdominal cavities of rats actively sensitized to ovalbumin. **a** and **b** The appearance of the isolated mastocytes under the phase-contrast microscope (**a**, before the addition of antigen; **b**, after the addition of antigen). The *arrows* indicate vacuolization in the cytoplasm. **c** and **d** Appearance of the mastocytes isolated after fixation and staining (**c**, before the antigen; **d**, after the antigen). Mota I, Dias da Silva W (1960) Nature 186:245

guinea pig mesentery demonstrated the possibility of passive sensitization of the mastocytes in vitro, followed by specific alterations of these cells provoked by subsequent contact with the specific antigen. The suggestion that the lesions of the mastocytes resulted from an antigen-antibody reaction at the level of the cell itself was reinforced by the observation that such cells were capable of responding to the antigen with morphologic alterations and liberation of active substances even when isolated. These experiments were performed with mastocytes collected from animals actively sensitized or after passive sensitization *in vitro*. In the rat, these alterations could be followed microscopically by phase contrast and were described as a "bubbling" of the surface of the cell accompanied by extrusion of the cytoplasmic granules (Fig. 9.8). Observed with an electron microscope after an anaphylactic reaction, the mastocyte membrane exhibited protrusions or spherical projections from the cellular membrane, measuring about 200 Å in diameter. It is possible that these projections represent vestiges of canals in the cellular membrane through which the granules are expelled to the exterior. In this respect, the expulsion of the mastocyte granules may be a particular case of exocytosis, i.e., the process by which particles are eliminated by the cell to the exterior. The first step in the mechanism that gives rise to the liberation of mediator (after the reaction of the antigen with the antibody molecule bound to the cell) may take place at the level of the cellular membrane. Recently, Behrendt studied the ultrastructure of sensitized mast cells after activation with antigen in several species. He described the anaphylactic degranulation process as characterized by sequencial exocytosis in the rat, by intracytoplasmatic chain formation in the guinea pig and by a unique channel formation and exocytosis in man.

The response of sensitized mastocytes to the antigen requires metabolically active cells maintained at physiologic temperature. For the cellular response to occur, Ca^{2+} and a thermolabile factor of unknown nature are indispensable. In addition to histamine, other mediators such as serotonin, SRS, and ECF-A also originate from the mastocytes in the anaphylactic reactions mediated by IgE.

Role of Mastocytes in the Anaphylactic Inflammatory Reaction. The location of mastocytes in cutaneous surface, in the mucosae and in the connective tissue around the venules suggests that these cells form a barrier sensitive to the penetration of allergens in the sensitized organism. The observation of mastocytes in the epithelium of the respiratory and digestive tracts admits the possibility of mediator liberation even before the antigen reach the subjacent connective tissue. As the mastocyte is practically the only connective tissue cell that possesses IgE receptors, its physiological role seems to be that of activating the defense mechanisms in order to prevent the establishment of a larger injury to the tissues after contact with the allergen. After triggering of the anaphylactic reaction, the mastocytes secrete mediators that cause the influx of plasma proteins (including complement factors and antibodies) and migration of polymorphonuclear leukocytes to the locality of the reaction. The mastocyte activity induces a biphasic response represented by an initial humoral phase and a final cellular phase.

The initial humoral phase is mediated by substances like histamine and SRS and come to a stop not only by local control mechanisms (histaminase and other factors that inactivate the mediators), but also by elements of the cellular phase such as the eosinophil. The cellular phase starts by migration of neutrophils and eosinophils attracted by chemotactic factors to the local of the reaction. These cells in presence of specific antibody and complement will help the local anaphylactic reaction to die away.

When the local humoral phase is not controlled, the mastocyte activation results in a patho-pharmacologic state described in the clinic as urticaria, angioedema, rhinitis or asthma. On the other hand, the incapacity of controlling the cellular phase lead to a severe inflammatory lesion such as there is in nasal polypos and bronchial allergic lesions.

The existence of a biphasic reaction in the anaphylactic reaction is shown by the observation that a subcutaneous injection of the allergen in atopic people induces an immediate wheal and flare that subsequently regresses and is followed a few hours later by an erythematous and pruritic swelling. In addition, it was also observed that the subcutaneous injection of F(ab')2 obtained from antihuman IgE antibody induces a local inflammatory lesion showing mastocyte degranulation and infiltration of eosinophils, but without deposition of immunoglobulins or complement factors. These observations indicate that mastocyte activation is by itself able to induce a biphasic anaphylactic reaction.

Inflammatory reactions mediated by mast cells may also have protective effects particularly in helminthic infections. The mastocyte seems to have a significant role in the immune and non-immune response induced by helminths. The immune response to these parasites are characterized by an increase of the specific and nonspecific IgE and by infiltration of the tissues by mastocytes and eosinophils. Recently, it was observed that mice depleted of mastocytes with compound 48/80 loose the immunity conferred by a previous infection with S. mansoni. For the specific as well as nonspecific resistance to S. mansoni there seems to be cooperation between mastocytes and eosinophils. In the non-specific resistance it seems that activation of the complement alternative pathway by schistosomules cause the production of anaphylatoxins that activate the mastocytes to produce ECF. This factor, besides attracting the eosinophils, increases the number of C3b receptors on these cells. The coating of the parasite with C3b via the alternative pathway permit C3b-dependent eosinophil mediated killing to occur in the non-immune response. In this way, the cytotoxicity mediated by eosinophils in the non-immune organism depends on the activation of the alternative pathway, production of anaphylatoxin and activation of the mastocytes and eosinophils. In the immune organism, the mastocytes sensitized with for the parasite antigens specific IgE, will be directly activated by these, secrete mediators including ECF, attract the eosinophils and duplicate the same mechanism described for the non-specific resistance. In addition, it is possible that the increase in capillary permeability, allowing the passage of IgG antibody specific for the parasit into the tissues, will facilitate the antibody dependent cytotoxicity caused by eosinophil, as it happens in humans. It is possible that the mastcell-IgE-eosinophil interrelationship may have been kept during phylogeny because of its advantage in immunity against some parasites.

According to Capron, immune resistance to S. mansoni may also be mediated by macrophages containing specific IgE antitbodies on their membrane.

Basophils. The polymorphonuclear cells of various species, including the human, are rich in histamine, which is localized principally in the basophils (50%–85%) and, in lesser quantities, in the neutrophils and eosinophils. Basophils are myeloid cells that otherwise are extremely similar to mastocytes, with both cell types possessing metachromatic granules rich in heparin and histamine (see also pp. 8 and 344). Addition of extremely small quantities of specific antigen (10^{-6} μg protein) to a suspension of sensitized leukocytes produces liberation of histamine without visible morphologic alterations of these cells. This type of reaction depends upon the reaginic antibody and does not depend upon complement. Greater quantities of antigen produce visible alterations of these cells.

It is now recognized that the basophils are the cells responsible for the histamine liberated by the antigen from leukocyte suspensions taken from atopic patients. This conclusion implies that basophils, in the same manner as mastocytes, must bind IgE molecules exclusively or preferentially. Actually, the addition of anti-IgE to a suspension of human leukocytes produces liberation of histamine and degranulation of the basophils. Moreover, autoradiography of human leukocytes previously incubated with anti-IgE labeled with ^{125}I has revealed localization of the IgE exclusively in the basophils. The presence of IgE in these cells also has been confirmed by electron microscopy. With the use of myeloma IgE labeled with ^{125}I, the number of receptors for this antibody on the membrane of the basophils was calculated to be 30,000–90,000 per cell.

The anaphylactic liberation of histamine by human leukocytes is used as a test to detect and study the sensitivity of allergic patients. For this purpose, the patient's leukocytes can be incubated directly with antigen, or normal leukocytes can be incubated with the allergic patient's serum and later transferred to the specific antigen. In both cases, the positivity and intensity of the reaction are measured through the liberation of histamine. The antibodies responsible for the sensitization of leukocytes in the human and rabbit are homocytotropic antibodies of the IgE class. As with mastocytes, in order for the cellular response to proceed, the leukocytes must be metabolically intact, and both Mg^{2+} and Ca^{2+} ions must be present.

Basophils accumulate in substantial numbers in certain biologically important forms of delayed hypersensitivity termed cutaneous basophil hypersensitivity that will be discussed later (see p. 344).

Platelets. Platelets are particles originating from the cytoplasm of megakaryocytes (see p. 13). Platelets contain organelles such as mitochondria, microtubules, lysosomes, and granules of unknown nature. When lysed, platelets liberate diverse substances including adenosine diphosphate (ADP), adenosine triphosphate (ATP), epinephrine, histamine, and lysosomal enzymes. The platelets do not synthesize the histamine and serotonin found within them; they are accumulated by an unknown mechanism. Contrary to what occurs with leukocytes and mastocytes, the liberation of active substances from the platelets does not depend upon an antigen–antibody reaction on the surface of these cells, since the platelets are incapable of fixing antibodies of any kind. Certainly, platelets of all species thus far studied are activated through antigen–antibody complexes or through immunoglobulin aggregates. In some species, though not all, complement is necessary for the activation of the platelets. For example, complement is necessary for the activation of rabbit platelets through antigen–antibody complexes; human pletelets are activated in the absence of complement.

In the human, as well as in several other species, platelets are activated mainly by two mechanisms: (1) a secretory mechanism initiated by the adherence of Fc pieces of antibodies that have bound antigen to the platelets; if an antibody binds an antigen or if an immunoglobulin aggregation results, conformational changes occur in the Fc pieces which permit adherence to the platelet; and (2) an indirect reaction that is induced originally by an antigen–antibody reaction on the surface of the leukocytes; platelet-activating substances are liberated as a result of this reaction.

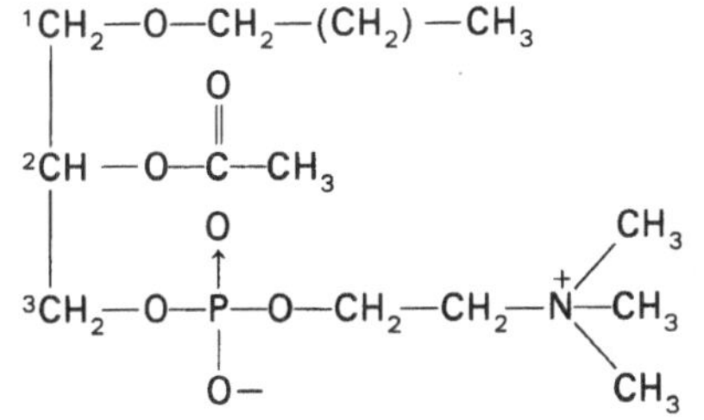

This mechanism was first demonstrated in experiments in which rabbit blood cells were added to (1) unsensitized platelets, (2) sensitized leukocytes, or (3) unsensitized platelets plus an equal quantity of the sensitized leukocytes present in (2). The amount of histamine liberated in (3) was much greater than that in (2), whereas none was liberated in (1). The leukocyte responsible for this phenomenon is the basophil sensitized with IgE. The cell is activated by the fixation of antigen to the IgE antibodies on the membrane and, in addition to histamine, it liberates a soluble factor that can activate platelets, called platelet-activating factor (PAF). Chemically, it is a phospholipid l-0-alkyl-2-acetyl-sn-glycosyl-3-phosphorylcholine with the length of the alkyl chain mainly C_{16} and C_{18} (Fig. 9.9). PAF has also been demonstrated in other species, and can be obtained from human mast cells. PAF causes aggregation of platelets.

The activation of platelets requires Ca^{2+}, uses energy, and is influenced by 3′,5′-AMP. Microtubules and microfilaments appear to play a role in the platelet-secretion mechanism. Platelet activation may play a significant role in the deposit of antigen–antibody complexes on the vascular wall. Basophils and/or mast cells sensitized with IgE lead to activation of platelets and this together with increase in permeability during an anaphylactic reaction appears to make possible or at least facilitate the deposit of complexes in the tissue.

Eosinophils. There is a well known increase in the number of eosinophils in the blood and other tissues in allergic conditions, parasitic infections (particularly helminths) and in some inflammatory and neoplastic conditions. The eosinophil functions and its role in the immune reactions began to be understood thanks to the development of technics to obtain purified suspensions of this cell and of biochemical and immunochemical methods applied to study its contents and its membrane receptors. The mechanism that regulate the generation of eosinophils in the bone marrow is becoming

$^1CH_2$—O—CH_2—(CH_2)—CH_3

^2CH—O—C—CH_3

$^3CH_2$—O—P—O—CH_2—CH_2—N$^+$—CH_3

Fig. 9.9. Chemical structure of platelet-activating factor (PAF)

to be clarified by the finding of a factor able to stimulate specifically the generation of eosinophil colonies *in vitro*. This factor is produced by lymphocytes activated by pokeweed or sensitized by antigens. It has been observed that the number of eosinophil colonies in bone marrow culture is significantly increased by the addition of the supernatant of a suspension of sensitized lymphocytes incubated with the specific antigen. Confirmation of the lymphocytic origin of the eosinophilopoiesis factor was established by *in vivo* experiments. It was observed that implantation in the peritoneal cavity of rats of cell-tight diffusion chambers containing lymphocytes sensitized to *T. spiralis* plus *T. spiralis* antigen induced an increase in the number of eosinophils in the recipient. Conversely, implantation of the chambers containing normal bone marrow in the peritoneal cavity of rats infected with *T. spiralis* resulted in a significant increase of the eosinophilopoiesis in the bone marrow contained in the chamber. Many experiments have demonstrated that this type of eosinophil increase is T cell dependent. For instance, the incrase in eosinophils in animals infected with *T. spiralis* is abolished by neonatal thymectomy, and nude mice do not show the increase in eosinophils that is usually present in normal mice infected with helminths. However, observations showing that the increase in eosinophils is not completely abolished by thymectomy suggest that there are other mechanisms independent of T cells that stimulate the production of eosinophils by the myeloid tissue. Eosinophils are usually attracted to the site of an allergic reaction mediated by IgE, appearing soon after activation of mast cells attracted by eosinophil chemotactic factors produced locally. There are many indications that the eosinophils act as a modulator of anaphylactic reactions. 25% of human eosinophils have IgE molecules in their membrane and can be activated by the specific antigen. Once activated these cells secrete prostaglandins that inhibit histamine release from mast cells by inducing an increase in their intra-cellular level of $3',5'$-cAMP. Furthermore, it has been shown that eosinophils preferentially engulf mast cell granules preventing the liberation of active substances present in the granule. Additional mechanisms through which eosinophils control anaphylactic reactions are inactivation of histamine by histaminase and secretion of a substance with anti-histamine activity. Eosinophils also produce phospholipase D that inactivates PAF.

There is some evidence that eosinophils have an important role in defense against parasites; most of the evidence is related to immunity to S. mansoni. Histopathologic studies have shown that a great number of inflammatory cells in granulomas around schistosomula are eosinophils probably attracted by an immunological mechanism. Injection of schistosomula directly into lung tissue results in an eosinophil infiltrate in animals immune to S. mansoni, but not in normal animals. Furthermore, monospecific anti-eosinophil serum injected in animals immune to S. mansoni before reinfection abolishes the protective effect of the previous immunity. *In vitro* studies have shown that destruction of schistosomula by antibody-dependent cytotoxicity is due to adherence of eosinophils to these parasites through their Fc receptors. Ramalho Pinto and coworkers have shown that in addition to the antibody-dependent cytotoxicity, activation of the alternative pathway by the surface of the schistosomula seems to contribute to lyse of the parasite mediated by eosinophils in rats. Deposition of C3b on schistosomula cause adherence of rat eosinophils through specific C3b receptors and damage of the schistosomula by the attached eosinophils.

Antibodies Involved in Anaphylaxis

In all species studied, both homocytotropic antibodies (IgG and IgE) are present in the serum of sensitized animals; however, the importance of the contribution of each in the in vivo anaphylactic reaction is difficult to evaluate. Homocytotropic antibodies of the IgG class (type I) are usually resistant to heat and to treatment with mercaptoethanol, reaching high concentrations in the serum, and are demonstrable in the skin after passive sensitization for a short time (24–48 h). Homocytotropic antibodies of the IgE class (type II), in contrast, are sensitive to heat and to mercaptoethanol, are present in serum in low concentration, and persist in the skin after passive sensitization for a long time (30–40 days) (see also p. 347). Data suggest that the type of mediator liberated does not depend upon the type of antibody bound to the cells. This implies that the anaphylactic phenomena, although possibly symptomatically similar, can be caused by intrinsically different mechanisms. A summary of the antibodies involved in anaphylaxis along with their characteristics is given in Table 9.2.

IgE Antibodies. IgE antibodies are responsible for immediate-type hypersensitivity and are important in immune resistance to parasites. They were first discovered in humans, initially in allergic patients and later in patients with myeloma in whom Johansson and Bennich characterized the first IgE secreting myeloma. The IgE antibodies were characterized as a new class of immunoglobulins by the Ishizakas. IgE antibodies were later detected by Mota in rats and mice sensitized with antigen plus *B. pertussis* and by Catty in guinea pigs infected with *T. spiralis*. Induction of IgE antibody production by artificial immunization of guinea pigs was later obtained by Mota and Perini.

The IgE antibodies are responsible for the anaphylactic and atopic phenomena in several species and in man. The serum concentration of IgE is very low and knowledge on its structure was obtained thanks to the finding of patients with IgE myeloma. The IgE molecule (see Fig. 4.19) originates from plasma cells and consists of two antigen-combining sites at the ends of the Fab pieces, and of the Fc piece formed by the carboxyterminal at the end of the two ε chains. The molecular weight of IgE is 188,000 daltons and the isolated ε heavy chain weights about 72,000 daltons. Electrophoretically, IgE migrates with the fast immunoglobulin fraction and it sediments as an 8S fraction in ultracentrifugation. The ε heavy chain possesses 5 domains (H_V, $C_\varepsilon 1$, $C_\varepsilon 2$, $C_\varepsilon 3$, and $C_\varepsilon 4$) but it does not possess a hinge region nor the nonadecapeptide of the carboxyterminal end of the μ chain. Studies comparing the primary structure of the constant region of the α, γ, and μ chains with that of the ε chain showed the greatest homology with the γ chain (33%).

As other immunoglobulins, the IgE molecule is also susceptible to the action of several enzymes. Pepsin produces one (Fab)2 fragment whereas papain breaks the molecule in monovalent Fab and Fc fragments. The Fc fragment possessed the domains $C_\varepsilon 2$, $C_\varepsilon 3$, and $C_\varepsilon 4$ and contains 2 antigenic determinants, ε_1 and ε_2 that are specific of the IgE molecule. The Fab fragment has a light chain and the Fd fragment of the heavy chain that contains the idiotypic determinants of the molecule. There are several characteristics proper of the IgE molecule. One is the presence of a double disulphide bridge in domain $C_\varepsilon 1$. Furthermore, the IgE molecule has 2 disulphide bridges limiting the $C_\varepsilon 2$ domain, one inter-chain bridge between $C_\varepsilon 1$ and $C_\varepsilon 2$ and another one between $C_\varepsilon 2$ and $C_\varepsilon 3$. The IgE molecule possesses 5 to 6 carbohydrate groups, one of which has a peculiar composition with 6 mannoses and 2 N-acetylglucosamines. As these groups are located near the carboxyterminal end of the chain, it is suggested that they may be important in the mechanism of fixation of the IgE to cell receptors.

The IgE molecule is very rich in cystein containing about 40 molecules of this aminoacid, 15 of which are located in the chains. The S–S bridges are important for the cytotropic properties of the molecule. The ability of IgE to fix to mast cells is lost after reduction and alkylation due to the breaking of some of the S–S bridges. It is believed that reduction of only 3 of these bridges is sufficient to destroy the IgE cytotropic property. The first S–S bridge to be dissolved on reduction is the bridge in position 318 that binds the 2 ε chains together, the next is the heavy-light S–S bridge and the last is the S–S bridge in the $C_\varepsilon 1$ domain.

The thermal sensitivity of the IgE molecule is well known. Studies with circular dichroism spectroscopy have shown that the changes that occur in IgE molecule when submitted to heating at 56° are restricted to the $C_\varepsilon 3$ and $C_\varepsilon 4$ domains.

The IgE level in serum of adult normal humans is about 250 ng/ml (1 ng $= 10^{-0}$ g) whereas in atopic individuals it may reach 700 ng/ml. In the blood of umbilical cord IgE level is of the order of 36 ng/ml. The elevation of the IgE level in children 1 year old or younger is almost always associated with some atopic disease.

Ontogeny of IgE B Lymphocytes. It is now well established that precursors of IgE B lymphocytes bear IgE molecules on their membrane and are derived from virgin B lymphocytes which have IgM or IgM and IgD molecules on their membrane. Expression of IgE molecules on either IgM or IgM-IgD double-bearing B lymphocytes occurs independently of either T lymphocytes or antigen during differentiation. Once IgE is expressed on the B lymphocyte membrane, these cells are committed for IgE synthesis. However, the differentiation of IgE B lymphocytes to IgE plasmocytes requires T lymphocytes and is controlled by a fine balance between T helper and T suppressor lymphocytes.

Biochemistry of Antigen-Induced Secretion of Mediators. When antibody molecules (IgE or IgG) fixed to the membrane of mast cells or basophils are bridged by antigen this causes aggregation of their receptors; this results in a membrane signal that is translated to the interior of the cell initiating a cascade of biochemical reactions that leads to the secretion of mediators: activation of a serine esterase, a simultaneous and transient increase in cAMP and methylation of phospholipids, increase of phos-

pholipid metabolism, oxydative glycolysis, protein phosphorylation and flux of Ca^{2+} to the interior of the cell (see Fig. 9.10). As many of these phenomena occur within seconds after cell activation, kinetics studies do not allow to distinguish parallel from sequential steps.

Activation of Serine Exterase. F. Austen and E. Becker observed many years ago that when antigens enter in contact with sensitized mast cells in the presence of diisopropylfluorophosphate (DFP) there is no mediator secretion but when DFP is removed before contact with antigen, it occurs a total mediator secretion suggesting that DPF acts on a serine proesterase that is activated only after antigen activation. Furthermore, the transfer of sensitized cells after contact with antigen in the presence of DFP into a DFP-free medium results in a release of mediators that is inversely proportional to the length of time of antigen contact in presence of DFP. Since DFP irreversibly inactives serine exterase, this result indicates that mediator release after removal of DFP reflects the continued activation of the remaining proesterase by antigen. It is possible that the first event in the cascade of biochemical reactions involved in mediator secretion is the activation of serine esterase since its inhibition by DFP prevents all the other reactions.

Phospholipid Methylation. IgE receptors are closely associated with methyltransferases and adenylate cyclase. Phospholipid methylation was studied incubating mast cells or their membrane with ^{3}H-labeled S-adenosyl-methionine. Activation of mast cells under this condition causes incorporation of methyl groups to phospholipids that reaches a maximum 15 seconds after contact of the cells with antigen and then decreases very rapidly. The phospholipid methylation is immediately followed by an influx of Ca^{2+} and by histamine liberation. Analysis of methylated phospholipids by thin layer chromatography shows that there occurs a considerable increase in the

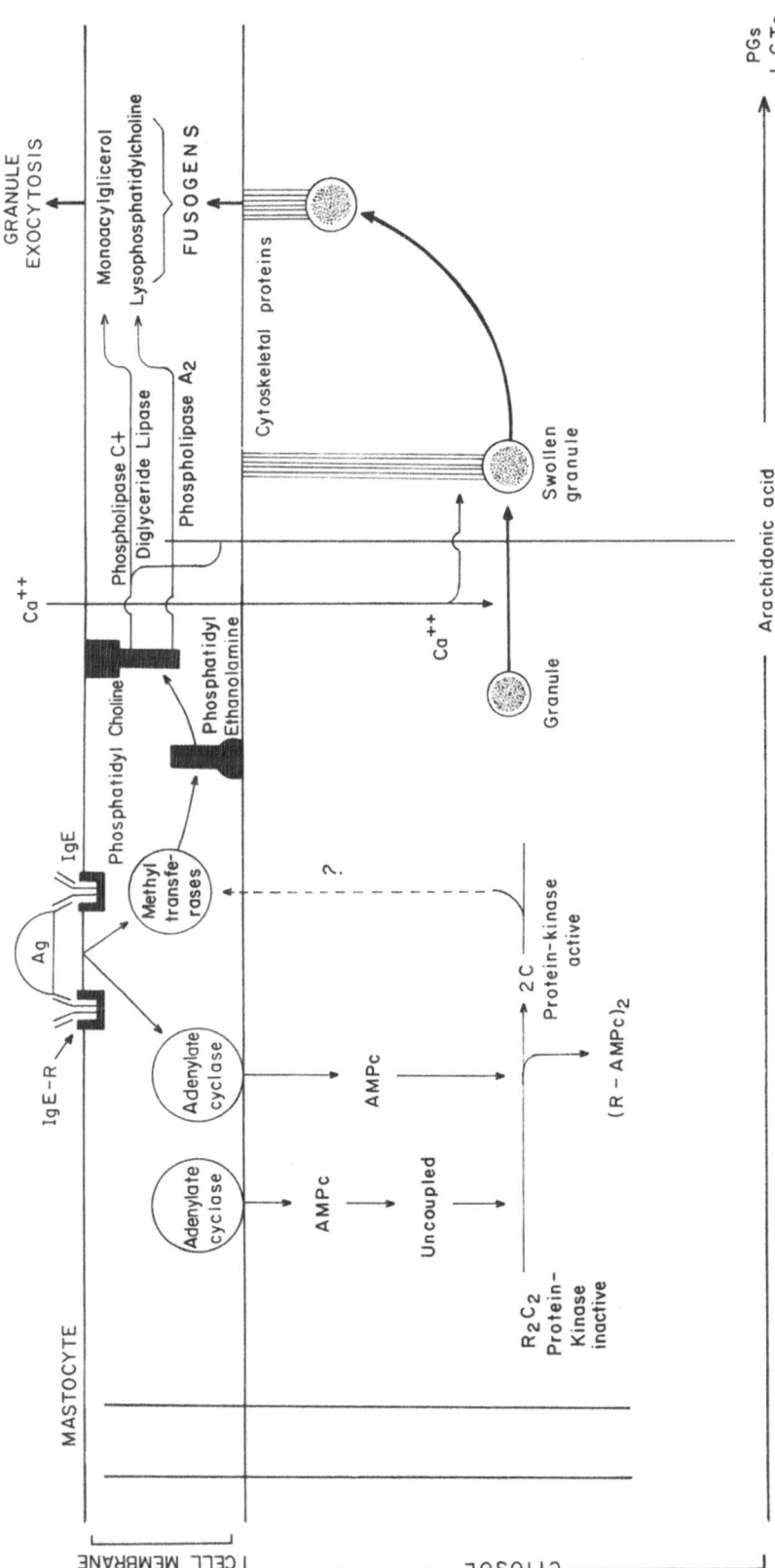

Fig. 9.10. Diagram for the biochemical events associated with IgE-dependent mediators secretion. (Adapted from Lewis et al., 1981)

synthesis of phosphatidylmonomethyletha-
nolamine, phosphatidyldimethylethanol-
amine and phosphatidylcholine. Phospholipid methylation is effected by methyltransferase I, located in the cytoplasmic
side of the cell membrane; the enzyme adds
one methyl group to phosphatidylethanol-
amine converting it to phosphatidylmono-
methyl-etanolamine. A second enzyme
methyltransferase II, located in the external
side of the cell membrane adds two further
methyl groups to phosphatidylmonometh-
ylethanolamine converting it to phosphatidylcholine. During the methylation process, displacement of the phospholipids occurs in such a way that they are translocated from the cytoplasmic to the external
side of the cell membrane. This re-orienta-
tion of the phospholipids within the cell
membrane increases the membrand fluidity
which may allow coupling of the IgE-recep-
tors to adenylate cyclase and formation of
calcium channels through which Ca^{2+}
enters the cell. The phospolipid methylation is essential for calcium influx and mediator's release. The increase in intracellular calcium ions activates phospholipase A2
which converts phosphatidylcholine to ly-
sophosphatidylcholine. Phospholipase C is
simultaneously activated and acts on membrane phospholipids producing diacygly-
cerol which is converted by diglyceride li-
pase to monoacylglycerol and fatty acids
including arachidonic acid. Lysophosphati-
dylcholine, diacylglycerol and monoacylglycerol are potent fusogens that promote
the fusion of the perigranular membrane
during the process of exocytosis.

Incrase in cAMP. A few seconds after
antigen stimulation there is a rapid and
transient increase in the level of mast cell intracellular cAMP. This increase in cAMP is
essential for mediator release and results
from adenylate cyclase activation. The
bridging of IgE receptors by antigen activates adenylate cyclase through a binding
protein that may be the serine esterase inhibited by DFP. The activation of adenylate cyclase depends upon a functional as-

sociation of a regulatory protein with a
catalytic protein. This association activates
the catalytic protein by causing a transient
exchange of GTP for GDP on the regulatory protein. The simultaneous activation
of an intrinsic GTPase converts GTP to
GDP and the balance of this reaction controls the activity of the catalytic protein.
Once activated and in the presence of Ca^{2+},
the catalytic protein converts ATP to
cAMP.

Protein Kinase Activation. In eukariotic
cells cAMP acts through activation of protein kinases. The increase in cAMP activates cAMP-dependent protein kinases
that function as intracellular biochemical
links between the transmembrane activation of adenylate cyclase by the extracellular Ige-receptor complex and the intracellular secretory events. The cAMP-dependent
protein kinases include type I and type II
isoenzymes according to their order of elution in NaCl gradient from diethylaminoethyl-cellulose. Both isoenzymes are tetramers made up of an inhibitory dimer
plus a dimer of catalytic subunits. Once activated the catalytic subunits transfer the
terminal phosphoryl group of ATP to the
hydroxyl groups of proteins. The protein
phosphorylation is probably responsible
for changes in the permeability of the perigranular membrane as well as for ATP-de-
pendent and actomyosin-dependent contraction of the microfilaments required to
bring the secretory granules close to the cell
membrane.

Calcium Influx. At the end of the fifties,
Mongar and Schild observed the absolute
requirement of calcium ions for the anaphylactic liberation of histamine. Absence of
calcium also prevented mast cell degranulation. Later, Foreman showed that activation of mast cells by antigen resulted in an
influx of calcium that was immediately followed by histamine release. One of the most
suggestive evidence that calcium influx
causes histamine liberation is the histamine
release induced by the divalent cation iono-

phores which cause a flux of Ca^{2+} to the interior of mast cells and basophils. There is evidence that Ca^{2+}, like cAMP, is an important intracellular regulator that functions as a second messenger for certain extra-cellular molecules. One of the first evidence for this came from experiments showing that the injection of a minute amount of Ca^{2+} into the striated muscle cell induced contraction of the muscle fiber. The total concentration of calcium ions is one thousand lower inside the cell. To keep the calcium concentration lower the cell pumps Ca^{2+} actively to the outside as well as to the interior of cell organelles such as mitochondria and the endoplasmic reticulum. Furthermore, various molecules bind to calcium gradient through the plasma membrane to translate extracellular signals. In the same way that some cell receptors are functionally associated to adenylate cyclase, others are associated with calcium channels and after receptor activation allows calcium flux to the interior of the cell through the plasma membrane. The formation of calcium channels is transitory and the intracellular calcium concentration is soon reestablished through calcium pumped to the outside of the cells. Calcium influx in activated mast cells occurs only after phospholipid methylation. Although the calcium influx or mobilization of the intracellular calcium is essential for the secretory process, the precise function of Ca^{2+} has not yet been established. It is possible that calcium acts through its association with calmodulin, a calcium-binding protein that has four high affinity Ca^{2+}-binding sites and suffers a large conformational change when it binds calcium. The allosteric activation of calmodulin by Ca^{2+} is similar to the allosteric activation of protein kinases by cAMP. Among the cellular enzymes regulated by calmodulin in a calcium-dependent way are adenylate cyclase, phosphodiesterases, membrand-bound ATPases, phosphorylekinase and the myosin light chain kinase of both muscle and non-muscle cells. The cellular activities regulated by cAMP and by calcium overlap

to a large extent and the intracellular concentrations of both molecules are often changed by some extracellular activating molecules. A Ca^{2+} and Mg^{2+}-dependent ATPase has been localized on the outer surface of rat peritonial mast cells as well as on the granule membrane. This membrane enzyme may act by hydrolysing ATP to provide energy for contraction of cytoskeletal elements that transports swollen membrane-bound granules to the plasma membrane for fusion and exocytosis.

In certain situations the influx of calcium is not a generalized phenomenon but is restricted to an activated site on the mast cell membrane. When sensitized mast cells are incubated in a physiological solution in which antigen is present, exocytosis occurs all over the cell membrane. However, if the stimulating antigen is attached to a solid bead so that it can interact only with a restricted region of the mast cell surface, exocytosis occurs only on the site where the cell actually contacts the bead. Thus, mast cells may not respond as a whole when they are activated. The activation of receptors, the resulting calcium influx and the subsequent exocytosis must all be localized in that particular region of the cell that has been activated.

Anaphylactoid Phenomena. In numerous situations artifically created in the laboratory, anaphylactic syndromes are observed similar to those classically obtained after introduction of antigen into a sensitized animal. These include Forssman shock and the shock induced by anaphylatoxin.

Forssman Shock. The Forssman antigen is a heterophilic antigen, i.e., it belongs to a group of antigenic substances of similar specificities, present in cells of widely different species. In 1911, Forssman observed that the immunization of rabbits with guinea pig kidney induced the production of antibodies that also reacted with sheep erythrocytes. This phenomenon is explained by the presence on sheep erythrocytes of antigenic determinants similar to those encountered on the cells of the guinea pig. Antibodies formed against the Forssman antigen are called Forssman antibodies. Forssman shock is obtained by injecting Forssman antibodies intravenously into the guinea pig, which produces a clinically acute symptomatology resembling anaphylactic shock. Postmortem examination, however, reveals lungs with minimal emphysema, but with severe edema and hemorrhage. The Forssman antigen occurs in the tissues of the guinea pig in particularly high concentrations on the endothelial cells of the blood vessels. Neither liberation of histamine nor alteration of the mastocytes occurs in this type of reaction. Forssman shock is the result of a typical cytotoxic reaction and as such requires complement.

Anaphylatoxin-Induced Shock. In 1910, Friedberger demonstrated that serum or plasma of the guinea pig incubated with antigen–antibody complexes in vitro and then centrifuged and injected intravenously into guinea pigs produced a shock closely resembling that of anaphylaxis. This indicated the formation of an anaphylatoxic substance by contact of the antigen–antibody complex with components of the serum. Friedberger named this substance anaphylatoxin. Many years later, it was verified that anaphylatoxin acted via the liberation of histamine and that, as in anaphylaxis, the histamine liberated by anaphylatoxin also originated from the mastocytes, which, upon contact with the anaphylatoxin, exhibited lesions identical to those produced by the antigen in the anaphylactic reactions. The liberation of histamine provided the explanation for the extreme similarity between the shock produced by anaphylatoxin and anaphylactic shock. Anaphylatoxin was also capable of contracting a isolated guinea pig ileum. Diverse substances such as agar, dextran, kaolin, and others, when incubated with serum or fresh plasma, also activate anaphylatoxin. An important observation made at an early date by Friedberger is that the heating of the serum or plasma to 56 °C destroys its capacity to form anaphylatoxin. Subsequently, it was shown that anaphylatoxin involves cleavage products of the complement system – specifically $C3a$, $C4a$, and $C5a$ (see Chap. 5).

Anaphylactic Phenomena in Man

Acute Anaphylaxis. Acute anaphylaxis in man is a rare though serious accident with possible fatal consequences. When serotherapy was at its zenith, acute anaphylaxis was usually produced by serum. Currently, it is produced more commonly by drugs, especially penicillin. The majority of drugs possess small molecules that require a covalent bond with tissue proteins in order to become capable of inducing an immunogenic response, as occurs, for example, with penicillin. Penicillic acid, which forms spontaneously in neutral penicillin solutions, is extremely active in the formation of a large number of derivatives with the amine and sulfhydryl groups from proteins. These derivatives behave as foreign substances, inducing the formation of antibodies directed against the haptenic penicillin group. Aside from penicillin, the most frequent causes of anaphylaxis in man are the bites of some insects (particularly bee stings), skin tests with antigens, and occasionally, heterologous serum. The symptoms appear some minutes after contact with the antigen; they consist of headache, precordial pain, sensation of heat, generalized pruritus, urticaria, apnea, hypothermia, and hypotension. Less frequently, the response is characterized by acute circulatory collapse. In fatal cases, autopsy reveals edema of the upper respiratory passage mucosae, particularly edema of the epiglottis, which could be the immediate cause of death.

Local Anaphylaxis. More frequently, anaphylaxis is evidenced by localized phenomena produced by contact of the antigen with specific organs or tissues. For example, anaphylaxis can be localized in the skin in the form of eczema or urticaria; in the respiratory apparatus, as with allergy to pollen or bronchial asthma; in the digestive tract with various functional perturbations due to the sensitization of the individual to certain foods, etc.

Atopy. Most people can be actively sensitized so as to exhibit typical anaphylactic symptoms when in contact with the antigen. However, there are certain individuals who are sensitized easily, even spontaneously, to a great number of environmental antigens, such as pollen, dust, dye, plants, and fungi. This facility in certain individuals to become allergic, termed atopy (Greek *uncommonness*), is familial and probably genetically controlled (see p. 270).

Tests for Detecting and Measuring IgE

Prausnitz-Küstner Test. In 1921, Prausnitz and Küstner described the test that today bears their names, commonly referred to as the PK test. This test, similar to the passive cutaneous anaphylaxis test, consists of injecting intradermally 0.1 ml of whole or diluted serum from an allergic individual into an unsensitized individual and, after about 24 h, injecting the antigen into the same site. A positive test produces local itching and formation of a papule surrounded by a zone of erythema. The reaction reaches a maximum within 10 min, persists for about 20 min, and gradually disappears. The antibody responsible for the Prausnitz-Küstner reaction was found at an early date to be thermolabile, losing its activity after heating to 56 °C for several hours; later, its sensitivity to reduction by sulfhydryl agents, such as

2-mercaptoethanol, followed by alkylation, was observed. The quantity of IgE present in the serum of an allergic patient is indicated by the highest dilution of serum still capable of producing a PK reaction. This test is now rarely used due to danger of transmission of viral hepatitis.

Liberation of Histamine. The addition of the specific allergen to a suspension of leukocytes obtained from an allergic patient liberates histamine which can be measured biologically or chemically. The quantity of histamine liberated is usually proportional to the degree of atopy exhibited by the patient and to the level of IgE in his serum.

Leukocyte Sensitization Test. Leukocytes obtained from nonallergic individuals are incubated with serum from an allergic patient and then washed and resuspended with the specific allergen. The quantity of histamine liberated is generally proportional to the quantity of IgE antibodies present in the serum.

Radioallergosorbent Test. This test, abbreviated RAST, is based on the absorption of IgE antibody by the insolubilized specific antigen and in the subsequent determination of the quantity of IgE antibody absorbed. In practice, the antigen is first combined by covalent linkage with particles of an insoluble substance (cellulose or activated Sepharose), and this combination is then added to the serum of the patient in a quantity that represents an antigen excess. After the particles are washed, the amount of absorbed IgE is determined with labeled anti-IgE antibody (Fig. 9.11).

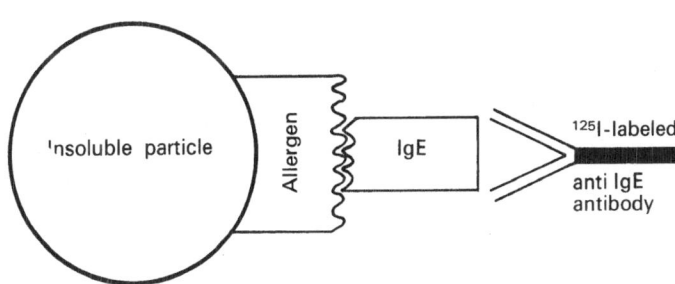

Fig. 9.11. Radioallergosorbent test

Radioimmunodiffusion. IgE also can be measured by the Mancini technique using specific anti-IgE antibody labeled with ^{125}I. The labeled anti-IgE antibody is suspended in agar in which, after solidification, wells are made into which is placed the serum of the subject whose IgE level is to be determined. Forty-eight hours later, the agar plate is washed, dried, and covered with a photographic film. After several days, the precipitation rings resulting from the reaction of IgE with the labeled anti-IgE, that have impressed the photographic emulsion, are then visible, and their diameters can be measured. With the help of a standard curve, one can determine the IgE concentration.

Biologic Activity of Human Reagin. Human reagin (IgE), aside from sensitizing homologous tissues, is also capable of sensitizing tissues of the higher primates. Experiments with rhesus monkeys have demonstrated that reactions similar to the PK reaction can be induced in the skin of this species with human sera obtained from atopic patients and that the sera lose this capacity after heating to 56 °C. It was also verified that segments of rhesus ileum could be passively sensitized with human reagin, producing Schultz-Dale reactions when placed in contact with the antigen. Neither cutaneous anaphylaxis (PK) nor the intestinal (Schultz-Dale) anaphylaxis could be reproduced with human antibodies of any other class of immunoglobulin. The anaphylactic phenomena produced in the tissues of the rhesus monkey with human reagin are accompanied by liberation of histamine. Skin sections from the rhesus monkeys sensitized with human IgE and treated with fluorescent antigen revealed selective fixation of human IgE in the mastocytes of these species. In addition, human reagin is capable of binding to homologous basophilic leukocytes and mastocytes. Morphologic alterations of the mastocytes were observed after incubation with lactic proteins of the mesentery of a patient sensitized to milk; furthermore, the passive sensitization of human lung by incubation *in vitro* with human reagin and subsequent contact with the specific antigen also resulted in morphologic alterations of the mastocytes, along with liberation of histamine and SRS.

In the passive cutaneous anaphylactic reactions of the guinea pig, homologous Ig and the Ig of certain other species blocked homologous sensitization by the IgG antibody. This blockage has been explained as being due to competition between the antibody and the nonspecific gamma globulin for the cellular receptors. It has been verified that nonspecific human IgE also blocks the binding of IgE antibody in the PK test (competitive inhibition at the cellular receptor level).

Effect of Heating and Alkylation-Reduction on the Cytotropic Activity of the IgE Antibody. One characteristic of the IgE antibody is that its cytotropic activity is destroyed by heating or by reduction and alkylation of the disulfide bridges. The capacity of the molecule to attach to the mastocyte and basophil membranes disappears when the antibody is heated to 56 °C, or when it is treated with a reducing agent (mercaptoethanol) and alkylated. Studies of the alteration of the circular dichroism spectrum of the IgE molecule and its fragments (Fab', Fc″, and Fc) indicate that only the two terminal domains of the molecule ($C_\varepsilon 3$ and $C_\varepsilon 4$) undergo irreversible alterations after heating to 56 °C. These results are in accordance with earlier observations indicating that, after heating, the IgE lost the skin-sensitizing property without loss of the ability to combine with the antigen. This same phenomenon occurred after reduction and alkylation of the molecule. The disulfide bridges responsible for the cytotropic properties are found between the Fd- and the hinge region of the heavy chains. Cleavage at this point considerably diminishes the cytoropic property of the molecule, but the capacity for fixation is totally lost only when one of the disulfide bonds between the ε chains of the N-terminal portion of the Fc fragments is cleaved.

Inverse Prausnitz-Küster Reaction. Since individuals not recognizable allergic possess IgE, it was expected that this type of immunoglobulin might be found under normal conditions in the target cells of normal organisms. Actually, an intradermal injection of specific antibody against IgE produces and inverse Prausnitz-Küstner ((PK) reaction. The minimum quantity of antibody capable of producing inverse PK is of the order of 10^{-5} µg N. The sensitivity of the skin to anti-IgE depends upon the quantity of IgE present in the skin. An allergic patients with an elevated concentration of IgE in the serum responds to 10^{-8} µg N of anti-IgE, whereas patients with a gammaglobulinemia cannot respond to 10^{-3} µg N of anti-IgE. Specific antibodies against IgG, IgA, IgM, and IgD do not produce any reaction when infected into the skin of the normal individual. $F(ab')_2$ fragments obtained from anti-IgE antibody also are capable of producing inverse PK, whereas the Fab fragment is not. These results suggest the necessity of bivalence for the induction of inverse PK and that the union of two molecules of IgE bound to the tissued is necessary to induce cellular damage (see Fig. 9.4). The fact that an inverse PK test also can be induced by the $F(ab')_2$ indicates that complement is not involved.

Mechanism of Immunotherapy in Atopic Diseases. If a sensitized guinea pig is injected repeatedly with small quantitities of antigen insufficient to cause death by anaphylaxis, the animal becomes desensitized; it loses, for as long as several days, reactivity to an antigen dose that in other conditions would be fatal. It is thought that the small, repeated doses of antigen exhaust the antibodies existing in the organism, thus impeding the shock that otherwise would be induced. The desensitization – or better, hyposensitization – is frequently used to render an atopic patient tolerant of a substance to which he is allergic (immunotherapy). In man, however, improvement of atopic symptoms induces by immunotherapy is attributed to the increase in IgE

class specific suppressor T cells and formation of blocking antibodies. These used to be detected and measured in the serum of allergic patients after prior heating of the serum to destroy the reaginic antibody. Different quantities of inactivated serum are mixed with constant quantities of antigen, and these mixtures are injected into previously sensitized skin locations on a healthy volunteer. The blocking antibody, if present, blocks the PK reaction, and the richer the serum of the patient is in blocking antibody, the less the quantity necessary to block the reaction. Atopic patients are commonly treated with injections of increasing doses of antigen, beginning with extremely small quantities, at proper intervals in order to avoid a possible systemic anaphylactic reaction. This treatment gives rise to the synthesis of blocking antibody. It is believed that these are nonanaphylactic antibodies which, although directed against the same antigen, do not possess the capacity of combining with the cells. However, the binding of the allergen via the blocking antibodies in the serum cannot always be correlated with improvement of the patient's symptoms.

IgE and IgG levels in sera from patients suffering from hay fever, in whom immunotherapy was being carried out, were examined. Immediately after the start of treatment, IgG and IgE levels rose noticeably, but the rise in IgG was much more pronounced. After long-term immunotherapy, the concentration of IgE antibodies decreased, wheras the IgG concentration continued to rise. Furthermore, there was no IgE secondary response in patients undergoing immunotherapy, which is normally observed in hay-fever sufferers during the hay-fever season. However, the increase in the concentration of IgG antibodies following immunotherapy cannot be entirely responsible for the repression of the IgE secondary response following immunotherapy.

Experiments in mice indicate that decreased IgE synthesis after repeated administration of antigen is dependent upon repression of the T-cell helper function, probably through the appearance of T suppressor cells. The positive effect of immunotherapy on increased production of blocking antibodies, has also been attributed to suppressor T cells. Thus, it seems that the beneficial effect of classical immunotherapy is both due to the formation of blocking antibodies as well as to the appearance of suppressor T lymphocytes specific for IgE antibodies. Immunotherapy has also been tried by the use of chemically modified antigens. Thus, weekly injections of a chemically modified antigen, E, which has lost the major antigenic determinants for B lymphocyte stimulation but has maintained the immunogenic determinants for T lymphocytes, depressed an ongoing IgE antibody response to native antigen E, and suppressed the secondary IgE response. These findings agree with the fact that this treatment diminishes the T lymphocyte helper function and suppresses the development of IgE-B lymphocytes specific for native antigen E. It seems reasonable to assume that the decline of IgE antibody synthesis and the depressed helper function by this treatment is probably due to generation of suppressor T cells. Since the differentiation of IgE-B lymphocytes to IgE plasmocytes is highly dependent on the T lymphocytes, it is possible to suppress IgE antibody formation either by reducing helper T cell activity or by inducing antigen-specific suppressor T cells. It is practicable to obtain this due to the fact that the immunogenic determinants recognized by T cells are not necessrily the same as the major antigenic determinants recognized by IgE-B lymphocytes. For instance, urea-denatured ovalbumin or ragween antigen E do not react with B lymphocytes specific for the major antigenic determinants and yet the same denatured antigens are able to stimulate T lymphocytes specific for the native antigens. Indeed, the injection of a large dose of the urea-denatured antigen without adjuvant can induce antigen-specific suppressor T lymphocytes that depress the IgE production. The same mechanism is responsible for diminution in IgE production induced by ovalbumin conjugated with polyethylene glycol. The OA-polyethylene glycol conjugate does not react with antibodies to the native OA but when injected without adjuvant can induce suppressor T cells specific for the native antigen. In both these situations the suppression is not confined to IgE class as there occurs also some suppression of IgG antibodies. On the other hand, multiple injections of OA-polyethylene glycol into sensitized animals enhance IgG level although decreasing IgE synthesis.

Some success in inducing specific suppression of the IgE class have been obtained by conjugating antigen to nonimmunogenic synthetic polymers. For instance, conjugates of ovalbumin or antigen E with a copolymer of D-glutamic acid and D-lysine (D-GL) when injected in mice under appropriate conditions induce a specific suppression of IgE antibody class with no change in IgG class. The suppressor mechanism in this situation is unknown since there seems to be no induction of suppressor T cells or B cells tolerance. An interesting approach to suppress IgE antibody production is the use of anti-idiotype antibodies. Blaser, Nakagawa and de Weck (1980) have reported that anti-idiotype antibodies are able to suppress the primary Ige antibody response as well as an ongoing IgE antibody formation to benzyl penicilloyl group. It is interesting to note that in these experiments the anti-idiotype antibodies suppressed the IgE production more efficiently than the IgG response. Some clinical findings have indicated that IgE production in humans is also under T cell control. Thus, in several clinical conditions in which there is impairment of cellular immunity, the patients have high IgE levels and atopic symptoms (such as in thymic alymphophasia and Wiscott-Aldrich syndrome). Katz has recently proposed an interesting concept of "allergic breakthrough." According to this concept the IgE antibody is maintained at low level in normal individuals by damping mechanisms specific to the IgE class. In experimental animals several treatments such as adequate dose of X-irradiation and cyclophosphamide can suppress temporarily the normal regulatory activity of T lymphocytes allowing an increased activity of the T-IgE helper cells. Contact of the organism with the allergen during the allergic breakthrough allows atopic sensitization. It has been demonstrated that once sensitization has occurred during the breakthrough the production of IgE specific for the sensitizing allergen remains elevated even after the damping activity has returned to normal. Control of the serum IgE level seems to be exerted through the activity of two soluble substances, with opposing activities, one enhancing and the other suppressing the IgE production. These factors would exist normally in serum, the ability to detect one vs the other requiring certain special manipulations. It is hoped that these findings on the mechanism of IgE antibody control will allow a better and more rational approach of the immunotherapy of atopic diseases.

Control of Anaphylactic Reactions. Anaphylactic phenomena can be blocked or attenuated by drugs that generally act by antagonizing the pharmacologic action of mediators or by impeding their formation and liberation. For example, antihistamines act by inhibition through competition, i.e., by blocking the pharmacologic action of the histamine at the receptor level. Numerous compounds with antihistaminic activity have been used in the treatment of allergies. Although these compounds may be effective in certain anaphylactic syndromes such as urticaria, they are relatively inefficient in other cases such as bronchial asthmapossibly because other mediators are implicated in these situations. In cutaneous anaphylaxis of the rat and mouse, it has been observed that the simultaneous application of an antihistamine and an antagonist of serotonin has a cumulative effect, with the use of the two drugs abolishing the reaction to-

tally, whereas the use of either drug singly produces only partial eradication of the reaction. In addition to inhibiting the action of histamine, the antihistamines, depending upon their concentration, not only can impede the anaphylactic liberation of histamine but, when used in excess, can actually produce the liberation of histamine. Diethylcarbazamine citrate (Hetrazan), a drug used as an anthelmintic agent, has a beneficial effect when used in asthmatic patients. Experiments with rat and monkey tissues have shown that this substance impeded the formation of SRS and histamine induced by the antigen-antibody reaction in anaphylaxis. Another substance, used clinically in asthma therapy, is sodium chromoglycate. This compound inhibits the anaphylactic liberation of histamine. Both of these drugs act subsequent to the antigen-antibody interaction. The inhibitory effect of chromoglycate appears to vary according to the type of antibody involved in the reaction and the tissue type or animal species used in the test. For example, PCA reactions induced by IgE in the rat are completely eradicated by chromoglycate, wheras the same reactions induced by the same type of antibody in the mouse are not affected by this compound.

Cromolycate apparently stabilizes mast cell membrane and thus prevents release of mediators.

The principal symptoms of anaphylaxis are due to vasodilation and to contraction of smooth muscle. Thus, compounds with pharmacologic activity contrary to these effects are used in the prevention of experimental and asthmatic anaphylaxis. Beta-adrenergic substances such as epinephrine and isoprenaline, which possess a strong bronchodilator effect, are beneficial in the treatment of anaphylaxis, particularly in guinea-pig anaphylaxis and human respiratory asthma, in which death is due to a respiratory deficit. In addition, the β-adrenergic compounds possibly owe their efficiency to their capacity to inhibit the liberation or formation of mediators through modulation of the level of 3′,5′-cyclic adenosine monophosphate (cAMP). The cAMP molecule is formed intracellularly from ATP by the action of an enzyme, adenyl cyclase encountered in the cellular membrane. Under normal conditions, the transformation of ATP into cAMP proceeds slowly. However, when a hormone is liberated into the blood, the hormone, acting as a primary messenger, binds to specific receptors on the cellular membrane and in this fashion augments the activity of adenyl cyclase, consequently accelerating the transformation of ATP into cAMP. This compound then acts as a second messenger, activating processes of synthesis and cellular secretion. For example, in hepatocytes, the augmentation of the reaction ATP → cAMP results in the conversion of glycogen into glycose. In the cells of the adrenal medulla, it results in the synthesis and secretion of the steroid hormones.

In various other conditions, however, an increase in the concentration of cAMP results in inhibition of the secretory mechanism. This appears to occur via the liberation of mediators of anaphylaxis. Normally, the level of cAMP depends on an equilibrium between the activity of the α- and β-receptors of the mastocytes (or basophils). Thus, stimulation of the β-receptors results in an increase of cAMP and in a consequent diminution of the enzymatic system responsible for the liberation of the mediators. Stimulation of the α-receptors produces a decrease of cAMP and an increase in activity of the enzymatic system. Thus, production and liberation of the mediators can be controlled with substances that stimulate or block the α- and β-receptors. Epinephrine and isoprenaline, which stimulate the β-receptors, cause an increase in cAMP levels and a decrease in the liberation of the mediators, whereas norepinephrine, which stimulates the α-receptors, has the opposite effect. Substances such as methyl-xanthines, which inhibit the action of phosphodiesterase (an enzyme that normally transforms $3',5'$-AMP into $5'$-AMP), also diminish the liberation of the mediators by causing an increase in cAMP. Some of the prostaglandins are capable of increasing the intracellular level of

cAMP and thus function as inhibitors of histamine liberation.

It has been shown that acetylcholine and carbamylcholine, in extremely small concentrations, enhance the anaphylactic liberation of mediators, independent of the $3',5'$-AMP cell level. There is evidence that the cholinergic receptor in the cell membrane is guanyl cyclase, which is activated through cholinergic substances and which transforms guanosyltriphosphate (GTP) into $3',5'$-guanosylmonophosphate ($3',5'$-GMP). In mast cells and basophils, intracellular increase of $3',5'$-GMP levels leads to an increase in the liberation of mediators. This liberation can be specifically inhibited with atropine. $3',5'$-GMP is transformed into its inactive form, $5'$-GMP, through a phosphodiesterase. Phosphodiesterase can be competitively inhibited by methyl-xanthine. Methyl-xanthines are much more effective on adenylphosphodiesterases than on guanyldiphosphodiesterases, which probably explains the previously discussed influence of methyl-xanthine on the $3',5'$-AMP system. The liberation of mediators from mast cells and basophils is apparently dependent upon equilibrium of the intracellular concentration of $3',5'$-AMP and $3',5'$-GMP.

The inhibition of mediator's secretion by compounds that increase the intracellular cAMP content seem contradictory to the required initial increase in cAMP for cell secretion. There seems to be no precise explanation for this but it has been suggested that:

a) cAMP pool may be different in each situation;

b) elevation of cAMP preceding immunological activation of the cell is inhibitory;

c) elevation of cAMP far above that induced by IgE-Fc receptor aggregation such as that induced by phosphodiesterase inhibitors have a negative effect on mediator's secretion;

d) cAMP-dependent protein kinases may exert selective biological effects as a function of their differential activation, regulation or concentration. Apparent opposite effects have been attributed to an activation of cAMP-dependent protein kinases type I and type II in cell proliferation. For instance, in lymphocytes, proliferation induced by ConA is accompanied by an activation of type I isoenzyme, whereas dibutyryl cAMP, which is inhibitory, activates simultaneously type I and type II isoenzyme, suggesting a negative effect of lymphocyte proliferation by either activation of both enzyme types or type II isoenzyme alone.

Microtubules are organelles that play a role in the cellular secretion mechanism. Apparently, they are important in the mechanism of mediator liberation. Study of the function of the microtubules has been facilitated by the use of drugs that specifically alter these structures. Colchicine, which binds to the subunits of the microtubules, producing dissociation and disappearance of these structures, inhibits the degranulation of the mastocytes and the anaphylactic liberation of the histamines from these cells and basophils. On the other hand, deuterium oxide induces the aggregation of the microtubule subunits, and in this way en-

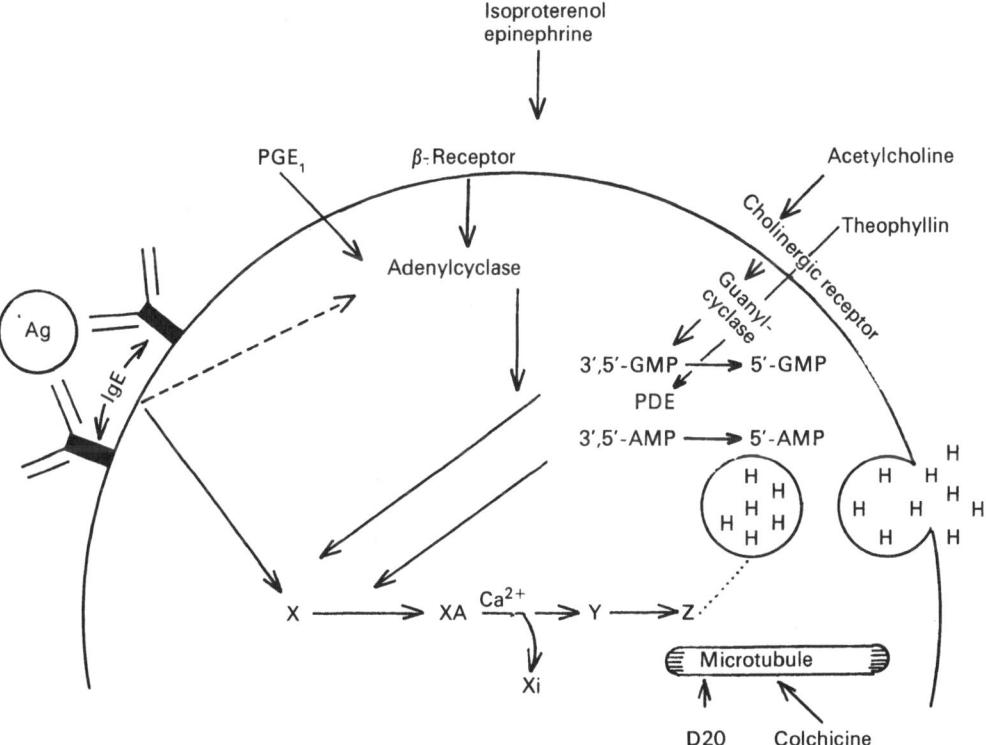

Fig. 9.12. Schematic representation of liberation of mediator (H), and the effect of different medications on the progression of this reaction. The anaphylactic reaction activates an enzyme system $(X \to XA \to Y \to Z)$ on the mast cell membrane that is responsible for the liberation of the mediator and whose activity appears to be controlled through the opposing effects of $3',5'$-AMP and $3',5'$-GMP (Yin-Yang hypothesis of biologic control). An increase in $3',5'$-AMP inhibits liberation of mediator, whereas a decrease in $3',5'$-AMP enhances liberation. Intracellular levels of $3',5'$-AMP can be increased through β-adrenergic substances like epinephrine and isoprenaline, (PGE$_1$), which activate adenylcyclases, or through methyl-xanthines (theophylline), which inhibit phosphodiesterase activity. Decrease in the $3',5'$-AMP level through α-adrenergic substances or through an increase of $3',5'$-GMP through cholinergic stimulation, enhances mediator liberation. Colchicine, which causes dissociation of microtubles, inhibits mediator liberation, whereas heavy water (D$_{20}$), which causes aggregation of microtubules, increases mediator liberation

hances the liberation of histamine. Figure 9.12 schematically summarizes the regulatory mechanisms of anaphylaxis.

Control of IgE Production. The induction of IgE antibody production depends primarily upon the manner in which the antigen is presented to the organism (dose, route of administration, adjuvant) and upon the genetic constitution of the individual. Since these conditions differ substantially from those that lead to the production of IgG and IgM antibodies, it is believed that the IgE antibody has a specific mechanism controlling its production at the cellular level.

When mouse inbred strains were immunized with different antigens, all produced IgE antibodies to one or more antigens but only some strains showed high or low IgE antibody response (Levine, 1974). Crossing between these strains showed that the genetic control for high or low IgE production was not linked to the MHC. Later studies have shown that some IgE non-responder mice (SJL and AKR) can be converted to high IgE producers through elimination of IgE T suppressor lymphocytes by X-irradiation or low dose cyclophosphamide. These findings showed that low IgE antibody production in these strains was not based on a genetic incapability to develop an IgE response but rather due to a genetic capability to suppress IgE production. These findings suggested that high IgE producers in mice and humans can result from a genetically controlled insufficiency of IgE T suppressor lymphocytes. Ir genes seem to be also implied in the control of IgE production. Levine and Vaz (1974) studied the responsiveness of mice to minute and repeated doses of antigen and observed striking differences in IgE production between different inbred strains. This difference in responsiveness was found to be correlated with the MHC of the strain. It must be pointed out that these differences in IgE response were not restricted to IgE production but were extended to the immune responsiveness in general to the studied antigen. Several studies have suggested that

a similar control of IgE production by *Ir* genes exists in man. According to various studies of serum IgE concentrations in unselected populations of adults, the distribution of values appears to be multimodal. This is probably due to a combination of genetic and environmental influences. Twin studies showed clearly the existence of a strong genetic determinant of basal total serum IgE level. Three different population studies suggested that the level of Ige in humans is controlled by two alleles at a single locus. Apparently high levels fo IgE are inherited as a recessive trait. Levine (1974) studied 7 families with a high incidence of hay fever to ragweed and observed that the occurrence of hay fever was highly correlated with a particular HLA haplotype in successive generations of allergic families. However, the associated haplotype varied from family to family and was different for each one of the families studied. Since some family members with the associated haplotype failed to manifest hay fever symptoms whereas none of the individuals lacking the haplotype had hay fever, it was concluded that the presence of a particular HLA haplotype within a family is necessary but not sufficient for a strong IgE response to ragweed. Other studies, however, did not confirm an HLA haplotype association for ragweed hay fever. Presently, the evidence for *Ir* genes controlling IgE production in man is still controversial. Furthermore, it is probable that many other genetic factors influence the expression of IgE-mediated allergic diseases.

Studies of IgE production under experimental conditions have shown that collaboration between T and B lymphocytes is essential for the production of IgE antibody. In addition, certain peculiarities of the IgE response may be explained by assuming the existence of IgE isotype specific helper and suppressor T cells. Several experiments in recent years have shown that there is dissociation between IgE and IgG production and that the IgE production is under a fine control by antigen specific and nonspecific T lymphocyte factors. For instance, low doses of X rays or pretreatment of mice with cyclophosphamide before immunization enhances IgE synthesis. On both these experimental conditions, the enhancement of IgE antibody is due to depletion of antigen non-specific suppressor T lymphocytes which selectively control IgE production. Some mouse strains (SJL) have a high number of T suppressor lymphocytes which depress IgE production without interfering with IgG production. Some treatments like the use of complete Freund's adjuvant increases the population of IgE T suppressor lymphocytes in mice. It was possible to demonstrate that serum from these animals contained a soluble factor that selectively suppressed IgE production. Other experimental conditions resulted in the production of antigenspecific suppressor T lymphocytes. Kishimoto and coworkers (1976) have shown that immunization of mice with DNP-coupled *Mycobacterium tuberculosis* induced the production of DNP-specific T suppressor lymphocytes which selectively regulate IgE production to DNP conjugated to a heterologous carrier such as DNP-ovalbumin. There are also examples of IgE regulation in which occurs a considerable enhancement of IgE without increase in IgG antibodies. For instance, rats immunized and subsequently infected with *Nippostrongylus brasiliensis* present high IgE antibody production to the immunizing antigen with no change in IgG antibody level.

In vitro experiments of Ishizaka's group have shown that T lymphocytes from *Nippostrongylus brasiliensis* infected rats produce two factors with affinity for IgE but differing in their biological activities, one having the ability to potentiate and the other to suppress IgE production. Both these factors have affinity for IgE, and both are produced by T lymphocytes and have similar molecular weight (10,000–20,000). The main difference between them is the presence of a carbohydrate moiety, the IgE potentiating factor having affinity for lentil lectin and ConA whereas the IgE suppressive factor does not. When T lymphocytes

are induced to synthesize IgE-binding factor in presence of tunicamycin, which inhibits protein glycosylation, this antibiotic does not suppress the synthesis of the IgE-binding factors but favors the synthesis of the IgE suppressive factor. Indeed, tunicamycin switches the synthesis of IgE potentiating factor to the synthesis of IgE suppressive factor. This same switching can also be induced by pretreatment of T lymphocytes with glucocorticoids, which thus favors the synthesis of IgE suppressive factor. Since glucocorticoids induce the synthesis of lipomodulin, a protein that inhibits phospholipase A_2, experiments were done in which T lymphocytes were induced to produce IgE-binding factors in presence of melittin or monoclonal antibody to lipomodulin, both of which activate cell surface phospholipase A_2. Under these conditions the factors formed had affinity for lentil lectin and potentiated the Ige response, suggesting that the same cells are able to form both IgE suppressive factor and IgE potentiating factor and the nature of the factor synthesized by the cells is decided by their evironment.

Mota observed many years ago that injection of *Bordetella pertussis* vaccine in rats induces preferentially the production of IgE antibody whereas complete Freund's adjuvant favored the production of IgG antibody. This observation was explained by recent findings of the Ishisaka group who showed that lymphocytes from rats treated with complete Freund's adjuvant produce the IgE suppressive factor whereas lymphocytes taken from *B.pertussis*-treated rats produce IgE-potentiating factor. Subsequent experiments on the mechanism of the preferential synthesis of the IgE suppressive or potentiating factors by these adjuvants revealed the cellular basis of this phenomenon. Studies on the cellular mechanism showed that both adjuvants induce macrophages to produce an interferonlike substance that can stimulate normal T lymphocytes to synthesize IgE-binding factors. However, Freund's adjuvant, in addition, stimulates suppressor T lymphocytes to produce a factor that prevents glycosylation of the IgE binding factor, inducing the formation of IgE suppressive factor. Conversely, *B. pertussis* stimulates T lymphocytes to produce a soluble factor that enhances glycosylation of the IgE-binding factor, favoring the production of IgE potentiating factor. Thus, the difference between Freund's adjuvant and B. pertussis is that different populations of T lymphocytes are stimulated to form either a glycosylation-inhibiting factor or a glycosylation-enhancing factor and these T cell factors determine the nature of the IgE-binding factor synthesized.

Katz and his group has also reported the presence of two different factors in serum of mice immunized with complete Freund's adjuvant, one of which, the enhancing factor of allergy (EFA) potentiates the IgE response whereas the other, the suppressive factor of allergy (SFA) inhibits the same response. Both factors are antigen non-specific and do not bind to IgE. The enhancing factor of allergy has high affinity for ConA which contrasts with the poor affinity for the same substance of the SFA.

Several groups have reported the presence of IgE-specific receptors (FcRε) on lymphocytes of rats, mice, and men. The role of these receptors in the regulation of IgE synthesis has been revealed with the discovery by Yodoi et al. in rats and by Chen et al. in mice, that when lymphocytes are exposed to high concentrations of IgE *in vitro* there occurs an increase in the number of FcRε in their membranes. This IgE induced FcRε expression is inhibited by both SFA and EFA. *In vivo* experiments suggest a physiological regulatory role for FcRε lymphocytes: when mice are neonatally exposed to IgE they fail to produce IgE when subsequently sensitized in adulthood and their lymphocytes are incapable of responding to IgE by expressing FcRε. Experiments *in vitro* have shown that exposure to IgE induces lymphocytes to express FcRε as well as to secrete soluble factors that modulate the expression of FcRε by other lymphocytes. These factors are designated IgE-induced regulants. According to Katz, B lymphocytes expressing FcRε initiate a cascade of cellular and molecular interactions which finally control FcRε expression and IgE synthesis. In summary, IgE would induce B lymphocytes to produce a soluble factor which in turn would induce B lymphocytes to express FcRε. These FcRε$^+$ lymphocytes would then interact either with Lyt-1$^+$ T lymphocytes to stimulate the production of SFA or with Lyt-2$^+$ to stimulate the production of EFA. In the first situation, SFA once produced would trigger Lyt-1$^+$ T lymphocytes to synthesize and secrete the final suppressive effector molecule which has the ability to inhibit the expression of FcRε by B lymphocytes (induced by exposure to IgE) or to suppress IgE antibody synthesis. In the second situation, FcRε$^+$ B lymphocytes would stimulate Lyt-2$^+$ T lymphocytes to secrete a soluble factor which would then act on other Lyt-2$^+$ T lymphocytes inducing them to express FcRε. During this process T lymphocytes produce the EFA (the precise subpopulation of T lymphocytes responsible for the EFA production is not yet known). One produced the EFA would stimulate FcRε$^+$ Lyt-2$^+$ T lymphocytes to secrete the final enhancing molecules which inhibits the expression of FcRε induced by IgE on B lymphocytes and is responsible for the marked enhancement of IgE synthesis both *in vivo* not *in vitro*.

Thus, both SFA and EFA inhibits FcRε expression by B lymphocytes but require T lymphocytes to exert their effects. SFA requires Lyt-1$^+$ T lymphocytes which produces the final suppressive effector molecule whereas EFA requires Lyt-2$^+$ T lymphocytes which produces the final enhancing effector molecules. These effector molecules would then act directly on B lymphocytes. In contrast with SFA and EFA which lack IgE-binding properties, both the final enhancing effector molecule and the final suppressive effector molecule are IgE-binding factors and may be identical ot IgE-binding factors described by the Ishizaka group.

A human T lymphocyte hybridoma has recently been obtained which produces large quantities of SFA that inhibits FcRε induction *in vitro* and IgE synthesis in vivo in the mouse model. Katz et al. has isolated messenger RNA from this hybridoma and in frog oocytes successfully translated SFA from this RNA which display comparable activity in both systems. The translation product of mRNA extracted from this hybridoma cell line shows identical biological activities as conventional human SFA. The fact that IgE-selective suppressor molecules can be obtained from human cells and human hybridomas give rise to hopes of a new therapy for IgE-induced allergic diseases.

Control of Anaphylactic Reactions in the Atopic Individual. The intensity of the anaphylactic reaction in the atopic individual depends, in addition to the nature and quantity of the antibody involved, upon other factors such as reactivity of the target cell, response of the anatomic structures sensitive to the mediators, and control of the autonomic nervous system. The reactivity of the target cells, such as mastocytes and basophils, appears to depend upon an equilibrium between the adrenergic α- and β-receptors that control the activities of the enzymes responsible for the formation and liberation of the mediators.

The intensity of the smooth-muscle response (as well as that of other structures) to the mediators also depends upon the equilibrium between their adrenergic α- and β-receptors. Stimulation of the α-receptors causes a diminution of 3′,5′-cyclic AMP, which enhances the contraction of the smooth muscle of the respiratory apparatus. Stimulation of the β-receptors produces an increase of cAMP that results in the opposite effect, i.e., relaxation of the smooth muscle and consequently bronchodilation.

In this way, β-adrenergic substances such as epinephrine and isoprenaline increase intracellular levels of cAMP through activation of β-adrenergic receptors, thereby inhibiting liberation of mediator and smooth-muscle contraction. For this reason, they have a favorable effect on bronchial asthma. Methyl-xanthines such as theophyllin exert a synergistically favorable effect when used together with epinephrine because they inhibit phosphodiesterases, thereby causing an increase in cAMP. Norepinephrine has the opposite effect because it causes a reduction in cAMP concentration by the activation of α-adrenergic receptors, which results in increased liberation of mediator and contraction of smooth musculature. Furthermore, equilibrium between the cAMP and 3′-5′-GMP systems, helps maintain homeostatic control of cell activity. This stimulation with acetylcholine causes an increase in 3′,5′-GMP, which leads to increased liberation of mediator as well as to intensified contraction of smooth musculature. The effect of cholinergic stimulation is blocked by atropine.

Atopic individuals exhibit excessive irritability of the smooth muscle of the bronchial tree and of other sectors of the organism due to blockage of the response of the β_α-adrenergic receptors. It is thought that atopic individuals lack the normal equilibrium between the α- and β-adrenergic receptors, which might also account for the therapeutic efficiency of drugs such as catecholamines, theophylline, and the corticosteroids, which enhance the effect of epinephrine and the β-receptors. Although a β-adrenergic receptor defective function may partially explain atopic symptoms, the same may also be explained by hyperactivity of the cholinergic receptors.

Cytotoxic Reactions (Type II)

Cytotoxic reactions are those in which the antibody combines with an antigen present in the tissues – either in the cells or in extracellular structures. The antigen can be a natural constituent of the tissues or it can be artificially bound to the cell surface. Transfusion reactions due to blood incompatibility, in which there is lysis of erythrocytes by antibodies against the ABO and other systems, are a good example of the cytotoxic reaction in which the antigen is a natural constituent of the cells. On the other hand, the lysis of platelets in purpura, induced by Sedormid or other drugs, exemplifies a cytotoxic reaction in which the antigen is not a natural component of the tissues. This type of cytotoxic reaction is due to the fact that numerous drugs are capable of binding to the cell surface, inducing the formation of antibodies that lyse the cells. Nephrotoxic nephritis, which results from antibodies against antigens present in the basement membrane of the renal glomerulus, represents a cytotoxic reaction in which the antibody combines with an extracellular structure. In most of these reactions, for there to be lesions of the tissues, fixation and activation of the complement system (see Chap. 5) are necessary.

Reactions by Antigen-Antibody Complexes (Type III)

Another type of immediate hypersensitivity reaction associated with complement activation is that of *vasculitis* mediated by antigen-antibody complexes (Fig. 9.13). Such forms of vasculitis occur when elevated concentrations of antigen–antibody complexes are formed in vivo, fix to walls of the arterioles, and then activate the complement system, generating chemotactic factors for leukocytes. Local types of vasculitis can be of great severity, producing localized hemorrhages and necrosis when the antigen is injected locally into an organism possessing a large quantity of circulating antibodies (Arthus reaction). There are also generalized forms of vasculitis, frequently involving the glomeruli (glomerulonephritis) observed when an organism is subjected to a dose of antigen sufficiently great that antigens are still present in the circulation at the time when antibodies begin to form. Large quantities of antigen–antibody complexes are formed in the blood, exceeding the clearing capacity of the reticuloendothelial system and localizing in the arteriolar networks throughout the organism. This type of phenomenon is common in persons injected with animal sera for the prophylaxis or

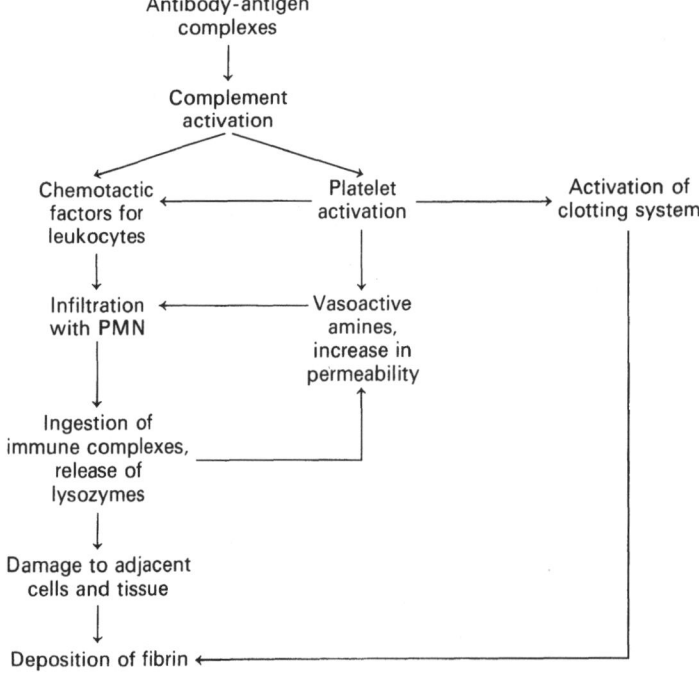

Fig. 9.13. Pathogenesis of inflammatory lesions due to immune complexes

Table 9.4. Diseases associated with immune complexes

Infections	
bacterial:	meningococcal (arthritis, vasculitis), gonorrheal, streptococcal (endocarditis, glomerulone-phritis), lepromatous leprosy, syphilis (glomerulonephritis) staphylococcal (shunt nephritis)
viral:	Dengue hemorrhagic fever, cytomegalovirus, hepatitis, infectious mononucleosis, subacute sclerosing panencephalitis, mumps, variola, varicella, adeno- and echovirus infections
parasitic:	malaria (nephropathy), trypanosomiasis, schistosomiasis (mesangia of glomeruli), toxo-plasmosis (glomerulonephritis) leishmaniasis, filariasis
Autoimmune diseases	rheumatoid arthritis (RF-IgG/M-IgG complexes), Felty's syndrom (RF-IgG-IgG complexes), systemic lupus erythematodes (antinuclear-anti-bodies and RF-IgM complexes), Sjögren syndrom (RF-IgM and other complexes), systemic sclerosis (RF and cryoglobulins), Hashimoto's thyroiditis
Other diseases	Crohn's disease (with extraintestinal manifestations), cystic fibrosis (secondary due to chronic and recurrent bacterial infections), sarcoidosis (in granulomas), multiple sclerosis (brain, kidney), myasthenia gravis, atopic diseases (IgE com-plexes), pemphigus (skin, autoantibody complexes), celiac disease, serum sickness, penicillamine nephropathy

treatment of infections (tetanus, diphtheria antisera) generating a syndrome called "serum sickness", but has also been recognized as a cause of many immunopathological effects in infectious, and autoimmune diseases (Table 9.4, and p. 391).

There are three general mechanism of antigen-antibody complexes: a) antibodies may react with structural antigens on the cell membrane or with other non-cellular tissue-structures. A structural non-cellular antigen against which antibodies are frequently formed is the basal membrane. Antibodies against the glomerular basal membrane usually produce glomerulonephritis; b) immune complexes may also result from interaction of antibodies with antigens introduced into the body or secreted by the body cells. The experimental example of this is the Arthus reaction that will be discussed later. Immunopathological ex-

amples are the deposition of immune complexes in thyroid follicles in autoimmune thyroiditis, around spermatogenic tubules after vasectomy and around parasites in tissues; c) antigen-antibody complexes may also result from the presence of soluble antigen in circulation such as it happens in serum sickness. Although most circulating Ag-Ab complexes are phagocytosed by polymorphonuclear leukocytes, monocytes, and macrophages, some may be retained in one or more of the vascular or filtering structures of the body and cause immune complexe diseases. Indeed, the rate of circulating Ag-Ab complexes depends in large part on the function of the body phagocytes. It has been observed in experimental serum sickness that over 99% of the immune complexes are eliminated by phagocytes and that the remaining 1% is responsible for the disease. Mantovani et al.

(1972) have shown the although attachment of immune complexes to macrophages is induced by C3b, ingestion requires in intact Fc of the IgG in the complex. It seems that immune complexes containing non-complement fixing antibody or antibody unable to interact with Fc receptors are more easily deposited in the tissues causing lesions.

The inflammatory activity of the antigen-antibody complexes depend on intrinsic and environmental factors. The nature of antibody and of antigen, for example, affect the immune complexe activity. In the case of antibody the most important properties are its isotype, valency, ability to fix to Fc receptor, to activate complement and its association constant with antigen. In regard to antigen, it is known that monovalent antigens produce small complexes (Ag1-Ab1 or Ag2-Ab1) that remain in circulation for long periods of time, without tissue deposition. On the other hand, multivalent antigens form complexes of varying composition depending on the molar ratio of the reactants.

The relationship Ag/Ab in the complexe is the most important factor that determines its biologic activity. In excess of multivalent antigen the resulting antigen-antibody complexes have their size inversely proportional to antigen excess.

In general, large complexes are more rapidly removed from circulation. Very small complexes formed in large excess of antigen usually do not activate complement and so are not efficient to cause inflammation. Immune complexes formed in large antibody excess are usually large and insoluble, being rapidly removed through phagocytosis. The most important immune complexes are those formed in slight antigen excess. These are of medium size and soluble, are not easily phagocytosed, are largely distributed in the body through circulation and, due to their ability to activate the complement system, are very pathogenic.

The intensity and persistency of the antigen contact with the body tissues are important in the establishment of the diseased induced by immune complexes. When the presence of Ag-Ab complexes lasts for a short time the induced lesions are transitory. However, when the contact with immune complexes is prolonged as it happens when there is a continuous supply of antigen, the lesions and symptoms of the disease tend to stay and to aggravate. This is a common situation in chronic infections and autoimmune diseases.

The mechanism of circulating Ag-Ab complexes deposition in tissues seems to depend in part on the release of vasoactive amines and the consequent increase of capillary permeability. In experimental serum sickness (see p. 285) seems to exist a leukocyte-dependent immune complexe deposition mechanism. Apparently, IgE sensitized basophils activated by antigen release vasoactive amines as well as PAF which increases the level of these mediators by releasing more vasoactive amines from platelets.

Immune complexes also induce an increase in capillary permeability through complement activation and formation of C3a, C4a, and C5a. These anaphylatoxins (see p. 128) acting on mastocytes and basophils release mediators that increase capillary permeability. In addition, C5a is also chemotactic for polymorphonuclear neutrophils. As a matter of fact, the inflammatory lesions induced by immune complexes depend to a large part upon the biological activities resulting from complement activation. These activities include also chemotaxis and immunoadherence. Chemotaxis is promoted by C5a and C5,6,7 and by anaphylatoxins that attract polymorphonuclears and activate mast cells to secrete more chemotactic factors. Lysosomal enzymes released from polymorphonuclear neutrophils are in great part responsible for tissue injury.

Complement seems to exert opposite effects on Ag-Ab solubility. Thus, activation of complement by the classical pathway and C1q fixation increase the precipitability of Ag-Ab complexes whereas precipitated immune complexes can be partially solubilized by complement factors. Nussenzweig et al.

(1975, 1976) have reported that Ag-Ab complexes solubilization is mediated by the properdin pathway since factor B, D, properdin, C 3, and Mg^{2+} must be present and apparently result from the association of C 3 b with the immune precipitates and formation of a C 3-convertase dependent on properdin and factor B. It has also been reported (Takahashi et al., 1978) that although the classical pathway does not solubilize the precipitated immune complexes, it greatly enhances the solubilizing activity of the alternative pathway.

Methods for Detection of Immune Complexes

The fact that numerous test have been described in the last past years to detect circulating immune complexes indicates that no single test is sufficient for all situations. Since the identity of the antigens is generally unknown particularly in the human, specific detection of the antigen is not possible – with some exceptions: nucleic acid antigen in systemic lupus erythematosus, drugs in drug sensitivity, and HB_sAg in some cases of polyarteritis nodosa.

Microcomplement Consumption Test. Presumptive evidence for the presence of immune complexes in sera is obtained by assessing the consumption of a standard amount of complement (C) added to heat-inactivated serum samples. Residual C activity is measured by the degree of lysis of IgM antibody-sensitized sheep red blood cells. Disadvantages of this test are that the serum samples have to be heat-inactivated, which may create immunoglobulin aggregates, and that not all human immunoglobulin classes activate complement (e.g. IgG_4), or they activate complement preferentially via the alternate pathway (IgE, IgA).

C1q Solid Phase Radioimmune Assay. C1q is adsorbed on plastic polystyrene tubes. The samples are incubated in the coated tube, then washed out. The amount of immune complexes bound to C1q is estimated by binding of radiolabeled or enzyme-linked anti-immunoglobulin antibodies or by binding of radiolabeled aggregated IgG onto free C1q. The sensitivity of the test is 1–10 µg Anti-Human-Gamma globulin (AHG) per ml.

Conglutinin Radioimmune Assay. Conglutinin is an unusual protein (mw 750,000) which occurs naturally in cattle serum (see p. 203). It has strong affinity for immune complex-fixed C3 fragment; it is not an immunoglobulin. Conglutinin produces strong agglutination of sheep red blood cells coated with IgM antibodies and C. The binding of conglutinin to immune complexes is complement and Ca^{2+} dependent and appears to be specific for the inactivated form C3bi of C3b. The assay is performed by placing serum samples in microtiter plates coated with conglutinin; the amount of bound IgG is then quantitated with a radiolabeled or enzyme-linked anti-IgG antibody. The sensitivity is in the order of 5–10 µg AHG per ml.

Platelet Aggregation Test. Platelets aggregate after their surface Fc-receptors interact with IgG-type immune complexes or aggregates. The test is sensitive (5–10 µg AHG per ml) but can give false positive results due to materials other than immune complexes (antiplatelet-antibodies, myxoviruses, enzymes).

Macrophage Inhibition Test. Immune complexes can be phagocytosed in vitro by macrophages. This is used in a *phagocytosis inhibition test*. Guinea pig peritoneal macrophages are incubated with the sample to be tested and with radiolabeled aggregated IgG. The presence of immune complexes in the sample is revealed by a decrease in the uptake of radioactivity by the cells compared to a control where incubation takes place with labeled aggregates alone.

Raji Cell Assay. B cells have surface receptors for C3 through which they can bind complement-fixing immune complexes. Cells of the cultured B-type lymphoblastoid cell line Raji possess high affinity C 3 receptors but lack surface immunoglobulins. Immune complexes bound to their surface can thus be estimated by secondary fixation of radiolabeled anti-Ig antibodies. The sensitivity of the test is 6–12 µg AHG per ml. Another cell line which is used in a similar way, is the cultured L 1210 murine leukemia cell, which binds immune complexes via Fc receptors with high affinity for the Fc portion of aggregated IgG.

Arthus Reaction

Shortly after the discovery of anaphylaxis, Arthus described another immunologic phenomenon dependent upon an antigen-antibody reaction; however, fundamental differences were noted between the mechanism of this reaction and that of anaphylactic reactions. Arthus observed that rabbits repeatedly inoculated intradermally with heterologous serum exhibited a local inflammatory reaction characterized by edema, erythema, hemorrhage, and in the more intense lesions, by necrosis.

The Arthus reaction can be elicited in practically any species with any antigen. It is distinguished from the anaphylactic reaction by many characteristics: (1) The anaphylactic reaction is rapid and transitory, whereas the Arthus reaction develops slowly, requiring hours to reach its maximum and hours or days to disappear. (2) Whereas in ana-

phylaxis the antibody involved is found fixed to the tissues and the reactions can proceed in the absence of circulating antibody, in the Arthus reaction binding of the antibody to the tissues is not necessary (hence absence of the latent period), and the reaction does not proceed in the absence of circulating antibody. (3) The type of antibody also is different in the two reactions in that the Arthus reaction requires precipitating antibody, whereas anaphylaxis does not. Furthermore, in the guinea pig, the IgG_1 antibody is highly efficient in producing anaphylaxis but inefficient in producing the Arthus reaction – with the contrary occurring with the IgG_2 antibody. This difference appears to relate to the fact that IgG_2 is capable of fixing complement whereas IgG_1 is not. IgG_1 induces an anaphylactic reaction effectively, but is hardly in a position to induce an Arthus reaction. There appears to be an interaction between IgG_1 and IgG_2 in the active Arthus reaction. (4) The Arthus reaction requires complement, which does not appear to be necessary in anaphylaxis (Fig. 9.14). (5) The Arthus reaction requires enormous quantities of antibody – about 10 mg when injected intravenously into rabbits and 0.1 mg when injected locally. In contrast, for a local anaphylactic reaction, fractions of micrograms (0.02 µg) are sufficient. (6) Polymorphonuclear leukocytes are necessary for the Arthus reaction. Depletion of circulating polymorphonuclear

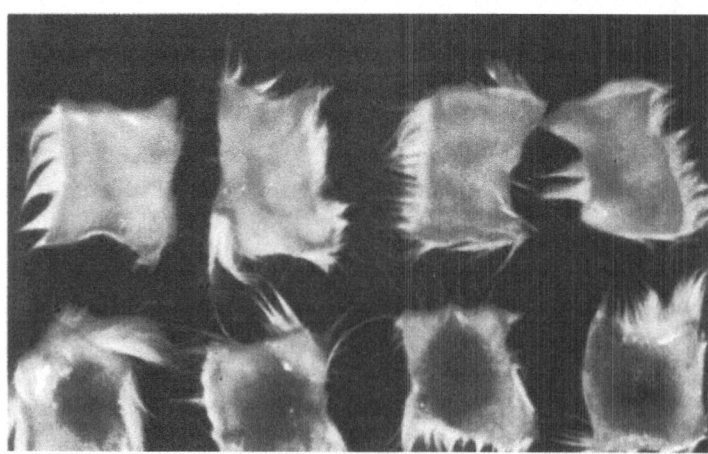

Fig. 9.14. Effect of decomplementation on the Arthus reaction. Lower row: decomplemented skin; upper row: control skin

cells reduces or suppresses the Arthus reaction but does not modify the anaphylactic reaction. (7) The Arthus reaction is characterized by formation and precipitation of antigen–antibody complexes in the affected vessels, which does not occur in anaphylaxis. (8) In anaphylaxis, the principal phenomenon is increase in capillary permeability; the Arthus reaction is much more complex, involving edema (generally intense), hemorrhage, cellular infiltration and, in more severe reactions, ischemia with necrosis and loss of tissue in the area affected. (9) The passive Arthus reaction does not require a period of sensitization as does the anaphylactic reaction.

Pathogenesis. Tissue modifications occurring in the Arthus reaction are the same as those occurring in the phenomenon of inflammation. Microscopic observations made with a transparent chamber adapted to the ear of an immunized rabbit have shown that the first modifications visible after contact with the antigen consist of constriction of arterioles, with decrease in blood flow, adherence of the polymorphs and platelets to the vessel walls, with formation of small clots, diapedesis of the leukocytes, and passage of plasma and erythrocytes to the interstitium . After several hours, edema and polymorphonuclear cell infiltration predominate. In more intense cases, there is ischemia due to thrombosis, producing necrosis of the affected tissues. Hemorrhage is a consequence of lesions of the blood vessels. It has been demonstrated by immunofluorescence that the first phenomenon to occur during the Arthus reaction is the deposition of antigen–antibody complexes. However, the formation of antigen–antibody complexes alone is not sufficient to produce the Arthus phenomenon. In fact, even given the formation of complexes, the reaction does not develop if the animal has previously been decomplemented (e.g., by injection of aggregated gamma globulin) or if it has been rendered leukopenic by the injection of antipolymorphonuclear serum. Thus the Arthus reaction depends upon the

following sequence of phenomena: (1) deposition of antigen–antibody complexes on the walls of the small vessels, between the endothelium and the basement membrane; (2) complement fixation; (3) having fixed complement, the complexes become chemotactic, provoking the migration of leukocytes to the site of the reaction; and (4) phagocytosis of the antigen–antibody complex and liberation of the lysosomal enzymes that aggravate the vasculitis, producing focal necrosis and other inflammatory alterations. The sequela just described is the principle pathogenic mechanism unterlying the development of autoimmune diseases (see p. 391).

Serum Sickness

From the beginning of this century until about 1940, various types of infections were treated with injection of relatively large volumes of heterologous antisera. After 1 or 2 weeks, patients subjected to this treatment generally exhibited a typical syndrome consisting of adenopathy, fever, erythematous or urticarial eruptions, and pain in the joints. This syndrome came to be known as serum sickness. Today, although serotherapy is not frequently used, the same syndrome may be produced by allergic reactions to penicillin or other drugs. The lesions generally disappear in a few days. In rare fatal cases, autopsy discloses vascular lesions resembling those observed in the Arthus reaction. The syndrome is easily reproduced experimentally, and its pathogenic mechanism is well known.

Cell Mediated Reactions

There is a group of immunological reactions mediated by T lymphocytes, collectively known under the designation cell-mediated reactions, which include delayed-type hypersensitivity reactions, allograft reactions, resistance to tumors and certain intracellular parasites, and the graft-VS-host reaction. All these reactions are mediated by two different populations of T lymphocytes. One population, the T_{DT} lymphocytes, is responsible for the delayed hypersensitivity reactions and when stimulated by antigen release lymphokines that attract and activate other cells particularly macrophages. These activated cells then act as non-antigen specific effectors of delayed hypersensitivity reactions. The second T lymphocyte population, represented by the cytotoxic T lymphocyte (Tc) is able to react with antigen located directly on the target cell membrane inducing its lysis. The two lymphocyte populations are probably more or less involved in all types of cell-mediated reactions.

Delayed Type Hypersensitivity, Type IV

Delayed hypersensitivity can be defined as slowly evolving (24–72 hs) mixed cellular reactions mediated particularly by lymphocytes and macrophages. These reactions are not induced by antibodies but by sensitized T lymphocytes and can be passively transferred in laboratory animals by these cells and not by serum.

Pathogenesis. In essence, serum sickness depends upon antigen–antibody interaction in the circulatory system, with formation of antigen–antibody complexes in the presence of antigen excess.
Experimental serum sickness is produced only with antigens capable of remaining in the circulation for long periods, such as the plasma proteins. These, when heterologous, are removed from the circulation by an elimination process that occurs in three successive stages. In an initial stage, 50% of the foreign protein disappears from the circulation within 24 h as a result of the passage of the protein to the extravascular spaces. The second step is represented by a constant decrease that follows an exponential curve; i.e., a constant aliquot is eliminated in a unit of time. This phase, which appears to represent the elimination of foreign protein by normal catabolic processes, lasts 6–7 days. This stage is followed by a third stage, sudden and accelerated, called the immune elimination phase. This phase results from the production of antibody against the foreign protein, giving rise to the formation of antigen–antibody complexes that are rapidly sequestered from the circulation by the activity of the reticuloendothelial system. The elimination curves of ^{131}I – labeled syngeneic and xenogeneic gamma globulins (bovine) injected in normal rabbits can be seen in Fig. 9.15. The complexes formed initially are small and originate in extreme antigen excess. These complexes of the Ag_2Ab type do not fix complement and can endure for a long time in the circulation. The size of the complexes or their antibody content increases proportionally to the increase in the quantity of antibodies produced. The complexes are of the $Ag_3–Ab_2$ type, fix complement efficiently, and are rapidly removed from the circulation. At this point, the exudative and inflammatory lesions of serum sickness are established in the tissues, particularly in the heart, arteries, joints, and kidneys. The glomerulonephritis is caused by the deposition of large quantities of anti-

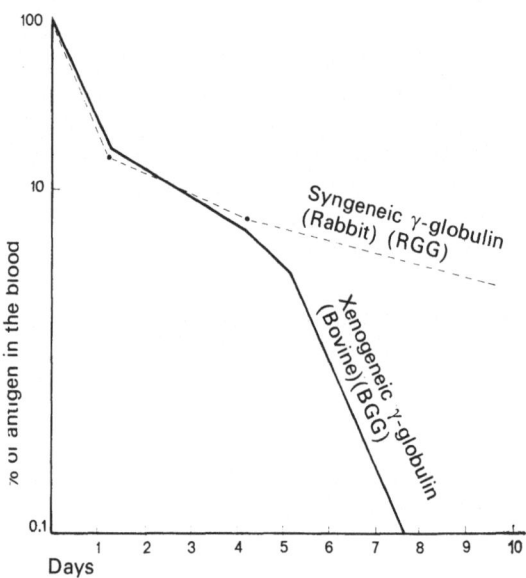

Fig. 9.15. Elimination curve of a xenogeneic protein (bovine gamma globulin) and a syngeneic (or allogeneic) protein (rabbit gamma globulin) in a normal rabbit injected with ^{131}I-labeled proteins

gen–antibody complexes on the epithelial side of the basement membrane. The events subsequent to deposition, include fixation of the complement components, production of chemotactic factors, attraction of leukocytes, liberation of proteolytic enzymes, and lesions of the endothelium, which cause the destruction of the glomerulus. A chronic form of glomerulonephritis can be produced experimentally by repeated injections of small quantities of antigen into an immunized animal or by injection of preformed antigen–antibody complexes. This type of mechanism occurs in glomerulonephritis associated with diseases such as diabetes mellitus (insulin-anti-insulin), thyroiditis (thyroglobulin-antithyroglobulin), and lupus erythematosus (DNA-anti-DNA) in which the individual produces antibodies against his own tissues. The lesions existing in these diseases are due primarily to the presence of complexes in the tissues (see Chap. 13). Such complexes are capable of activating C 1, giving rise to the production of fibrinolysin, anaphylatoxin, and vasoactive oligopeptides such as bradykinin. The role of these substances in the establishment of serum sickness lesions has not yet definitely been proved. After the complete elimination of the complexes, the lesions disappear rapidly and the recuperation of the tissues is as complete as possible. The dependency of the antigen–antibody complexes, the participation of complement, and the similarity of the histologic lesions raise the inference that serum sickness is a type of systemic Arthus reaction. In this case, the same dose of the substance injected would serve initially as immunogen and later as antigen. However, since the immune response is complex, homocytotropic antibodies are also formed and are possibly responsible for some lesions of the anaphylactic type, such as urticaria. Serum sickness is considered a mixed syndrome in which phenomena common to the Arthus reaction and the anaphylactic reaction coexist.

In clinic, a condition similar to Arthus reaction is produced by organic particles of diverse nature, that when repeatedly inhaled attain the lung tissue and induce the production of precipitating antibodies. These antibodies on reaction with the antigen in the lung tissue, causes a local hypersensitive reaction, similar to Arthus reaction, named extrinsic allergic alveolitis. This disease is characterized by fever, dispnea and cough a few hours after inhalation of the allergen. The sera of virtually all patients with clinically demonstrable allergic alveolitis have high serum levels of complement-fixing IgG antibodies. The prototype of this group of disease is the farmer's lung disorder.

Reaction to Tuberculin

The prototype of the delayed reaction is the reaction to tuberculin, exhibited by an individual sensitized to *Mycobacterium tuberculosis*. Koch observed that tuberculous guinea pigs inoculated with live tuberculosis bacilli responded with a local inflammatory reaction much more rapidly and intensely than did noninfected guinea pigs (Koch's phenomenon). Subsequently, it was verified that the same phenomenon could be reproduced by injection of tuberculin or of a filtrate of heated, concentrated *Mycobacterium tuberculosis* cultures. Currently, the proteins present in tuberculin are precipitated with ammonium sulfate and the product, known as PPD (purified protein derivative), is used in place of the tuberculin. When a sensitized individual is injected intradermally with tuberculin or PPD, no modification is observed at the site. After about 6–10 h, a small firm papule appears at the site, accompanied by erythema. This papule grows slowly, becoming considerably larger during the next 24–72 h, and then disappears slowly over several days. In the more intense reactions, hemorrhaging and necrosis can occur. A positive tuberculin test indicates that the individual has or has had a *Mycobacterium tuberculosis* infection.

In human beings the reaction can be obtained with extremely small quantities of PPD (of the order of 0.02 µg), whereas guinea pigs require larger quantities (0.5 µg) for an appreciable reaction. In rats and mice, the reactions are much weaker and sometimes require microscopic examination to identify the response. In man, the tuberculin reaction also can be provoked by percutaneous application, i.e., by direct application to the skin of pieces of filter paper (or other tissue) imbedded with tuberculin (patch test). The percutaneous reaction is not possible in the guinea pig, which does not possess sweat glands. It is positive in man only in the areas of the skin that contain sweat glands. The antigen may penetrate the skin through the ducts of these glands.

Systemic Reaction to Tuberculin

In sensitized persons or guinea pigs, the injection of relatively large quantities of tuberculin can provoke a generalized reaction, tuberculin shock. In the guinea pig, tuberculin shock is characterized by prostration and hypothermia, which appears within 2–3 h and can cause death. In extremely sensitive individuals, intradermal inoculation of tuberculin can produce, after a few hours, indisposition, headache, and prostration, and rarely death. If the individual is tuberculous, the inflammatory process in the pulmonary lesions or other locations can be exacerbated. Similar systemic reactions can be provoked with other antigens obtained from infectious agents in sensitized individuals. For this reason, it is advisable in performing the tuberculin test (Mantoux test) always to use only small quantities of tuberculin or PPD.

Delayed Reaction to Proteins

Delayed hypersensitivity reactions to simple proteins such as ovalbumin and serum albumin can be obtained using special sensitization methods. The method used initially was to inject the protein directly into the lesions of tuberculous guinea pigs. Currently, the more common method is the intradermal injection of small quantities of protein (of the order of micrograms) emulsified in complete Freund's adjuvant or of small quantities of antigen in the form of antigen–antibody complexes obtained in antibody excess.

Contact Sensitivity

Many natural substances and relatively simple chemical products are responsible for an allergic illness commonly encountered in patients – so-called contact dermatitis. The reaction typically is of the delayed type and, in this case, the sensitizing and unleashing doses are applied in the same fashion by contact with the skin. A great variety of substances can be responsible for the ailment; among the most common are certain plants, such as the primrose, cotton seed, citrus fruits, tomatoes; diverse drugs; and other commonly used chemical products (herbicides, insecticides, dyes, and cosmetics). These substances have two characteristics in common: They are nonimmunogenic, and they easily form conjugates with proteins. It is believed that such substances penetrate the epidermis and combine with the tissue proteins, which then become recognized as foreign. On many occasions an isolated contact with these substances is sufficient to establish contact sensitivity, whereas in other cases more frequent contact is necessary to obtain the same effect. About a week after the sensitizing dose, contact between any region of the skin and the antigen provokes, after 10–12 h, erythematous papules, which later transform into small blisters that burst, leaving erythematous areas without epidermis. Later still, there is extensive formation of crusts along with hyperkeratosis. In the guinea pig, the same reaction is observed, but without the formation of blisters. At the site of the reaction, the dermis is invaded by inflammatory mononuclear cells – especially around the blood vessels and the sweat glands. This cellular infiltrate is indistinguishable from those observed in other types of delayed reactions.

Many of the substances that cause contact dermatitis in man are also capable of producing contact hypersensitivity in the guinea pig. Of these, picryl chloride, dinitrofluorobenzene, and dinitrochlorobenzene are most often used. As with the delayed hypersensitivity reaction, contact hypersensitivity is more specific than the serologic reactions. For example, guinea pigs sensitized with 2,4,6-trinitrochlororbenzene (picryl chloride) react with this substance, yet they do not react with 2-4-dinitrochlorobenzene. In this case, the specificity conferred by the carrier protein is important, a phenomenon to be discussed more extensively later.

Transfer of Delayed Hypersensitivity

Numerous attempts at passive transfer of the delayed reactions by antisera have consistently failed. On the other hand, viable lymphoid cells obtained from sensitized guinea pigs conferred upon normal recipients the capacity to respond to the antigen with the typical delayed reaction, as indicated in Fig. 9.16. Transfer by cells is termed adoptive sensitivity. Adoptive sensitivity persists only while the transferred cells survive in the recipient. If the adoptive sensitivity occurs between genetically differ-

ent individuals, the sensitivity is of short duration (about a week), but if occuring in syngeneic animals it persists for a long time. Dead lymphoid cells or lymphoid cells with damaged mechanisms for protein synthesis do not produce adoptive sensitivity. It should not be forgotten that adoptive sensitivity also transfers immediate hypersensitivity that is dependent upon the transfer of antibody-forming cells or those involved in the production of antibodies.

Transfer Factor. Whereas in laboratory animals, adoptive sensitivity has been obtained only with viable lymphoid cells, Lawrence observed that the sensitivity of the tuberculin type in man can be transferred by means of extracts of leukocytes obtained from sensitized individuals. The retarded reaction appears in the recipients a few hours after the intradermal injection of the leukocytic extract, although it usually requires 2–3 days for maximum sensitivity. Sensitivity thus conferred persists for years and can be transferred in series, i.e., the cells

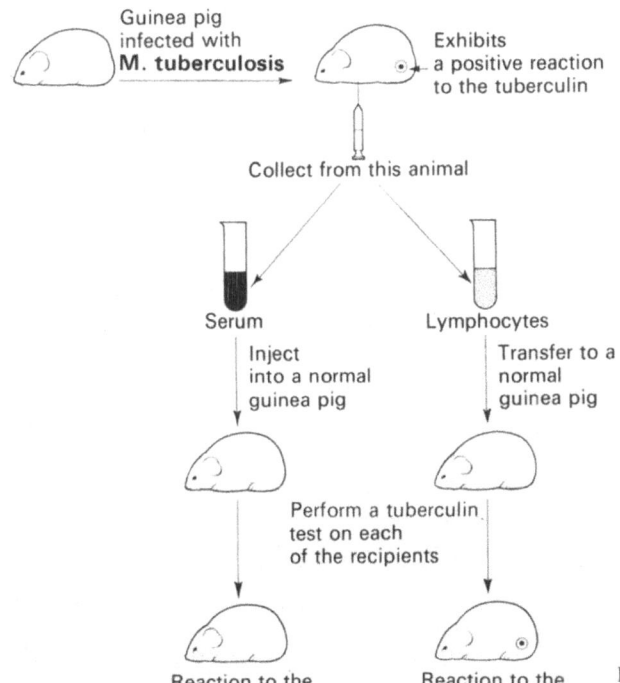

Fig. 9.16. Transfer of cellular or delayed hypersensitivity

of the first recipient are capable of transferring sensitivity to a second and from this to a third recipient, suggesting that the factor is capable of self-replication. The active component of these extracts is called the transfer factor; it can be liberated from lymphocytes incubated with the antigen. The material is stable, dialysable, and has an absorption spectrum in the nucleic acid zone, but is not inactivated by ribonuclease or by deoxyribonuclease. The nature and operative mechanism of transfer factor are unknown.

The Effector Cell
in Delayed Hypersensitivity

The fact that the capacity to transfer delayed hypersensitivity is limited to lymphoid cells, together with the observation that at the site of delayed reactions there exists an infiltration of cells morphologically similar to lymphocytes, suggested that the cells transferred were totally responsible for the cellular infiltration of delayed hypersensitivity. However, transfer experiments with sensitized cells labeled with tritiated thymidine showed that these cells constituted only 5%–10% of the cells present at the site of the reaction. Moreover, when the cells of the recipient were labeled beforehand with tritiated thymidine, 80%–95% of the cells present in the infiltrate were labeled cells. Thus, it became clear that the transferred cells modified the behavior of the cells of the recipient, conditioning them to migrate to the locality of the reaction. Experiments with animals whose lymphoid and myeloid tissues had been destroyed by irradiation demonstrated that the local inflammatory reaction site in delayed hypersensitivity was comprised almost exclusively of macrophages originating from the bone marrow. In these experiments irradiated animals, incapable of exhibiting a delayed reaction to tuberculin, were divided into four groups, inoculated respectively as follows: (1) bone marrow cells of sensitized donors; (2) bone marrow cells of nonsensitized donors; (3) lymph node cells of sensitized donors; and (4) bone marrow cells of nonsensitized donors plus lymph node cells of sensitized donors. The results of these experiments are illustrated in Fig. 9.17. The animals of group (1) developed delayed reactions similar to those found in the nonirradiated control group. At the reaction site there was intense infiltration by mononuclear cells, many of which appeared to be lymphocytes. Delayed reactions with cellular infiltration identical to these were obtained in the animals of group (4), but not in the animals of groups (2) and (3), which did not react to the tuberculin tests. These results demonstrated that the cells of the lymph nodes as well as of the bone marrow are capable of migrating to reaction sites. Apparently, the lymphoid cells condition the macrophages of the bone marrow, inducing them to migrate to the reaction site, thus showing the existence of cooperation between the bone marrow cells and the lymphocytes. The exact mechanism by which the macrophages accumulate in the site of the reaction is not known.

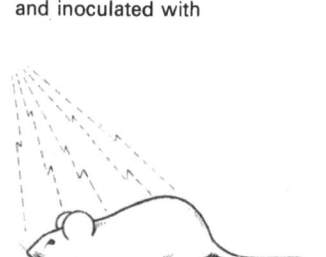

Recipient irradiated and inoculated with

		Delayed Reaction
(1)	Cells from the bone marrow of sensitized donor	+
(2)	Cells from the bone marrow of unsensitized donor	0
(3)	Lymph node cells from sensitized donor	0
(4)	Bone marrow cells from unsensitized donor plus lymph node cells from sensitized donor	+

Fig. 9.17. Protocol of experiment showing cooperation between cells of the bone marrow and lymph node cells in the establishment of delayed reactions

Cellular Interaction in the Development of Delayed Hypersensitivity T Cell

The subclass of T lymphocytes responsible for delayed type hypersensitivity was identified by adoptive transfer experiments in which T lymphocytes taken from a sensitized donor were transferred to a syngeneic recipient. The injection of the specific antigen in the footpad of the adoptively sensitized recipient induced a delayed hypersensitivity reaction as shown by a local measurable swelling. In this condition, when the T lymphocytes to be transferred were previously treated with anti-Lyt-1[+] or anti-Lyt-2,3[+], it was verified that T lymphocytes responsible for delayed hypersensitivity reactions were of the same phenotype than helper T lymphocytes, that is Lyt-1[+].

The observation that pretreatment of mice with a low dose of cyclophosphamide or X-irradiation increases delayed hypersensitivity reactions, have suggested that T helper lymphocytes are involved in differentiation of delayed hypersensitivity T lymphocytes (T_{DH}). The interpretation of this observation is that cyclophosphamide or X-irradiation destroys T suppressor lymphocytes that normally regulate the activity of T helper lymphocytes. Recently, Leung and Ada (1981) have studied the establishment of specific delayed hypersensitivity to influenza virus, in vitro. These authors observed that when Lyt-1[+] lymphocytes are added to the in vitro cultures they increase the generation of delayed hypersensitivity. In addition, Nash et al. (1981) have reported that intravenous injection of avirulent mutant strain of herpes simplex virus produces tolerance to the virus that is restricted to delayed hypersensitivity, both antibody response and generation of cytotoxic T lymphocytes being normal. This state of split tolerance (that is, inhibition of delayed hypersensitivity with normal antibody response) was long-lasting and not transferable with spleen cells in the first week after priming but easily transferable from the second week on, presumably as a con-sequence of T suppressor lymphocyte appearance. Taken together, these studies suggested that differentiation of T_{DH} lymphocytes from precursors cells is balanced by the activity of helper and suppressor T lymphocytes. There is evidence that both precursors and committed T_{DH} lymphocytes are susceptible to the inhibiting effect of Ts lymphocytes.

Interaction in Vitro of the Antigen with Sensitized Lymphoid Cells. Many types of tests have been developed to detect delayed reactions in vitro. One most often used is inhibition of macrophage migration by specific antigen. In performing this test, capillary tubes open at one end and filled with cells obtained from abdominal cavity exudates from sensitized animals (such exudates, produced experimentally by intraperitoneal injection of mineral oil, contain a large proportion of lymphocytes and macro-

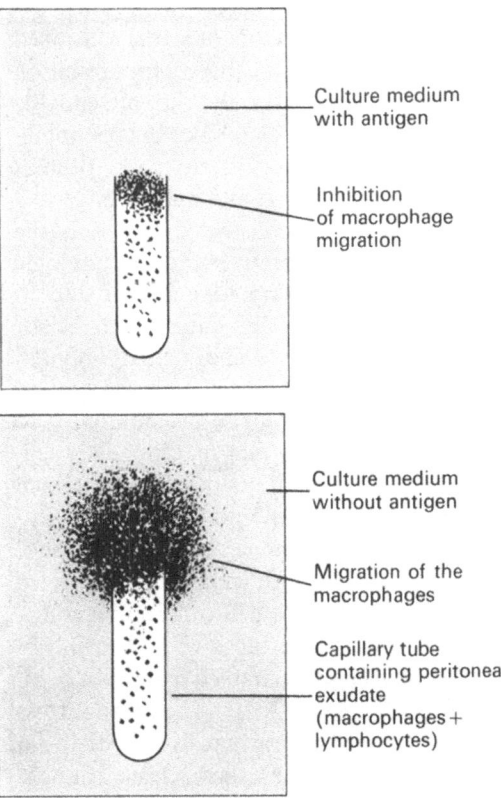

Fig. 9.18. Macrophage inhibition test

Culture medium with antigen

Inhibition of macrophage migration

Culture medium without antigen

Migration of the macrophages

Capillary tube containing peritoneal exudate (macrophages + lymphocytes)

phages) are immersed in culture medium in special chambers. Usually, two preparations of this type are made, but only one of them receives the antigen to be tested. Then the chambers are incubated at 37 °C for 24–48 h. Microscopic observation after this period demonstrates that in the control preparation the macrophages migrate to the exterior of the open end of the capillary tube, invading the culture medium, whereas in the preparation to which the antigen was added, this macrophage migration does not occur (Fig. 9.18). This inhibition of migration is specific, being produced only by the antigen capable of inducing a delayed reaction in the animal from which the cells were obtained. Cells of a nonsensitized animal do not respond to the antigen in the manner. If cells from nonsensitized animals are mixed with cells (1% is sufficient) from sensitized animals, the former become responsive to the antigen as if they also had come from sensitized animals. This transfer of sensitization requires live cells; dead cells or cellular extracts are ineffective. Moreover, sensitized cells only transfer the capacity for inhibition to nonsensitized cells when they are capable of synthesizing proteins, since the phenomenon is inhibited by mitomycin C. Studies with pure lymphocyte and macrophage suspensions have demonstrated that it is the lymphocyte that possesses the immunologic information necessary for transmission to the macrophage of the capacity to be inhibited by the antigen. The fact that only 1% of sensitized lymphocytes are sufficient to transfer the property of antigen inhibition to a population of normal macrophages suggests that the inhibition does not result from direct cell-to-cell interaction. Various experiments have demonstrated that lymphocytes sensitized and incubated with antigen synthesize and liberate into the ambient medium a soluble substance of unknown nature, which has been named macrophage inhibitory factor, or MIF. The substance is dialysable, thermoresistant, is not destroyed by treatment with ribonuclease or deoxyribonuclease, but is destroyed by proteolytic enzymes. Its operative mechanism is

unknown. The test for inhibition of macrophage migration has also been attempted with human cells. The addition of antigen to lymphocytes obtained from the peripheral blood of patients with delayed hypersensitivity liberates a factor inhibitive of the migration of both human and guinea pig macrophages. This observation suggests that the MIF is not species-specific. Aside from MIF, other substances may be produced upon contact between sensitized lymphocytes and antigen: These are collectively termed lymphokines. For example, in the supernatant of cultures of sensitized lymphocytes stimulated by the antigen, there is a factor that possesses a chemotactic effect on macrophages. Moreover, intradermal injection of MIF into nonsensitized animals induces the appearance of a local reaction resembling delayed hypersensitivity. The various lymphokines and their activities are summarized in Table 9.5. Whether or not each of these activities corresponds to a specific substance has not yet been established.

Table 9.5. Properties of the lymphokines[a]

Lymphokine	Biologic activity
Macrophage activation factor	Augments motility and the phagocytosis of macrophages
Skin reactive factor	Produces inflammation in the skin
Chemotactic factor for macrophages	Attracts macrophages
Chemotactic factor for lymphocytes	Attracts lymphocytes
Chemotactic factor for neutrophils	Attracts neutrophils
Chemotactic factor for eosinophils	Attracts eosinophils
Mitogenic factor	Induces lymphocyte transformation (blast transformation)
Lymphotoxin	Destroys cells in a fashion identical to that of sensitized lymphocytes
Macrophage inhibitory factor (MIF)	Impedes migration of the macrophages in vitro
Macrophage aggregation factor	Causes aggregation of the macrophages
Transfer factor	Transfers human cellular hypersensitivity

[a] See also pp. 330–331

Mechanism of Target-Cell Destruction

Histologically, the delayed hypersensitivity reaction is characterized by accumulation of inflammatory cells in the site where the antigen was inoculated, initially represented by polymorphonuclear cells, but later by mononuclear cells, with lymphocytes and macrophages predominating. Microscopically, one can observe the formation of perivascular islets of mononuclear cells resembling large lymphocytes, monocytes, or macrophages. These are the cells responsible for the local inflammatory phenomena. In fact macrophages are involved in two steps in delayed hypersensitivity (as well as any type of cell mediated reactions). In the inductive or afferent stage the macrophages present to lymphocytes the conventional antigen associated with MHC products on their membranes; in the effector or efferent stage the effector T_{DH} lymphocytes recognize antigen associated with the same MHC produce of the inductive stage, and are activated. The fact that T lymphocytes only see antigen when associated with MHC products is responsible for the MHC restriction phenomenon. T_{DH} lymphocytes or their precursors recognize antigen associated with class II MHC products whereas Tc lymphocytes recognize antigen associated with class I MHC products.

Activation of T lymphocytes involved in cell-mediated reactions requires two signals provided by the macrophages. The first, which we have already mentioned is the presentation of antigen plus the MHC product on the macrophage membrane. This implies that the macrophage needs to have the proper quality and quantity of MHC products to be able to present antigen in an effective way to the T lymphocytes. The second signal involves the synthesis and secretion of IL-1 by the macrophage. Among other properties, IL-1 induces antigen-activated T lymphocytes to produce IL-2 that allow T lymphocyte full differentiation to effector cell.

In general it is thought that cell destruction during delayed reactions may occur through any of four different mechanisms;

(1) Activated Macrophages. Effector T_{DT} lymphocytes activated by antigen release lymphokines that activate the macrophages. Once activated these cells will release proteolytic enzymes that destroys cells and other tissues components (see Fig. 9.19).

(2) Contact Lysis. Sensitized T cells come in direct contact with target cells and destroy them. Although the exact procedure is unknown. If sensitized lymphocytes are mixed in in vitro culture with target cells, they adhere to the target cells by fine cytoplasmic protruberances, the "uropods." By electron-microscopic examination, one can observe wide areas of surface contact with narrow interstices between the lymphocytes and target-cell membrane, with long, fine projections from the cell surface and microvilli and microtubules in the cytoplasm in the area of the contact side. Some time after cell contact, the target cell swells, stops moving, and lyses. The recognition and adherence to the target cell probably occur via killer-cell receptors. If killer cells are added to a mixture of cells containing only one type against which they are sensitized, only the specific target cell is lysed, which suggests that lysis occurs because of a specific mechanism and does not depend on the liberation of a soluble, cytotoxic factor. Because a linear relationship exists between the number of added lymphocytes and the number of lysed target cells, one can postulate a reaction of the "one-hit" type.

(3) Lymphotoxin-Mediated Destruction. Sensitized lymphocytes, activated by a specific antigen, or nonsensitized lymphocytes, non-specifically stimulated by mitogens, liberate a toxic substance (lymphotoxin) that kills cells. In these cases, the reaction with the antigen of the target cell is specific, but the destruction is nonspecific.

(4) Antibody-Dependent Cell-Mediated Cytotoxicity (see Chaps. 2 and 10). In this case, lymphocytes can destroy cells that have antibodies bound to their surfaces. However, the active cells are not only lymphocytes, but adherent cells, probably B cells, macrophages, or K cells (adherent

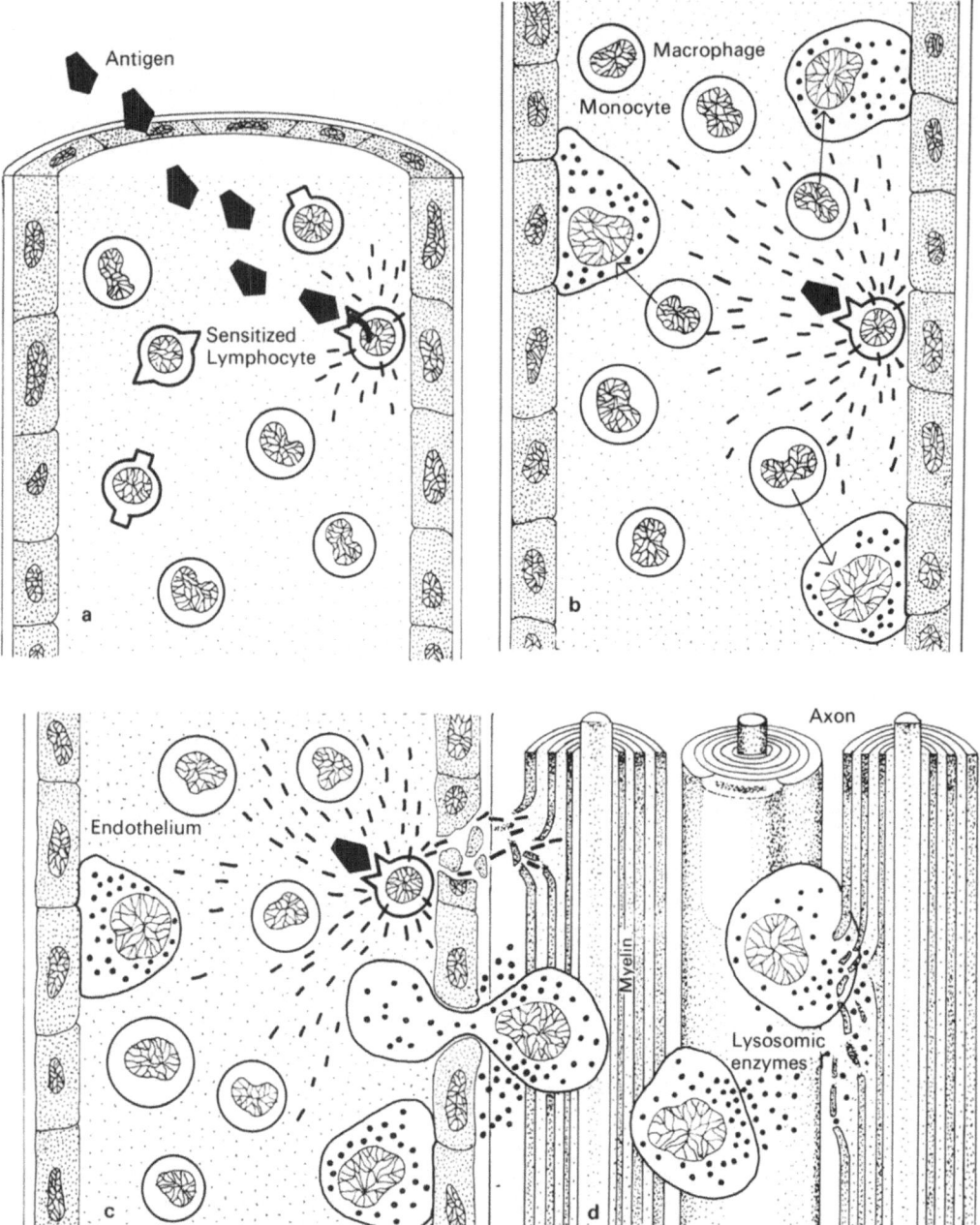

Fig. 9.19 a–d. Sequence of a delayed hypersensitivity reaction. **a** Sensitized lymphocytes activated by antigen release lymphokines including MIF. **b** Lymphokines activate the macrophages some of which adhere to endothelium. **c, d** The activated macrophages liberate enzymes, attack the vessel walls, and invade the local parenchyma, i.e., in this case, the myelin in experimental encephalomyelitis. Adapted from Waksman BH (1971) Delayed hypersensitivity: immunologic and clinical aspects. In: Good, Fisher (eds) Immunbiology. Sinauer Ass, Stanford, p 83

lymphoid cells of unknown origin), which have surface receptors for immunoglobulin-Fc fragments. Complement plays no role in this reaction.

Antigen Recognition by Cytotoxic T Cells

It is generally recognized that cytotoxic T cells are a normal component of the immune response to cell associated antigens. Indeed, cytotoxic T cells recognize conventional antigens only when associated with products of the H2-K or H2-D loci of the mouse MHC or products of the HLA-A, HLA-C or HLA-B of the human MHC.

Delayed Hypersensitivity and Histocompatibility. Intercellular reactions are restricted by the genes of the major histocompatibility complex. In the case of delayed hypersensitivity reactions this exigency results from the fact that such reactions depend on interactions between T lymphocytes and macrophages. It has been observed that parental macrophages containing antigen in their surface are capable of inducing T lymphocytes of the F1 generation to differentiate in T_{DTH} (T lymphocytes effector of delayed hypersensitivity) but that these last are able to transfer delayed hypersensitivity only to individuals whose *I* region is the same as that presented by the macrophages that initially contact the T lymphocytes originated the T_{DTH}. Thus, it seems that the T_{DTH} lymphocytes recognize the antigen on the cellular surface only when associated with the same product of the *I* region with which the antigen was associated during the induction phase of the T_{DTH} lymphocytes.

Cutaneous Basophil Hypersensitivity. Under certain experimental conditions a form of delayed cutaneous hypersensitivity reaction can be induced with characteristics that differentiate it from a typical delayed reaction. The reaction also called Jones-Mote reaction, is characterized by the presence of an infiltration with basophil leukocytes which represents 20 to 60% of the infiltrating cells. The cutaneous basophil hypersensitivity is usually induced by immunizing the animal with antigen in incomplete Freund's adjuvant or in saline. T lymphocytes seem to be essential for the induction and expression of this type of delayed reaction. Animals presenting this reaction show an increase of the paracortical areas of the draining lymph nodes and the reaction is passively transferred by T lymphocytes. Activated T lymphocytes produce a lymphokine chemotactic for basophils. The functional significance of this type of delayed hypersensitivity is not known.

Role of Mast Cells in Delayed Hypersensitivity. In addition to their role in anaphylaxis, mast cells seem to play an important functional role in delayed hypersensitivity. Askenase (1980) has shown that delayed hypersensitivity reactions in mice are preferentially elicited in skin sites richer in mast cells and that depletion of serotonin by reserpine abolishes delayed hypersensitivity. Furthermore, ultrastructural and radioautographic studies indicated that mast cells are activated and release serotonin in delayed hypersensitivity. Released serotonin induces formation of gaps in the endothelium of postcapillary venules allowing passage of leukocytes into the extravascular tissues. Mast cell degranulation and formation of endothelial gaps in delayed hypersensitivity reactions have also been observed in humans.

References

Askenase PW (1980) Effector cells in late and delayed hypersensitivity reactions that are dependent on antibodies or T cells. Fougereau M, Dausset J (ed) Progress in Immunology IV. Academic Press, London, p 829

Austen KF, Wassermann SI, Goetzl EJ (1976) Mast cell derived mediators: Structural and functional diversity and regulation of expression. In: Johansson SGO, Strandberg K, Uvnas B (eds) Molecular and biological aspects of the acute allergic reaction. Plenum Press, New York

Behrendt H (1979) Zur Morphologie sensibilisierter und stimulierter Mastzellen. Allergologie 4:136

Bennich H, Bahr-Lindstrom H (1974) Structure of immunoglobulin E (IgE). Prog Immunol 1:49

Blaser K, Nakagawa T, Weck AL (1981) Suppression of antihapten IgE and IgG antibody responses by isologous anti-idiotypic antibodies against purified anti-carrier (ovalbumin) antibodies in Balb/c mice. J Immunol 126:1180

Braun W, Lichtenstein NW, Parker CW (eds) (1974) Cyclic AMP, cell growth and the immune response. Springer, Berlin Heidelberg New York

Buckley RH (1980) IgE antibody in health and disease. In: Bierman CW, Pearlman DS (eds) Allergic diseases of infancy, childhood and adolescence. Saunders Company

Capron A, Dessaint JP, Capron M (1975) Specific IgE antibodies in immune adherence of normal macrophages to Schistosoma mansoni schistosomules. Nature 252:474

Coombs RRA, Gell PGH (1975) Classification of allergic reactions responsible for clinical hypersensitivity and disease. In: Gell PGH, Coombs RRA, Lachmann PJ (eds) Clinical aspects of immunology. Blackwell, Oxford

Gupta S, Good RA (eds) (1979) Cellular, molecular, and clinical aspects of allergic disorders. Plenum, New York

Ishizaka K (1981) Regulation of the IgE antibody response. Int Arch Appl Immunol 66 (Sup 1):1

Ishizaka K, Ishizaka T, Okudaira H, Bazin H (1978) Ontogeny of IgE-bearing lymphocytes in the rat. J Immunol 120:655

Ishizaka K (1984) Isotype-specific regulation of the IgE response. Progress in Immunology V. Academic Press, London, p 455

Johansson SGO, Foucard T, Dannaeus A (1974) IgE in human disease. Prog Immunol 4:62

Kaliner M, Austen KF (1973) A sequence of biochemical events in the antigen-induced release of chemical mediators from sensitized human lung tissue. J Exp Med 138:1077

Kanellopoulos JM, Rossi G, Metzger H (1979) Preparative isolation of the cell receptor for immunoglobulin E. J Biol Chem 254:7691

Kanellopoulos JM, Liu TY, Poy G, Metzger H (1980) Composition and subunit structure of the cell receptor for immunoglobulin . E J Biol Chem 255:9060

Katz DH (1978) The allergic phenotype: Manifestation of "Allergic Breakthrough" and imbalance in normal damping of IgE antibody production. Immunol Rev 41:77

Katz DH, Marcelletti JF (1984) Regulation of the IgE antibody system in humans and experimental animals. Progress in Immunology V. Academic Press, London, p 465

Kay AB (1980) Dynamics, role and function of eosinophils. In: Ochling, Glazer, Mathov, Arbesman (eds) Advances in Allergology and Applied Immunology. Pergamon Press, Oxford

Kitamura Y, Go S, Matsuda M, Hatanka K, Seki M (1979) Distribution of mast cells precursors in hematopoietic and lymphoietic tissues of mice. J Exp Med 150:482

König W, Pfeiffer P, Speralski A, Bohn A (1981) Membrane biochemical events in mast cell and basophil activation and secretion. Behring Topics in Allergology. Behring Inst Mitt 68:30

Kulczycki A, Parker CW (1979) The cell surface receptor for immunoglobulin E. E. The use of repetitive affinity chromatography for the purification of a mammalian receptor. J Biol Chem 254:3187

Levine B (1974) Genetics of atopic allergy and reagin production. In: Clinical Immunology and Allergy in Paediatric Medicin. Blackwell, Oxford, p 49

Levine B, Vaz N (1970) Effect of combinations of inbred strain, antigen and antigen dose on immune responsiveness and reagin production in the mouse. A potenital mouse model for immune aspects of human atopic allergy. Ing Arch Allergy Appl Immunol 39:156

Lewis RA, Austen KF (1981) Mediation of local homeostasis and inflammation by leukotrienes and other mast cell-dependent compounds. Nature 293:103

Lewis RA, Holgate ST, Roberts LJ, Oates JA, Austen KF (1981) Preferential generation of prostaglanding D_2 by rat and human mast cells. In: Becker, Simon, Austen (eds) Biochemistry of the acute allergic reactions. Alan R Liss, New York

Marssh DG, Meyers DA (1980) Genetics of human immune response to allergens. J Allergy Clin Immunol 65:322

Metzger H, Kinet JP, Perez-Monfort R, Rivnay B, Wank SA (1984) A tetrameric model for the structure of the mast cell receptor with high affinity of IgE. Progress in Immunology V. Academic Press, London, p 493

Mossman H, Possart-Schmitz P, Hammer OK (1981) Early molecular events in mast cell and basophil activation. Behring Inst Mitt 68:19

Mota I (1953) Mast cell damage by anaphylaxis, peptone shock and compound 48/80. MD Thesis University of S. Paulo, Brazil

Mota I (1963) Mast cells and anaphylaxis. Ann NY Acad Sc 103:264

Mota I (1964) The mechanism of anaphylaxis. I. Production and biological properties of mast cell sensitizing antibody. Immunology 6:681

Mota I, Catty D (1974) Biological actions of anaphylactic antibodies. Prog Immunol 4:306

Nash A, Gell PGH (1981) The delayed hypersensitivity T cell and its interaction with other T cells. Immunology Today, August

Nash A, Phelan J, Wildy P (1981) Cell-mediatd immunity in herpes simplex virus-infected mice: H-2 mapping of the delayed-type hypersensitivity response and the antiviral T cell response. J Immunol 126:1260

Ramalho-Pinto FJ, McLaren DJ, Smithers SR (1978) Complement-mediated killing of schistosomula of Schistosoma mansone by rat eosinophils in vitro. J Exp Med 147:147

Riley JF, West GB (1953) The presence of histamine in tissue mast cells. J Physiol 120:528

Schartz LB, Austen KF (1982) Mast cells and mediators. In: Lachman PJ, Peters DK (eds) Clinical Aspects of Immunology, 4th ed. Blackwell, London, p 130

Sehon AH (1984) Down regulation of IgE antibodies by suppressogenic conjugates. Progress in Immunology V. Academic Press, London, p 483

Tada T (1975) Regulation of reaginic antibody formation in animals. Prog Allergy 19:122

Tada T (1981) Regulation of antibody formation. A sociobiological circuit. Behring Inst Mitt 68:1

Taurog JD, Fewtrell C, Becker EL (1979) IgE mediated triggering of rat basophil leukemia cells: Lack of evidence for serine esterase activation. J Immunol 122:2150

Theofilopoulos AN, Dixon FJ (1979) The biology and detection of immune complexes. Adv Immunol 28:89

Vaz NM, Levine B (1971) Persistent formation of reagins in mice infected with low doses of ovalbumin. Immunol 21:11

Wilander O (1938) Studien über Heparin. Skand Arch Physiol (Suppl) 81:1–89

Winslow CM, Austen K (1982) Enzymatic regulation of mast cells and secretion by adenylate cyclase and cyclic AMP-dependent protein kinases. Fed Proceedings 41:22

Chapter 10　Transplantation

Dietrich Götze and Ivan Mota

Contents

Terminology 297
Transplantation Reactions 298
  Host-Versus-Graft Reaction 298
  Graft-Versus-Host Reaction 299
Genetics of Rejection 299
  Host-Versus-Graft Reaction 299
  Graft-Versus-Host Reaction 300
Mechanism of Graft Rejection 301
  Recognition Phase 301
  Proliferation and Differentiation 301
Destruction Phase . . . . : . . 302
Mixed Lymphocyte Culture 302
  Reaction Partner 302
  Specificity of MLR 303
  Number of Allogenic Reactive Cells 304
  Genetics of MLC Reactivity 304
  Cell-Mediated Cytotoxicity 305
Specific Absence of Reaction Against
  Allogenic Tissue 307
Organ Transplantation 311
  Serologic Typing 311
  Cellular Typing 311
Clinical Organ Transplantation 312
  Kidneys 312
  Bone Marrow Transplant 314
  Thymus 315
  Blood Transfusion 315
References 316

Terminology

Transplantation is defined as the transfer of living cells, tissues, or organs from one site to another in the same individual (*syngeneic* transplantation) or from one individual to another – of the same (*allogeneic* transplantation) or another (*xenogeneic* transplantation) species. The terminology used to characterize the genetic relationship between recipient and donor was presented in Table 6.1 (see pp. 140). If a transplant is transferred to the same site, i.e., to its normal anatomic location, it is termed an *orthotopic* graft; if it is implanted in a location other than its normal one, it is termed a *heterotopic* graft. The fate of the graft is determined by the genetic relationship between donor and recipient. Grafts exchanged between genetically identical individuals are *accepted*. Grafts exchanged between genetically different individuals are *rejected*, i.e., they are destroyed. Rejection is the result of a specific immune response to histocompatibility antigens. Under certain conditions, the recipient can be rendered incapable of reacting to the transplant, a state called *immunologic tolerance*. If the capacity for an immunologic reaction is suppressed by circulating antibodies ("blocking antibodies"), one speaks of *enhancement*. If only the recipient is capable of a reaction, one speaks of a host-versus-graft reaction; however, if the graft consists of immunocompetent cells – or contains such cells – there is a graft-versus-host reaction. The former is the case with organ transplants such as skin, kidney, heart, liver, etc.; the latter occurs after transplantation of bone marrow, spleen, lymph node, or thymus cells. The structures responsible for the transplantation reaction are controlled by histocompatibility genes. These include those that control 1) erythrocyte alloantigens, 2) lymphocyte alloantigens, and 3) transplantation antigens. This subdivision is based on the methods of their identification. Erythrocyte alloantigens are demonstrated primarily by agglutination (see Chap. 7, p. 187), lymphocyte antigens primarily by the lymphocytotoxicity test, and transplantation antigens by tissue (skin) and tumor grafts.

Approximately 60 such genes (or loci) are known in the mouse, of which a little more than half belong to the third category. On the basis of the strength of the induced immune response, one can divide the H genes into two groups: 1) those that cause an acute reaction, in vivo and in vitro (major histocompatibility complex, MHC), and 2) those that cause a delayed, chronic reaction (minor histocompatibility genes, non-MHC). In addition to the different forms of reactivity in relation to a graft, there are additional characteristics that differentiate the two groups: 1) The MHC is extremely polymorphic, with more than 50 alleles in the mouse (also in man, see Tables 6.4 and 6.8) in comparison to the non-MHC genes, in which a maximum of three alleles are known. 2) The MHC is closely linked with genes that control the immune response. 3) The MHC plays a decisive role in the graft-versus-host reaction and the mixed lymphocyte reaction. 4) It is much more difficult to induce tolerance to MHC antigens than to non-MHC antigens. 5) Immunosuppression is more effective for non-MHC antigen differences than for MHC-antigen differences.

In man, two groups of histocompatibility genes can be distinguished: genes that control 1) lymphocyte alloantigens (HLA = MHC) and 2) blood-group antigens (ABO, P).

In general, MHC antigens cause acute rejection of transplanted organs or tissue, such as skin, heart, bone marrow, kidney, and liver. Two organs appear to be exceptions to this rule. Cases of kidney transplant have been described in which the transplanted kidney was accepted despite different MHC antigens between the recipient and the donor; in many of these cases, however, the skin of the kidney donor was normally rejected, without affecting the function of the transplanted kidney. Such occurrences are observed regularly in experimental kidney transplants in the rat and dog. This phenomenon may be dependent upon "enhancing" (blocking) antibodies.

The second organ that deviates from this rule is the liver. In experiments in pigs, an unexpectedly large number of animals that received a liver allograft survived for a long period even without immunosuppressive therapy. However, not only did the liver transplant survive longer (and here the liver transplant differs from the kidney transplant), but organs from the same donor animal that were simultaneously or later transplanted (skin, kidney, heart) were protected from normal rejection (also in pigs, these organs were immediately rejected by untreated animals). However, animals that tolerated skin or kidney transplants after liver transplantation normally rejected grafts from a second, different donor. This tolerance can also be achieved through intraperitoneal or intraportal injection of liver extract. The basis of this protective effect is not yet understood, but perhaps the liver releases antigens in a tolerogenic form.

Transplantation Reactions

Host-Versus-Graft Reaction

The sequence of the host-versus-graft reaction of a skin graft between allogenic mice can be summarized as follows: The transplant first appears pale; after 2–4 days, the transferred skin becomes vascularized and appears pink. A difference between allo- and autografts is visible after 4–7 days: With an autograft, the pink color (circulation) remains and epithelialization of the grafted area progresses; the graft is integrated into the skin of the recipient (hair growth occurs after about 12 days). The allograft, on the other hand, turns cyanotic and later necrotic, and falls off after 10–12 days (rejection).

Histologically, around the fifth day, one can observe in the allografts perivascular infiltration by mononuclear cells (lymphocytes, histiocytes), an increase in mitoses in the basal layer of the epidermis, and a little later, vascular thrombosis – a microscopic index of rejection that precedes macroscopic rejection.

The time of rejection is determined by four principal factors: the quantity of tissue engrafted, the immunogenicity of the transplantation antigen of the donor, the degree of genetic difference between the donor and the receptor, and the immune status of the recipient.

In recipients that receive a second graft from the same donor, the rejection, instead of taking 10–12 days (first set rejection) occurs in 5–7 days (second set rejection). In hyperimmunized animals that have antibodies in their blood against the transplantation antigens of the donor, the rejection is even more rapid and proceeds before the graft has had time to vascularize (white graft rejection).

Graft-Versus-Host Reaction

Such a reaction is caused by immunocompetent cells implanted in a recipient that itself is not immunologically reactive. This is the case 1) when a newborn is the recipient and the result is runt disease, or 2) when an adult recipient is rendered immunologically nonreactive by immunosuppression (accidental, therapeutic or experimental chemotherapy or radiation), or by existing immune deficiency diseases (primary, Chap. 12, or secondary, by the presence of neoplastic processes or treatment with immunosuppressives), or finally 3) by the transplantation of immunologically competent homozygous parental cells in F_1 hybrids. The syndrome caused by the reactions of the transplanted cells is called secondary disease (the primary disease is one of those named above) or "wasting" syndrome or disease.

The graft-versus-host (GVH) reaction can be studied experimentally by three principal methods:

1. *Lethally irradiated* (900 r) *adult animals* (e.g., mouse) receive, 1 day after irradiation, several million lymphoid cells intravenously. If spleen, lymph node, or thymus cells are injected, a GVH reaction occurs between the 8th and 20th days and the animals die, whereas control animals (which are lethally irradiated but receive syngenic cells) survive; animals that are irradiated but receive no cells die between the 5th and 9th day. If bone-marrow cells are transferred, a GVH first occurs after the 20th day and exhibits a protracted course.

2. *The splenomegaly test according to Simonson*, whereby newborn F_1 mice (less than 24 h old) are injected intraperitoneally with several million spleen cells from an allogeneic (parental) donor. The animals are killed 10 days later; their body (B_{exp}) and spleen (S_{exp}) weights are measured and compared to those of the control animals (which received syngeneic cells):

$$\frac{S_{exp}/B_{exp}}{S_{con}/B_{con}} = \text{spleen index (SI).}$$

Depending upon the standard deviation of the ratio S_{con}/B_{con}, a GVH reaction is positive with values of $SI > 1.0$ or > 1.3.

3. *The local lymph node weight test according to Ford* whereby F_1 animals or animals treated with anti-lymphocytic globulin and lethally irradiated (stimulator) receive 20×10^6 cells of a parental (or allogenic) donor (responder) in the foot pad; as a control, syngenic cells are injected in the other foot pad. Five days later, the popliteal lymph nodes are removed, freed from fat tissue, washed in acetone, and dried overnight. The next day the lymph nodes are weighed. Depending on the standard deviation, a quotient (stimulation index) of ≥ 2.0 between the weight of the allogenically stimulated and the syngenically stimulated lymph nodes indicate a positive GVH.

Genetics of Rejection

Host-Versus-Graft Reaction

The genetics of histocompatibility in general has been described in Chap. 6. Here, we shall give a more detailed picture. The most important genes which induce a graft reaction (rejection) are those of the major histocom-

Table 10.1. Survival time of skin grafts exchanged between siblings as a function of the HLA genotype[a]

Recipient genotype	Donor with HLA genotype			
	1	2	3	4
	B/D[b]	A/D	B/D	A/C
1 B/D	∞[c]	14	22	13
2 A/D	14	∞	13	13
3 B/D	20	16	∞	13
4 A/C	12	14	13	∞

[a] Used with kind permission of Ceppellini R (1968). The genetic basis of transplantation. In: Rapaport FT and Dausset J (eds) Human transplantation. Grune and Stratton, New York
[b] A/B are the paternal genotypes, C/D, the maternal genotypes.
[c] Autotransplant.

Table 10.2. Skin graft survival times for differences for individual loci of the major histocompatibility complex in the mouse and in man

MHC locus difference between recipient and donor	Average survival time in days
A. Mouse	
−	∞
Non-H-2	Between 25 and >200
H-$2K$	<11
H-$2I$-A	10–14
H-$2I$-E	18–>200
H-$2S$	>200
H-$2G$	?
H-$2D$	<16
B. Man[a]	
−	∞
Non-HLA	≥16
HLA-A	14
HLA-B	13,3
HLA-D	11,5
HLA-A, HLA-B and HLA-D	10

[a] From van Rood JJ et al. (1975) LD typing by serology. IV. Description of a new locus with three alleles. In: Kissmeyer-Nielsen F (ed) Histocompatibility testing 1975. Munksgaard, Copenhagen, pp. 629–636; and Dausset J et al. (1970) Skin allograft survival in 238 human subjects: Role of specific relationships at four gene sites of the first and second HL-A loci. In: Terasaki PI (ed) Histocompatibility testing 1970. Munksgaard, Copenhagen, pp. 381–397

patibility complex, MHC (Table 10.1). Disparity in MHC alleles between recipient and donor leads to an acute reaction; differences in several of the MHC linked loci have a cumulative effect on the speed of the reaction (Table 10.2). (The fact that skin grafts exchanged between HLA identical individuals are also rejected eventually is due to various non-HLA allelic differences which are not linked to the HLA complex and, therefore, are inherited independently of these.)

Among the MHC genes in the mouse, differences for the K, D, and I alleles cause rejection reactions (Table 10.2). The I region appears to harbor at least two histocompatibility genes, one that is identical with or closely linked to the I-A locus, and the other located between the I-A and S locus. The former is a strong histocompatibility gene, the latter a weak one. Disparity for the S locus does not cause graft rejection.

In man, differences for individual HLA loci lead to an accelerated rejection, i.e., HLA-A, B, and D represent strong histocompatibility genes (whether HLA-C is a histocompatibility gene has not yet been determined). The survival time of skin grafts with HLA-D differences shows a direct correlation to the magnitude of the stimulation between donor and recipient (Fig. 10.1).

Graft-Versus-Host Reaction

A graft-versus-host (GVH) reaction is caused by differences in MHC alleles as well as in non-HLA alleles between recipient and donor. The time course and severity of a GVH in combinations differing for minor histocompatibility alleles depends upon the "strength" of the minor locus(i) in question, and upon the number of injected cells, the route of administration, and the preimmunization. In general, the strength of the reaction parallels that of the HVG reaction for the same H-gene differences. With individual minor-H-gene differences, the reaction is delayed and is in most cases chronic, even if spleen cells have been injected.

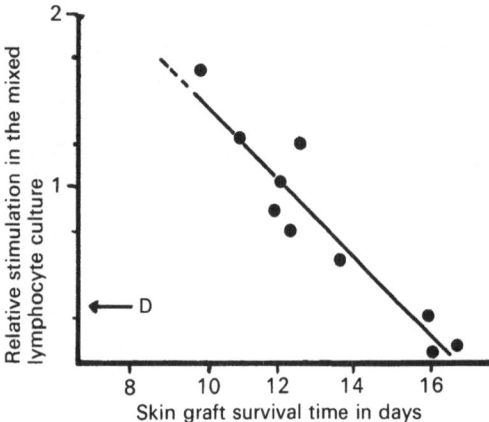

Fig. 10.1. Survival times for skin grafts between HLA-A and B identical, HLA-D different donor-recipient pairs (Summarized from Koch CT et al., 1973). The relative importance of matching for the MLC versus HLA loci in organ transplantation. In: Dausset J and Colombani J (eds) (1972) Histocompatibility testing, Munksgaard, Copenhagen; pp 521–524; and Thorby E, Jorgensen F (1973) Skin graft survival time and MLC response in four HLA seroidentical unrelated combinations, ibid, pp 525–526

When there are differences for MHC genes between recipient and donor, there is always an acute graft reaction after injection of lymphoid cells. This leads acutely to death when spleen, lymph node, thymus, or peripheral blood cells are injected. However, a chronic course is displayed if bone-marrow cells are transferred. Clearly, the strongest reaction occurs with differences for the *I* genes; but also differences for *K* or *D* alleles cause an acute reaction. Within the *I* region, several loci have been identified that can elicit a graft-versus-host reaction and that appear to be identical to those that cause an MLR in vitro.

Mechanism of Graft Rejection

Graft rejection is a complex process, and the mechanism that leads to rejection can be different for different organs, e.g., for skin, kidney, or bone marrow (lymphoid tissue). The process can be differentiated into three principal phases: recognition, proliferation and differentiation, and destruction. The recognition and destruction phases occur directly on the graft, whereas proliferation and differentiation phases take place in the regional lymph nodes that drain the graft bed.

Recognition Phase

Immediately after transplantation, antigen from the donor organ is shed into the systemic circulation of the recipient, or resides on the cells of the vascular endothelium of the graft; they are exposed to the recipient's immune cells in the circulation. The effector component of the immune response consists of lymphocytes, macrophages, and polymorphonuclear cells, each with an individual role to play but in many instances either cooperating with or suppressing one or another component of the system.

The recognition of the alloantigens is achieved by T lymphocytes which have the characteristics of T helper cells ($Ly-1^+2^-3^-$). Receptors of T cells recognize the alloantigen in association with self (see p. 164). The antigens are either recognized by T cells passing through the graft, or after being "collected" by macrophages in the graft or out of the tissue fluid (lymph), and presented to T cells in the lymph node (macrophage–T cell cooperation).

Proliferation and Differentiation

After contact and recognition of the antigen(s), the lymphocytes apparently return – if they have recognized the antigen(s) as cells passing through the graft – to the regional lymph nodes, proliferate, and stimulate additional effector precursor cells, such as T effector cells and B lymphocytes. The majority of the newly sensitized cells leave the lymph node and via the blood reach the graft where they directly or with the help of other systems (K cells – see below, polymorphonuclear leukocytes, specific antibodies with or without complement) destroy the graft. A certain number of lymphocytes remain in the circulation as memory cells .

Destruction Phase

The destruction of the graft is effected by several pathways, every one of which may act alone or in combination:
1) Activated T killer cells (with the characteristic markers Ly-$1^-2^+3^+$) bind via specific cell-bound receptors to the cells of the graft and lyse them; T cells also release factors, such as macrophage migration inhibition factor (MIF) which accelerate the rate of mononuclear cell infiltration.
2) Activated B lymphocytes differentiate to plasma cells and produce antibodies specific for the graft's antigens; they may bind directly and activate complement which then attracts polymorphonuclear leukocytes (PMN). Disruption of PMN causes the release of lysosomes and proteolytic enzymes with resulting destruction of graft tissue. Vasoactive peptides cause vasospasm, which slows blood flow and facilitates accumulation of both PMN and monocytes, and thereby produces diffuse ischemic changes. Accumulation of platelets also occurs, with resulting activation of clotting mechanisms and the formation of thrombi.
3) Recently, a type of lymphocyte has been identified – K lymphocytes – which recognize humoral antibodies (IgG) against specific donor antigens, react with the Fc portion, and destroy the target cells to which they are attached. This system is known as antibody-dependent, cell-mediated cytotoxicity (ADCC) (see pp. 45 and 306).
The first of the three outlined pathways appears to be the primary mechanism of graft destruction in unsensitized recipients, in which the two latter mechanisms come into play only to complete the rejection. In sensitized recipients (sensitized by preimmunization, e.g., blood transfusion or pregnancy), all three mechanisms may contribute equally to the graft's destruction.
Individual phases can be studied in in vitro experiments: the mixed lymphocyte culture

reaction appears to represent an in vitro equivalent of the recognition and proliferation phases. The destruction phase can be studied in the form of a primary or secondary response in vitro using the cell-mediated lympholytic reaction (CML).

Mixed Lymphocyte Culture

The principles of the mixed lymphocyte culture (MLC) reaction were discussed on pp. 150. Only the reaction partner and the possible mechanism are briefly discussed here.

Reaction Partner

Stimulator. In the one-way reaction, the cell whose proliferation is blocked by treatment with mitomycin C or by irradiation (2,500–5,000 r) is termed the stimulator. To stimulate the untreated cell, the stimulator must be alive and able to be metabolically active; RNA or protein synthesis inhibitors or germicidal ultraviolet irradiation cause a loss of stimulating ability.
Lymphatic cells exhibit good stimulation, however, stimulation can also be observed with epidermal cells but not with kidney cells. Of the lymphoid cells, primarily B cells appear to cause stimulation; although, stimulation by T cells and macrophages has also been demonstrated. In addition to B lymphocytes, T lymphocytes also stimulate, depending upon the genetic differences for certain I-subregions between responder and stimulator.

Responder Cell. It is generally agreed that the cells in a MLC that proliferate in response to a stimulus are T cells (Thy-1^+ cells). With the additional T-cell markers Ly-1,2, and 3, it was shown in the mouse that the transforming cells are derived from Ly-$1^+,2^+,3^+$ cells and that among the proliferating cells, Ly-$1^+,2^-,3^-$ as well as Ly-$1^-, 2^+, 3^+$, cells are found.

The following findings in the mouse were obtained from selection experiments (i.e., pretreatment of the responder cell population with anti-Ly-1 or anti-Ly-2,3 serum plus complement): Responder T cells stimulated by K or D molecules exhibit primarily the markers Ly-2 and Ly-3; responder cells stimulated by I molecules are composed of both T-cell populations. These findings by Cantor and Boyse, and results obtained from studies by Wagner and colleagues, suggest the following: After contact with allogeneic cells differing for the H-2 K, D, and I molecules, T precursor cells (Ly-1$^+$, 2$^+$, 3$^+$) are stimulated by the I molecules to differentiate to T helper cells (Ly-1$^+$, 2$^-$, 3$^-$), and by the K and D molecules to differentiate to T effector cells (Ly-1$^-$, 2$^+$, 3$^+$). The generated T helper cells augment the production of T effector cells reacting specifically with K or D molecules, and initiate the formation of T effector cells reacting specifically with I molecules (T–T cell interaction) (see also below, CML). At the same time, T helper cells also affect B cells and bring about their differentiation into antibody-secreting plasma cells (T–B cell interaction). If there is no difference between the responder cell population and the stimulator cell population for I-gene-controlled molecules, the antigen apparently must first be processed by macrophages before it is in the position to bring about the formation of T helper cells (macrophage-T cell cooperation).

Whether T helper cells and T effector cells derive from the same T precursor cells or whether both types of cells originate from different precursor cells that develop before contact with the antigen, i.e., independently of the antigen, from common precursor cells, is still unknown.

Specificity of MLR

Although it is generally accepted that the T-cell response to antigens is clonal like that of B cells, there is as yet no direct proof. This does not mean that no specificity can be shown. Selection experiments have indi-

cated that stimulated cells in a specific allogenic combination react specifically:

1) *Negative selection:* One obtains negatively selected cells by injecting lymphocyte cultures at the time of maximal proliferation into previously lethally irradiated animals of a strain from which the stimulator cells are derived; a few hours later, the ductus thoracicus is drained; it contains only those responder cells that were not stimulated in the allogenic culture because the stimulating cells were absorbed in the host.

2) *Positive selection.* Positively selected cells are obtained by injecting proliferating cells of an MLC into syngenic (to the responder), thymectomized, lethally irradiated animals that have been reconstituted with anti-Thy-1 serum plus complement treated bone marrow (B animals). The cells can be "parked" in such animals for weeks.

Positively and negatively selected cells can also be obtained by an in vitro process: If cells in the proliferative phase are separated in a serum gradient at 1 g (1 g velocity sedimentation), two cell populations are obtained: One consists of lymphoblasts, the other of lymphocytes. Lymphoblasts are the positively selected cells, whereas the lymphocyte fraction contains the nonstimulated (negatively selected) cells. Both cell fractions can be maintained in culture for weeks and can be used to test their reactivity to allogenic cells. Negatively selected cells no longer react to allogenic cells that originate from the donor used for the first stimulation; their ability to react to other allogenic donors is, however, in no way influenced. Positively selected cells react much faster and more vigorously to cells of donors used for the first stimulation. However, they also react (in various degrees) to cells that are unrelated to the original cells, which can be explained by the considerable cross-reactions exhibited by alloantigens.

Immunologic specificity can also be demonstrated by specific tolerance: Lymphocytes of tolerant rats do not react to cell antigens of the strain used to induce tolerance, but they react with a normal proliferative response to "third party" stimulator cells.

Furthermore, it has been shown that anti-bodies against receptors that recognize the alloantigens of the specific stimulator can destroy these lymphocytes, and the remaining cell population no longer shows reactivity against these stimulator cells; however, it can react unimpaired against cells of other allogenic donors.

Number of Allogenic Reactive Cells

The number of cells in the allogenic MLR has been calculated to be about 3%–6% of the T cells used. Different methods are employed for this calculation, including the following: Hydroxyurea in appropriate concentrations (10^{-2}–10^{-3} M) leaves blast formation untouched but can reversibly block DNA synthesis. This substance can be used to arrest the reacting cells in the blast stage. By counting the blasts at the time of maximal transformation, one can easily calculate the number of stimulated cells.

The percentage of cells that react to an allogenic stimulus is, at first glance, high. Assuming that only two or three antigenic determinants per haplotype lead to stimulation, one must conclude that not more than

about 20–50 different determinants occur in one species. This is, however, obviously not the case. It appears, therefore, that allogenic stimulation occurs via a large number of determinants, whereby unrelated haplotypes share a large though variable number of determinants. This would also explain why there is a clear proliferative response of positively selected cells toward third-party stimulator cells. This hypothesis is also substantiated by the linear proportionality of the relative reactivity due to the presence of 0, 1, or 2 HLA-D antigen differences (Fig. 10.2) between the responder and the stimulator.

Genetics of MLC Reactivity

In allogenic combinations in man, the capacity to stimulate is almost entirely linked to the *HLA-D* region.

In the mouse, variations in individual non-MHC histocompatibility genes between responder and stimulator lead in some cases to stimulation (*H-1*, *H-3*, and *H-4*), whereas in other cases no stimulation is observed (*H-7*, *H-8*, *H-9*, and *H-Y*). Differences for several non-MHC genes in general lead to stimulation. The *H-2* haplotype also influences the reactivity in the MLC. Thus, the reaction against non-MHC determinants is strong in the presence of the *H-2*ᵃ haplotype; however, the difference for the same non-MHC determinants causes weak stimulation in the presence of almost all other *H-2* haplotypes, particularly the *H-2*ᵇ haplotype.

Relatively strong stimulation has been described in cases of differences in the Thy-1 locus; in comparison, the Ly antigens 1 and 2 and the TLa antigen apparently lead to no stimulation. Festenstein described a locus (*M*) with four alleles, M_1, M_2, M_3, and M_4, which is not linked to genes of the *H-2* complex but causes stimulation that is comparable in strength to that observed with *H-2* disparity. (An *M* locus disparity leads neither to an HVG nor to a GVH reaction, and M-locus-controlled determinants cannot be serologically demonstrated but are apparently expressed on B lymphocytes.)

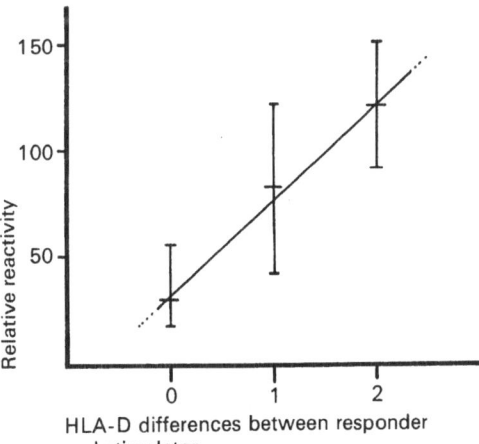

Fig. 10.2. Reactivity in the mixed lymphocyte culture between unrelated cells that differ in the 0, 1, or 2 HLA-D determinants (From Thorsby E et al., 1975). Human MLC activation determinants. In: Kissmeyer-Nielson F (ed) (1975) Histocompatibility testing 1975. Munksgaard, Copenhagen; pp 502–508

H-2 disparity leads to strong stimulation in the MLC. In the MLC, disparity in the *I* region clearly causes the strongest reactions, primarily dependent upon determinants controlled from *I-A* genes. However, also the *I-E* region controls determinants that lead to clear but weak reactions. A disparity for K and D antigens also causes stimulations which are, however, clearly weaker. Other findings support the supposition that the lymphocyte-activating structures are identical with Ia antigens (in the mouse) or B-cell-specific *HLA-D* linked antigens in man: 1) The tissue distribution of Ia antigens is the same as that of the stimulating antigens. 2) The stimulation can be inhibited by antisera that react specifically with Ia antigens. Finally 3), the gene loci that control stimulation in the MLR, are found in all species examined thus far on the same chromosome region as that which controls the Ia antigen (or Ia-like antigens).

The ability of lymphocytes to react in xenogeneic combinations was also tested. In certain combinations, stimulation reaches the magnitude of HLA-D or H-2 disparate allogenic combinations; however, reactivity appears to decrease as the phylogenetic relationship becomes more and more distant.

Cell-Mediated Cytotoxicity

Cell-mediated cytotoxicity can occur in two ways: 1) through direct interaction between target cells and specific sensitized lymphocytes in the absence of antibodies and complement (cell-mediated cytolysis, CML) and 2) through antibody-dependent, cell-mediated cytotoxicity (or lysis) (ADCC).

Direct Cell-Mediated Cytolysis. Cell-mediated, antibody-independent cell lysis (CML) can be considered as the effector phase of MLR. Lymphocytes stimulated by alloantigens in vitro or in vivo lyse cells of the same donor when they are offered to them as target cells. Culture cell lines, mitogen-stimulated lymphoblasts (LPS, PHA or con A) or macrophages are suitable target cells in vitro. The destruction of the target cells is

usually measured by the release of ^{51}Cr, with which the target cells were previously labeled.

Sensitized or nonsensitized lymphocytes are co-cultivated with stimulator cells for 5 days; then the activated lymphocytes are added to ^{51}Cr-labeled target cells in different proportions to the number of effector cells. The cell mixture is incubated for 6–16 h at 37 °C, and after removal of the cells by centrifugation, the radioactivity in the supernatant is measured. The specific lysis is given as a percentage of the maximum release of radioactivity (measured by lysis with water or NP 40) after subtraction of the spontaneous release.

In this reaction in the mouse, the effector cell is an Ly 2^+, 3^+-T cell. For the destruction of the target cell, neither B cells nor macrophages need be present. The effector cells are either still in the blast stage or have, after stimulation, already transformed back into small lymphocytes. Upon a second contact with the antigen (e.g., 10–30 days), effector cells need not go through a proliferative phase; they are completely effective lytically. However, it appears that effector cells are short-lived, because one no longer observes lysis when primary stimulated cells come into renewed contact with the antigen after a few weeks, although an accelerated proliferative response can still be seen; this proliferative response is probably dependent on T helper cells (Ly-1$^+$), which accordingly survive longer. Direct contact between effector cells and target cells is required for lysis.

Specificity and Genetics. From studies of families with children who exhibit recombinant *HLA* haplotypes, the following results were obtained:

1) *Responder-stimulator combinations which differ* for HLA-A, HLA-B, and HLA-D, show a good proliferative reaction, and generate cytotoxic effector cells that specifically destroy target cells carrying the same *HLA* haplotype as the stimulator; likewise, target cells that have only the HLA-A and/or HLA-B antigens in common with the stimu-

lator cell are destroyed. Target cells that share the HLA-D determinants with the target cell but whose HLA-A and HLA-B antigens differ from those of the stimulator cell are not destroyed.

2) *Responder-stimulator combinations which are identical* for HLA-A and HLA-B antigens, but differ for HLA-D determinants, exhibit a good proliferative reaction but no formation of effector cells, i.e., target cells that are identical with the stimulator cells are not destroyed.

3) *Responder-stimulator combinations which differ* only for the HLA-A and/or HLA-B antigen, but not for HLA-D determinants, show no or only a weak proliferative reaction and no cytotoxic effector cells; i.e., target cells with HLA-A or HLA-B antigens identical to those of the stimulator cells are not destroyed.

From these findings one can conclude that (1) for the induction of cytotoxic effector cells, the stimulator cell population must differ for the HLA-A and/or HLA-B antigens as well as for the HLA-D determinants from the responder cell population, and (2) the specificity for the effector cells produced is only directed against the HLA-A and HLA-B antigens of the stimulator cells, not against HLA-D determinants.

Further studies have shown that for the formation of specific anti-HLA-A or anti-HLA-B effector cells, the A or B antigen on the one hand and HLA-D determinants on the other need not be present on the same stimulator cells; rather, the latter (or the former) could be offered through a third cell. In principle, these results can be substantiated by studies with cells from unrelated donors. However, one finds here – in contrast to families in which phenotypic identity signifies also genotypic identity – a more or less strongly expressed cross-reactivity, i.e., effector cells that are induced against specific HLA-A or HLA-B antigens of a stimulator cell usually lyse not only target cells that have the HLA-A or HLA-B antigens of the stimulator cells, but also target cells that carry other HLA-A or HLA-B antigens. These

findings are explained by the high cross-reactivity of the HLA antigen known from serologic studies.

In the mouse, it has been found that all three loci, K, D, and I, can independently of each other induce a proliferative response as well as effector cell generation with specificity for K, D, and I molecules. It could be shown that the effectivity for the induction of K or D antigen-specific effector cells is significantly increased if, in addition to the K or D molecule disparity, a difference for I loci controlled determinants exists, i.e., in the proliferative reaction, Ly-1^+ (helper) cells as well as Ly-$2^+, 3^+$ (effector) cells are generated; the former enhance the recruitment of the latter (see above, MLR).

The different results obtained in studying man and the mouse might be explained on methodological grounds: In man, PHA stimulated cells are generally used as target cells; these cells do not express readily detectable DR antigens. In mice, usually LPS or ConA stimulated cells serve as target cells which express Ia antigens; if PHA target cells are employed, Ia-antigen-specific effector cells cannot be easily detected.

Antibody-Dependent Cell-Mediated Cytotoxicity. In addition to direct, cell-mediated cytolysis, another type of cell-mediated lysis can be observed, particularly in man: antibody-dependent, cell-mediated lysis (lymphocyte antibody lympholytic interaction, LALI, or antibody-dependent, cell-mediated cytotoxicity, ADCC). Human lymphocytes that are not specifically sensitized have the capacity to lyse target cells such as chicken erythrocytes, sheep fibroblast monolayers, Chang liver cells, a human liver-cell line, human erythrocytes, when these are charged with a xenogeneic or allogeneic antibody that reacts specifically with determinants of the target cell. For cell lysis to occur, the antibody must be complete, i.e., without the Fc fragment, no lysis occurs. Complement is not necessary for the reaction. Different mononuclear cells apparently can be used as effector cells, whereby different target cells from different effector cells are lysed:

1) *K cells* (killer cells) are nonadherent, nonphagocytic cells that exhibit neither B- or T-cell characteristics (Ig$^-$, Thy-1$^-$) and have the appearance of small to medium-sized lymphocytes. K cells carry receptors for the Fc fragment of immunoglobulin as well as for C3b and C3d. K cells lyse human lymphocytes that are coated with anti-HLA antibodies, chicken erythrocytes but not human erythrocytes, numerous cell lines, and some tumor cells, if they are sensitized with corresponding antibodies.

2) *B cells* also appear able to lyse coated chicken erythrocytes.

3) *Macrophages and monocytes* can lyse different sensitized target cells.

In addition to the cells mentioned here, other cells can affect sensitized target cells cytolytically, including fetal liver cells, lymphoid human cell lines, and long-term, non-lymphoid mouse culture tumor-cell lines.

It is not known whether this reaction plays a role in vivo, but there are a large number of K cells in mononuclear infiltrates of transplanted kidneys in patients who exhibit a chronic rejection reaction. There is also experimental evidence that this type of antibody-dependent cell-mediated cytotoxicity may play a role in virus infections and in certain types of neoplasms (melanoma, virus-induced and methylcholanthrene-induced tumors).

Specific Absence of Reaction Against Allogenic Tissue

Enhancement. Under certain conditions, allogeneic tissue, after it is transferred, induces no rejection reaction. One such situation will be discussed in detail below: specific immunologic tolerance. This form of lack of reaction is maintained by a cellular mechanism. Another form of the specific lack of reaction is enhancement. Enhancement can be transferred by serum and leads to prolonged or permanent survival of a tissue (or tumor) graft that normally would be rejected.

Enhancement can be achieved through active or passive immunization. The mechanism of immunologic enhancement is still unclear; however, it appears that antibodies that are not cytotoxic (i.e., cannot activate complement) bind with alloantigens on the surface and thus prevent the induction of a specific cellular immune response (afferent enhancement) or, by covering the alloantigen, obscuring the target for the cytotoxic killer cell (efferent enhancement).

In the rat, the preferred animal model in enhancement studies, it is also observed that during the production of alloantisera by repeated injection of lymphatic cells the recipient produces antibodies directed against idiotypes of its own anti-alloantigen antibodies (auto-anti-idiotype antibodies). Thus, antibodies with the specificity for this alloantigen disappear from the serum, as do probably also lymphocytes with the receptors that possess these idiotypes. The result of this reaction is also a specific lack of reaction to corresponding allogeneic tissue, a state in which the border between enhancement and tolerance begins to disappear.

Immunotolerance. Immunotolerance is a state of immunologic inactivity that is specific in regard to antigens or cells that, in normal animals, would induce an immune response. The most notable example of immunologic tolerance is the incapacity of the organism to be stimulated by its own constituents, even though these elicit immunogenic activity when transferred to other organisms. To explain this phenomenon, Ehrlich postulated the existence of a mechanism that he named "horror autotoxicus," by virtue of which the organism was incapable of producing antibodies against its own antigenic constituents.

The first clarifications regarding the phenomenon of immunotolerance originated from what could be classified as an experiment of nature: When dizygotic bovine twins occur, there is an anastomosis of the placental vessels. Each twin is born possessing not only red cells belonging to its own blood group, but also those of the sibling. Curiously, such red cells do not behave as antigens, that is to say, they are not recognized as foreign. Such twins possess a state of acquired immunologic tolerance which has been called chimerism [in Greek mythology, the chimera (Lat. *chimaera*, Gr. *chimaira*) was a fabulous monster with a lion's head, a goat's body, and a serpent's tail]. On the basis of these observations, made by Owen in 1945, Burnet and Fenner sought to explain why the organism did not form antibodies against its own constituents. They suggested that during embryologic development the organism "learned" to recognize its own constituents and thus predicted that if an embryo were injected with an antigenic substance, the organism would, as an adult, become tolerant to that particular antigen. The theory of Burnet and Fenner encouraged Medawar and his collaborators in England to extend the experiments of Owen, showing that dizygotic bovine twins failed to reject skin grafted between them, yet rejected in normal fashion grafts from other siblings.

The prediction of Burnet and Fenner was thus verified; corroboration followed by the Hašek group in Czechoslovakia. By joining in developing chicken embryos the chorioallantoid membranes, which are extremely rich in blood vessels, Hašek and his colleagues achieved an intense interchange of cells between the embryos (parabiosis). Under these circumstances, after hatching, neither bird was capable of producing antibodies against the antigens of its partner or of rejecting grafts of its skin.

In the experiments of Medawar, schematized in Fig. 10.3, embryos of strain A mice were injected on the 17th day of fetal life with a suspension of cells obtained from strain CBA mice[1]. Two months after birth, the strain A mice, having received skin from the strain CBA mice, were unable to reject such grafts, which remained viable for the entire life of the recipient animal. Meanwhile, these same animals retained the capacity to reject, in a normal period of time (10–14 days), grafts from other donors. This state of tolerance could be abolished by transfer of lymphoid cells from a normal strain A mouse, or from an animal of the same strain, immunized by previous contact with cells of the CBA strain. The breaking of tolerance required a longer period of time and a much greater number of cells in the first case. These observations demonstrate that tolerance represents an inherent form of reaction of the immune response and that the graft maintains its immunogenicity in the tolerant animal.

---

1 The cells of the lymph nodes and spleen are more efficient in inducing tolerance than those of the thymus or bone marrow

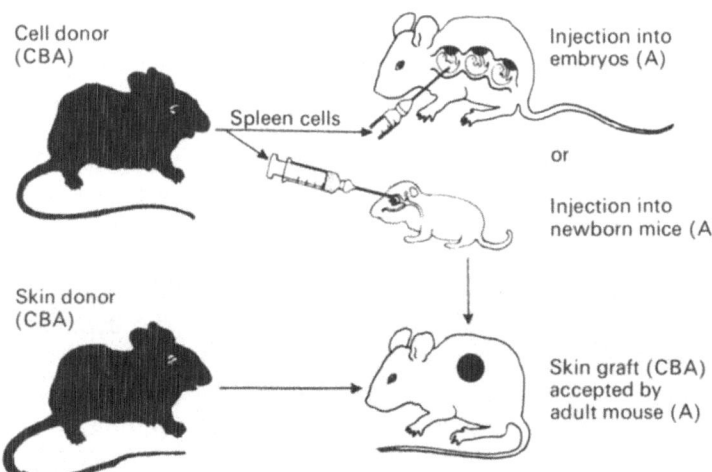

Cell donor (CBA)

Spleen cells

Skin donor (CBA)

Injection into embryos (A)

or

Injection into newborn mice (A)

Skin graft (CBA) accepted by adult mouse (A)

Fig. 10.3. Induction of immunologic tolerance (Medawar's experimental procedure). Embryos or newborn strain A mice are injected with spleen cells from strain CBA mice; the donor cells are not rejected because the immune system of the recipient is still undeveloped. Subsequently adult strain A mice, whose lymphocytes have acquired tolerance to the H antigen of strain CBA mice, accept skin grafts from them

The prediction of Burnet and Fenner was corroborated by numerous immunologists, who demonstrated, soon after the experiments of Medawar and Hašek, that the injection of numerous antigens into neonate animals produced a state of specific immunologic tolerance that persisted for a limited time (months or years) and disappeared gradually. A state of permanent tolerance nevertheless could be obtained by repeated injections of the same antigen. To maintain such a state of tolerance, the constant presence of the antigen appears to be indispensable.

In all species, there exists a period in fetal or postnatal life in which tolerance can easily be induced. The existence of this period, called "the period of tolerization," should not be seen as implying the existence of a period outside of which tolerance cannot be induced. Actually, contrary to what initially was maintained, it is possible to make even adult animals tolerant to allografts. To realize this possibility, however, it is necessary to repeatedly inject large numbers of the donor's cells into the recipient, or to maintain the two animals united by parabiosis for a determined period before performing the graft. The degree of genetic difference between the donor and the recipient determines the magnitude and the duration of contact with the donor antigens required to render the recipient tolerant.

Tolerance to "dead" antigens may be established with large or small doses. Tolerance for large doses, or "high-dose tolerance," requires quantities of antigens several times greater than those normally necessary to induce a perceptible immune response. Tolerance for small doses, or "low-dose tolerance," requires the continuous or repeated injection of quantities of antigen considerably smaller than those necessary to induce high-dose tolerance. The tolerogenic capacity of antigens is highly variable; however, generally speaking, weak antigens, i.e., poorly immunogenic antigens, are highly tolerogenic whereas strong antigens are poorly tolerogenic.

The induction of tolerance in adult animals is facilitated by diverse treatments that temporarily diminish the immunologic reactivity of the animal. Through the use of antimetabolic substances such as cortisone, X-rays, antilymphocytic serum, depletion of the lymphocytes by lymphatic drainage, etc., it is possible to achieve tolerance using a quantity of antigen that normally would induce an immune response. With certain antigens, such as serum proteins, it is possible to induce tolerance in adult animals using highly soluble *antigens*, which through ultracentrifugation, are rendered aggregate-free.

Animals that are already sensitized against an antigen and therefore have memory cells, can be made tolerant to this antigen only with great difficulty. In such cases, contact even with an extremely small quantity of a weak antigen stimulates a vigorous immune response, and it has not been possible to induce low-dose tolerance under such conditions. In special circumstances (e.g., in animals that have received an immunosuppressive agent and when large doses of a weak antigen are used), it is possible to induce high-dose tolerance even after a primary response.

It should be noted that immunologic tolerance may be partial as well as total. In the former condition, only part of the cellular population is rendered tolerant. Every time the lymphoid system enters into contact with an antigen, two alternatives are presented to each cell whose specificity is directed against this antigen: Either the cell proliferates, or it is blocked. In the first case, an immune response occurs, whereas in the second, tolerance results. It should further be noted that at the cellular level, cellular activation and tolerance are opposed phenomena; in the organism as a whole, the two phenomena may occur simultaneously, the dominance of one or the other depending upon conditions not yet understood.

As we have noted, two types of immunocompetent cells evolve during the response of the organism to a large number of antigens. One of these, the B lymphocyte, possesses on its membrane receptors for antigens similar to those of serum antibodies – these being direct precursors of the plasma cells. The activation of these cells requires, or is greatly accentuated by, the cooperation of one other cellular type, which itself is incapable of producing or of differentiating into cells forming antibodies: T helper cells. Studies regarding the mechanism of tolerance have demonstrated that both cellular types can be involved in this phenomenon. Thus, tolerance can, in comparison to thymus-dependent antigens, be determined by the absence of either a T-cell or a B-cell response. It was shown that T and B cells can be made tolerant, but that the induction mechanism, the duration, and the loss of tolerance are different for both cell types.

If T and B cells from animals tolerant to human γ-globulin are administered at various intervals, after induction of tolerance, to irradiated, syngeneic mice and the capacity of recipients to produce antibodies is then tested, it can be shown that T-cell tolerance can be induced with low doses of antigen and that it occurs more quickly (24 h in contrast to 15–20 days in B cells) and lasts longer (> 100 days) than B-cell (~ 45 days) tolerance. The findings suggest that natural tolerance to self-antigen is probably dependent upon T cells.

For thymus-dependent antigens, B- or T-cell tolerance is sufficient to make the entire organism tolerant. Because the threshold of tolerance for T cells is considerably lower than for B cells it is difficult in vivo to obtain exclusive tolerance for B lymphocytes, at least with protein antigens. However, this difficulty can be circumvented through the use of haptens conjugated to molecules that do not stimulate T cells. For example, specific tolerance of B cells for haptens has been produced by the introduction into the organism of haptenic groups conjugated to nonimmunogenic synthetic copolymers, to autologous proteins, or even to syngeneic erythrocytes.

Mechanisms of Tolerance. From the experimental data available, it appears unlikely that clonal deletion ("forbidden clones"), i.e., tolerance resulting from the elimination of lymphocyte clones specific for the tolerogen, as proposed by Burnet, is the underlying mechanism to induce and maintain tolerance. It has been demonstrated that lymphocytes can be sensitized against syngeneic tissue under appropriate conditions (e.g. in vitro) indicating that immune cells specifically reacting with self-determinants are not eliminated but present in normal animals; however, they appear to be inactivated or suppressed.

On the basis of experimental data, several mechanisms have been proposed for the induction and maintenance of tolerance which either result in the prevention of T-helper-cell activation, or the predominant activation of T suppressor cells:

(1) small amounts of soluble antigens which may interact with antibody and surface receptors, thereby preventing cooperation of macrophages, T helper cells and B cells; (2) large amount of soluble antigen, which lead to activation of T suppressor cells: high dose-tolerance (see above) induction is accompanied by an increase in DNA synthesis in thymocytes which proliferate and differentiate to T suppressor cells; (3) antibodies especially in small quantities have been shown to be immunosuppressive (see p. 334, anti-D antibodies in preventing fetal erythroblastosis); it is thought that antibodies prevent interaction of the sensitizing antigens with host lymphocytes by (a) forming soluble (antigen excess) complexes and, therefore, preventing the formation of stimulating aggregates on macrophages (B cells), and/or (b) covering antigens so that they cannot be recognized by T cells, and/or (c) acting as feedback inhibitors blocking the activation of suppressor cells specific for B cells or antigen specific T helper cells, or causing the formation of anti-idiotypic antibodies (see Chap. 6); and (4) antibody-antigen complexes, the effects of which are discussed in more detail in Chap. 9 (pp. 279).

It is now recognized that each individual possesses very low levels of autoantibodies in the serum, and the presence of T suppressor cells, preferentially in thymus and spleen, has been ample demonstrated: after transfer of thymocytes from mice tolerant to sheep red blood cells (SRBC) into normal mice the formation of anti-SRBC antibodies is blocked in the recipient. Mice treated with anti-T cell serum show an enhanced antibody response to pneumococcal polysaccharide; this augmented response can be abrogated by reconstitution with thymocytes. Experiments with carrier-hapten conjugates suggest that the T suppressor cell effect is mediated through carrier recognition like that of T helper cells; thus, thymocytes of carrier-tolerant mice suppressed the anti-hapten response after transfer to normal mice; however, when hapten-tolerant T cells are transferred to normal mice, B cells are able (allowed) to produce anti-hapten antibodies.

Thus, it appears that tolerance is the result of an actively maintained balance between help and suppression and requires the continuous presence of low levels of antigen and antibodies.

Organ Transplantation

The transfer of tissue and organs from one individual to another is not a discovery of our time. In the Middle Ages, attempts were made to heal wounded surfaces with skin grafts (Tagliacozzi). As early as 1800, Baroni carried out successful autografts on sheep. Paul Bert in 1860 described the different behavior of auto- and allografts. The first kidney transplants were carried out around 1900 by Carrel and Guthrie in cats. In different places, attempts were made to treat uremia with xenogenic kidney transplants. The biologic factors responsible for the failures remained unknown until the studies of Little, Loeb, Gorer, and Snell produced the first evidence of an immunologic rejection process. Medawar and his colleagues then carried out a series of classic experiments (1944–1946) that served as the basis for the progress in transplantation immunity observed today. The successful series of clinical kidney transplants between identical twins by Murray and Merril in Boston (1955) gave clinical transplantation a lasting impetus.

Today it is known that the prerequisite of a successful tissue graft is histogenetic conformity between recipient and donor. The methods of choice are the serologic typing of lymphocytes (HLA-A, HLA-B, HLA-C, and HLA-DR antigens) and erythrocytes (AB0 and P blood groups) and the mixed lymphocyte culture reaction for determination of histogenetic relationship.

Serologic Typing

Although clinical findings clearly indicate that the degree of serotypic identity and the graft survival time are directly proportional, there is the limitation that serotyping for unrelated pairs does not permit a prediction concerning the fate of the graft. The following factors support this statement: (1) antigens still unknown; (2) cross-reactions; (3) different individual reactions to HLA antisera and HLA antigens; and (4) the fact that serotyping encompasses only some of the structures responsible for the immunologic reaction.

Serotyping has a completely different value for family members in the phenotype and genotype are identical and whom the limitations just described play almost no role.

Cellular Typing

The MLC reaction has achieved a particular significance for compatibility testing because it can uncover differences for the major histocompatibility complex that cannot as yet be serologically recorded: HLA-D. In contrast to serologic typing, in which testing is based on identity, in cellular typing, differences between donor and recipient are uncovered. If stimulation by the donor cells is weak or nonexistent, then the graft function is usually good. The disadvantage of this method is that 5 days are necessary before the results are available, so that, in general, it can be carried out only for bone marrow grafts and organs from living donors. An accelerated but not yet routinely used modification of the MLR is the PLT (primary lymphocyte typing) test. In this test, specifically sensitized lymphocytes are used as reference cells. The cells are stimulated only by lymphocytes that possess determinants identical to those used for the first stimulation (see p. 152). The secondary proliferation occurs after 24 h. Cross-reactions represent a certain uncertainty factor, as does the fact that donor and recipient cells are not tested in direct contact with one another, but in relation to a third cell.

Clinical Organ Transplantation

Organ transplantation is an ideal therapy for many pathological conditions. However, histogenetic matching is only one of several factors that have to date prevented widespread application of most organ transplantations. Organ transplantation is, with few exceptions, still in its pioneer stages. Therefore, we shall restrict the discussion here to transplantation of kidneys and bone marrow, where substantial progress has been made in the last decade, and the thymus because of the theoretical importance.

Kidneys

The kidney was the first internal organ whose transplantation was attempted. The large number of patients who died from uremia was the stimulus for these attempts. The primary diseases are chronic glomerulonephritis and pyelonephritis, diabetic nephropathies, cystic kidneys, malignant hypertonia, and amyloidosis. Because hemodialysis now offers the anephric patient an alternative treatment, transplantation is no longer urgently indicated in all cases of terminal kidney failure. However, absolute indications include progression of uremic complications, hypertension, and the side effects of dialysis such as osteoporosis and polyneuritis. Patients with antibodies against the glomerular basal membrane are not suitable recipients for a graft because they often experience recurrence of the glomerulonephritis that necessitated the transplant in the first place.

Patients should be taken into a transplantation program early, because a graft as a last resort, i.e., when dialysis is no longer effective, represents a worse prognosis that an early transplant. In other words, it should be decided early whether a graft or dialysis should be used.

The large number of successful kidney transplantations – in contrast to most other organ transplantations – results partially from the organ's relative resistance to ischemia. This and the development of nationally and internationally organized exchange systems (Eurotransplant) and efficient conservation methods over recent years permit large-scale use of cadaver kidneys for implantation into the best-matching (ABO, HLA) patient. In addition, the kidney is the only organ (except bone marrow) that can be obtained from living donors.

Suitable donors are people killed in accidents and victims of subarachnoid hemorrhage or heart infarcts. Kidneys from living donors should only be considered if there is histogenetic identity. Kidneys from living donors who are identical for one haplotype (parents, siblings) and that show only minimal stimulation in the MLC reaction provide approximately the same chance of survival as kidneys from unrelated serotypic- and *HLA-D*-identical donors.

In general, the kidney is implanted heterotopically in the fossa iliaca. Immediately after the vessels are unclamped, the transplanted kidney becomes pink and achieves its normal turgor. When the kidney is not damaged, urine production begins immediately. Even though the chances of survival appeared slim (in 1963, only 6 of 176 people receiving a transplant survived longer than a year) in the early years of allogenic kidney transplantation, the chances of survival have increased considerably in the last 15 years. Today, the chances of survival for the recipient of an HLA-identical kidney

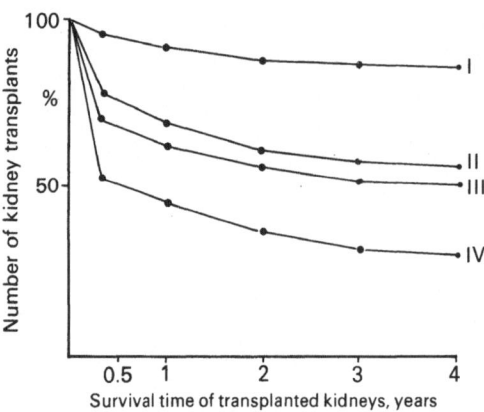

Fig. 10.4. Survival time of kidney transplant in relation to tissue compatibility between recipient and donor. *I*, Transplants from HLA-identical siblings; *II*, transplants from one haplotype-identical siblings; *III*, transplants from HLA-identical, unrelated donors; *VI*, transplants from HLA-different, unrelated donors. [From Hors et al. (1974) France-transplant: kidney transplantation as guide for bone marrow grafting. Transplant Proc 6:421]

from a relative is over 90% after 1 year and 85% after 4 years, those of recipients of an HLA-identical, unrelated kidney greater than 60% after 1 year and ca. 50% after 4 years (Fig. 10.4). Most deaths occur in the first 6 months. The survival rate of patients (not of the kidney) is today increased through (1) early removal of the graft when rejection occurs, with subsequent hemodialysis (or a second graft) and (2) reduced immunosuppressive treatment (see Chap. 14), which renders the recipient less sensitive to infection.

A hyperacute rejection reaction is rarely observed: When it does occur, immediately after resumption of blood flow, the kidney is irreversibly damaged due to intravascular thromboses. It is thought that circulating antibodies were present even before the transplant.

Acute rejection reaction is expressed as a decrease in bodily functions, swelling, pain, fever, tachycardia, general malaise, lymphocytosis, thrombopenia, lymphocyturia, and increase in blood pressure. An immediate,

intensified treatment with immunosuppressives can render the rejection reaction milder or cause it to stop.

Chronic rejection reactions are first manifested clinically as proteinuria. There is progressive obliteration of the vascular lumina and thus decreased renal perfusion. Tertiary hyperparathyroidism with bone dystrophy can occur as a result of disturbance in kidney function.

Specific complications accompanying kidney transplants include recurrence of glomerulonephritis in the transplanted kidney and metabolic disturbances. Immediately after transplantation, there can be intense diuresis and hypokalemia that result in severe dehydration and sometimes lead to shock or even death of the patient. Whereas secondary hyperparathyroidism is found in almost all patients with chronic kidney failure, after successful transplantation the parathyroidial function usually normalizes again – if not, a parathyroidectomy is necessary. Osseous alterations in children with hyperparathyroidism usually do not, in the case of a kidney transplant, re-form. Skeletal alterations and growth disturbances are therefore frequent causes of invalidism in young kidney transplant recipients. Heterotopic implantation of the kidney in the pelvis in general is not a contraindication for a pregnancy. The influence of immunosuppressive substances on the pregnancy and/or the fetus is not yet completely clear; normal children have been borne by recipients of kidney transplants undergoing immunosuppressive treatment. The immunosuppressives azathioprine and prednisolone do not appear to have any damaging influence on spermatozoa. Donor kidneys should not be obtained from patients with malignant disease, because tumor cells present in the transplanted kidney may be transferred, and the recipient dies from metastases. The infectious diseases that can be transferred from donor to recipient include in particular viral hepatitis and histoplasmosis. Thrombocytopenic purpura and hypersensitivity reaction also can be transferred.

Bone Marrow Transplant

In contrast to organ transplants, bone marrow transplants consist of the transfer of immunocompetent cells or their precursors. If the recipient and donor are not identical histogenetically, the transplant can lead to a further complication: the graft-versus-host reaction. Therefore bone marrow transplant assumes a particular place among the organ transplants.

Cases for bone marrow transplants include immune-deficiency diseases, aplastic anemia and severe hemoglobulinopathies, leukemias, and radiation damage. According to results thus far, identical twins (syngenic transplant) or HLA-A, HLA-B, HLA-C, and HLA-D identical siblings (allogenic transplantation) are acceptable as donors.

Recipients of syngenic bone marrow do not need any pretreatment with immunosuppressives (however, they may undergo cytoreductive treatment); the same is true for patients with severe, combined (total) immune deficiency who are recipients of syngenic or allogenic bone marrow. All other recipients of allogenic bone marrow must be pretreated with immunosuppressives in order for the bone marrow to be "taken." Patients with aplastic anemia are usually pretreated with cyclophosphamide, 50 mg/kg/day on each of 4 days followed 36 h later by the marrow infusion.

Acute leukemia is pretreated with chemotherapeutic (antileukemic) and total-body irradiation:

Six and five days before irradiation, patients receive 60 mg/kg cyclophosphamide in addition to antileukemic treatment. Irradiation is applied as total-body irradiation with 1,000 rad from two opposing sources (^{60}Co, two sources are necessary to achieve homogeneous irradiation).

With the donor under narcosis, the bone marrow is taken from the iliac crest by multiple aspirations, usually 400–800 ml. Using filtration through a sieve, a single-cell suspension is produced. The number of cells transferred intravenously can vary between 10^8 and 10^9 per kg. In the presence of severe immunodeficiency, purified stem cells in small but repeated doses might be infused. Whether the purification of stem cells is necessary and advantageous for the success of a bone marrow transplant is strongly affirmed by some (van Bekkum) but questioned by others.

The acceptance of a transplant is evident from the fast increase in the numbers of granulocytes, reticulocytes, and thrombocytes in the blood between the 10th and 30th day after transplantation. Chimerism, i.e., the survival of the donor's cells, can be verified by the presence of donor blood group markers, immunoglobulin allotypes, blood cell enzyme allotypes, or chromosomal markers (sex chromosome).

Acute graft versus host reactions are characterized by hepatomegaly with increase in transaminase level and jaundice, intestinal disturbances, decreased in blood cell counts, and erythematous eruptions. Chronic graft-versus-host reactions cause autoimmune-like symptoms, i.e., scleroderma-like skin alterations (see p. 395), sicca-syndrome (see p. 390), and chronic aggressive hepatitis (see p. 385).

Prophylactic immunosuppressive therapy post-transplantation consists of administration of corticosteroid, cyclophosphamide, methotrexate, or cyclosporine A for the first 100 days; with the occurrence of an acute graft-versus-host reaction, corticosteroid doses are increased and anti-lymphocyte serum (or gamma globulin) is additionally administered. In cases of chronic graft-versus-host reactions, a long-term therapy with steroids and azathioprine is necessary. Whether a germ-free environment (gnotobiotic unit, lamina flow) is an advantage for the survival of the patient after transplantation, except for the presence of immunodeficiency, is not yet clear.

The prognosis of bone marrow transplantation has improved considerably since the first operations at the end of the 1960s. In most transplant centers, up to 80% of patients with aplastic anemia who had received syngeneic bone marrow had been cured. Patients with aplastic anemia who had received transfusions prior to the marrow graft of allogeneic, HLA-identical donors, and were conditioned for engraftment by the administration of cyclophosphamide recovered to about 50%. In contrast, about 95% of the patients who had never received blood transfusion have been cured under the same regimen.

The prognosis for leukemia is not as good as for aplastic anemia. In the Seattle group, 37% of leukemic patients pretreated with cyclophosphamide and total body irradiation (TBI), and who had received syngeneic (identical twins) bone marrow, survived in remission more than 7 years following transplantation.

After allogeneic (HLA-identical) bone marrow transplantation, approximately 25% of those with acute lymphatic leukemia (ALL), and about 17% of those with acute myeloic leukemia (AML) survived more than 2 years. More than half of patients with acute myeloic or lymphatic leukemia who had received a bone marrow graft during remission showed long-term survial.

The causes of death in bone marrow transplantation in the presence of aplastic anemia or leukemia are rejection reactions, graft-versus-host reactions, infections (general, and specific as cytomegalovirus and pneumocystis carinii), recurrent leukemia (but not aplasia!), and immunodeficiency (humoral as well as cellular, of unknown etiology).

Of 14 patients in the Minnesota Group (Good) with severe immunodeficiency (autosomal recessive, sex-linked immunodeficiency and Swiss-type agammaglobulinemia) who received bone marrow transplants, five survived more than 2 years; of these, three patients were able to lead a normal life for 3, 4, and 5 years, respectively. In most cases, the cause of death was a combination of graft-versus-host reaction and infection (sepsis).

Thymus

The effects of neonatal thymectomy were cured experimentally by thymus implant.

As a result, thymus transplants were performed in patients with immunologic insufficiency syndrome (see Chap. 12). A thymus implant is considered for patients suffering from decreased or failed thymus function, i.e., those with Di George's syndrome and Swiss-type agammaglobulin anemia. In some cases, considerable improvement was achieved after transplantation of a histogenetically almost identical thymus, in some cases combined with bone marrow transplant. In one case with an isolated T-cell defect, clear improvement was achieved by implantation of a fetal thymus. A possible alternative is the administration of purified thymus hormone (thymosin, see Chap. 1). In patients with primary (thymus aplasia) or secondary (lymphatic leukemia and other neoplasms) immune insufficiency, noticeable improvement in immunologic capacity was achieved by administration of a thymosin fraction (from calf thymus). However, it appears that long-term therapy is necessary to maintain this effect. In contrast, one patient with combined immune deficiency exhibited no improvement of immunologic function after administration of thymosin. This finding may indicate that in certain cases of immune deficiency later steps in differentiation are not disturbed and that developmental disturbances exist at the level of the lymphopoietic stem cells or prolymphocytes.

Blood Transfusion

Repeated transfusion leads to the formation of leukagglutinating and lymphocytotoxic anti-HLA antibodies. The presence of such antibodies in polytransfused patients can lead to nonhemolytic, febrile, and urticaria-accompanying reactions. However, there is no absolute correlation between antibody titer and the intensity of the reaction.

To prevent such reactions with antileukocytic antibodies patients can receive leukocyte- and platelet-free blood. In this way, the numbers of leukocytes and thrombocytes are sharply reduced by mechanical methods.

Thrombocyte Transfusion. In patients who have antibodies against HLA antigens – even when clinically no transfusion reaction occurs – the survival time of leukocytes and thrombocytes is sharply reduced because they are destroyed and eliminated. Antibodies against platelet-specific antigens (Zw, Ko, and Pl[e]) in general play a minimal role in this reaction, although severe cases of incompatibility with the Pl[A] system due to the presence of anti-Pl antibodies have been observed.

It is therefore advantageous for patients who need regular platelet transfusions to use HLA-identical, at best related, donors.

Leukocyte Transfusion. Leukocyte transfusions are used primarily as preventive or curative measures for infection in severe aplasia or agranulocytosis. Because the survival time of granulocytes and monocytes is short (half-life less then 6 h), the transfusion must be repeated frequently at short intervals in order to be effective. Also in these cases donors should be HLA-typed and only those who are most similar to the recipient should be chosen. Whether alloantigens are significant on neutrophilic leukocytes (NA, NB, and the 9 system) is unknown. However, it is known that neutropenia in a newborn can result from maternal antibodies against NA or NB.

For a more detailed description of erythrocyte and plasma transfusions, see Chap. 8.

References

Albert ED, Baur MP, Mayr WR (eds) (1984) Histocompatibility Testing 1984, Springer, Berlin Heidelberg New York Tokyo

Burnet FM (1969) Self and non-self. Cambridge University Press, Cambridge

Cantor H, Boyse EA (1975) Functional subclasses of T lymphocytes bearing different Ly antigen. I. The generation of functionally distinct T cell subclasses is a differentiative process independent of antigens. J Exp Med 141:1376

Cantor H, Boyse EA (1975) Functional subclasses of T lymphocytes bearing different Ly antigens. II. Cooperation between subclasses of Ly[+] cells in generation of killer cell activity. J Exp Med 141:1390

Dresser DW, Mitchison NA (1968) The mechanism of immunological paralysis. Adv Immunol 8:129

Eisen HN (1974) Immunology. In: Introduction to molecular and cellular principles of the immune response. Harper and Row, New York

Feldman M, Nossal GJ (1972) Tolerance enhancement and the regulation between T cells, B cells and macrophages. Transplant Rev 13:3

Floersheim GL (1971) Transplantationbiologie. Springer, Berlin Heidelberg New York

Götze D (ed) (1977) The major histocompatibility system in man and animals. Springer, Berlin Heidelberg New York

Gold P (1971) Organ transplantation. In: Freedman SO (ed) Clinical immunology. Harper and Row, New York, pp 419–464

Hašek MA, et al. (1962) Mechanisms of immunological tolerance. Pub House Czechoslovac Acad Sci, Prag

Heimpel H, Gordon-Smith EC, Heit W, Kubanck B (eds) (1979) Aplastic anemia. Springer, Berlin Heidelberg New York

Howard J, Mitchison NA (1975) Immunological tolerance. Prog Allergy 18:43

Klein J (1975) The biology of the mouse histocompatibility-2 complex. Springer, Berlin Heidelberg New York

Landy M, Braun W (eds) (1969) Immunological tolerance. A reassessment of mechanisms of the immune response. Academic, New York

MacLennan ICM, Harding B (1974) Workshop report: Non-T cytoxicity in vitro. In: Brent L, Holborow J (eds) Progress in immunology II, vol 3. North-Holland, Amsterdam, pp 347–350

Medawar PB (1961) Immunological tolerance. Nobel lecture. Nature 189:14

Nossal GJV (1971) Recent advances in immunological tolerance. In: Prog Immunol Academic, New York, p 666

Rood J van, van Leeuwen A, Termijtelen A, Kuening JJ (1976) B cell antibodies, Ia-like determinants, and their relation to MLC determinants in man. Transplant Rev 30:122

Santos GW, Elfenbein GJ, Tutschka PJ (1979) Bone marrow transplantation. Transplant Proc 11:182

Snell GD, Dausset J, Nathenson S (1976) Histocompatibility. Academic, New York

Thomas ED, Storb R, Clift RA, Fefer A, Johnson EL, Neiman PE, Lerner KG, Glucksberg H, Buckner D (1975) Bone marrow transplantation. Part I. N Engl J Med 292:832; ibid Part II. N Engl J Med 292:895

Voisin G (1971) Immunological facilitation, a broadening of the concept of the enhancement phenomenon. Prog Allergy 15:328

Weigle WO (1973) Immunological unresponsiveness. Adv Immunol 16:61

Chapter 11   Immuity

Dietrich Götze and Wilmar Dias da Silva

Contents

Mechanisms of Immunity 317
Natural Immunity 317
   Polymorphonuclear Cells 320
   Macrophages 326
   Interaction of Microorganisms
     with Phagocytes 329
Adaptive Immunity 330
Immune Response to Infections 331
   Special Aspects of Bacterial Infections . . . 334
   Special Aspects of Viral Infections 334
   Special Aspects of Protozoal
     and Metazoal Infections 339
Acquisition of Immunity 350
   Passively Acquired Immunity 350
   Actively Acquired Immunity 355
References 357

Mechanisms of Immunity

The resistance to infections is based on several defense lines erected at different levels of specificity: natural or nonspecific immunity, and adaptive, acquired, or specific immunity.

In simplified terms, natural resistance refers to the ability of an individual to resist infections through normal body functions. Natural resistance does not include resistance resulting from a previous exposure to the pathogenic organism or its toxic products; this is adaptive resistance. Natural resistance relies on nonadaptive or normal activities of an organism that are always present. On the other hand, natural resistance and adaptive immunity are intimately connected and operate together; deficiencies on

either part will result in a marked increase in frequency and severity of infections (see Chap. 12).

Natural Immunity

The first lines of defense are skin and mucosa. They are not a mere physical barrier: desquamation and other forms of epithelial cell turnover at body surfaces remove large numbers of adherent microbes; in addition, it is known that lactic acid in sweat and unsaturated fatty acids from sebaceous glands are microbiocidal: skin and mucosa produce chemical disinfectants. Salivary glycolipids prevent attachment of potentially cariogenic bacteria to oral epithelial cell surfaces. Saliva and milk contain a lactoperoxidase-$SCN-H_2O_2$ system that possesses antibacterial activity. Mucosal tissue produces a gelatinous-like bioadhesive slime; microorganisms impinging on this film are caught and swept away by the cilial activity of the cell layer beneath the mucous film. Nasal mucus, tears, saliva, and also urine contain lysozyme (muramidase, see below) in high concentration, which cleaves a β-1,4-glycosidic bond that unites N-acetylglucosamine and muramic acid, a substrate accessible in the cell wall of gram-positive bacteria (in gram-negative bacteria, the enzyme substrate is also present, but shielded from the enzyme by lipid). In the stomach, a very acid (pH 1.0) environment is not favorable for the growth of microorganisms. Bile acids are excreted as glycine and taurine conjugates and are deconjugated by intestinal anaerobes. Deconjugated intestinal bile salts are inhibitory for a number of microorganisms (e.g., *Cl. perfringens*, lactobacilli, enterococci). The small and large intestines are heavily colonized with the normal flora, basically noninvasive bacteria, which, however, produce certain acid end products and antibiotic-like substances. In addition, almost all secretions contain (preformed, natural) antibodies, which are produced in response to many different, continuously present bacterial antigens, primarily of the intestinal flora.

Acidity of skin and vaginal secretions retards local colonization by potential pathogens. Spermine, a polyamine present in prostatic secretions, is a potent inhibitor of gram-positive microorganisms. Seminal fluid also possesses potent bactericidal activity.

Intact skin is not easily penetrated. For many pathogens, the first step in initiating infections is attachment to epithelial or mucosal cell surfaces. This is in part a function of the microbial surface, e.g., pili of *gonococci*, *shigellae sp.*, *vibrios*. Many viruses have surface components which allow them to attach to specific cell membrane receptors, e.g., influenza agglutinin attaches specifically to N-acetylneuraminic acid residues on cell membranes; human cells have receptors for poliovirus. Attachment by itself need not be followed by penetration of the microbe into the cell; thus, *Mycoplasma pneumoniae*, *C. diphtheriae*, and *B. pertussis* remain on the epithelial surface. Other penetrate into epithelial cells, stay there (e.g., shigellae), and do not spread further. Staying inside cells, particularly in those which do not have bactericidal systems (which phagocytes possess), protects the microorganisms from antibodies (and antibiotics), and very often from ingestion and killing by phagocytes (see below).

The host defense against these activities is manifold: (a) the above-mentioned "chemical factory" of outer and inner dermis may prevent effective attachment; (b) rapid turnover of the outer cell layer sweeps away attached or even penetrated microbes; (c) antibodies at the local mucosal level play a significant role in the interference with possible infections. The antibody response at mucosal surfaces is mediated primarily by secretory IgA. Mucosal immunity appears to be highly localized: elevated antibody titers in salivary secretions may not be associated with similar activity in the tears. This local activity is also suggested by the anatomical situation, i.e., the high number of lymphoid nodules of the tonsillary ring of Waldeyer, of the ileum (Peyer patches), and the diffuse lymphoid tissue in the lamina propria of the trachea, small intestine, and vaginal mucosa, all of which are directly fed by capillary lymph vessels coming from the mucosal surface.

It appears that secretory IgA has major importance in protection from many virus infections (e.g., poliomyelitis) by neutralizing infectious microbes on the mucosal surface. Of course, some microorganisms have developed mechanisms to prevent the action of IgA: thus, *N. gonorrhoeae* and *N. meningitidis* possess IgA proteolytic activity in vitro, cleaving and so inactivating IgA. This game of effect and countereffect played by invaded and invading participants is the essence of resistance and susceptibility (see below).

Pathogens successfully penetrating these barriers will be confronted with the internal armour of defense. The polymorphonuclear (PMN) leukocytes are generally considered to be the first to fight against bacterial invasions, reflecting the fact that these cells are the first to arrive at the scene. The PMN is thus the hallmark of the acute inflammatory process. If the bacterial invasion is sufficiently strong such that the PMN are unable to cope with the swarms of invaders, the second in line, the macrophages, will take over, giving rise to the condition of chronic inflammation. The third line of defense, the adaptive immunity, becomes established only after lymphocytes have been stimulated and activated by "activated and antigen-presenting" macrophages (Fig. 11.1).

Polymorphonuclear cells and macrophages have been termed "professional" phagocytes, because their membranes possess specialized receptors for the Fc portion of IgG

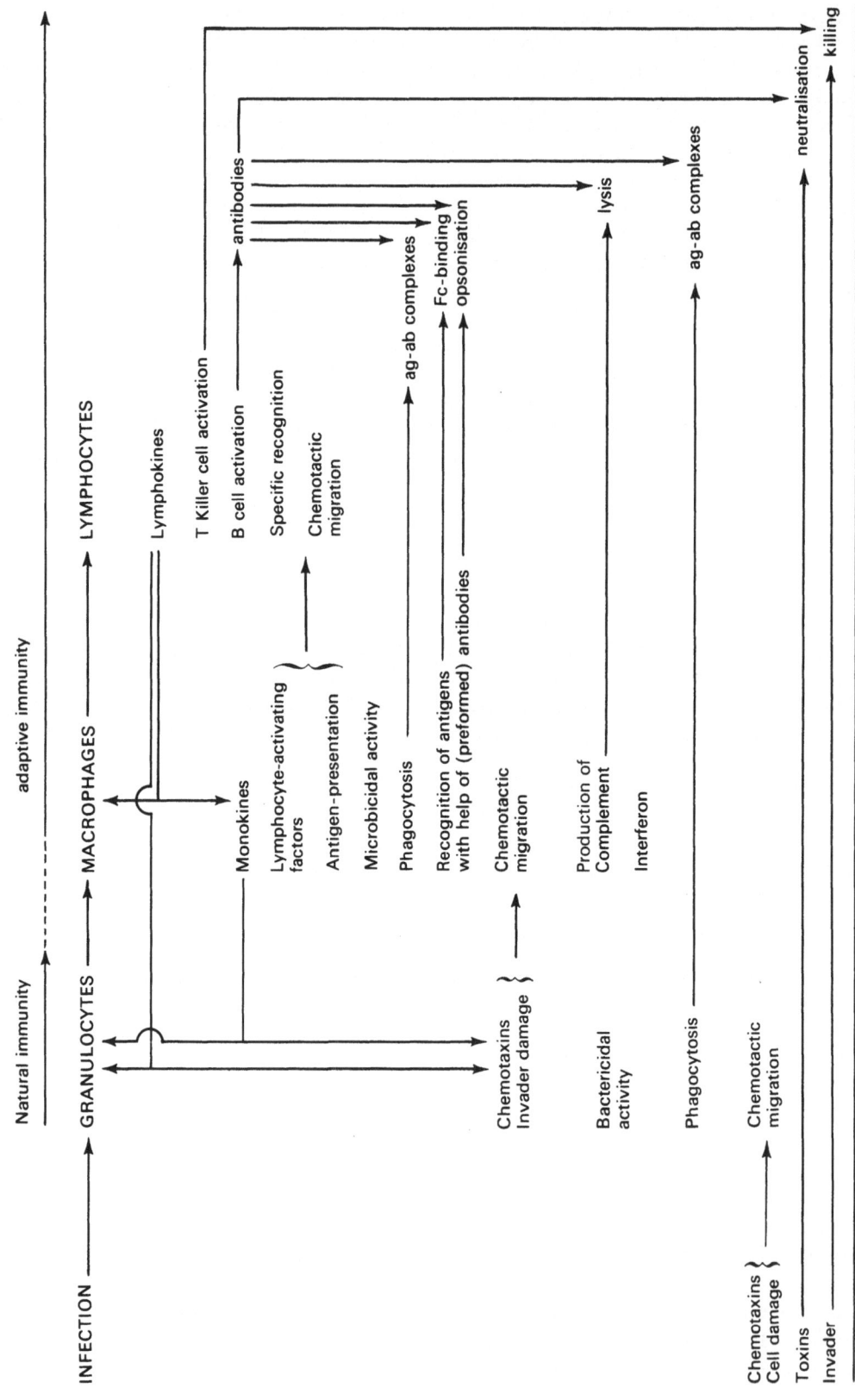

Fig. 11.1. Sequence of defense actions against infectious agents

molecules (IgG$_1$ and IgG$_3$ subclasses in man), and for activated C3. Nonprofessional or facultative phagocytes include endothelial cells, epithelial cells, fibroblasts, and other cells which will ingest microorganisms under specialized conditions but which do not possess receptors for IgG and C3.

Polymorphonuclear cells are concerned principally with the destruction of microorganisms which rely upon the evasion of phagocytosis for survival, i.e., extracellular pathogens; their prototype is the pneumococcus. Mononuclear cells are concerned with the control of microorganisms which are able to survive intracellular residence and against which neutrophils are ineffective.

Natural immunity does not only rely on the activity of the two phagocytic cell systems but is supported by factorial systems present in the blood. These are the pool of so-called natural or *preformed antibodies*, the *complement systems*, and certain proteins such as *betalysin, lysozyme*, and *C-reactive protein*.

Natural or *preformed antibodies* are actually not "natural" but have been formed by specifically stimulated antibody-secreting cells. We do not know their specificity in terms of which particular material induced their formation. They are formed primarily against microbial antigens of the intestinal flora and other "commensal" microorganisms, and against any other microbes which happen to come in close contact with the immune system, but are not necessarily pathogenic. Animals which have been delivered by caesarean section into a germ-free environment, and further raised under germ-free conditions, have a less well-developed immune system; the immunoglobulin synthesis is drastically reduced in comparison to animals raised conventionally. The factors and activities of the *complement system* have been described in detail in Chap. 5.

Betalysin is a highly reactive heat-stable cationic protein; it is released from platelets and destroys nonenzymatically the cell membrane of gram-positive microorganisms, except pneumococci. The characteristics and mechanisms of action of lysozyme, which is present in serum in a concentration of 1–2 µg/ml, will be discussed below.

C-reactive protein (CRP) is a nonimmunoglobulin acute-phase protein which appears in increased amounts in sera during infection and tissue damage; it is synthesized in the liver and released into the blood. CRP forms calcium-dependent precipitating complexes with somatic C-polysaccharide of pneumococcus, and of several other bacteria and fungi; it induces increased (random) migration of leukocytes, promotes phagocytosis, and activates complement through the classical pathway.

Polymorphonuclear Cells

After infection, PMN cells detect the pathogen and migrate out of the blood stream and into the tissue area where the intrusion occurred. This sequence of events involves an *increase in the permeability* of the capillary wall, *migration* through the endothelial gap of the vessel, and directed movement of the cell toward the pathogen in the tissue (*chemotaxis*). The initial "trigger mechanisms" that initiate these changes are not known with certainty but probably the bacterial surface and bacteria-produced substances are the activating components.

Migration

Permeability. Alteration in vascular permeability after the onset of the acute bacterial infection has a biphasic character; the initial phase of increased permeability begins immediately and lasts for no more than 1 h. A delayed second phase starts after about 2 h and reaches a peak after 4–6 h before subsiding. The first increase is almost certainly due to a release of histamine (serotonin in mice and rats) from basophils and mast cells. The mediators of the delayed permeability response are not identified with certainty, but kinins appear to be the most likely candidates; they are generated as indicated in Fig. 11.2. Possible other mediators are prostaglandins and the slow-reacting substance (see p. 253).

Migration. Concomitant with increased permeability, neutrophils adhere to the endothelium of blood vessels, extend pseudopodia, and penetrate the endothelium at or near the cell junction. The signal for adherence and emigration of cells has not been documented but it is assumed that the cells are responding to some type of chemotactic stimulus (see below). The cell movement is due to microfilaments and microtubules. The microfilaments are composed of contractile proteins; actin, myosin, and actin-binding protein have been demonstrated in neutrophils and macrophages. The actin in leukocytes is capable of reversible polymerization which is thought to underlie cellular locomotion. Also, microtubules have been implicated in the normal process of directed cell movement.

Chemotaxis. Substances with chemotactic activity have been collected from bacterial growth culture supernatants in which they have been released; these are peptides containing hydrophobic N-formylmethionin at the amino terminus, and lipids. In contrast to mammalian proteins, bacterial protein synthesis is universally initiated by incorporation of N-formylmethionin and as such is bacterial specific and a possible candidate for the "recognition molecule" to which phagocytes can respond. Perturbations of cell membranes lead to the mobilization from membrane phospholipids of the prostaglandin precursor arachidonic acid; oxidized compounds of this acid, HHT (12-L-hydroxy-5,8,10-heptadecatrienoic acid) and HETE (12-L-hydroxy-5,8,10,14-eicosatetraenoic acid) are potent chemotactic factors for both eosinophils and neutrophils. Other chemotactic factors, generated by the interaction of bacteria with host components, derive from the activation by immune complexes of the classical, and by bac-

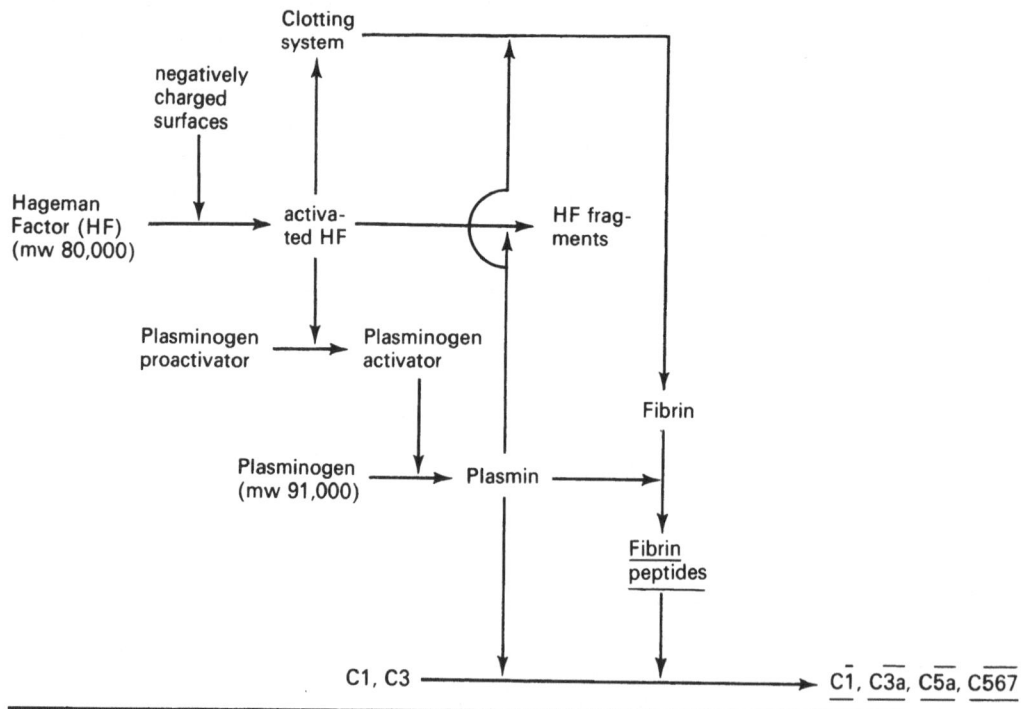

Underlined substances possess chemotactic activity

Fig. 11.2. Generation of chemotactic substances by the combined action of clotting and the complement system

terial polysaccharides of the alternative, complement pathway, as well as from activation by negatively charged surfaces of Hageman factor of the clotting system (see Fig. 11.2). Stimulated host cells, e.g., mast cells, release chemotactic factors for neutrophils and eosinophils. The eosinophil chemotactic factor (ECF-A) is a family of 300–500 mol. wt. peptides. ECF-A extracted from human lung was extensively purified and was shown to contain two acid tetrapeptides of amino-acid sequence Ala-Gly-Ser-Glu and Val-Gly-Ser-Glu. Both highly purified ECF-A were maximally chemotactic for eosinophils at concentrations of 10^{-7} to $10^{-6} M$. Analysis of analogues of the tetrapeptides revealed that a hydrophobic amino terminus is required for interaction with the eosinophil, while an anionic carboxy terminus is required for chemotactic activation.

The mechanism whereby the various factors (summarized in Table 11.1) elicit a directed migration of the cell is obscure. It has been demonstrated that chemotactic factors cause activation of an esterase that contains a serine residue at its active site. Cells that have previously been incubated with serine inhibitors are unable to respond chemotactically to either complement components or bacterial factors. Likewise, once the serine esterase has been completely activated, the neutrophil is no longer capable of further chemotaxis. One might expect increased activation of the enzyme as it comes closer to the source of chemotactic factors. Once the neutrophil has made its way from the site of origin in the bone marrow to the area in the tissue where bacterial infiltration has occurred, the cell begins to phagocytoze or ingest viable microbes with subsequent destruction of the microorganism within the cell. This process consists of several stages: opsonization, adherence of neutrophils to bacteria, and ingestion.

Phagocytosis

Opsonization. The rate and extent of phagocytosis depends on a number of factors, particularly the nature of the particle. Not all bacteria are equally susceptible to phagocytosis; cells have special difficulty in ingesting encapsulated organisms. To counter this

Table 11.1. Chemotactic factors for human eosinophil and neutrophil polymorphonuclear leukocytes[a]

Chemotactic factor	Source	Structural characteristics
C5a	Classical and alternative complement pathways	17,000 mol. wt. basic protein
C$\overline{567}$	Classical and alternative complement pathways	435,000 mol. wt. protein complex
Fibrinopeptides and fibrin fragments	Coagulation and fibrinolytic pathways	30,000–50,000 mol. wt. 1,000 mol. wt. proteins and peptides
C$\overline{3bB}$	Alternative complement pathway	234,000 mol. wt. protein complex
Bacterial soluble factors	Bacterial culture supernatants	300–1,000 mol. wt. peptides
Eosinophil chemotactic factor of anaphylaxis (ECF-A)	Mast cells	300–500 mol. wt. peptides
Histamine	Mast cells and basophils	111 mol. wt. amine
Crysta-induced chemotactic factor	Neutrophil lysosomes	8,400 mol. wt. glycoprotein
Lymphokines	Lymphocytes	12,500–60,000 mol. wt. proteins
Bacterial lipids	Bacterial culture supernatants	lipoproteins and lipids
HHT	Arachidonic acid cyclooxygenase pathway	280 mol. wt.
HETE	Arachidonic acid lipooxygenase pathway	330 mol. wt.

[a] After Valone FH (1980) Modulation of human neutrophil and eosinophil polymorphonuclear leukocyte chemotaxis: An analytical review. Clin Immunol Immunopathol 15:52

"armor coat" higher organisms have developed serum factors, opsonins, that attach to the bacteria and thus render them susceptible to phagocytosis. Two general classes of opsonins are known to exist (see also p. 197): (a) heat labile, derived from the complement system, involving activated components C 1, C 4, C 2, and C 3; and (b) heat stable, in serum of animals previously exposed to bacteria (immune opsonins). These are antibodies, primarily of the IgG_1 and IgG_3 subclasses.

A third factor stimulating phagocytosis was recently described and called "tuftsin" – because it was discovered at Tufts University in Boston. It is not really an opsonin but activates neutrophils to increased phagocytosis. Tuftsin is a tetrapeptide (threonine-lysine-proline-arginine) cleaved from gamma globulins (leukokinin) by the combined action of two proteolytic enzymes, one present in the spleen, and the other localized in the membrane of neutrophils (leukokininase, see p. 379).

Adherence is a prerequisite of subsequent ingestion but is not, in itself, sufficient. For example, mycoplasma adheres to human or rabbit neutrophils and this interaction leads to alterations of the metabolism in a manner similar to that observed with phagocytosis of particles, and yet no ingestion occurs. The adherence is thought to be mediated by receptors (Fc, complement), and appears to act as a trigger mechanism to initiate the biochemical events that accompany phagocytosis and bacterial killing by the cell. Concurrent with the attachment of a particle to the cell is a marked stimulation of the cellular metabolism including increase in oxidative metabolism and in lysosomal enzyme secretion.

Ingestion. Immediately following the attachment of the bacteria to the neutrophil under normal conditions, the phagocyte extends pseudopodia around the particle, eventually meeting and fusing to form the phagocytic vacuole (phagosome); the lining of the phagosome, therefore, is inverted plasma membrane. The phagosome buds off from the cell periphery and moves centripetally, apparently through the mediation of microtubules. The ingestion proceeds more readily if the particle is more hydrophobic than the membrane of the neutrophil; opsonization increases hydrophobicity. Parallel to these events, the phagocytic cells show an increased rate of glycolysis, a decrease in pH within phagocytic vacuoles – probably due to lactic acid accumulated as a result of increased glycolysis – and an increased turnover of lipids. The increased metabolism of lysophospholipids is of special interest since these compounds have detergent-like properties. Neutrophils possess a phospholipase-A activity that can remove a fatty acid from a phospholipid to yield the corresponding lysophospholipid. The presence of such enzymes in the plasma membrane may explain the turnover of membrane-lipid fatty acids and indicate the mechanism by which the cells reseal themselves. It has been suggested that membrane fusion might be facilitated by the presence of lysophospholipids in the membrane leading to the formation of micellar structures allowing fusion.

Bactericidal Activity

After ingestion, killing of bacteria depends upon two factors: *degranulation* of lysosomal constituents into the phagocytic vacuole, formation of phagolysosomes, and an alteration in oxygen metabolism referred to as *"respiratory burst."*

Degranulation proceeds by an unknown mechanism. At first, the specific granules with an optimal activity at neutral pH, containing lysozyme, lactoferrin, collagenase, and alkaline phosphatase, fuse with the phagosome. Only then, azurophilic granules (lysosomes) operating optimally at an acid pH and containing lysozyme, myeloperoxidase, acid hydrolases, neutral proteases, cationic proteins with bactericidal activity, and NADPH-oxidase, fuse with the phagosome; the activation of each type of granule is independent of the other. The net effect is that the contents of the various granules are brought into direct contact with the ingested particle. Frequently, the process of degranulation begins before the phagocytic vacuole is completely sealed; this results in the extrusion of granule constituents outside of the cell. This extrusion is selective, as only lysosomal enzymes accumulate in the medium during phagocytosis while cytoplasmic enzymes such as lactate dehydrogenase do not. This release of hydrolytic enzymes to the exterior of the cell may be responsible for much of the tissue damage that accompanies acute inflammation.

Oxygen-dependent Bactericidy. Concomitant with the ingestion and formation of phagolysosomes alterations in the oxidative metabolism, respiratory burst occurs. Cells that are unable to mount a normal respiratory burst show defective ability to kill many strains of bacteria; it appears, therefore, that these metabolic changes are necessary for the bactericidal activity. The respiratory burst is characterized by a marked increase in oxygen consumption which is cyanide independent, and therefore, mitochondrial-enzyme independent; an increase of glucose oxidation (via hexosemonophosphate shunt); and generation of high amounts of H_2O_2, and of highly reactive hydroperoxy radical (HO_2) and superoxide anions (O_2^-). The described appearance of chemiluminescence during phagocytosis is a reflection of superoxide anion generation since superoxide dismutase (SOD)[1] inhibits this chemiluminescence. Another reaction employed for the estimation of phagocytic activity, the reduction of nitroblue tetrazolium dye (NBT) to the insoluble blue formazan during phagocytosis, also shows an absolute requirement for oxygen and is inhibited by the addition of SOD; this reaction also reflects the formation of superoxide (see p. 363).

---

[1] Two molecules of superoxide anions interact in a dismutation (or disproportionation) reaction to form oxygen and H_2O_2: $O_2^- + O_2^- + 2 H^+ \rightarrow H_2O_2 + O_2$. This reaction is catalyzed by the enzyme superoxide dismutase

Since H_2O_2 can penetrate into the cytoplasm, the presence of catalase and coupled glutathione is important for its extra-vacuolar destruction. Similarly, superoxide dismutase may function to protect the cell cytoplasm from superoxide anions.

The biochemical basis of the respiratory burst is the initial activation of NADPH-oxidase. NADPH is generated by the hexosemonophosphate shunt (Fig. 11.3). In this reaction, superoxide anions occur as intermediates and can spontaneously give rise to singlet oxygen ($^1O_2$).

A large number of mechanisms have been considered to explain the actual killing of microbes by neutrophils. It is clear that multiple interlocking microbicidal systems are present, providing considerable redundancy in host defense mechanisms. The antimicrobial mechanisms of human neutrophils may be divided into two general categories: oxygen dependent and oxygen independent (Table 11.2).

Table 11.2. Microbicidal mechanisms and substances operating in neutrophils

Oxygen dependent
Peroxidase dependent: oxidizable cofactors (halides)
Peroxidase independent: H_2O_2, free radical forms of oxygen
Oxygen independent
Lysozyme
Lactoferrin
Hydrolytic enzymes
Hydrolysases
Cationic proteins
Nuclear histones

The oxidative mechanisms of killing may be divided into those which are myeloperoxidase (MPO) mediated, and those which are not. Peroxidase-mediated processes are: iodination, formation of hypochloride (OCl^-) or Cl_2 with subsequent formation of hypochlorous acid, and singlet oxygen generation (Fig. 11.3).

The myeloperoxidase, present in the azurophilic granules, catalyzes optimally at an acid pH, a condition which is met in the pha-

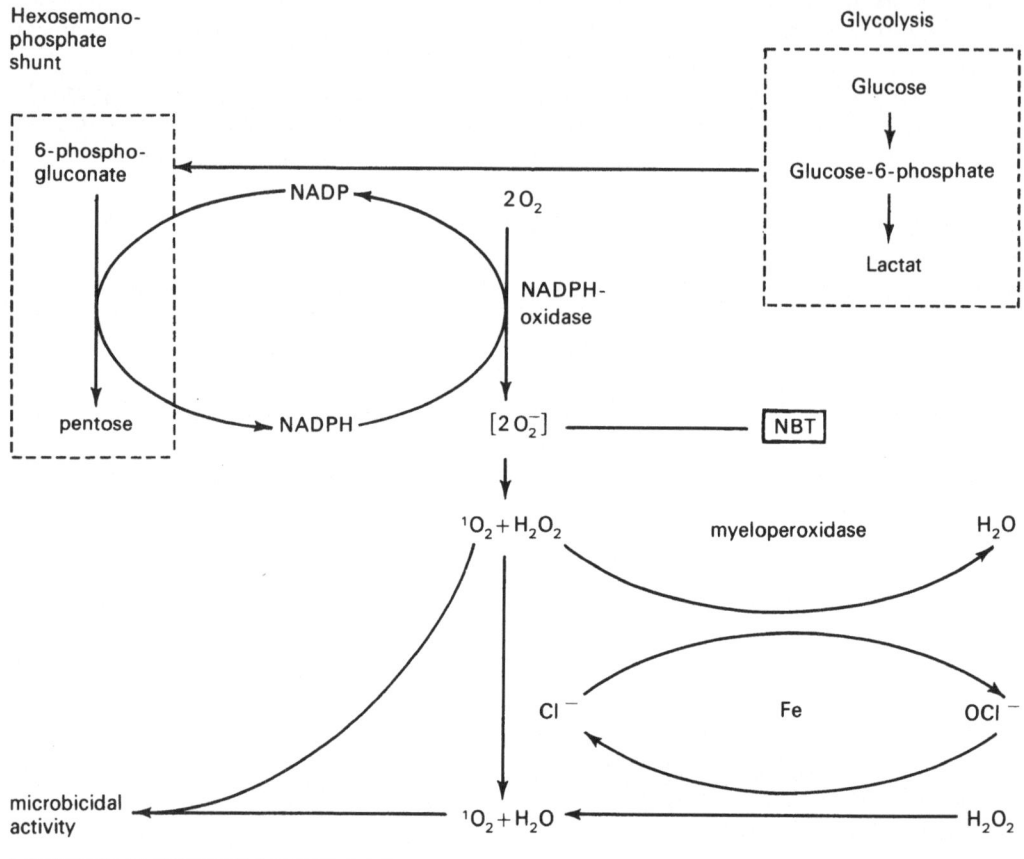

Fig. 11.3. Oxidative metabolism for the generation of H_2O_2, and its action with microbicidal mechanisms in polymorphonuclear cells

gocytic vacuole. In the presence of iodide (present in the serum in a concentration of < 1 µg/100 ml) or T_3 and T_4 which are membrane bound both to neutrophils and bacteria, microbial damage may occur through direct iodination of bacterial proteins, oxidation of sulfhydryl groups of enzymes or lipid peroxidation. Covalent attachment of activated iodide to tyrosine residues of external proteins of bacteria disrupts the protein's structure and results in alteration in permeability that causes the death of the microorganism.

Activated chloride might damage microorganisms by a number of mechanisms: oxidation of sulfhydryl groups, with enzyme inactivation; formation of aldehyde, which is known to be bactericidal,

$$H_2O_2 + \underset{\underset{R}{\overset{|}{\underset{|}{C}}}-NH_3}{\overset{COOH}{\overset{|}{}}} \xrightarrow[Cl^-]{MPO} CO_2 + NH_4 + R-CHO;$$
$$(HOCl)$$

and chloramine formation. Chloramines are amines, amides, or imides containing an N-chloro substituent; they are unstable in water, and release chlorine. It is thought that this reaction results in cleavage of proteins. Singlet oxygen is generated as a metastable oxygen intermediate during peroxide generation (see Fig. 11.3). It can react with compounds at areas of high electronic density such as unsaturated carbon-to-carbon bonds, to form oxygenation products

$$\underset{/}{\overset{\backslash}{C}}=\underset{\backslash}{\overset{/}{C}} + {}^1O_2^* \longrightarrow \underset{|}{\overset{O-O}{\underset{|}{\overset{|}{C}-\overset{|}{C}}}} \longrightarrow \overset{O}{\overset{\|}{C}} + \overset{O}{\overset{\|}{C}}.$$

A number of individuals have been identified whose leukocytes carbonyl products contain no MPO. The bactericidal activity of MPO-deficient leukocytes is characterized by a lag period, but the killing of most ingested microorganisms is eventually complete. Thus, MPO is required for optimal microbicidal activity but its absence from phagocytes is not totally disabling. Obviously, there are MPO-independent oxygen-requiring mechanisms for the destruction of invading pathogens. These are the generation of hydrogen peroxide itself, and the formation of free radical forms of oxygen, superoxide anion, and hydroxyl radicals resulting from the interaction of superoxide and hydrogen peroxide (Haber-Weiss cycle)

$$O_2^- + H_2O_2 \rightarrow OH + OH^- + O_2.$$

It has been demonstrated that this reaction occurs in human neutrophils during phagocytosis and that superoxide in combination with H_2O_2 results in products highly toxic to a number of bacterial species.

Oxygen-Independent Bactericidy. The preponderance of evidence suggests a major role for oxidative processes in the neutrophilic killing of most bacteria. Most studies suggest that H_2O_2 derived from dismutation of O_2 is the lethal species rather than the superoxide itself. In addition to these oxygen-dependent processes, nonoxidative microbicidal mechanisms are of obvious importance because certain microorganisms can clearly be killed by neutrophils under anaerobic conditions.

The simplest nonoxidative mechanism involves the decrease in pH (~ 4.5) that occurs within the phagocytic vacuole: some bacteria are very sensitive to acid (e.g., pneumococci); furthermore, a low pH provides optimal conditions for a variety of enzymes. *Lysozyme* was the first antibacterial substance to be discovered in leukocytes. It is a cationic (pI ~ 11), low molecular weight (14,000 daltons) protein consisting of a single polypeptide chain of 129 amino acids. Its substrate is the peptidoglycan portion of the bacterial cell wall (see p. 317).

Lactoferrin is a large protein (77,000 daltons) that is contained entirely within the specific granules of the cells. It may exert an antimicrobial function by binding and withholding iron required as an essential nutrient by the bacteria ingested, thus suppressing bacterial growth.

Some *hydrolytic enzymes* with different pH optima, e.g., alkaline phosphatase (pH optimum ~ 10), proteases, esterases (pH optimum ~ 7), are highly active in digestion of elastin, a particularly refractory substrate for proteolysis. Hydrolases, e.g., acid phosphatase, nucleases, a wide variety of carbohydrases, proteases, phospholipases, β-glucuronidase, neuraminidase, and aryl-sulfatase are released from azurophilic granules in large numbers. Cationic proteins are also released from azurophilic granules, also called "phagocytin" and "leukin." They bind to bacteria within the phagosome and damage microbial membrane barriers. Nuclear histones are substances which are released into surrounding tissue by death and autolysis of cells. They have a direct antimicrobial activity.

The intracellular killing of viable particles takes only a few minutes. Shortly after the microbes are digested, the membrane of vacuoles disintegrates and their contents are released into the cytoplasm causing the self-digestion (autolysis) of the neutrophil.

Macrophages

The mononuclear phagocyte system has its origin in the bone marrow monoblast and promonocyte (see p. 9). Only the intermediate stage cell, the monocyte, is ordinarily encountered in the circulation. Not nearly as much is known about macrophages as about neutrophils. Work with mononuclear cells is still in a more descriptive phase and biochemistry of these cells has been less precisely correlated with their antimicrobial and immunologic functions. The reasons for this deficiency lie in the fact that mononuclear phagocytes are functionally much more heterogeneous than granulocytes; unlike polymorphonuclear cells which are end cells and die when they have left the circulation, monocytes live for long periods (months, in man) and continue to differentiate after they have left the marrow, enter the tissue, and come under the influence of phagocytable particles and of lymphocytes. They cannot easily be obtained in bulk.

In general, it appears that mononuclear phagocytes ingest and kill microbes with mechanisms similar, or perhaps in some instances identical to those employed by PMN. They show less locomotion, they are sensitive to chemotactic factors which are different from those active for neutrophils. Chemotaxins for macrophages are C3a and C5a, C567 as well as lymphokines released by lymphocytes. They do not contain bactericidal cationic proteins and the MPO-peroxide-halide system as do neutrophils. On the other hand, macrophages are able to divide, produce a variety of active compounds involved in the immune response, including lymphocyte-activating factor(s) (interleukin-1) (see p. 170), monokines (Table 11.3), and can be activated by lymphocytes. After phagocytosis of

Table 11.3. Secretory products of macrophages, monokines

Regulator substances
    Interleukin-1 (lymphocyte activating factor, LAF)[a]
    Inhibitor of lymphocyte proliferation
    Colony-stimulating factor
    α_2-macroglobulin
    Prostaglandins
Effector substances
    Complement components: C2, C4, (C5?)
    Interferon
    Pyrogen
    Cytolytic, cytotoxic, cytostatic factors
Enzymes
    Acid hydrolases
    Neutral proteases
        Plasminogen activator
        Collagenase
        Elastase
    Lysozyme (muramidase)

---

[a] Acronyms are: MP, mitogenic protein; HP-1, helper peak-1; TRF-III, T cell replacing factor; TRF$_M$, T cell replacing factor from macrophages; BAF. B cell activating factor: BDF, B cell differentiation factor

microbial materials, processed immunogenic substances are presented to neighboring T lymphocytes; those which possess receptors for the presented antigenic determinants are stimulated. Stimulated T lymphocytes, in turn, release factors (lymphokines) that activate macrophages but also other T cells and B lymphocytes. Activated macrophages develop increased phagocytic and digestive power; they show increased attachment to and spreading on surfaces, a greater than normal number of lysosomes and mitochondria, an increased metabolic activity, and they are larger than normal macrophages.

Activated macrophages are not encountered in all stages of an infection. They occur rather late and reach a maximal concentration at a certain stage of the infection which depends upon species and number of infecting microorganisms. For instance, infection with *Listeria monocytogenes* causes an early appearance of activated macrophages in contrast to infections with *brucellae* in which activated macrophages appear much later. Macrophages are activated by immunological mechanisms; that can be demonstrated by adoptive transfer studies. Peritoneal cells of mice which have recovered from a sublethal infection of *L. monocytogenes* and which are therefore resistant to this organism are able to transfer this resistance to normal noninfected mice. Resistance cannot be transferred by serum from resistant mice. Parallel to the transferred resistance a delayed hypersensitivity to *L. monocytogenes* develops.

The activation of macrophages by lymphokines follows an immunologically specific interaction between lymphocytes and microbial antigens (presented by macrophages), but the expression of this reactivity is nonspecific against a wide range of microorganisms. Thus, macrophages activated by *M. tuberculosis* also show increased ability to digest and destroy other intracellular bacteria such as *L. monocytogenes* and protozoa such as leishmania. These and similar findings indicate that the acquired cellular resistance involves a heightened nonspecific microbicidal power of macrophages; this declines with increasing time after immunization perhaps parallel with the decline in amounts of persisting microbial antigen. Nonspecific resistance can be specifically recalled by the reexposure of the original pathogen. In persistent infections such as tuberculosis, macrophages can remain activated for longer periods, probably because of the continued expression of antigen.

Macrophages are also activated during the course of certain virus infections, particularly those in which macrophages are themselves infected, and can express this reactivity against unrelated microorganisms. For instance, when mice are infected with ectromelia virus and 6 days later injected intravenously with listeria, the spleen macrophages show an increased ability to ingest and destroy the bacteria. Less is known about macrophage activation in protozoal infections: in a resistant host, leishmania parasites are destroyed after phagocytosis by activated macrophages, and unrelated microorganisms such as listeria are also killed. Nonactivated macrophages, in contrast, generally support the growth of both leishmania and listeria. Mice primarily infected with protozoa *Toxoplasma gondii* or *Besnoitia jellisoni* become resistant to *L. monocytogenes*, *S. typhimurium*, and the fungus *Cryptococcus neoformans*. There is some evidence that activated macrophages in the presence of antibodies (to promote phagocytosis) give protective immunity in malaria; they ingest erythrocytes more extensively than normal macrophages.

Not much is known about the reactivity to metazoan parasites because of the enormous diversity in their structure, behavior, and habitat. But it appears that in cases of *Litosomoides carinii* infection macrophages are the major effector cell. After development from infective larvae, the adult worms reside in the pleural cavity and give rise to microfilariae that enter the blood stream. The termination of microfilaremia (onset of latency) is associated with adhesion of mononuclear cells to microfilariae in the pleural cavity. In vitro, cells from animals with latent infections were found not to adhere to microfilariae, but cells from normal or latent-infected animals adhered strongly in the presence of serum from latent-infected animals. Adherence is followed by death of the microfilariae. Furthermore, treatment of animals with antimacrophage serum led to the breakdown of latency.

In shistosomia infection, granuloma form around eggs in the lung; they contain macrophages but also lymphocytes and eosinophils. The relative roles of each cell type in egg destruction is not known, but eosinophils from infected animals are the most potent effectors of egg destruction in vitro (see p. 346).

The way in which activated macrophages exert their microbicidal activity is almost unknown. Increased phagocytosis per se is an inadequate explanation because intracellular killing does not necessarily follow phagocytosis. Actually, many pathogens "seek" phagocytosis to grow and multiply (Table 11.4). Phagolysosome formation with discharge of the content of lysosomes into phagosomes as described for PMN certainly contributes a great deal to the microbicidal activity. However, there is other evi-

Table 11.4. Microorganisms that multiply in macrophages

Protozoa	Leishmania
	Trypanosomes
	Toxoplasma
Fungi	Cryptococcus neoformans
	Coccidia
	Candida albicans
	Histoplasma capsulatum
Bacteria	M. tuberculosis
	M. leprae
	L. monocytogenes
	Brucellae
Rickettsia	R. rickettsi
	R. prowaẓeki
Viruses	Psittacoses
	Herpes-type viruses
	Measles
	Arbovirus (Dengue)
	Poxvirus
	Lymphochoriomeningitis

dence indicating that microbicidal activity cannot be explained solely on the basis of lysosome activity. There is a lack of correlation between antimicrobial activity and lysosomal content of activated macrophages; by electron microscopy studies it could be observed that in rabbit alveolar macrophages infected with several bacteria (*L. monocytogenes, S. typhi, S. aureus*) there was no fusion of large electron-dense, lysosome-like bodies with the phagosome, but there was fusion of smaller vesicles with the phagosomes. The bacteria rapidly showed signs of damage. Around the phagosomes there was the appearance of nonmembrane-bound granular or fibrillar dense material, which also appeared in the phagosomes.

Interaction of Microorganisms with Phagocytes

Pathogens successfully interfere with the antimicrobial activities of polymorpho- and mononuclear cells. As pointed out above, the sequence of events in natural resistance after penetration of the outer surface by microbes starts with the migration out of the circulation attracted by chemotaxins of granulocytes and macrophages to the site of invasion; they attach to the microorganisms, ingest, and kill them. Disturbance of any of these events results in a less efficient or even no reaction of leukocytes against invaders.

The most straightforward antiphagocytic approach of microorganisms is to kill phagocytes. This is, indeed, the case in infections with pathogenic streptococci which release hemolysins (streptolysines). As the name indicates, these substances lyse red blood cells, but have even more profound effects on phagocytes. Within a few minutes of addition of streptolysin O to polymorphonuclear cells, their granules "explode" and their content is discharged into the cytoplasm with resulting autolysis. Some pathogenic staphylococci also release various hemolysins. In addition, staphylococci also produce a nonlytic leukocidin; this protein acts on the leukocyte membrane and causes discharge of the lysosomal content into the

cytoplasm. *L. monocytogenes* releases similar toxins. In general, polymorphonuclear cells are more sensitive to these toxins than macrophages, possibly because their lysosomes are more easily discharged. In addition to the lytic activity, streptolysin in low concentrations has been shown to suppress chemotaxis.

A prerequisite for phagocytosis is adherence or adsorption of the microbe to the surface of phagocytes. *Mycoplasma hominis* prevents in some unknown manner adsorption to the polymorph surface. Streptococci possess on their surface M proteins which are responsible for their attachment to the surface of epithelial cells in sites of infection, yet they do not adhere to macrophages. Under the electron microscope, these proteins are identifiable as a fine hairy layer on the outer surface. It has been suggested that this coat permits the bacteria to slither off the surface of macrophages. Similarly, pneumococci, but also *Hemophilus influenzae* and *Klebsiella pneumoniae* owe their resistance to phagocytosis to their polysaccharide capsule; these bacteria are readily phagocytozed when decapsulated by hyaluronidase. The cell walls of gram-negative bacteria contain a lipopolysaccharide complex (endotoxin) with the somatic (O) antigen in the polysaccharide side chain (see p. 189). This structure causes inhibition of phagocytosis; gram-negative bacteria lacking this antigen are normally phagocytozed. Anthrax and plague bacteria possess a thin acidic polysaccharide capsule which causes inhibition of phagocytosis. All these microbes are readily phagocytozed when they are coated with antibodies, except *Staphylococcus aureus*. These bacteria possess a Protein A that attaches to the Fc portion of IgG and, therefore, prevents binding of the Fc portion, and thus the opsonized bacteria, to the Fc receptor on phagocytes. They may attach, however, to macrophages by the C3b receptor.

There are microbial parasites that do not mind being phagocytozed but then start to interfere with the normal killing and digestive processes. Actually, phagosomes can be seen as a cordon of forts protecting their "residents" from any attack from the outside, i.e., antibody, complement, toxins, phagocytic cells, cytotoxic cells, if by some means the formation of phagolysosomes is prevented or the discharged content inactivated. This strategy is indeed applied by some microorganisms which multiply in phagocytic phagosomes and eventually kill the macrophage (Table 11.4). *Mycobacterium tuberculosis* produces sulfatides that inhibit fusion of phagosomes and lysosomes. *Toxoplasma gondii, Aspergillus flavus, psittacosis chlamydia,* and *staphylococcus aureus* are all phagocytozed but have developed mechanisms that prevent fusion; nothing is known about these mechanisms. Another way around the antimicrobial activity is resistance to killing, of which we know almost nothing. It is, however, likely to depend on the nature of the outer surface of microorganisms, and the production of lytic enzyme inhibitors. Thus the outer surface of *Mycobacterium lepraemurium* contains waxes which are not readily digested by lysosomal enzymes; these bacteria grow in phagocytic vacuoles even after extensive fusion with lysosomes.

Viruses fuse with the cell membrane and enter the cytoplasm. If they are trapped in phagosomes, the membrane of which is derived from the plasma membrane, they also reach the cytoplasm by fusion, usually before lysosomes have fused. In case of reoviruses, exposure to lysosomal enzymes is necessary to "uncoat" the virus particle and thus help the virus to multiply.

Adaptive Immunity

One of the most important properties of the macrophage is its mediator function linking the natural and adaptive parts of the immune system. The carriers of specific immunity, the lymphocytes, do (almost) nothing on their own unless being told by macrophages. Highly purified populations of committed lymphocytes do not respond to antigens, nor do purified normal lymphocytes respond to allogeneic cells in mixed lympho-

Table 11.5. Lymphocyte mediators, lymphokines

Mediators affecting macrophages
Migration inhibition factor (MIF)
Macrophage activating factor (MAF, indistinguishable from MIF)
Chemotactic factors for macrophages
Mediators affecting polymorphonuclear leukocytes
Chemotactic factors
Leukocyte inhibitory factor (LIF)
Eosinophil stimulation promoter (ESP)
Mediators affecting lymphocytes
Interleukin 2[a]
B cell suppressing factor
Mediators affecting other cells
Lymphotoxin (LT)
Osteoclast activating factor (OAF)
Collagen-producing factor
Colony-stimulating factor (CSF)
Interferon
Immunoglobulin binding factor (IBF, probably identical to IgG-Fc receptor on T cells)
Procoagulant (tissue factor)

[a] Acronyms are: TSF, thymocyte stimulating factor; TMF, thymocyte mitogenic factor; TCGF, T cell growth factor; Co-stimulator; KHF, killer cell helper factor; SCIF, secondary cytotoxic T cell-inducing factor

cyte reaction or to unspecific mitogens. Without being told (stimulated) they do not produce lymphokines either.

The reactivity of committed lymphocytes to antigen requires the presentation by macrophages of processed antigen to them suitably associated with class II (Ia) molecules of the MHC (see p. 169), and the stimulation by a factor, interleukin-I, produced by macrophages. The first lymphocytes activated in this process are T helper cells, possessing receptors which can bind the antigen in association with Ia molecules. These cells then activate, in turn, B lymphocytes, T suppressor cells, and cytotoxic T lymphocytes,[2] which proliferate and differentiate to effector and memory cells. The activation of these effec-

---

2 It is not known with certainty whether macrophages and/or T helper cells are needed to generate cytotoxic T cells in cases of virus infections or allogeneic transplantation; it might be that cytotoxic T cells are able to recognize the viral or allo-antigen in association with class I molecules directly. T helper cells certainly augment the recruitment of cytotoxic T cells

Table 11.6. Physicochemical properties of lymphokines (see Table 9.5, p. 291)

Property	Lymphokine				
	MIF[a]	CTF[a, b]	$\alpha-$LT[a, c]	LMF[a]	IBF[d]
Molecular weight	23,000–55,000	12,000	75,000–100,000	20,000–50,000	140,000–300,000
Sensitivity to chymotrypsin/ trypsin	Sensible	Sensible	Stable?	Sensible	Sensible
neuraminidase	Resistant	Resistant	Resistant	Resistant	Sensible
Temperature (56 °C, 30 min)	Stable	Stable	Stable	Stable	Labile
Isoelectric point (pI)	4–6	10.1; 5.6	6.8–8.0	6.5–7.5	6.3
Electrophoretic mobility	Albumin	Albumin	α_2, β-globulin	–	–
Buoyant density (CsCl)	Protein	–	–	–	–

MIF, migration inhibition factor; CTF, chemotactic factor; LT, lymphotoxin; LMF, lymphocyte mitogenic factor; IBF, immunoglobulin binding factor
[a] From human
[b] Monocyte/macrophage chemotactic factor
[c] Two smaller components found in addition to $\alpha-$LT: $\beta-$LT, with a molecular weight of approximately 45,000, and $\gamma-$LT with a molecular weight of 10,000–15,000. These are not distinct substances but heterogeneous groups of unstable compounds
[d] From mice

tor cells requires the presence and binding of antigen by the interacting cells as well as the action of factor(s), lymphokines (Table 11.5), which are produced by lymphocytes. These factors, in turn, regulate the activity of macrophages and polymorphonuclear cells but also that of other lymphocytes.

Most of these factors are not, or not well, characterized, and it is not clear whether the numerous functional effects which distinguish them are caused by many distinct products or by only few substances displaying several effects depending upon the experimental conditions (Table 11.6).

Immune Response to Infections

In the immune response to infections usually all parts of the defense system participate, i.e., the natural and the adaptive system.

However, since the natural system does not confer immunity (or only in a very restricted sense), i.e., specific resistance to repeated infections by the same pathogen, the term immune response refers primarily to the response of T and B lymphocytes against infectious agents. For practical reasons, these two parts of the immune response are distinguished as humoral (antibody-mediated) and cellular (cell-mediated) immunity. Both types of the immune response are only efficient when adequately supported by the two other important adjuncts, the complement systems and the polymorphonuclear-monocyte systems.

The participation of the two arms of the specific immunity is revealed by several activities: antibodies enhance phagocytosis due to opsonization; they neutralize microbial toxins; they neutralize viruses; they form immune complexes with subsequent activation of the complement system resulting in lysis of microorganisms and cells, and the

Table 11.7. Tests for detection of antibodies in infectious diseases (see Chap. 7)

Test	Antigen	Positive result	Microorganisms
In vitro			
Hemagglutination inhibition	Hemagglutinin on the surface of viruses	Inhibition of agglutination	Rubella, influenza, mumps, measles, variola, vaccinia, arbovirus encephalitis, adeno- and rheoviruses
Hemagglutination	Microbial antigens adsorbed to erythrocyte surface	Agglutination	Rhinoviruses, serum hepatitis (HB$_s$Ag) brucellosis, leptospirosis, leprosy, typhus (Felix reaction), infectious mononucleosis (Paul-Bunnell), toxoplasmosis, American trypanosomiasis, schistosomiasis, malaria, amebiasis, tuberculosis, metazoa
Hemolysis	Streptolysin – anti-streptolysine	Inhibition of erythrolysis	Streptococcal infections
Latex test	Microbial antigen adsorbed to latex	Agglutination	Serum hepatitis B(HB$_s$Ag), leptospirosis, echinococcosis
Complement fixation	Microbial antigen reacts with antibody and fixes complement	Complement depletion	Most microorganisms
Precipitation, agglutination, gel diffusion	Antigen on surface of microbe, soluble microbial antigen	Visible agglutination or precipitation, precipitin line in gel	Salmonella (Widal), brucella, diphtheria (Elek), leptospirosis, histoplasmosis, aspergillosis
Immobilization	Antigen on locomotor organ (flagellum, cilium)	Inhibition of mobility	Treponema pallidum (TPI)
Immunofluorescence antibody test	Antigen on microorganism or antigen formed in infected cells	Binding of fluorescein labeled antibody (direct) or labeled anti-Ig (indirect)	T. pallidum, respiratory syncytial virus, malaria, leishmaniasis, trypanosomiasis, toxoplasmosis, trichinosis, filariasis, schistosomiasis
Radioimmune assay, ELISA	Microbial antigen	Binding of radiolabeled or enzyme bound antibody	Serum hepatitis (HB$_s$Ag)
Capsular swelling	Capsules on surface of bacteria	Swelling of capsule	Pneumococcus Klebsiella
Immunelectrophoresis	Soluble antigen	Precipitin line	Amebiasis, echinococcosis
Flocculation	Antigen (cardiolipin) adsorbed to surface of cholesterol crystals	Agglutination	T. pallidum (VDRL), trichinosis, echinococcosis, schistosomiasis
Methylene blue	Microorganism	Antibody and C cause loss of affinity of cytoplasm for methylene blue	Toxoplasmosis (Sabin-Feldmann)
In vivo			
Intradermal (immediate hypersensitivity)	Toxin, microbial extract	Erythematous induration within 24–48 h	Streptococcus (Dick), diphtheria (Schick), lymphogr. venereum (Frei), Echinococcosis (Casoni), filariasis, schistosomiasis, trichinosis
Neutralization	Virus; multiplication in experimental animal or cell culture	Antibody inhibits multiplication and prevents pathologic lesions or death	Most viruses

liberation of kinins; they render microbes nonmotile and inhibit their growth by coating them. The ways in which antibodies can be detected and assayed have been described in detail in Chap. 7 and are briefly summarized in Table 11.7.

It is, however, not sufficient for the diagnosis of a present infection to demonstrate that antibodies against a certain infectious agent are in the serum; such antibodies could have been the result of an earlier infection a long time ago. Usually, the activity must have a certain strength above a "normal" threshold, and must increase with time in order to indicate an ongoing infection. Antibodies do not appear immediately after beginning of an infection, but only after a few days or even weeks; thus, antibodies against the H agglutinins and Vi agglutinins in typhoid infections appear rather late (Fig. 11.4). In other infectious diseases, antibodies appear only after the disease is resolved (cutaneous leishmaniasis, see below). Thus, in many cases, the determination of antibody formation is not helpful in the early diagnosis of an infection, but usually extremely valuable in the assessment of the development of protective immunity – or its failure to develop.

Cell-mediated immunity might be detected by several means: In vivo, by the induction

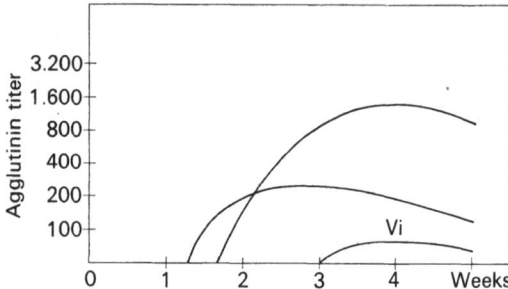

Fig. 11.4. Appearance of the anti-O, anti-H, and anti-Vi agglutinins during untreated typhoid fever [Adapted from Faure M et al. (1964) Les réactions sérologiques, 2éme ed. Albert de Visscher, Paris]

of inflammation and mononuclear cell infiltration by application of antigen into skin (see p. 286, tuberculin test). In vitro, by the proliferative response (incorporation of tritiated thymidin) of lymphocytes after exposure to the antigen; migration inhibition of macrophages (see p. 290); migration of macrophages and polymorphonuclear cells through millipore filters due to chemotactic factors; and destruction of cells bearing microbial antigens (e.g., virus) on their surface by cytolytic T lymphocytes, measured by the release of ^{51}Cr incorporated previously in the target cells (Table 11.8).

Table 11.8. Test system for assaying cell-mediated immunity

Test system	Outcome
In vitro	
Lymphocyte stimulation	^{3}H-thymidine incorporation of sensitized lymphocytes
Migration inhibition	Inhibition of macrophage migration (see Fig. 10.16)
Chemotaxis	Migration of macrophages into millipore filter (Boyden's chamber, see Fig. 5.8)
Blastogenic factor	Transformation of normal lymphocytes
Lymphotoxin	Cytotoxicity for certain cultered cells
Interferon	Protection of cells against virus infections
Cell-mediated cytotoxicity	Destruction of cells bearing antigens, e.g., viral antigens or haptens on the cell surface
In vivo	
Skin reactive factor	Induction of delayed hypersensitivity in guinea pig skin
DTH skin test	Delayed type hypersensitivity after injection of antigen (e.g., PPD, lepromin, parasite antigens)

The delayed hypersensitivity reaction in the skin does not become positive until several weeks in infections such as tuberculosis, brucellosis, and leishmaniasis, but after smallpox vaccination it is positive within 1 week. If the individual has been previously exposed to the antigen, the response takes a shorter time to develop, i.e., 1 or 2 days.

Special Aspects of Bacterial Infections

Bacteria owe their pathogenicity to two basic properties: invasiveness and toxicity. The invasiveness causes lesions at the areas of entry and metastases thereof; the formation of toxins leads to damages in areas far from the point of entry, sometimes systemic. Some bacteria are particularly invasive, e.g., pneumococcus and *B. anthracis;* others are pathogenic primarily because of toxin formation such as the diphtheria bacillus, *Clostridium tetani*, *Clostridium botulinum*, and the clostridia of gas gangrene. Frequently, invasive and toxicogenic properties are found together, e.g., in the case of *Staphylococcus* and *Streptococcus pyogenes*. The properties and effects of bacterial exotoxins are summarized in Table 11.9.

There are two mechanisms that lead to immunity in bacterial infections: the destruction of the microorganisms by lysis or phagocytosis-facilitating antibodies (antibacterial immunity), and the neutralization of toxins (antitoxic immunity). The mechanisms by which bacteriolysis and phagocytosis occur have been described in detail above. It is sufficient to indicate that the destruction of microorganisms inside the phagocytes takes place through distinct processes depending upon whether the bacteria in question are capable of multiplying outside the cell, e.g., pneumococcus, streptococci, and *B. anthracis*, or inside the macrophages, e.g., *M. tuberculosis*, *brucellae*, and *L. monocytogenes*. In the former case, the bacteria are opsonized by circulating antibodies acting together with $C1$ to $C5$ complement components. In the latter case, immunity is not mediated by circulating antibodies, but rather by sensitized lymphocytes which, upon being stimulated by the antigen, liberate a chemotactic factor which attracts macrophages, and a macrophage-activating factor. Antibacterial immunity mediated by cells depends upon mechanisms described as delayed hypersensitivity (Chap. 9. pp. 284–294). In diseases such as tuberculosis, brucellosis, and others in which the organisms persist inside the macrophages, allergy and immunity not uncommonly develop parallel.

Antitoxic immunity depends upon the formation of antibodies (antitoxins) capable of neutralizing the bacterial exotoxins. The mechanisms for the neutralization of exotoxins have been described in Chap. 7 (pp. 209–212).

Special Aspects of Viral Infections

The kind of immunity which develops after viral infections depends to a large extent upon the way a virus spreads and replicates. At the cellular level, three types of viral transmission have been defined: (1) extracellular, infectious virions are released from the cell to spread in the extracellular space, and infect new cells; (2) intercellular, the virus spreads from cell to cell through desmosomes of intercellular bridges without contact with the extracellular milieu. The surfaces of infected cells often contain viral antigens (e.g., herpes virus); and (3) nuclear, the viral genome is latent or incorporated into the host genome and is passed from parent cells to progeny during mitosis (e.g., C type oncornaviruses). The first two modes are also called horizontal transmission, the latter is called vertical transmission.

It is obvious that antibodies are most efficient in the first mode; and they may be able to act in the two other forms if viral antigen is expressed on the surface of infected cells; here, cell-mediated immunity might be most efficient.

At the level of the host, two general types of viral spread are distinguished: (a) local, the viral infection is largely confined to a mucosal surface or organ (e.g., rhinoviruses on

Table 11.9. Bacterial toxins and their properties

Microorganism	Disease	Toxin	Mol. wt.	Action	Symptoms	Toxicity[a] LD$_{50}$ (kg)/ml
Bacillus anthracis	Gas gangrene	Complex of toxins		Chelating agents, increase in vascular permeability	Edema, hemorrhagia	
Bordetella pertussis	Whooping cough	Toxin	82,000	Ciliary damage	Necrosis of epithelial cells, leukocyte infiltration	
Clostridium botulinum	Botulism	8 type-specific neuro-toxins	Type A 70,000	Blocks release of acetylcholine	Neurotoxic signs, paralysis	20×10^6 (M)
Clostridium tetani	Tetanus	Tetanospasmin	67,000	Blocks action of inhibitory neurons	Overaction of motor neurons, muscle spasm	6×10^6 (M)
Clostridium welchii (perfringens)	Gas gangrene	α-toxin enterotoxin	90,000	Lecithinase Activates adenyl cyclase and raises cAMP levels	Loss of water and electrolytes, block of Na resorption; diarrhea	
Corynebact. diphtheriae	Diphtheria	Toxin	62,000	Inhibits cell protein synthesis	Cell necrosis, nerve paralysis	3.5×10^3 (GP)
Escherichia coli	Dysentery	Enterotoxin	24,000	Activation of adenyl cyclase, raises cAMP level	Diarrhea	
Shigella dysenteriae	Dysentery	Entero- and neurotoxin		Activation of adenyl cyclase Vascular endothelial damage (brain)	Diarrhea Neurological disturbance	1.2×10^6 (R)
Staphylococcus aureus	Scalded skin syndrome food poisoning	α-hemolysine, enterotoxin	$3 \times 10,000$ 40,000	Cytotoxic, acts on cell membrane Acts on the vomiting center in the brain	Necrosis of site of infection, Systemic toxic nausea, vomiting, diarrhea	
Streptococcus pyogenes	Scarlet fever	erythrogenic toxin	29,000	Vasodilatation	Scarlet fever rash	
		Streptolysine leukocidin streptokinase	60,000	Lysis of phagocytes and erythrocytes Lysis of fibrin	Phagocytolytic, hemolytic Promotes spread of bacteria in tissue	
Vibrio cholerae	Cholera	Enterotoxin	2 subunits A: 27,000 B: 14,000	Attaches to ganglioside receptors on epithelial cells Activates adenylcyclase and raises cAMP level	Water and electrolyte loss, block of Na resorption; diarrhea	

[a] M, mouse; GP, guinea pig; R, rat

respiratory epithelium); and (b) systemic, either primarily when viruses are inoculated directly into the blood stream with subsequent organ dissemination (arbovirus, hepatitis B virus), or secondary, when the viral infection and replication initially occur on a mucosal surface and invasion into the blood stream or the tissue occurs afterwards (e.g., poliomyelitis, mumps).

The first type of infection elicits predominantly a humoral response whereby local plasma cells produce IgA, and immunity is not long lasting. The immune response to the second group of infections involves both humoral and cellular reactions; immunity is strong and long lasting; the predominantly produced antibodies are of the IgG type. IgA antibodies are, however, also produced which interfere with virus implantation at the site of entry (respiratory system, intestinal mucosa).

Antibodies probably constitute one of the more important mechanisms of host resistance to viral infections, but in most cases they appear to play no role in recovery from established infections. The following virus-antibody reactions have been identified in vitro and they presumably operate also in vivo. (1) Complement-independent neutralization by specific antibodies to virus coat protein (arbovirus, enterovirus, pox, herpes, and arena viruses); the antibodies prevent cellular adsorption and penetration of the virus. The exact mechanism of neutralization is unclear but probably it involves changes in surface structure configurations since only a few antibody molecules per virion are sufficient for neutralization. Of course, the reaction is only possible if the virus spreads extracellularly. (2) Complement-dependent neutralization. "Natural" IgM and early immune antibodies to several viruses enveloped with an outer lipoprotein coat neutralize virus more efficiently in the presence than in the absence of complement components (e.g., rubella, herpes, Newcastle disease virus). Complement may participate in neutralization in several ways: it stabilizes virus-antibody complexes, it causes lysis of enveloped viruses by mechanisms analogous to bacterio- or cytolysis, it prevents attachment of the virus to susceptible cells, and it promotes uptake of the virus by polymorphonuclear and mononuclear phagocytes. Complement-dependent host cell lysis may occur in cases in which viral antigen is expressed on the surface of infected cells (e.g., herpes virus, myxovirus).

Cell-mediated immunity can be demonstrated in many virus infections. Thus, macrophages are important in preventing spread of viruses from primary sites of infections to highly susceptible cells (e.g., hepatitis virus, herpes virus); they play an important role in collaboration with lymphocytes in controlling pox virus, herpes virus, measle, and cytomegalovirus infections. The antiviral mechanisms may include: lymphocyte cytotoxicity mediated by cytolytic T cells recognizing viral antigens expressed on the virus envelope (e.g., myxo-, paramyxo-, rhabdo-, arena-, togaviruses which mature by budding from the cell surface) or the surface of infected cells (e.g., pox and herpes virus), or with the help of cytophilic antibodies to which killer cells attach (see pp. 45 and 306) and release of lymphokines of which some are toxic (LT, see p. 331), others attract macrophages and polymorphonuclear cells, and still others which interfere with virus propagation and replication such as interferons.

Interferons are a family of low molecular weight proteins (16–25,000) discovered by Isaacs and Lindenmann in 1957. There are three antigenetically and chemically distinct types of interferon (IFN), now known as α, β, and γ. For IFN-α several subtypes has been found in man. The molecular weight of human interferons is in the range of 16–23,000 daltons. IFN-β and γ, but generally not α, are glycosylated. The production of interferon α and β are induced by any virus, multiplying in virtually any type of cell, and in any species of vertebrates. On the other hand, IFN-γ is produced only by lymphocytes and only, following antigen or mitogen stimulation. Some IFNs display a degree of species specificity, e.g. most murine interferons are ineffective in primates.

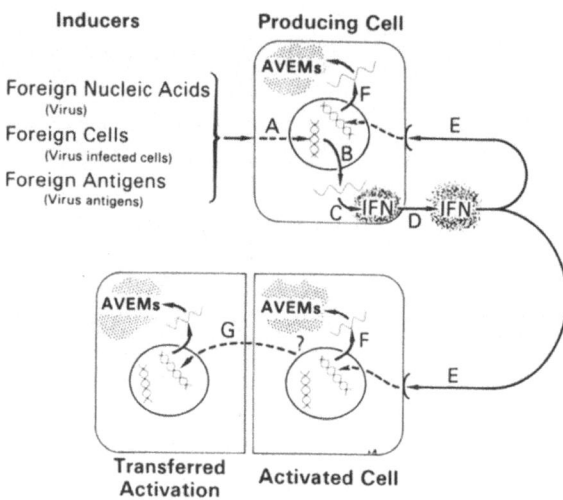

Inducers

Producing Cell

Foreign Nucleic Acids
(Virus)

Foreign Cells
(Virus infected cells)

Foreign Antigens
(Virus antigens)

Transferred
Activation

Activated Cell

Fig. 11.5. Cellular events of the induction, production, and action of interferon (IFN). Inducers of IFN react with cells to derepress the IFN gene(s) (A). This leads to the production of mRNA for IFN (B). The mRNA is translated into the IFN protein (C) that is secreted into the extracellular fluid (D) where it reacts with the membrane receptors of cells (E). The IFN-stimulated cells derepress genes (F) for antiviral effector molecules (AVEMs) that are required to establish antiviral resistance eventually. The activated cells also stimulate contacted cells (G) by a still unknown mechanism to produce AVEMs. (With kind permission reproduced from Notkins and Oldstone, 1984)

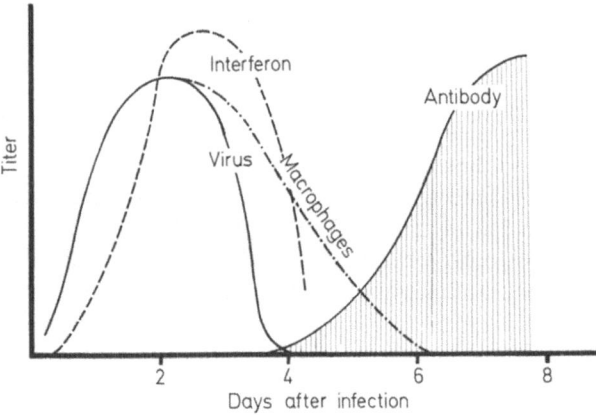

Fig. 11.6. Appearance of interferon, macrophages, and antibodies in virus infections; also shown is the increase of the virus load at the beginning of the infection. With increasing amounts of interferon produced, the virus titer decreases

The mechanism of antiviral action of interferons has not been clearly elucidated. After IFN reacts with a specific receptor on a cell membrane, an induction process involving secondary cell "signal molecules" is initiated (Fig. 11.5). The signal molecules induce the synthesis of antiviral effector molecules (AVEMs). The functions of the AVEMs that result in the development of an antiviral state are not yet understood. An intriguing and unresolved aspect of the AVEMs' mechanism of action are their ability to inhibit viral mRNA translation significantly more than cell mRNA translation.

Interferons are formed within hours after infection. The IFN system appears to be the earliest of the known host-defense mechanisms. Its importance is suggested by the large numbers of subclinical virus infections that occur and the significant exacerbation of virus infections in animals when the IFN defense is deleted, as in the young embryo or by treatment with antibodies to interferon.

Escape from Immune Defense Mechanisms.
There are a number of viruses which have developed the ability to evade the immune defense mechanisms of the infected host or which interfere with the immune response in such a way that it becomes ineffective in eliminating or controlling the infection. This happens in cases when infections occur at in-

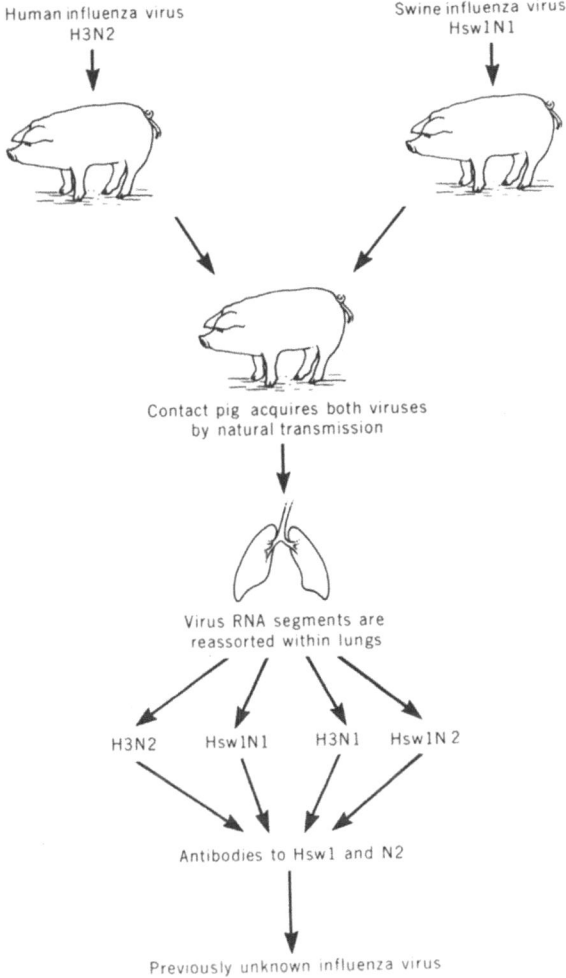

Human influenza virus
H3N2

Swine influenza virus
Hsw1N1

Contact pig acquires both viruses
by natural transmission

Virus RNA segments are
reassorted within lungs

H3N2   Hsw1N1   H3N1   Hsw1N 2

Antibodies to Hsw1 and N2

Previously unknown influenza virus
H3N1

Fig. 11.7. Experiment by Webster demonstrating recombination of human and swine influenza viruses to produce a virus with a new combination of hemagglutinin and neuraminidase antigens. The "new" virus was also shown to be pathogenic and transmissible in a stable form [reproduced from E. J. Shillitoe and F. Rapp (1979) Virus induced cell surface antigens and cell-mediated immune responses. Springer Sem. Immunopathol 2:237]

accessible sites, when viruses reside within cells and do not express viral proteins in the membrane, or when they are able to change their antigenic makeup, or when they are able to avoid the induction of an immune response.

Some viruses are shed to the exterior via saliva (herpes, cytomegalovirus, rabies in vampire bats), milk (cytomegalovirus in man), or urine (polyoma virus in man). Others are only formed on the lumenal surface of cells or in the keratosquamous layer of epidermis (human wart virus), and there is no way in which lymphocytes or antibodies can reach these sites and eliminate the infections.

Herpes simplex or varicella virus persistently infect dorsal root ganglion cells, Epstein-Barr (EB) virus resides in circulating lymphocytes. Herpes and measles virus spread progressively from cell to cell, and are protected in this way from the action of immune cells or antibodies.

Another major way to escape the immune reaction is antigenic variation. Influenza and human rhinoviruses, and foot-and-mouth disease virus develop variants outside the host. Influenza B virus shows repeated small antigenic changes over the years (antigenic drift). A given individual can be reinfected later in life by an antigenic

Table 11.10. Pandemic influenza A virus strains

Pandemic	Influenza A virus strain[a]
1889	? $(A_2?)$
1918/1919	H_0N_1 (A_0)
1933	H_0N_0 $(PR-8)$
1946	H_1N_1 (A_1)
1957	H_2N_2 $(A_2$, Asian flu)
1968	H_3N_2 (Hong Kong flu)
1976	Hsw_1N_1(swine flu)

[a] Old designation in parentheses

variant that has been gradually generated in other groups of individuals. Influenza A shows in addition to slight variations drastic antigenic changes (antigenic shift) in intervals of 10–15 years. The major antigenic changes involve one or both of the surface components of the virus, either hemagglutinin (H) or neuraminidase (N). New variants are thought to develop by recombination of nonhuman and existing human viruses when they infect a host at the same time (Fig. 11.7). Thus, in 1976 a new variant of influenza appeared with the neuraminidase of the 1946 pandemic strain combined with the hemagglutinin from pig influenza virus (Hsw 1 N 1) (Table 11.10). Whenever a new major variant appeared, major global outbreaks of flu occurred, since a large proportion of the population had not been exposed to such a virus and was, therefore, highly susceptible. Thus, antibodies against A_2, the pandemic strain appearing in 1957 (Asian flu) could be found only in individuals who had experienced the 1889 epidemic. The simplest way for an agent to achieve a progressive infection is to elicit *no* immune response at all. There is indeed a group of viral microorganisms that multiply, persist, and spread in the infected host, giving pathological changes only after very long incubation periods. These microorganisms multiply in the brain and cause a neurological disease that is always fatal. To this group of "slow viruses" infections belong scrapie, transmissible mink encephalopathy, and in man, Kuru and Creutzfeld-Jacob disease. Scrapie has been best studied, and no indica-

tion for antibodies or cell-mediated responses after infection has been found. In mice, neonatal thymectomy or thymectomy, lethal irradiation, and reconstitution with fetal liver cells (T lymphocyte depletion) had no effect on the incubation period or pathology of scrapie. The infection neither induces nor is susceptible to the action of interferons. Other persistent viruses like lymphochoriomeningitis and leukemia virus in mice and human adenoviruses do not induce the production of interferon in spite of continued multiplication of virus. Presumably, infected cells do not recognize the virus nucleic acid as foreign.

Special Aspects of Protozoal and Metazoal Infections

Protozoa (plasmodia, amebia, leishmania, toxoplasma, and trypanosoma) and metazoa (trematedes, cestodes, and nematodes) are highly complex organisms; they represent a mosaic of antigens; their life cycle may consist of many different morphological forms, possibly bearing different antigenic structures; and they may be present simultaneously or sequentially within the same host. Therefore, immune responses to parasites have diverse manifestations, which are, additionally, modified ·by interactions of the parasite. In general, there are four possible results of immunological host-parasite interactions: (1) development of immunity with complete protection to reinfection (cutaneous leishmaniasis), (2) exaggerated hypersensitivity causing an immune disease (tropical eosinophil syndrome in filariasis, hepatic granulomae in schistosomiasis, antibody-mediated anaphylactic shock of a ruptured hydatid cyst), (3) absence of an effective immune response (malignant or diffuse cutaneous and mucocutaneous leishmaniasis, primary amebic meningoencephalitis, African trypanosomiasis, American trypanosomiasis), and (4) a balanced "immunity" which prevents large numbers of parasites from overwhelming the host but the response is generally ineffective at eliminating parasites (as in the majority of protozoan and metazoan infections).

Quite certainly, the last, "homeostatic" situation has to be the most favored by the parasite since it will secure its survival, and indeed, one key feature of most protozoan and metazoan infections is their chronicity. A number of mechanisms are invented by parasites to achieve this stage of "adaptive tolerance": anatomical inaccessibility, seclusion into host cells, antigenic variation, molecular masking, interference with the host's immune response such as inhibition of macrophage function, polyclonal B cell stimulation, induction of T suppressor cells, and immunosuppression (see p. 348). Resistance to homologous parasitic reestablishment is often seen in already parasitized individuals. The term "concomitant immunity" has been used to describe this situation, where parasitized hosts are already highly or completely resistant to reinfestation or reinfection with the same parasite (e.g., schistosomiasis, fascioliasis). This type of immunity, in which *establishing* parasites are susceptible to immune responses which are ineffective against *established* parasites, has also been termed nonsterilizing immunity or premunition.

For some parasitic infections (e.g., malaria, filariasis), residents of endemic regions show less severe disease symptoms and the progression of the pathology is slower than in "immigrants." This suggests that there must be a modulating influence on the pathogenesis of infections in endemic areas, the source of which may extend back even into intrauterine, prenatal immunologic experience of the host: maternal-fetal transfer of (partially) protective IgG antibodies, infections at times at which the immune system or parts of it have not acquired complete maturity. Depending upon the stage of the development of the immune system and the presence of antibodies, the first encounter with a pathogenic parasite may direct the course of the disease in future infections: strong reactions with elimination of the parasite and subsequent immunity (cutaneous leishmaniasis) to weak, inadequate, or no

reaction with extensive pathological effects (diffuse cutaneous leishmaniasis) to the same parasite in different individuals. Also in filariasis, various clusters of immunologic responses to the same parasite can be observed: immunologic hyperresponsiveness in tropical eosinophilia syndrome at the one extreme and asymptomatic microfilaremia at the other extreme; between these two lie states characterized by lymphatic inflammation and/or damage.

Protozoal Infections. In general, both the humoral and the cellular immune system, finely tuned, are needed to control the infection. In most cases, chronicity and pathogenesis of the parasite infection appear to be the result of an inadequate or impaired macrophage (*L. donovani* and *braziliensis*, *T. gondii* infections, *Tr. cruzi*), T cell (*Plasmodium*, *L. donovani* and *braziliensis*, *T. gambiense* and *rhodesiense* infections) and/or B cell response (*L. donovani* infections), which is most probably due to interference of the parasite with the activity of the immune system (see below).

The antibody response to parasites has captured most of the attention in the past, whereas the cellular immune response to parasites has just started to be explored and not much detailed knowledge is available for most of the parasitic diseases at the present time. From experiments in mice with parasites, which are "natural" to these animals (Table 11.11), it has been demonstrated that athymic nude (T cell deficient) mice develop a more severe picture of these diseases: parasite burdens are higher, infections persist longer, resistance to reinfections are not seen, or the mice are killed by infections which are not lethal in normal mice. The importance of cell-mediated immune responses in leishmaniasis is very clearly demonstrated by the fact that in cutaneous leishmaniasis an early and strong cellular reaction with almost no antibody present confers healing and sterile immunity, whereas visceral leishmaniasis (a generally fatal disease if not treated) is characterized by a conspicuous

Table 11.11. „Natural" protozoan and metazoan parasites of mice

---

Plasmodium yoelii
Babesia microti
Leishmania tropica
Trypanosoma musculi
Giardia muris
Mesocestoides corti
Taenia taeniformis
Hexamita muris
Hymenolepis nana
Nematospiroides dubius
Aspicularis tetrapetra
Syphacia obvelata

---

absence of any cellular reaction; in animals, T cell depletion (neonatal thymectomy, ALS treatment, see p. 427) leads to a prolonged course of infections with *L. tropica*, which, in normal animals, is self-healing. Most of the aggravations appear due to a lack of T helper cell activity. Thus, in filariasis blast transformation in vitro is observed in the case of lymphocytes from young children exposed to the nematode, but this response is then "damped down" in chronic infections. The T cell dependency has been demonstrated to extend to macrophage activation, eosinophil activation in metazoan infections, and IgG response as well as fibrotic encapsulation, all of which are T helper cell functions. Delayed type hypersensitivity (skin test) in human parasitic infections is found in amebiasis, cutaneous leishmaniasis, *Tr. cruzi* infections (although only in the late stages), toxoplasmosis, schistosomiasis, echinococcosis, trichinosis, but not in malaria, diffuse cutaneous and mucocutaneous leishmaniasis, and *Tr. brucei* infections. Evidence for the presence of cytotoxic T cells against cells harboring parasites (malaria, toxoplasma, leishmania, *Tr. cruzi*) or parasites *(schistosoma)* has been found in mice: *Leishmania enriettii* infected macrophages are susceptible to lysis by T cells; splenocytes from *Tr. cruzi* infected mice were found to destroy infected fibroblasts in vitro. It is, however, not at all

clear whether or not these mechanisms also operate in vivo.

Activated (by T cells) macrophages play an important role in controlling parasitic infections, and their effectiveness is impaired in malaria, toxoplasmosis, *L. donovani* and *braziliensis*, and *Tr. cruzi* and *brucei* infections. Unspecific activation of macrophages (e.g., by BCG) renders mice resistant to otherwise fatal infections of *Plasmodium winckei;* activated macrophages release mediators which produce degeneration of parasites within circulating erythrocytes; the mechanism of this effect is unknown. In toxoplasma infections, lymphokines are released which inhibit toxoplasma replication in macrophages; it has been demonstrated that the lymphokine interacts with a trypsin and neuraminidase sensitive receptor on the surface of macrophages. In addition, activated macrophages synthesize proteins which inhibit toxoplasma replication within their parasitic vacuole. In immunologically impaired individuals infected with toxoplasma parasites, there appears to be an impaired activation of macrophages by lymphocytes. On the other hand, blood forms of *Tr. cruzi* possess an antiphagocytic substance on their surface; removal of this substance by trypsin treatment in vitro renders them phagocytable for macrophages.

In protozoan infections, the predominant immune response appears to be the formation of specific IgG antibodies, which is under the control of T helper cells. In general, they confer only partial protection to reinfections and are not efficient in eliminating existing infections, but only keep the extent of parasitic burden at a low level. They are usually not directed against, or do not affect, the adult, replicating parasite: thus, in malaria, IgG antibodies are produced against merozoites which confer protection against reinfection of the same strain; they are complement independent and apparently neutralize merozoites in a way comparable to virus neutralization; they are specific for glycoproteins on the surface coat of the parasite. This surface coat can undergo variations, thus eluding the action of antibodies (see below). There are no protective antibodies against the gametocyte in erythrocytes or the trophozoite (replicating stage) in liver parenchyma cells. In amebiasis, high titers of circulating antibodies can be demonstrated, yet there is no indication of acquisition of resistance to reinfections (colitis); however, recurrence of amebic liver abscesses after cure are rare. In diffuse cutaneous and visceral leishmaniasis high titers of specific antibodies in addition to generally elevated immunoglobulin levels are detected, but they are not protective. Since in the cutaneous form, the specific antibody titer is low, it is assumed that immunity in leishmania infections is established by cellular mechanisms (see above). In *Tr. brucei* infections, complement-activating antibodies are formed against predominant blood variants; however, new variants escape their actions (see below). Complement-activating and opsonizing IgG antibodies are produced in the course of *Tr. cruzi* infections, which confer in collaboration with cellular mechanisms a certain degree of immunity. Lytic and opsonizing IgG antibodies are demonstrable in toxoplasmosis; however, they appear to be protective only in the presence of (lymphokine) activated macrophages; in immunologically impaired individuals, this necessary activation of macrophages by sensitized lymphocytes is apparently absent or inefficient.

Metazoal Infections. Metazoan infections are characterized by eosinophilia and the production of specific (and unspecific) IgE antibodies, in addition to IgG antibodies, as well as local infiltration of macrophages, basophils, mast cells, and eosinophils at the site of infection. These reactions occur against tissue invasive and penetrating larvae forms of the parasites: schistosomiasis, fascioliasis, paragonimiasis, echinococcosis (hydatid cyst disease), ascariasis (particularly the pulmonary phase), strongyloidiasis, trichinosis, and filariasis. Parasites which neither enter the host tissue, i.e., remain in the intestinal tract, nor induce per-

sistent inflammatory responses do not usually elicit eosinophilia, e.g., enterobiasis, *Trichuris* infections, hookworm infections, and tapeworm *(Taenia)* infections, or only locally at the site of their fixation. In addition to IgE antibodies, IgG (particularly IgG_1) antibodies are formed usually against developmental (molting fluid in filariasis) and metabolic by-products, enzymes (acetylcholinesterase in nematodes), or other secretory products rather than structural components. In addition to specific immune responses, some metazoa activate independent of antibodies the properdin system (see p. 127), which by activation of the late complement components kills the parasites.

IgE Response. High levels of IgE have long been considered a feature of *chronic* metazoan parasitic infections. This potentiated IgE response is T cell dependent as no IgE response are obtained in athymic nude mice. The underlying reasons for the IgE response is unknown, but it has been suggested that antigen persistence in mucous membranes and subcutaneous tissue and disruption of such structures by migrating or resident metazoa might be (one of) the reason(s). It has been shown that soluble factors present in cell-free culture supernatants of mesenteric lymph node cells from parasite-infected rats *(Nippostrongylus brasiliensis)* induce the conversion of IgM-bearing cells to IgE-IgM-double-bearing cells when added to normal bone marrow cell cultures. The effect of the factor is specific as it does not increase either IgM-bearing or IgG-bearing cells. There are some indications that this factor is derived from B cells rather than from T cells. However, the differentiation from IgM-IgE-bearing B cells to IgE memory cells and IgE-secreting plasma cells requires the interaction of specifically sensitized T helper cells.

IgE antibodies sensitize selectively basophilic granulocytes and mast cells, both of which possess receptors with high affinity for the Fc portion of IgE immunoglobulins. Binding of IgE-antigen complexes leads to bridging of these receptors, which in turn triggers

Table 11.12. Immunologic features of protozoal infections in man

Disease	Vector	Host	Prepatency	Duration of infection	Infected tissue	Cellular activities	Humoral activities	Comments
Malaria (*Plasmodium vivax, ovale, falciparum, malariae*)	anopheline mosquitoe	Human only	24 h	3 years / 1 year / indef.	Liver parenchymal cells, erythrocytes	CMI present; increase of phagocytic activity; T helper cell activation	IgG against merozoite antigens (partially protective)	Exoerythrocyte stages do not induce antibody formation; hypergammaglobulinemia, autoantibodies, immunosuppresion; immunopathology (nephrosis due to immune complexes and autoantibodies)
Amebiasis (*Entamoeba histolytica*)	Primates, domestic animals		8–35 days	Indefinitely	Intestinal cell wall, portal circulation, liver	CMI present	IgG, IgM, IgE; Arthus reaction	No evidence that Igs are protective
Leishmaniasis Cutaneous L. (*L. tropica*) Oriental Sore	Phlebotomus (sand fly)	Rock hyrax	Days to months	6 Months	Cutis macrophages	Early and strong delayed hypersensitivity	Little antibody response	Cell-mediated protection; development of immediate hypersensitivity coincides with healing
Viscerale L. (*L. donovani*) Kala-Azar	"	Hamster, gerbil, dog		Indefinitely	Dermis, macrophages, RES, liver, spleen	No CMI; only after spontaneous recovery or treatment	Polyclonal Ig response; circulating L. antigens	CMI suppressed (defective host response); immune complexes. CMI plays role in resolution of disease
Mucocutaneous L. (*L. braziliensis*) Espundia	"	Sloth hamster, opossum		Indefinitely		CMI present, but inadequate	Elevated Ig levels	Immunopathology (immune complex deposits)
Toxoplasmosis (*T. gondii*)	Mammals, partic. cats, birds		2–4 weeks	Indefinitely	All cells and tissue	DTH develops late; if trophozoite is exposed to antibody and C macrophages kill parasite	IgG, IgM, IgA; non-specific Ig elevated	Ig not protective; immune complexes in kidney
Trypanosomiasis (*T. cruzi*) Chagas disease	Reduviidae bugs (*Triatomae*)	Mammals (dogs)	2–3 weeks	Indefinitely	RES cells, macrophages, glia cells cardiac muscle cells	No effective CMI	Polyclonal antibody response	Reconvalescent sera confer some protection; experimentally: transfer of protective immunity by spleen cells; immunopathology
(*T. brucei*) Sleeping sickness	Tsetse fly (*glossina*)	Human, domestic oxen, antelope	1–3 weeks	1 year	Blood, lymph circulation, cerebral fluid	Increased phagocytic activity	Polyclonal (IgM) + specific antibodies, antibody-antigen complexes	Systemic Arthus-reaction, immune complex deposits, autoantibodies; immunosuppression; >20 antigenic variants with predictable sequence

the release of granules from basophils and mast cells. Furthermore, it has been demonstrated that macrophages are able to adhere via their Fc receptor to IgE antibodies, which react with metazoan antigens, and kill the parasite in a complement-independent reaction (see p. 250, and 262).

Mast Cell and Basophil Activity. Two types of mast cells are distinguished (see p. 8, 255): connective tissue mast cells and mucosal mast cells.

The activity and activation of *connective tissue* mast cells are thymus independent. Thus, nude mice have normal numbers of typical connective tissue mast cells in their skin and these cells function normally in passive cutaneous anaphylactic (CPA, see p. 247) reactions.

Mucosal mast cells are capable of rapidly increasing in numbers, especially in primary immune responses of the intestine to infections with parasitic nematodes. When animals are reinfected with the same intestinal nematode, the number of mucosal mast cells increases with a reduced latent period and with heightened magnitude. This effect is not seen in athymic nude mice; however, this response can be restored with subcutaneous thymic grafts from normal syngeneic adults. This mucosal mast cell response can be transferred by hyperimmune sera from nematode infected donors, but not by 56 °C-heat-inactivated hyperimmune sera. It appears, therefore, that the activation, proliferation, and accumulation of mucosal mast cells is induced by IgE antibodies, the formation of which is strictly T cell dependent. Upon activation of mast cells by IgE-antigen complexes which bind with the Fc portion to the IgE specific Fc receptor, the mast cells release their granules, containing, among many substances (see below) involved in the acute inflammatory process, chemotaxins for basophils and eosinophils. Mast cells appear to have several important functions in the inflammatory reaction toward metazoan parasites: damage of parasites by the release of granules containing

pharmacologically active components and enzymes; recruitment of local accumulation of effector cells such as eosinophils and lymphocytes; and activation of and cooperation with effector cells (see below). Mast cells are probably required in immunity to some metazoa (e.g., schistosomiasis).

Basophils are normally present in the blood and not in the extravascular tissue space (see pp. 8 and 259). Basophils are recruited to enter the tissue as part of specific immune-inflammatory processes guided by soluble factors including antibodies. Basophil-rich immune-inflammatory reactions are rather restricted to the skin and the gut. In the skin these reactions are called cutaneous basophil hypersensitivity (CBH). In guinea pigs, the accumulation of basophils in cutaneous hypersensitivity reactions is mediated by small amounts of low affinity 7S antibodies, IgG_1. The antibody acts via Fc receptors. The mechanism of this antibody-mediated reaction may initially involve antibody-coated mast cells that release mediators when exposed to antigen. Among the mediators are chemotactic factors for intravascular basophils.

Upon binding of antigen to the Fc-receptor-bound IgE antibody, basophils release mediators such as histamine, and morphologically demonstrate anaphylactic degranulation (see p. 259) via exocytosis. Basophils may also demonstrate "piecemeal" degranulation: this consists of progressive dissolution of the granules, without fusion of granule-containing vacuoles with each other, or extrusion of granules from cytoplasm.

Eosinophilia. The fact that eosinophils are involved in allergic reactions and metazoan parasitic infections has been documented for a long time. Irrespective of the specific time course of the hypersensitivity (inflammatory) reaction, eosinophils arrive *after* the humoral phase. The activation of eosinophil proliferation in the bone marrow is T cell dependent: allergogenic and certain metazoan antigens, or substances released from

11.13. Human pathogenic metazoa

Metazoa	Vector	Host	Tissue infected	Life span of adult in man	Prepatency
Trematodes					
Schistosoma hematobium	Snails	Human	Venes of urogenital tract; eggs penetrate wall of bladder		3–6 weeks
S. mansoni	Snails	Rodents, human	Mesenterial venes; eggs penetrate wall of colon or disseminate	10 years or more	5–10 weeks
S. japonicum	Snails	Cattle, domestic animals, man			5–10 weeks
Fasciola hepatica	Fluke snail	Herbivore mammals, occ. man	Bile duct (fibrotic capsule)	Several years	7–8 weeks
Paragonimus	(1st) snail (2nd) shrimp	Canides, felides; accid. man	Lung, also dissemination (fibrotic cyst)	Several years	2–3 months
Cestodes					
Diphyllobothrium latum	Fishes	Dog, cat, pig, bear, man	Intestinal lumen	Several years	3 weeks
Taenia saginata	Cattle	Human	Intestinal lumen	10 years	2–3 months
T. solium	Pig, man	Man	Cysticercosis; striated muscle, lymph nodes, occ. brain, eye	20 years or more	2 months
Echinococcus granulosis	Sheep, pig man	Canides	Liver; lung, brain (hytatide cyst)	Life span of host	2 months
E. multilocularis	Rodents, rhesus m., man	Fox, dog, cat	Liver	Life span of host	35–47 days
Nematodes					
Without vector, oral infection					
Trichuris trichiura			Wall of colon	3–3.5 years	6 weeks
Trichinella spiralis			Striated muscle, encapsulation	Life span of host	6 days
Ascaris lumbricoides			Liver, heart, lung (eosinophil infiltrate)	12–18 months	2–3 months
Toxocarna canis			Larvae migrans visceralis	5 years	5–6 weeks
Without vector, percutaneous infection					
Ancylostoma duodenale			Lung		
Necator americanus			Lung		
Strongyloides stercoralis			Lung	Because of self-infection 30 years or more	15 days
With vector, oral infection					
Dracunculus medinensis	Crab	Human	Lymph; subcutaneous tissue	12 months	12 months
Arthropod-borne					
Wucheria bancrofti	Mosquitoes	Vertebrates except fishes	Lymph nodes and vessels	10–15 years	1–2 years
Loa loa	Horse fly	Human	Subcutaneous connective tissue	5–15 years	2–4 years
Onchocerca volvulus	Mosquitoes		Connective tissue (eye!), fibroid capsules (Onchocercosis)	15 years	15–18 months

cells or tissue in contact with allergens or metazoa, induce T cells to produce an eosinophilic colony-stimulating factor (CSF) which augments the generation of eosinophils. The eosinophils are then attracted to migrate to the site of inflammation by chemotactic factors released from tissue which the parasite invades. IgE-dependent activation of fragments of human lung tissue have been shown to release an array of eosinophilic chemotactic stimuli from mast cells and basophils, including histamine and low molecular weight peptide eosinophil chemotactic factors of anaphylaxis, ECF-A (see pp. 254 and 322). But in addition to those mediators, T lymphocytes are critical to the stimulation by eosinophil chemotactic lymphokines, e.g., eosinophil stimulation promotor (ESP) (see p. 330). The T cell dependency of eosinophilia and tissue eosinophil accumulation during parasite infections has been demonstrated in experimental animal models; thus, eosinophils are present in hypothymic nude mice, but such mice fail to mount a response to infections involving eosinophilia or accumulation in localized sites.

Eosinophils have been found to act in two ways in parasitic inflammatory reactions: (1) antibody-dependent parasitocidal, and (2) mediating tissue repair by neutralizing the products of mast cells and basophil degranulation in immediate hypersensitivity reactions, and by limiting the extent of fibrotic encapsulation (e.g., in *Fasciola hepatica, Paragonimus, Onchocerca,* and *Trichinella* infections), wound repair, and granuloma formation during parasitic infections. Human eosinophils can damage schistosomula (invading larvae of schistosomes) in vitro in the presence of sera from schistosome-infected patients, through an opsonizing, IgG-antibody-dependent, and complement-independent reaction (ADCC): IgG antibodies attach to antigenic determinants on the parasite and then eosinophils adhere via surface Fc receptors for IgG. The attached eosinophils spread out along the surface of the parasite, degranulate, and damage the underlying tegument of larvae; after

degranulation, eosinophils are autolytically destroyed. One of the factors damaging to the metazoa was identified as eosinophilic major basic protein. Mast cells are required for the parasitocidal activity of eosinophils, since depletion of mast cells in eosinophil-rich effector cell populations significantly decreases the cytotoxicity. However, when purified mast cells which by themselves show no cytotoxicity are added to purified eosinophils, there is a significant augmentation in antibody-dependent, eosinophil-mediated cytotoxicity compared to the effect of purified eosinophils alone (mast cell-eosinophil cooperation). The mast-cell-mediated augmentation of eosinophil cytotoxicity seems to depend, in the mouse, on IgG_{2a} antibody or its Fc fragment. The mast cell effect can be replaced by supernatants of mast cells that have released mediators in response to IgE or IgG_{2a}. Eosinophil-IgG-mediated cytotoxicity develops in the early phase of the immune response; macrophage-IgE-mediated cytotoxicity occurs most effectively in the later phase of the infection (Fig. 11.8).

The prominent protective role of eosinophils in the host response to a variety of helminth, has been amply demonstrated: larvae of *Schistosoma* migrating in immune animals are damaged as they penetrate the skin and the histopathology of the infiltrates around them are predominantly eosinophils. Similarly, when larvae are introduced into the lungs without penetrating the skin, the intensity of local eosinophil infiltration is greater in immune animals (rats) than in those not sensitized previously. Administration of monospecific antieosinophil serum to immune mice prior to reinfection with *S. mansoni* abolishes the protective effect of active antimetazoan immunity. Depletion of other leukocytes by specific antisera did not affect the level of protection. Utilizing the release of ^{51}Cr from prelabeled larvae of *S. mansoni* as a measure of cytotoxicity, complement-independent metazoicidal activity of human leukocytes in the presence of opsonizing IgG antibodies has been demonstrated; the reaction was ablated by

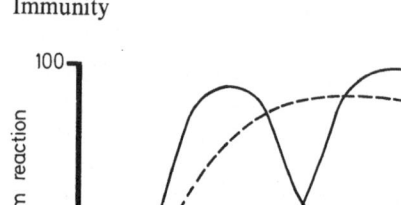
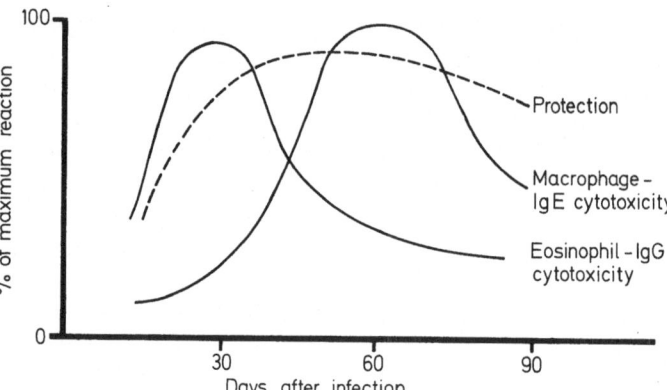

Fig. 11.8. Development of eosinophil-IgG and macrophage-IgE mediated immunity in *S. mansoni* infections in the rat

antieosinophil serum, and was not dependent on the presence of monocytes. The cytotoxic effect was inhibitable by the addition of immune complexes which block eosinophil Fc receptors and prevent adherence of eosinophils to the parasite. Eosinophil-mediated cytotoxicity has also been demonstrated for epimastigotes of *Tr. cruzi*. The second function, containment of inflammatory reactions, is deduced from the fact that eosinophils are known to produce and release prostaglandins E_1 and E_2, which inhibit histamine release from mast cells and basophils by increasing the intracellular cyclic AMP level. They also contain in their granules histaminase, arylsulfatase B, phospholipase D, lysophospholipase, enzymes which degradate histamine, SRS-A (slow reacting substances of anaphylaxis, see pp. 254), platelet lytic factor (PLF, which causes release of serotonin from platelets), and lysophospholipids, all substances which are released by cells others than eosinophils in an inflammatory reaction. In addition, eosinophils phagocytose extruded mast cell granules containing heparin and cationic proteases. Part of their postulated repair function may, therefore, be to limit the pathological consequences of chronic inflammation or even the extent of acute inflammations resulting from tissue penetration and damage by parasitic larvae. Thus, at certain stages of schistosomula egg-induced hepatic granuloma formation, eosinophils compose approximately 50% of the

cells within the lesion. In *Ascaris lumbricoides* infections, there is a heavy eosinophil cell infiltration in the lung alveoles in which the parasite resides. In nematode infections *(Ancylostomatidae)*, there is a local infiltration of eosinophils, basophils, and mast cells at the site of parasitic fixation in the intestinal mucosa.

Escape from Immune Defense Mechanisms. In many protozoan and metazoan infections, a specific immune response is clearly detectable and yet parasites evade these possible attacks of the immune system. Apparently, parasites have developed mechanisms which permit them to escape the host's protective responses. Demonstrated or postulated mechanisms are listed in Table 11.14.

Anatomical Inaccessibility. It appears that some parasites, particularly *D. latum* and *T. saginata*, are inaccessible for immune mechanisms since they stay in the luminal space of the intestine. However, they are fixed to the mucosa at one point. The immune system is principally able to mount an effective reaction against the parasite as demonstrated in rats with *Nippostrongylus*; the parasite is rejected by a locally elicited immune response within 2 weeks after primary fixation. That some parasites escape such an attack can only mean that they have developed mechanisms which protect that part of their tissue in close contact with the host mucosa; the nature of these mechanisms is not known.

Other parasites such as *Fasciola hepatica*, *Paragonimus*, *E. granulosus*, *T. spiralis*, and *O. volvulus* are more truly inaccessible although they are in the tissue of the host; they provoke the formation of fibrotic capsules around them which protect them from even most vigorous immune responses (e.g., particularly *Echinococcus*).

Seclusion Inside Host Cells. All human pathogenic protozoa except *Tr. brucei* are intracellularly replicating parasites, and they are protected from the activity of antibodies and cellular immune reactions by the host's cell membrane, as long as infected cells do not express parasitic antigens on their surface. Some of the parasites have, additionally, developed mechanisms to avoid the microbicidal activity of macrophages after phagocytosis by or penetration into these cells: *L. donovani* is resistant to the activity of lysosomal enzymes, *T. gondii* inhibits phago-lysosomal fusion, trypomastigotes escape into the extravacuole space (cytoplasm) after phagocytosis.

Antigenic Variation. It has been shown that malarial parasites and *Tr. brucei* protozoa have a repertoire of intrastrain variants which appear sequentially during infections. It appears that the change from one variant to the next is independent of the immune (antibody) response. Since the sequence of variation occurs in a predictable pattern, it is assumed that the antigenic variants are genetically determined. It is not known which mechanism(s) effect(s) the sequential predominance of one variant above the

Table 11.14. Mechanisms of evasion of host-protective responses by parasites

Mechanism	Parasite
Anatomical inaccessibility	Intestinal parasites, encapsulated or encysted parasites (*Echinococcus*, *F. hepatica*, *Paragonimus*, *T. solium*, *T. spiralis*, *T. gondii*)
Seclusion inside host cells	*Plasmodium* (trophozoites in liver parenchymal cells), *Leishmania* (macrophages and cells of the RES), *Tr. cruzi* (macrophages, muscle cells), *T. gondii* (virtually all cells)
Antigenic variation	*Plasmodium*, *Tr. brucei*
Molecular masking	*Schistosoma*
Loss of MHC antigens	*Leishmania*
Immunosuppression	
Disruption of lymphoid tissue	Trypanosomes
Antigen competition	*Plasmodium*, trypanosomes, schistosomes, microfilaria
Mitogenic exhaustion of B cell clones	?
Vigorous antibody response blocking T cell recognition (?)	Leishmania
Lymphotoxic factors	*T. spiralis*, *F. hepatica*, *Tr. brucei*
Lymphocyte suppressive factors	*Tr. brucei*

Soluble antigens
  Effector cell blockade
  Feedback inhibition
  Suppressor T cell activation (?)
  Clonal abortion by toxic
Antigens
	Plasmodium, *L. donovani*, trypanosomes, filariae, toxoplasma, and schistosomes

others. The variable surface layer induces in the host the formation of specific antibodies which are toxic for the parasites. This response is T cell dependent, and there are some indications from experimental studies that T helper cells recognize strain specific antigens (carrier) common to all antigenic variants, thus helping B lymphocytes to react in an anamnestic fashion to antigens specific for each successive variant. However efficient the immune response might be, it will be defeated by the extreme plasticity these parasites exhibit: the parasite will be always ahead of the "floundering" immune response.

Molecular Masking. Adult schistosomes are living and reproducing in the blood stream; although an infection confers strong immunity to reinfection (concomitant immunity, see above), the established parasites are unharmed by this immune response. In a series of very elegant experiments, Smithers, Terry, and Hockley could demonstrate that schistosomes a few days after host invasion have coated themselves with host material containing blood group glycolipids and major histocompatibility gene products. It has been thought that the masking of parasite antigens by host-derived material serves as a disguise preventing any effect of the immune response. However, it has recently been shown that schistosomes acquire resistance also in macromolecule-free solutions; the proposed mechanism of antigen masking in order to escape the host's immune response appears, therefore, at least doubtful.

Loss of MHC Antigens. Experimental studies show marked differences of susceptibility between mouse strains to infections with *L. tropica*. BALB/c mice are highly susceptible and develop persistent expanding ulcerated lesions similar to diffuse cutaneous leishmaniasis in man. In contrast, CBA mice develop lesions that resolve within a few weeks like oriental sore in man. Uninfected macrophages from these strains can be used as efficient in vitro blockers of alloreactive cytolytic T cells. When BALB/c macrophages are infected with *L. tropica*, they are no longer efficient blockers of alloreactive killing, but macrophages from CBA mice infected with *L. tropica* remain effective blockers. This suggests that *L. tropica* infections in susceptible BALB/c cause a decrease in the surface expression of MHC coded molecules which may result in defective T cell recognition of parasitized macrophages.

Immunosuppression. Reduced responses to nonparasite antigens have been demonstrated in *Plasmodiae*, *Babesia*, trypanosome, toxoplasma, leishmania, and some metazoan (schistosome, fasciola, *T. spiralis*) infections. The immunosuppression is in general not complete but rather selective and results in partial inhibition of certain immune responses (so as not to threaten the survival of the host). Immunosuppression may have several causes: disruption of lymphoid tissue (trypanosome infection); antigenic competition in infections with high antigen load due to destroyed parasites (e.g., malaria, trypanosomiasis, schistosomiasis, microfilaria) resulting in a blockage of the macrophage-reticulo-endothelial system; parasite-derived mitogens which lead to an exhaustion of B cell clones – thus far, no mitogen has been identified; induction of an early and strong antibody response as in visceral leishmaniasis, which may prevent T cell activation or effectiveness by covering target antigens normally recognized by T cells; lymphocytotoxic factors such as agglutinins produced by *T. spiralis* and trypanosomes, or secretory and excretory products of *Fasciola hepatica,* which in addition to being toxic inhibit attachment of adherent cells to flukes in the presence of serum. Similarly, trypanosomes cover themselves with sialoglycoprotein from the host's serum which impedes the attachment of antibodies and antigen recognition by T cells; parasite-derived lymphocyte suppressive factors such as tryptophol, a substance synthesized by *Tr. brucei*, which suppresses thymidine incorporation, and a low molecular weight, heat-stable factor produced by schistosomes, which suppress B as well as T cell proliferation.

Soluble Antigens. Soluble antigenic material is present in the serum after infections with *Plasmodiae*, *L. donovani*, trypanosomes, filariae, toxoplasma, and schistosomes. There are several effects soluble antigens may have on the antiparasite immune response: (1) lymphocyte (effector cell) blockage by antigens; (2) feedback inhibition by antibody (see p. 109), (3) "weak" immunogenic antigens may stimulate suppressor T cells (thus far, there is no evidence for suppressor cells in parasitic infections); and (4) clonal abortion of specific B and T cells. Thus, trypanosomes release from their surface coat exoantigens (filopodia), which in addition to blocking antibodies are toxic for cells which absorb them; if the cells are lymphocytes specifically binding these antigens, a depletion of these specifically reacting clones might be the result. (5) Formation of antibody-antigen complexes can lead to immunosuppression in several ways: (a) Immune complexes may block antibody formation at the B cell level through interaction with both antigen and Fc receptors of antigen-reactive cells. Cross-linking of antigen receptors (surface Ig) and Fc receptors by immune complexes has been shown to be a direct blocking signal for B cells without participation of T cells or macrophages. (b) Immune complexes may suppress the immune response via activation of Fc-receptor-bearing suppressor T cells (see pp. 42, 55, 361). (c) Immune complexes can lead to effector cell blockage, i.e., inhibition of antibody secretion from terminally differentiated B cells after interaction with small amounts of antigen complexed to antibodies. (d) Immune complexes bound to Fc receptors on B cells can block the immune response nonspecifically, probably by inhibition or "freezing" of the movement of surface molecules necessary for the activation of the cells. (e) Immune complexes induce the release of soluble factors from T cells combining with the Fc portion of antigen-complexed IgG and inhibiting C′ fixation.

Acquisition of Immunity

An organism may acquire immunity through a passive process, by transfer of antibodies synthesized in another organism, e.g., maternal antibodies, reconvalescent antisera, immune sera of animals, or transfer of immune cells (adoptive immunity). It also may acquire immunity through an active process, i.e., natural infections, which leads to the formation of its own protective antibodies and sensitized cells, or artificial infection with attenuated or killed microorganism (vaccination). Hence, different forms of acquired immunity are classified according to the following scheme; their differences are summarized in Table 11.15:

1. Passively acquired immunity
   a) natural (congenital)
   b) artificial (serotherapy, adoptive immunity)
2. Actively acquired immunity
   a) natural (postinfection)
   b) artificial (vaccination).

Passively Acquired Immunity

Maternal-Fetal Transfer. Passively acquired immunity occurs under normal conditions by passage of maternal antibodies to the fetus (passive congenital immunity). The mechanism of this transfer varies according to the species under study. In man, the placenta, which is of the hemochorial type, permits the transfer of IgG antibodies; these enter the circulation of the fetus and provide protection to the newborn during the first weeks of life. In other species, the passive transfer of immunoglobulins occurs only after parturition, through the colostrum of the milk, which contains appreciable quantities of IgG, IgA, and IgM. In this case, immunoglobulins are taken up at the level of the intestinal mucosa, which at this time is not yet fully developed. In primates, the milk possesses a certain amount of IgG and IgA, but the newborn resorbs hardly any; thus in primates, the principal manner of transfer is

	Active immunity	Passive immunity
Origin of the antibodies	Same organism	Other organism
Intensity	High	Moderate to low

Mode of acquisition	1) Disease
	  a) Clinical
	  b) Subclinical
	2) Vaccination
	  a) Killed or attenuated
	    vaccines
	  b) Toxoids
		Administration of antibodies:
		1) Through placenta
		2) Via colostrum
		3) Serotherapy

Time required for development	5–14 days	Immediately after injection
Duration	Months to years	Days to weeks
Reactivation	Easy via booster doses	Risk of anaphylactic shock
Use	Prophylactic	Prophylactic, therapeutic

Table 11.15. Comparison between active and passive immunity

Table 11.16. Alternative paths of maternal-fetal transfer of immunoglobulins

Species	Yolk sac	Placenta	Colostrum
Birds	+		
Rodents	+	−	+
Swine	−	±	+
Cattle	−	±	+
Sheep	−	−	+
Primates	−	+	−

whereas IgM quickly attains such values, especially in the event of a neonatal infection. The initial decline of the immunoglobulin concentration (Fig. 11.9) is due to the degradation of the maternal immunoglobulins, and the ascent reflects the rate of immunoglobulin synthesis in the newborn. The greater or lesser rapidity with which this portion of the curve reaches normal values reflects the state of development of the immune system and the number and nature of antigenic stimuli experienced.

Ontogenic Development of Immunologic Capacity. Generally speaking, the reactive capacity of the immune system, measured by the production of circulating antibodies, is less in the fetus and in the newborn than in the adult. The majority of fowl, for example, only reach a state of immunologic maturity 5 weeks after hatching. Similar results have been obtained for the majority of mammals. This is why newborns are practically without isoagglutinins for the AB0 system and also do not respond to certain antigens such as antityphus vaccine. Influenced by these observations, some pediatricians think vaccination to be indicated only after the sixth month or even later. In fact, if certain vaccines, for example that against poliomy-

transplacental. Nevertheless, the immunoglobulin present in the colostrum and in the milk can be important in the local protection of the gastrointestinal mucosa. The principal routes of maternal-fetal transfer in different species are listed in Table 11.16.
Regardless of the path of maternal-fetal transfer, the immunoglobulin levels in the newborn diminish considerably in the first weeks of extrauterine life (Fig. 11.9). Between the first and the tenth week, a slow but continuous increase begins in the immunoglobulin level, now due to the individuals own immune system, establishing normal adult levels (6–16 mg/ml of plasma) within 1–4 years of age.
The IgG and IgA immunoglobulin concentrations gradually approach normal levels

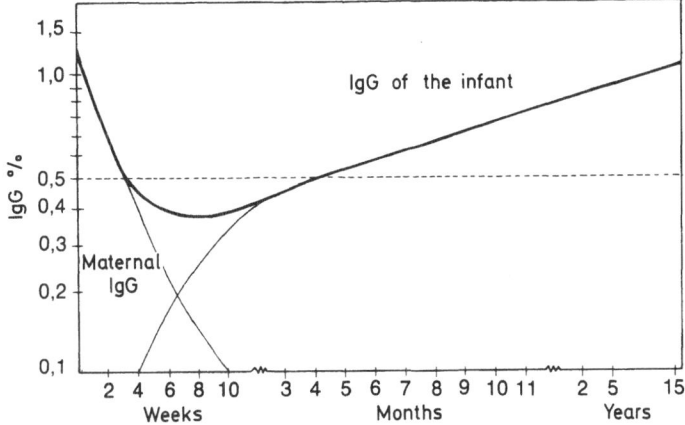

Fig. 11.9. Variation of the serum levels of IgG after birth. The dotted line parallel to the abscissa indicates the lower limit of normal gamma globulin. There is a physiologic hypogammaglobulinemia between the first and fifth months

elitis with attenuated virus, are applied within the first 10 weeks, 95% of those vaccinated produce antibodies for type two, 75% for type three, and only 25% for type one. However, when this vaccine is given to infants over 1 year of age, it induces antibodies for the three types of poliovirus in nearly 100% of those vaccinated. For other vaccines such as against whooping cough, tetanus, and diphtheria, this does not occur; infants vaccinated even in the first weeks of life can be effectively protected.

Immunotherapy. Passive artificial immunity is in general achieved through injection of hyperimmune serum, particularly of antitoxin sera (against snake venom, diphtheria toxin, tetanus toxin, and others, see below), that is either produced in animals (e.g., horse) or obtained from hyperimmunized human (either postinfection or after vaccination, e.g., rabies).

Although active vaccination is long term, the protection conferred by serum is immediate but of short duration because the foreign immunoglobulins are quickly eliminated from the organism (see Fig. 9.13, p. 285).

In man, the metabolic elimination of allogeneic immunoglobulin corresponds to a half-life of 20–30 days[3] – which means that

in this period of time the concentration of antibodies is reduced by one-half. The allogeneic immunoglobulins, because of their gradual elimination, are capable of conferring passive immunity for relatively long periods, affording better prophylactic and therapeutic prospects than xenogeneic immunoglobulins; evidence for that are the particularly favorable results observed in the treatment of certain virus diseases (e.g., measles, hepatitis, rabies) and in the prophylaxis of newborn hemolytic disease.

Xenogeneic and Allogeneic Serotherapy. Because of the availability of chemotherapeutic agents and antibiotics for the treatment of bacterial infections, serotherapy today is restricted to treatment of toxic infections, accidents with venomous animals, and to treatment of virus infections.

Two classes of products are utilized for passive immunization: (a) hyperimmune, xenogeneic sera, generally obtained from horses, and (b) human gamma globulin concentrates from normal donors (measles, infectious hepatitis, hepatitis B, vaccinia, varicella) or hyperimmunized donors (rabies, tetanus) (Table 11.17).

The methods for purification of horse antitoxins and the fractionation technique with cold ethanol (Cohn's fractionation) used for obtaining human gamma globulin in concentrates were described in Chap. 4 (p. 83). The antitoxins are measured in international units (IU), and the human gamma

---

3 The half-life of gamma globulin (IgG), up to a certain point, is proportional to the size of the animal: 15–20 days for sheep, 5–7 days for rabbits and guinea pigs, and 3–4 days for mice

Table 11.17. Serotherapeutic materials used in human diseases

Disease	Product	Dosage[a]	Comment
Toxic infections			
Botulism	ABE polyvalent anti-toxin from horse	1 vial iv, 1 vial im	Repeat if symptoms persist
Diphtheria	Antitoxin from horse	Prevention: 1,000 IU Treatment: 30,000–60,000 IU	
Tetanus	Immune globulin from human	Prevention: 1,000 IU Treatment: 3,000–6,000 IU	Recommended only for exposed individuals who have fewer than two doses of toxoid at any time in the past
Viral infections			
Hepatitis B	Immune globulin from human	0.06 ml/kg	As soon as possible after exposure up to 7 days
Measles	Immune globulin from human	0.25 mg/kg	As soon as possible after exposure
Rabies	Immune globulin from human	20–40 IU/kg	Give until 72 h after exposure
Vaccinia	Immune globulin from human	Prevention: 0.3 ml/kg Treatment: 0.6 ml/kg	
Varicella	Immune globulin from human	3–5 ml	Within 72 h of exposure
Poisonings			
Black widow spider bite	Antivenin from horse	1 vial im or iv	
Snakebite	Coral snake or crotalide antivenin from horse	3–5 vials iv	
Others			
Fetal erythroblastosis	Anti-D gamma globulin from human	300 µg antibody	Give within 72 h of exposure

[a] Passive immunotherapy or immunoprophylaxis should always be administered as soon as possible after exposure; antisera are always given intramuscularly (im) unless otherwise stated. iv, intraveneously

globulin concentrates generally are adjusted to a protein concentration of not more than 15%.

Special mention should be made of the prophylaxis of fetal erythroblastosis by postpartum administration of anti-D gamma globulin. Rh$^+$ red cells of the fetus in the Rh$^-$ mother do not stimulate an immune response in the first pregnancy because of the insufficient quantity of fetal blood that passes into the maternal circulation through the intact placenta. At the time of parturition, however, transplacental hemorrhage can deliver the necessary immunogenic stimulus leading to the occurrence of fetal erythroblastosis in subsequent pregnancies. The injection within 72 h postpartum of only 300 µg of anti-D is effective in preventing erythroblastosis through two nonexclusive mechanisms: (1) the elimination of opsonized fetal erythrocytes; and (2) repression of the formation of maternal anti-D antibodies through passively inoculated anti-D antibodies that prevent the binding of the antigen to the receptors of the corresponding maternal lymphocytes.

In a well-controlled study in the United States with two groups of approximately 600 women treated or not treated with anti-D, the formation of antibodies was observed in 76 individuals in the control group and in only one in the treated group – indicating a protection index of 99.8%. Failures have been recorded, however, and they can be attributed either to massive transplacental hemorrhage or to intense secondary stimuli in repeated pregnancies.

Serotherapy Accidents. The administration of horse serum can cause serum sickness and, in rare cases, anaphylactic shock. To avoid the latter, which can be extremely severe, especially in individuals who have previously been injected with serum or who have a history of allergies, it is advisable first to perform a sensitivity test. This is done by intradermal injection of 0.05 ml of serum at a dilution of 1:10. If there is a positive reaction (development of an urticarial papule within 15 min), it is expedient to adopt the following precautions: (1) Injection of an antihistamine ½ h before injection of the serum, (2) injection of fractionalized doses of serum subcutaneously, starting with 0.1 ml and increasing progressively, with 15 minutes intervals between successive doses, (3) conceivably, intravenous injection of the serum. In any case, it is always safe to have on hand a solution of 1:1,000 of epinephrine to inject (0.5 ml intramuscularly) in the event of peripheral collapse.

Table 11.18. Types of vaccines currently in general use or only used occupationally, or in experimental stage

Type	Live vaccine	Killed vaccine
Viral	Smallpox	Poliomyelitis
	Rubella	Influenza
	Measles	Rabies
	Rabies (veterinary use)	Foot-and-mouth disease (veterinary use)
	Yellow fever	Typhus
	Mumps	
	Newcastle's disease (veterinary use)	
Bacterial	Tuberculosis (BCG)	Cholera
	Brucella (veterinary use)	Typhoid
		Whooping cough
Bacterial toxoids	Diphtheria	
	Tetanus	
	Cl. welchii (veterinary use)	
Helminths	Cattle lung worm	
	Sheep lungworm	
	Dog hookworm } veterinary use	
	Bovine babesia	
	Schistosoma bovis	

Occupational use or experimental:
Adenovirus (attenuated oral virus), arborvirus (equine encephalitis, occupational use), cytomegalovirus (live attenuated vaccine), hepatitis B (experimental), herpes virus hominis (experimental), influenza (live attenuated, orally administered, experimental); anthrax (protein antigen extracted from culture filtrates, occupational use), cholera (purified heat- and formalin-inactivated toxin), streptococci (dental caries, experimental), gonococci (experimental), typhoid (live attenuated oral); malaria (falciparum merozoites, experimental)

As with sera, gamma globulin preparations should be injected intramuscularly and only exceptionally intravenously. In the latter case, it is indispensable to use preparations that do not contain aggregates, for these produce anaphylactoid reactions resulting from the formation of kinins and of anaphylatoxins due to activation of the complement system.

Adoptive Transfer. Adoptive immunity is that which the organism acquires through the transfer of lymphocytes from a sensitized individual to a normal individual. Attempts have been made to transmit cell-mediated immunity, e.g., to vaccinia virus in immunologically incompetent hosts; to *Coccidioides immitis* in patients with disseminated coccidioidomycosis; and to *M. leprae* in lepromatous leprosy. Whole blood, leukocyte-rich buffy coat, and leukocyte-derived transfer factor have been used. The value of the therapy is uncertain, and these procedures are still rather experimental.

Actively Acquired Immunity

The first known method for active artificial immunization (vaccination) was immunization against smallpox, discovered by Edward Jenner in 1796. Jenner having noted the popular observation that dairymaids became immune to smallpox after being infected with the cowpox virus (vaccinia), concluded that a cross-immunization had occurred, and decided to inoculate the vaccinial pustule from a milkmaid (Sara Nelmas) into the skin on the arm of an English youth, James Philipp. The latter acquired a localized pustule like that seen today when the vaccine "takes," and upon being inoculated 6 weeks later with the smallpox virus, was

Table 11.19. Scheme of active immunization

Vaccine	First immunization				Revaccination or booster; comments
	Age	Route[a]	Doses	Interval	
BCG	Until 3 months After 3 months	id id	1×0.05 mg 1×0.1 mg	– –	Revaccination in absence of allergy
DTP	2 months to 5 years	im	3×0.5–1.0 ml	1–2 months	1 and 5 years after the 1st dose
DT	5–7 years	im	2×0.5–1.0 ml	1–2 months	Annually until age of 7; thereafter only tetanus (T)
Measles[b]	6 months to 4 years	sc	1×0.5 ml	–	May prevent natural disease if given less than 48 h after exposure
Mumps[b]	After 1 year	sc	1 dose	–	Reimmunization if given before 1 year of age
Rubella[b]	After 1 year (usually girls at age 10–12)	sc	1 dose	–	Contraindicated during pregnancy; women must prevent pregnancy for 3 months after immunization
Sabin[c] (trivalent)	3 months and after	oral	3×1 drop	2 and 6 months	5 years after the first dose
Smallpox[d]	2 years	id	1 drop	–	Revaccination after 5 years
Tetanus	Only after 7 years	im	2×0.5–1.0 ml	1–2 months	In the event of exposure

[a] id, intradermally; im, intramuscularly; sc, subcutaneously
[b] available as combination vaccine (MMR)
[c] Can be combined with first and second dose of DTP
[d] No vaccination if child or contacts have eczema or (any) skin disease

Table 11.20. Additional vaccines against infectious microorganisms

Disease	Vaccine	Route of administration[a]	First immunization	Duration of effect	Comments
Cholera	Killed bacteria	sc, im	2 doses 1 week or more apart	6 months	Only partially protective
Influenza	Killed whole or split virus A and/or B (chick embryo)	im	1 dose	1 year	Vaccination in November; composition of the vaccine varies depending upon epidemiologic circumstances
Meningo-coccus	Meningococcal polysaccharide group A or C	sc	1 dose	Permanent	Recommended in epidemic situations
Plague	Killed bacteria	im	3 doses 4 weeks or more apart	6 months	Only occupational exposure and residents of endemic areas
Pneumo-coccus	Pneumococcal polysaccharide, polyvalent	sc, im	1 dose	At least 3 years	Recommended for patients with cardiorespiratory diseases and sickle cell disease
Rabies	Killed virus (duck embryo)	sc	Preexposure: 2 doses 1 month apart; 3rd dose 6–7 months later. Postexposure: always give human rabies immune globulins. 23 doses: 2 doses for the first 7 days, then 7 daily doses, and boosters on days 24 and 34	2 years	
	(Human diploid)	im (m. deltoides)	Preexposure: 3–4 doses. Postexposure: immune globulin; 6 doses: days 0, 3, 7, 14, 28, and 90		
Typhoid	Killed bacteria	sc	2 doses 4 weeks or more apart	3 years	Recommended only for exposure from travel, epidemic or carrier
Typhus	Killed virus	sc	2 doses 4 weeks or more apart	6–12 months	Recommended only for occupational exposure
Yellow fever	Live virus (chick embryo)	sc	1 dose	10 years	Recommended for residence in or travel to endemic areas

[a] sc, subcutaneous; im, intramuscular

found to be immune: the "humanized" cow-pox virus was effective in imparting immunity to smallpox.

Experimenting further, Jenner in 1798 inoculated into a youth named Summers material taken directly from the vaccinia pustule of a cow. The pustule resulting from this inoculation material was passed by vaccination to a second child and so on, until the process had been repeated for a fifth time: the cowpox virus could be artificially humanized by serial inoculations (passages) into human skin.

These experiments resulted in the general use of the Jennerian vaccination with humanized (attenuated) vaccinial viruses. The procedure rapidly spread from country to country, with the vaccinia lymph passed from arm to arm. Soon it was realized, however, that the humanized vaccinia virus tended to weaken, losing its immunizing effectiveness; for this reason, the direct animal vaccine later came into use.

Eighty-five years later, Pasteur discovered vaccination with artificially attenuated germs (fowl cholera, hematic anthrax, rabies). In deference to Jenner and his fundamental discovery, he proposed that the name vaccine (Lat. *vacca*, cow) be given to the suspensions of attenuated germs utilized to produce active immunization.

Later, when it was verified that in certain cases, suspensions of dead germ or products derived from bacterial toxins (anatoxins or toxoids) are both capable of conferring immunity, the word vaccination was used as a synonym for active, artificial immunization.

Vaccines. The vaccines available today and used in human medical and veterinary practice are summarized in Table 11.18. A scheme for active immunization is found in Table 11.19, and vaccines used in special cases (occupation, travel, accidents, epidemics) are summarized in Table 11.20. For obvious reasons, the use of live vaccines in man has been restricted as much as possible; with the exception of the tuberculosis vaccine (BCG) they are used only in the prevention of certain virus diseases. In veterinary practice, however, live vaccines are used in the prophylaxis of bacterial infections, virus infections, and parasitic infections. Attenuation of microorganisms for the use of vaccines can be achieved by passages and selection of less pathogenic variants (viruses), and by irradiation (protozoa and metazoa).

References

Allison AC (1974) On the role of mononuclear phagocytes in immunity against viruses. Prog Med Virol 18:15

Cline MJ (1975) The white cell. Harvard University Press, Cambridge/Mass.

Cohen S, Sadun EH (eds) (1976) Immunology of parasitic infections. Blackwell, Oxford

Dixon FJ (ed) (1979) Viral immunopathology. Springer Sem Immunopath 2:233

Dönges J (1980) Parasitologie. Thieme, Stuttgart

Fudenberg HH, Stites DP, Caldwell JL, Wells JV (1980) Basic and clinical immunology, 3rd ed. Lange Medical Publications, Los Altos/Calif.

Gadebusch HH (ed) (1979) Phagocytosis and cellular immunity. CRC Press, Boca Raton, Fla.

Goodwin LG (1974) Pathology of african trypanosomiasis. In: Trypanosomiasis and leishmaniasis. Ciba Foundation Symposium, Elsevier-North Holland, Amsterdam

Gupta S, Good RA (eds) (1979) Cellular, molecular, and clinical aspects of allergic disorders. Plenum, New York

Jawetz E, Melnick JL, Adelberg EA (1978) Review of medical microbiology, 13th ed. Lange Medical Publications, Los Altos/Calif.

Klebanoff SJ, Clark RA (1978) The neutrophil. Function and clinical disorders. North-Holland, Amsterdam

Kraus R (ed) (1980) Immunopathology of parasitic diseases. Springer Sem Immunopath 2:355

Mims CA, White DO (1984) Viral pathogenesis and immunology. Blackwell, Oxford

Mitchell GF (1979) Responses to infections with metazoan and protozoan parasites in mice. Adv Immunol 28:451

Möller G (ed) (1974) The immune response to infectious diseases. Transplant Rev 19

Najjar VA, Schmidt JJ (1980) The chemistry and biology of tuftsin. Lymphokine Rep 1:157

Nelson DS (ed) (1976) Immunobiology of the macrophage. Academic, New York

Notkins AL, Oldstone MBA (eds) (1984) Concepts in viral pathogenesis. Springer New York

Rocklin RE, Bendtzen K, Greineder D (1980) Mediators of immunity: Lymphokines and monokines. Adv Immunol 29:56

Steward II WE (1979) Interferon. Springer, Wien New York

Stossel TP (1974) Phagocytosis. N Engl J Med 290: 717, 774, 833

Theofilopoulos AN, Dixon FJ (1979) The biology and detection of immune complexes. Adv Immunol 28:89

Zinkernagel RM, Doherty PC (1979) MHC restricted cytotoxic T cells: Studies on the biological role of polymorphic transplantation antigens determining T cell restriction-specificity, function, and responsiveness. Adv Immunol 27:52

Chapter 12   Immunodeficiencies

Wilmar Dias da Silva and Dietrich Götze

Contents

Evaluation of the Immune System Functions . 359
  Immunoglobulins and Antibodies 359
  B Lymphocytes 360
  T Lymphocytes 361
  Phagocytes 362
Classification of Immunodeficiencies 364
  B Cell Deficiencies 364
    Hypo- and Agammaglobulinemias 364
    Selective, Variable
      Hypogammaglobulinemias 366
    Hypergammaglobulinemias, Disorders
      of Ig-Secreting Cells 367
  T Cell Deficiencies 370
    DiGeorge's Syndrome 370
    Mucocutaneous Candidiasis 370
    Hodgkin's Disease 371
  Combined T, B Cell Deficiencies 371
    Severe Combined Immunodeficiency
      Syndromes (SCID) 371
    Wiskott-Aldrich Syndrome 372
    Ataxia Telangiectasia 372
  B and T Lymphocyte Proliferation Disorders 373
    Lymphomas 373
    Cutaneous T Cell Lymphomas 375
    Leukemias 375
  Phagocyte Deficiency Diseases 377
    Neutropenias 377
    Chemotactic Deficiencies 378
    Ingestion Deficiency 378
    Bactericidal Deficiency 379
  Complement Deficiencies 381
References 382

Control of infectious diseases by immunotherapy and chemotherapy has made possible the survival of individuals genetically predisposed to a series of diseases including immunodeficiencies that formerly resulted in death before the individual reached reproductive age. As a result, today, rare genes are expressed, which formerly were the exception. Thus, immunodeficiencies may cease to be rare diseases in the not too distant future.

The immunodeficiencies, conceptualized as aberrations in immunologic functions, might be considered as experiments carried out by nature, which immunologists have (also) studied in order to elucidate important aspects of the immune response.

As described in previous chapters, the immune response is made up of several subsystems: B lymphocytes and their immunoglobulin-secreting descendants, the plasma cells, and their products in the serum: IgM, IgG, IgA, IgE, and IgD; T lymphocytes, which help or suppress the function of B or other T lymphocytes, release lymphokines, and destroy specifically target cells upon stimulation; macrophages and polymorphonuclear cells, which are very effectively involved in the defense against infections and in enhancing the activity of lymphocytes (see Chap. 11). Deficiency of any part of the defense system will result in disturbance of the whole system.

Evaluation of the Immune System Functions

The first stage in the identification of immunodeficiencies is to evaluate the functional state of each of the components of the immune system: immunoglobulins, B and T lymphocytes, polymorphonuclear cells and macrophages, and the complement system.

Immunoglobulins and Antibodies

The immunoglobulin level is evaluated by serum electrophoresis and immunoelectrophoresis of the total serum; the concentration of immunoglobulin classes is assessed by the Mancini test (IgG, IgM, IgA, and IgD) or radioimmune assay (IgE) (see p. 275). Furthermore, the following parameters are usually determined: (1) the titer of IgM isoagglutinins and heteroagglutinins to rabbit and sheep erythrocytes as well as against *B. pertussis;* (2) the titer of IgG antibodies after immunization with diphtheria toxoid using the Schick reaction (see p. 332) or the quantification of diphtheria antitoxin in guinea pigs; (3) neutralizing antibody titer for measles by hemagglutination inhibition, and (4) the quantification of complement-fixing antibodies against mumps, and other previous infections or immunizations.

Under normal conditions, the immunoglobulin levels remain relatively constant due to an equilibrium between synthesis, distribution in the vascular and tissue compartment, and degradation. The synthesis of immunoglobulins has preference over that of other proteins in relation to the utilization of the essential amino acids available; more over, as mentioned already, the synthesis of immunoglobulins is normal even in cases of extreme malnutrition. It has been calculated that each IgG-producing plasma cell synthesizes 2,000 molecules of immunoglobulin per second, which corresponds to 1.5–2.5 g per day in an individual weighing 70 kg (154 lb). With these values, it was possible to determine the number of functioning IgG-producing plasma cells which, under normal conditions, is of the order of 5.5×10^{10}. For IgM and IgA, the median synthesis values are of the order of 0.4 g and 3.0 g per day, respectively, in the adult.

The distribution of immunoglobulins in the organism is not homogeneous. IgG is equally distributed in the intravascular and interstitial spaces and in such a way that variations in serum levels are reflected in the interstitial spaces. A similar distribution is observed for IgA, although it should be noted that IgA is most abundant in the secretions. IgM is found almost exclusively in the intravascular spaces, whereas IgE is de-

tectable in the blood only in cases of increased synthesis (allergic conditions and IgE myeloma).

The catabolic elimination of the immunoglobulins that are not combined with antigens occurs principally in the digestive tract, the liver, and the lungs. In man, the half-life of the immunoglobulins is 26 days for IgG, 6 days for IgA, 5.1 days for IgM, 2.8 days for IgD, and about 2 days for IgE. When the immunoglobulins are combined with antigens in the form of immune complexes, the elimination is rapid and occurs through phagocytosis by macrophages.

To evaluate the capacity for the formation of antibodies in vivo, the commonly employed antigen is diphtheria toxoid, and the intensity of the humoral response is verified by the Schick test.

B Lymphocytes

Under normal conditions, about 10%–30% of the lymphocytes in the peripheral blood are B lymphocytes expressing surface immunoglobulins. Their fraction among lymph node lymphocytes is about 20%, in tonsils about 40%, and in the spleen about 35%. Pre-B cells in the bone marrow have no surface immunoglobulins (Ig) but cytoplasmic IgM which can be assayed by fluoresceinated anti-immunoglobulins. Mature B cells possess, in addition to surface IgM, receptors for C 3 b and the Fc portion of IgG, and surface IgD. Antigen-stimulated B cells, mostly memory cells, express instead of IgD IgA or IgA together with IgM (see Chap. 1, pp. 12–13).

B cell function can be assayed in vitro by pokeweed mitogen stimulation, which induces normal B lymphocytes to proliferate (thymidine uptake) and to differentiate into mature antibody-secreting plasma cells of all classes. For this response to occur, B cells have to be co-cultured with helper T cells which are purified from healthy donors. Ig production is assessed at the end of the culture period by radioimmune assay of the culture supernatant fluid, or by the determination of uptake of labeled amino acid precursors, or by the demonstration of cytoplasmic Ig with fluoresceinated antisera.

T Lymphocytes

Human T cell function is evaluated by (1) enumeration of circulating T cells and T cell subpopulations, and (2) in vivo and in vitro testing of T cell functions.

The percentage and absolute numbers of T cells in the peripheral blood can be assessed by their ability to form rosettes with neuraminidase-treated sheep red blood cells (SRBC). Normally, about 75% of the circulating lymphocytes are T cells, in absolute numbers: 1,600–4,300 per mm^3 until 18 months of age, and 600–3,000 per mm^3 thereafter. Subpopulation of T cells can be distinguished by using T cell specific monoclonal antibody reagents (see p. 55). The functional tests for T cells comprise (a) delayed type hypersensitivity skin tests, (b) proliferation assays, (c) demonstration of release of soluble factors (lymphokines, see p. 330), and (d) assessment of killer, helper, and suppressor activity.

The following skin tests are usually applied: mumps, trichophytin, PPD, Candida, and streptokinase-streptodornase. Patients with no positive skin test to recall antigens are stimulated with 2,4-dinitrochlorbenzene or keyhol limpet hemocyanin.

Proliferation assays employ either unspecific mitogens such as PHA, ConA, and PWM, or antigens. Commonly used antigens are: PPD, Candida, tetanus, diphtheria. Cells of patients who had no prior encounter with these antigens do not proliferate. In stimulation experiments with allogeneic cells (MLR, see p. 150), B cell lines or T cell depleted normal cells, irradiated or mitomycin treated, should be used as stimulators to avoid the release of blastogenic factors.

The production of lymphokines (MIF, interferons, lymphotoxins, see p. 49, 331, and 336) can be by B and T cells; therefore, purified cell populations have to be used in determining the capacity of T or B lymphocytes to release these substances.

In order to assess helper and suppressor activity of T cells, the pokeweed mitogen-induced maturation of B cells into Ig-secreting plasma cells is used (see above). Normal peripheral B cells and monocytes are rigorously depleted of T cells and cocultivated with T cells of patients. Two cultures are run simultaneously, one with irradiated (1,000–2,000 r) T cells (T suppressor cells are radiosensitive), and the other with nonirradiated T cells. The ability to generate cytotoxic T cells is best studied after in vitro allogeneic stimulation as described in Chaps. 2 (p. 45) and 6 (p. 150 and 170).

Table 12.1. B and T lymphocyte specific characteristics

Characteristics	T cells	B cells	K cells	Method of detection
SRBC receptor (E rosettes)	+	−	−	Binding of sheep red blood cells
HT1	+	−	−	Cytotoxicity, fluorescence
Receptor for rabbit IgM	+ (Tμ)	−	−	Rosette formation with ox erythrocytes
Receptor for rabbit IgG	+ (Tγ)	−	+	coated with rabbit IgM or IgG, respectively
Receptor for Ig-Fc	−	+	+	Aggregated Ig; immunofluoresence
Receptor for C3b (EAC rosettes)	−	+	?	Binding of complement and IgM-coated sheep or ox red blood C.
CD antigens (see Tab. 2.2, p. 55)	+	+	?	Monoclonal antibody reagents
Surface Ig	−	+	−	Immunofluorescence
Proliferation to PHA	+	−	?	Thymidine up-take
Proliferation to ConA	+	−	?	
Proliferation to PWM	+	+	?	
Radiosensitivity	Tμ−, Tγ+ +	+	?	PWM induced plasma cell maturation

Phagocytes

Polymorphonuclear and mononuclear cell functions in a defense reaction can be, for practical purposes, separated into distinct operations: chemotactic (directed) and random movement, adherence to microbes, ingestion of microbes, degranulation of lysosomes into phagosomes or exterior, and killing of microbes (Fig. 12.1).

Motility. Random motility can be tested for by the capillary tube migration test. Purified neutrophils (5×10^6/ml in 0.1% albumin solution) are placed in siliconized microhematocrit tubes; the tubes are heat sealed at one end and centrifuged at 1,500 rpm for 10 min. The tubes are then severed at the top of the leukocyte pellet and the truncated capillary tube is placed horizontally in a Petri dish containing a suitable medium at 37 °C. During this incubation, the cells migrate out of the tube in a fan-shaped manner (see Fig. 9.16, p. 290).

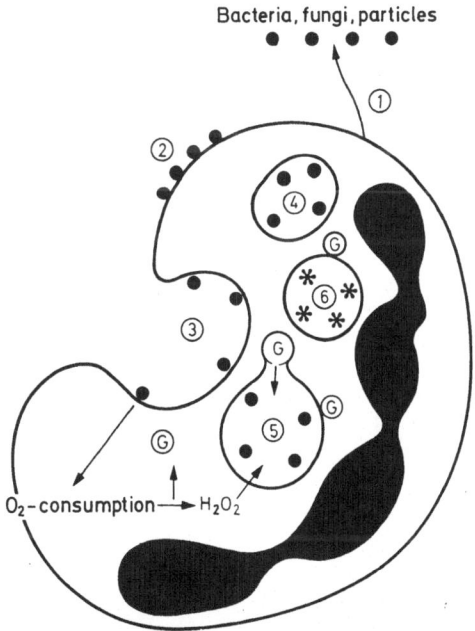

Fig. 12.1. Functional steps of phagocytosis in neutrophils: *1*, chemotaxis; *2*, opsonization; *3*, ingestion; *4*, phagosome; *5*, degranulation (phagolysosome formation); *6*, bacteriolysis. *G*, granules containing lytic enzymes

Chemotactic movement is tested by the use of Boyden's chambers (see Fig. 5.8). Cells to be tested are placed in the upper chamber and are separated from the lower chamber containing a chemotactic substance by a millipore filter (pore size usually 3 µm). Neutrophils can enter the filter membrane but are trapped in transit through the membrane. After several hours of incubation at 37 °C, the filter is removed and stained, and the underside is microscopically examined for the presence of neutrophils.

Another technique, migration under agarose, permits the determination of random and chemotactic movement at the same time. Wells are cut in an agarose medium. The center well is filled with a suspension of purified cells while two peripheral wells are filled with medium and chemotactic material, respectively. The cells respond to the chemotaxin and migrate in a tear-drop fashion toward that well. By measuring the distance of migration from the leading edge to the center well, one can quantitate the intensity of the chemotactic stimulus. The random migration is measured by the degree of migration toward the control well.

Adherence. Neutrophil and monocytes adherence is evaluated by their ability to spread on certain surfaces (glass, plastic).

Opsonization. Opsonization is measured in terms of increased phagocytosis of microorganisms coated with antibodies and complement in comparison to noncoated microorganisms.

Ingestion. Methods for quantitation of ingested material include direct counting of ingested microbes by light microscope, estimation of cell-bound radioactivity after ingestion of labeled microbes, and measurement of stained particles after ingestion.

In the first procedure, cells are mixed with appropriate bacteria; after a suitable incubation time (usually 30–60 min), the cells are fixed. Internalized bacteria are directly counted with the light microscope from stained smears.

The second procedure uses bacteria which have been grown on ^{14}C-amino acids or ^{3}H-thymidine. The opsonized, labeled bacteria are incubated with cells for varying periods of time and the reaction is terminated by the addition of cold buffer containing an inhibitor of glycolysis (NaF). Free bacteria are removed from ingested bacteria by repeated washings. The cell-associated radioactivity is then measured.

The third method utilizes paraffin oil emulsions containing a dye, oil red O. Following incubation of the neutrophils with the test emulsion and removal of noningested paraffin, the amount of cell-associated dye is quantitated spectrophotometrically.

Degranulation. Degranulation is tested by "frustrated phagocytosis": heat-aggregated γ-globulin or immune complexes are fixed to the plastic surface of a Petri dish so that they cannot be ingested. Neutrophils are placed in Petri dishes with and without attached γ-globulin. They are stimulated and discharge

their intralysosomal content, particularly β-glucuronidase and acid phosphatase, into the suspending medium. Nonspecific cell death or cytolysis can be estimated by measuring the discharge of lactate dehydrogenase, a cytoplasmic (nongranule) enzyme into the medium.

Intracellular Killing. Intracellular killing is assessed by two methods: the nitroblue tetrazolium dye reduction test (NBT) and the intraleukocytic killing test.

Nitroblue tetrazolium is a clear, yellow, water-soluble compound that forms formazan, a deep blue dye, on reduction. Neutrophils can reduce the dye following ingestion of latex or other particles subsequent to the respiratory burst. The reduced dye can be easily measured spectrophotometrically at 515 nm after extraction from neutrophils with the organic solvent pyridine. For the mechanism of dye reduction, see p. 324.

In the intraleukocytic killing test, bacteria (about 5 per neutrophil in the final test) and

Table 12.2. Additional tests for the evaluation of the white blood cell status

Tests	Comments
Special stainings	
Myeloperoxidase	*Negative:* neutrophils with toxic granulation during severe infections
	Positive: neutrophils and eosinophils
Acid phosphatase	*Negative:* normal plasma cells; *positive:* plasmocytoma cells
PAS reaction (periodic acid Schiff reaction)	*Negative:* myeloblasts; *positive:* lympho- and monoblasts
Esterase reaction with α-naphthyl-acetate	*Positive:* monocytes
Functional tests	
Rebuck skin window test	Chemotaxis in vivo
H$_2$O$_2$ generation	Evaluation of different ingestive and bactericidal functions
O$_2$-consumption	during phagocytosis
Glucose-1-^{14}C-oxidation	
Formate-^{14}C-oxidation	
Superoxide production	
Iodination of phagocytosed particles	
Leukocyte survival time with DF ^{32}P or ^{51}Cr	
Adrenaline test	Evaluation of marginated pool
Endotoxin-, etiocholanolon- and prednisolone test	Evaluation of granulocyte pool in the bone marrow
Serum lysozyme (muramidase)	Leukocyte turnover
Anti-neutrophil antibodies	
Radiological examination	Thymus aplasia, thymom, a.o.

opsonins are incubated with neutrophils for 1, 2, or 3 h at 37 °C. After incubation, extracellular bacteria are killed by the addition of antibiotics. Intracellular bacteria are liberated by lysis of neutrophils by sterile water, and the number of viable bacteria is estimated from the number of bacterial colonies after plating. Additional tests for the evaluation of the status of leukocytes are listed in Table 12.2.

Classification of Immunodeficiencies

The defense system consists of several distinct functional complexes, the cooperation of which confers protection against the constant assault by viral, bacterial, fungal, protozoal, and noninfectious agents (see Chap. 11). Dysfunction of any of these systems, i.e., T lymphocytes, B lymphocytes, phagocytes, and complement, will result in an overall deficiency, usually expressed in enhanced susceptibility to infections. The known deficiencies can be classified according to the system(s) involved:
1. B cell deficiencies
   Hypo- or agammaglobulinemias
   Transient hypoglobulinemia in infants
   Congenital Bruton-type (X chromosome) agammaglobulinemia
   Acquired primary and secondary hypogammaglobulinemias
   Selective, variable hypogammaglobulinemias
   Hypergammaglobulinemias, disorders of Ig-secreting cells
   Monoclonal gammopathies
   Polyclonal gammopathies
2. T cell deficiencies
   DiGeorge's syndrome
   Chronic cutaneous candidiasis
   Hodgkin's disease
3. Combined T, B cell deficiencies
   Severe combined immunodeficiencies (SCID)
   Lymphoid stem cell defect (Swiss type)
   Adenosine-deaminase deficiency
   Purine nucleoside phosphorylase deficiency

Transcobalamin II deficiency
   Nezelof's syndrome
   Ataxia telangiectasia
   Wiskott-Aldrich syndrome
4. B and T lymphocyte proliferative disorders
   Lymphomas
   Cutaneous T cell lymphomas
   Leukemias
5. Phagocytic dysfunctions
   Neutropenias
   Chemotactic deficiencies
   Ingestion deficiency
   Bactericidal deficiencies
6. Complement deficiencies.

B Cell Deficiencies

Hypo- and Agammaglobulinemias

Transient Hypogammaglobulinemia in Infants. A full-term neonate possesses approximately 1 g IgG per 100 ml of maternal origin, whereas IgM and IgA are practically absent. In the first weeks of life, the IgG level falls progressively, reaching concentrations of 2,5 mg per ml at the third month of age. By this time, the infant begins to synthesize its own immunoglobulin, first IgG and IgM, then a little later IgA; by the fourth month, a progressive elevation of immunoglobulin levels to approximately 5,6 mg per ml has occurred. The period of depression of serum immunoglobulin levels in the third month coincides with the elimination of maternal IgG and generally signals the onset of synthesis of the infant's own immunoglobulins. In certain cases, however, this synthesis of immunoglobulins is retarded; during such a phase, the infant exhibits increased susceptibility to infections such as pneumonia, otitis media, and pyoderma. This abnormal condition is called transient hypogammaglobulinemia. This period is characterized immunoelectrophoretically by a shortening of the IgG anionic arc. The restoration of normal serum levels of immunoglobulins generally occurs between the third and the 30th month of life.

Fudenberg proposed an interpretation for transient hypogammaglobulinemia in infants of both sexes that is distinct from congenital autosomal agammaglobulinemia which is discussed later. Transient hypogammaglobulinemia may represent the isoimmunization of the mother against fetal IgG carrying different Gm allotypes that give rise to the formation of antigen-antibody complexes that can be eliminated rapidly by the mononuclear phagocytic system.

Congenital and Hereditary and Acquired Agammaglobulinemias. The term agammaglobulinemia is restricted to cases in which the total serum level of immunoglobulins is less than 100 mg per 100 ml; above this level the expression hypogammaglobulinemia is used. Agammaglobulinemias customarily are separated into two groups: congenital and acquired. The former appear in the first two months of life, whereas the latter appear later in puberty or adulthood. At times it is difficult to decide whether an agammaglobulinemia manifesting itself at puberty is in fact an acquired form, or whether it represents the delayed appearance of a hereditary disease.

Congenital Hypogammaglobulinemia Bruton-Type. This type of X-linked, infantile hypogammaglobulinemia is due to a regulatory gene defect that affects pre-B cell differentiation (see Fig. 12.4). In general, patients lack B cells, although normal numbers of pre-B cells (approximately 0.6% of nucleated bone marrow cells) are observed in bone marrow samples. The cellular immunity appears to be normal. The number of circulating lymphocytes is usually normal, but the thymus-dependent areas of the lymphoid organs are poorly delimited, and there are hardly any follicles or plasma cells. There is a scarcity or absence of pharyngeal lymphoid tissue. The latter phenomenon can be shown radiographically by the increased size of the nasopharyngeal space (Newhauser's space). The thymus is generally normal; however, there can be a scarcity of Hassal's bodies. Successive and recurring

gram-positive infections occur insidiously from the sixth month onward in distinct locations (e.g., otitis media, pyoderma, and pneumonia). It is believed that the resistance in these patients to gram-negative bacterial infections and to viruses is due to the properdin system and the cellular immunity, which appear to be unaffected. The frequency of autoimmune diseases and malignant tumors of the lymphoid tissue in such patients is relatively high. This form of immunodeficiency exhibits a pattern of anomalies of the immune system similar to those observed in the experimental model resulting from bursectomy in the chicken.

Acquired Primary Hypogammaglobulinemias. These hypogammaglobulinemias appear after a period of normal functioning of the immune system. The age at which the disease appears varies between 30 and 50 years, and generally precedes by some years the appearance of malignant tumors of the lymphoid tissue. Those afflicted exhibit low levels of IgG, IgM, and IgA; they respond poorly to antigenic stimulation, although they are capable of producing delayed hypersensitivity reactions and rejection of allografts. The number of circulating lymphocytes is normal, these cells being capable of producing a normal blastogenic response to stimulation by phythemagglutinin. The peripheral lymphoid organs are practically devoid of plasma cells, the number of lymphoid follicles being sharply reduced. In some cases, lymphoid hyperplasia occurs, especially in the small intestine; the resultant picture is that of intestinal malabsorption and loss of proteins. There is a correlation in about 10% of all cases between this immunodeficiency and tumors of the thymus; in those cases, an excessive activity of T suppressor cells have been found, and Tγ cells are increased.

Acquired Secondary Hypogammaglobulinemias. This group includes all forms of hypogammaglobulinemias associated with processes that do not directly affect the lymphoid organs.

Selective,
Variable Hypogammaglobulinemias

These are selective deficiencies of one or more classes of immunoglobulins that are always accompanied by a deficient response to certain antigens. These disorders are attributed either to the absence of synthesis of a particular class of immunoglobulins or to the production of functionally abnormal immunoglobulins. From the innumerable combinations of immunoglobulin deficiencies possible, only a few types have been studied extensively. Almost all patients exhibit recurring infections – principally in cases of IgG deficiency. Cellular immunity remains normal.

Selective IgM Deficiency is characterized by a selective lack of IgM in the serum. In some cases, B cells with IgM on their surface are present in normal numbers; apparently, IgM cannot be secreted probably because of a defect in the secretory peptide (see p. 104). In other cases, suppressor T cell activity specific for the IgM class has been demonstrated. Clinical observation reveals sudden episodes of septicemia caused in general by gram-negative bacteria. This disease illustrates the biologic role of IgM as an immunoglobulin with intravascular protective activity.

Selective IgG Deficiency involves imbalances in the production of IgG subclasses, and has been defined as inherited structural gene defects by using allotype markers specific for each subclass. In a few patients, B cells are able to synthesize IgG upon stimulation by a T-cell-derived mitogenic factor but can not secrete it. The secretory defect of these cells has been associated with a failure in glycolyzation of newly synthesized IgG; this process normally occurs just before secretion of IgG. Clinically, such patients exhibit repeated pyogenic infections, the occurrence of which is extremely similar to those in patients with Bruton-type agammaglobulinemia.

Selective IgA Deficiency is the most common immunodeficiency disorder, and occurs in two forms: in one, there is a deficiency in serum as well as in secreted IgA, and in the other, there is only a deficiency in secreted IgA. The first form is autosomal dominantly or recessively inherited, but sometimes occurs sporadically. In a few patients it is observed together with one of the following disorders: ataxia-telangiectasia, malabsorption syndrome, and recurrent respiratory infections; an increased incidence of autoimmune diseases has also been observed.

In patients with serum and secreted IgA deficiency, B cells are normal and express IgA on their surface; however, the differentiation of the B$^\alpha$ cells to plasma cells is defective. In some patients, an increase of suppressor T cells specific for IgA has been demonstrated. In other patients, a deficiency in the helper function of T cells specific for IgA-B cells has been suggested.

Patients who lack IgA in their secretions, but who have normal IgA serum levels, have a deficiency in the formation of the secretory piece in the intestinal mucosal cells; the number of IgA-B cells in the blood is often elevated. Clinically, infections of the respiratory tract, otitis media, and recurrent pneumonias are observed.

Selective IgG and IgA Deficiency is often accompanied by elevated (normal) IgM levels (1.0–1.5 mg/ml). In some case, the deficiency is X-linked inherited, but apparently the deficiency can also be acquired in later life, and then affects both sexes. It is assumed that the underlying mechanism, at least in the inherited form, is a regulatory gene defect resulting in the inability of mature B cells to switch from IgM to IgG and IgA production, maybe primarily to IgG production (see p. 13 and 104). Clinically, recurrent pyogenic infections of the lungs occur. Transient neutropenia is common during severe septicemic infections. In addition to infections, these patients also exhibit autoimmune diseases (thrombocytopenia, neutropenia , hemolytic anemia). Histologic examination of the spleen and lymph nodes indicates an increase in IgM-producing plasma cells characterized histochemically by intense staining with periodic acid (Schiff's reaction) due to the high level of IgM carbohydrates.

Selective IgA and IgM Deficiency is characterized by a simultaneous IgM and IgA deficiency, along with normal concentrations of IgG. The ratio of male to female among affected patients is 4:1. In some patients, the produced IgG appears to be inert, i.e., functionally defective. Patients exhibit recurrent bacterial infections, and have a reduced capacity to respond adequately to a large number of antigens.

Secondary Immunologic Deficiencies are defects in the immunologic activity associated with other pathologic entities. They may derive from exaggerated catabolism of immunoglobulins, e.g., in the nephrotic syndrome, or in enteropathies with protein loss, or from dysfunction of the bone marrow due to toxic factors (e.g., renal insufficiency, drugs), or they may be due to reticuloendothelial neoplasias such as reticulosarcoma, Hodgkin's disease, lymphosarcoma, chronic lymphocytic leukemia, and thymoma.

Hypergammaglobulinemias, Disorders of Ig-Secreting Cells

Monoclonal Gammopathies. These result from the abnormal proliferation of a particular clone of plasma cells, with production of elevated quantities of immunoglobulins of one class, one type, and one specificity. Included among these are multiple myeloma (plasmocytoma), Waldenström's macroglobulinemia, heavy chain diseases, and light chain diseases.

Monoclonal gammopathies can involve any class of immunoglobulin. They consist of a paraprotein generally called the "M" (myeloma) component. In certain cases, light chains (λ or κ) are encountered free in the serum and in the urine (Bence Jones protein).

Multiple myeloma is characterized by malignant proliferation of plasma cells in de-

lineated regions of the bone marrow. The M component can be demonstrated electrophoretically. The component can belong to any class of immunoglobulins: in about 16% of cases, Bence-Jones protein can be demonstrated in the urine. Functional hypogammaglobulinemia (relative!) and deficiencies of other immunoglobulins are almost always present, making the patient singularly susceptible to infections, pneumococcal pneumonia in particular.

In parts a, b, and c of Fig. 12.2, the electrophoretic diagrams of a normal individual, of a patient with hypogammaglobulinemia, and of one with polyclonal hypergammaglobulinemia, respectively, are shown; parts d, e, and f correspond to profiles of IgG, IgA, and IgM, respectively (Waldenström's macroglobulinemia) myelomas.

Figure 12.3 shows electrophoretic diagrams of normal serum and of IgA (a), IgG (c), IgD (e), and IgM (f) myeloma sera as well as that of urine containing the Bence Jones protein (g). IgG and IgA myelomas are relatively more frequent, especially the former, whereas those of IgD and IgE are exceptional.

The myeloma proteins possess structural and antigenic properties similar to those of corresponding normal immunoglobulins. Antibody-type activity, such as that of cold agglutinin, antiglobulin, antistreptolysin, and others, has been demonstrated for myeloma proteins. Exceptions include the paraproteins encountered in heavy chain disease and Deutsch's paraproteins.

Waldenström's Macroglobulinemia is a proliferative disorder of IgM-producing cells. Serum levels of IgM are significantly elevated (β_2-globulins); due to the high molecular weight of this immunoglobulin, a great increase in the viscosity of the serum of these patients occurs. Antibody activity has been detected in these monoclonal IgM-immunoglobulins (e.g., antierythrocyte and anti-IgG activity), responsible for hemolytic anemia and for glomerular lesions that usually appear in association with this disease. Figure 12.2 f and 12.3 f show the electrophoretic

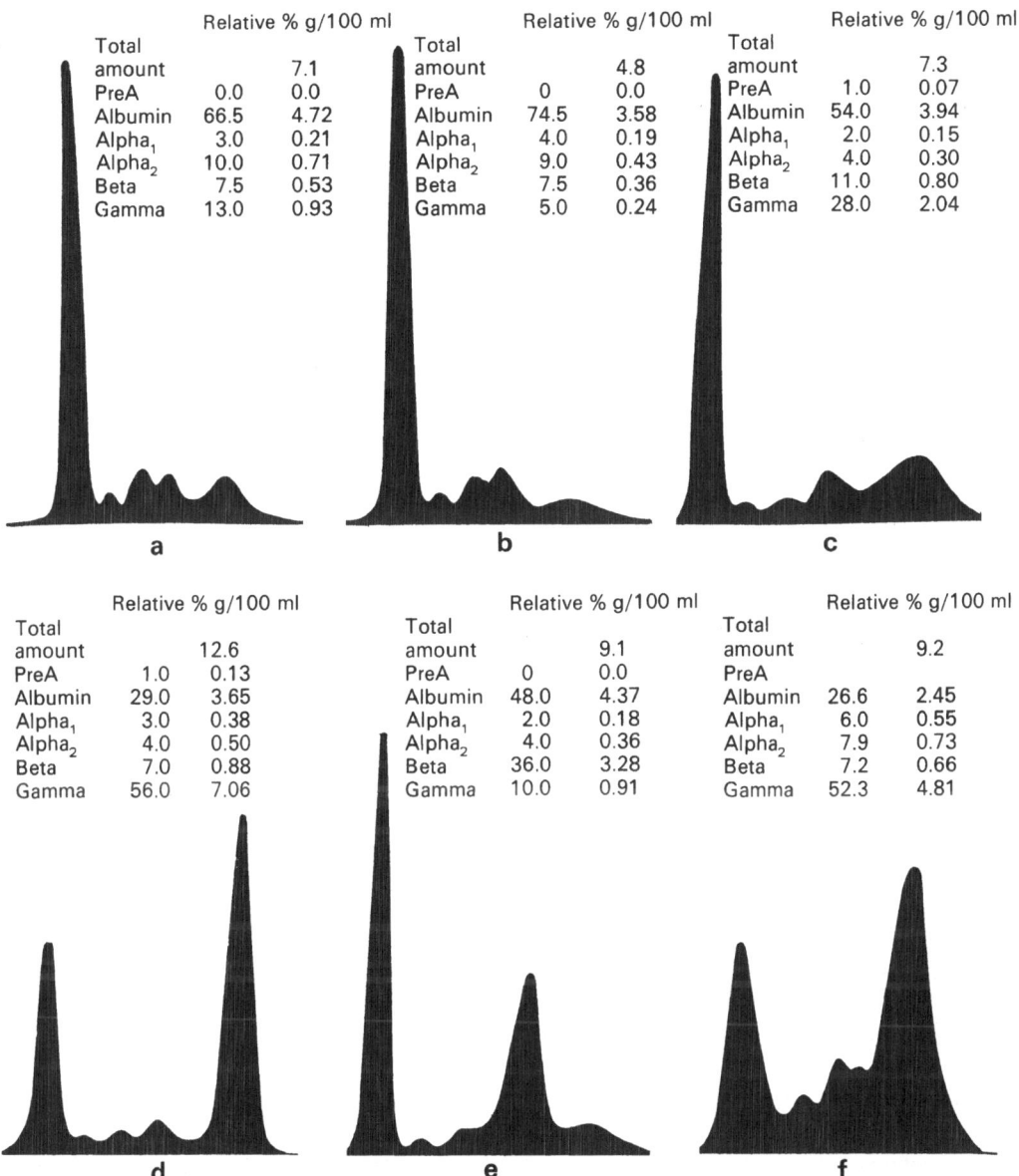

	Relative %	g/100 ml
Total amount		7.1
PreA	0.0	0.0
Albumin	66.5	4.72
Alpha$_1$	3.0	0.21
Alpha$_2$	10.0	0.71
Beta	7.5	0.53
Gamma	13.0	0.93

a

	Relative %	g/100 ml
Total amount		4.8
PreA	0	0.0
Albumin	74.5	3.58
Alpha$_1$	4.0	0.19
Alpha$_2$	9.0	0.43
Beta	7.5	0.36
Gamma	5.0	0.24

b

	Relative %	g/100 ml
Total amount		7.3
PreA	1.0	0.07
Albumin	54.0	3.94
Alpha$_1$	2.0	0.15
Alpha$_2$	4.0	0.30
Beta	11.0	0.80
Gamma	28.0	2.04

c

	Relative %	g/100 ml
Total amount		12.6
PreA	1.0	0.13
Albumin	29.0	3.65
Alpha$_1$	3.0	0.38
Alpha$_2$	4.0	0.50
Beta	7.0	0.88
Gamma	56.0	7.06

d

	Relative %	g/100 ml
Total amount		9.1
PreA	0	0.0
Albumin	48.0	4.37
Alpha$_1$	2.0	0.18
Alpha$_2$	4.0	0.36
Beta	36.0	3.28
Gamma	10.0	0.91

e

	Relative %	g/100 ml
Total amount		9.2
PreA		
Albumin	26.6	2.45
Alpha$_1$	6.0	0.55
Alpha$_2$	7.9	0.73
Beta	7.2	0.66
Gamma	52.3	4.81

f

Fig. 12.2 a–f. Electrophoretic profiles of human sera: **a** normal; **b** hypogammaglobulinemia; **c** polyclonal hypergammaglobulinemia. Monoclonal hypergammaglobulinemias: **d** IgG myeloma; **e** IgA myeloma; **f** IgM myeloma. (Courtesy of Dr. Rubens G. Ferri)

and immunoelectrophoretic diagrams of the serum of a patient with Waldenström's macroglobulinemia.

Monoclonal Gammopathies with Abnormally Structured Immunoglobulins. Gammopathies associated with abnormally structured immunoglobulins appear under certain pathologic conditions of immunocompetent cells, as in heavy chain disease, light chain disease, and Deutsch's paraproteinemia.

Heavy Chain Disease (γ-chain or Franklin's disease) involves a lymphoma that preferentially affects the cervical, axillary, mediastinal, and abdominal lymph nodes. Among

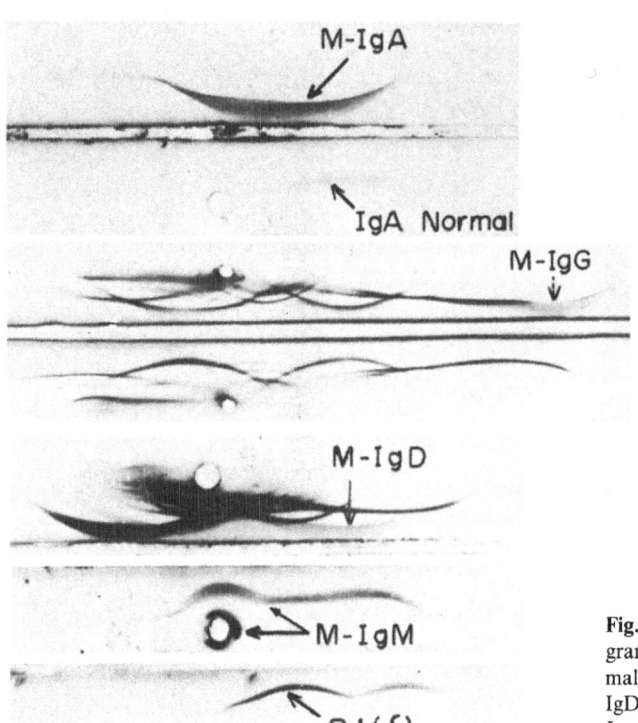

Fig. 12.3 a–g. Immunoelectrophoretic diagrams of human sera: **a** IgA myeloma; **b** normal IgA; **c** IgG myeloma; **d** normal serum; **e** IgD myeloma; **f** IgM myeloma; **g** Bence Jones-protein (urine). (Courtesy of Dr. Rubens G. Ferri)

the cases described, the male-female ratio is 3:2, with greatest prevalence around 50 years of age.

There is an abnormal production of a paraprotein with a molecular weight of 55,000 daltons, containing IgG antigenic determinants. Basically, this involves a deletion in the Fc fragment of the heavy chain so that no disulfide bridges can be formed between the light and the heavy chains. It is not known whether these proteins represent intact products of genes with deletion of the codifying nucleotides of the N-terminal region, or whether they are products of postsynthetic degradation of a heavy chain polypeptide. In some of the proteins in which the amino acid sequence has been determined, the N-terminal sequences were normal, extending from the V region to the greater part of the C_H-1 region and always terminating at position 216. These observations suggest that the proteins represent the product of aberrant synthesis and not that of a degradation process. The majority of patients

do not exhibit positive reactions to a test for Bence-Jones proteins. The heavy chain excreted in the urine possesses high carbohydrate levels.

Alpha Chain Disease (Mediterranean Lymphoma) is characterized by an infiltrative lymphoma involving the small intestine and the mesenteric lymphoid nodules. It occurs preferentially in young individuals, and there appears to be a close relationship between the incidence of this disease and endemic intestinal parasitosis. Also in this case, the disturbance is in the Fc fragment, however, in the heavy chain of IgA.

Mu Chain Disease. Thus far, only one case has been described. In that case, light chains appeared in the urine along with the heavy chains, although they were not combined.

Deutsch's Paraproteinemia is characterized by the appearance of paraproteins containing IgG_1 antigenic determinants with a deletion in the region of the heavy chains in which the Gm factor is localized. Since normal IgG molecules of the same patient possess the same genetic marker, Deutsch's protein must be a product of abnormal synthesis by a specific cellular clone.

Light Chain Abnormalities have been described in a few immunodeficient patients who completely fail to produce antibodies with kappa light chains. Circulating B lymphocytes, which were examined for light chain expression and surface immunoglobulins, were exclusively lambda chain in type. Since the kappa chain family contains its own set of variable region genes, it is worth noting that kappa-chain deficient patients have an important gap in their antibody repertoire. Another patient, whose serum Ig and plasma cells were virtually all of the lambda chain type, had a normal κ/λ ratio for surface bound Ig on circulating B lymphocytes and cytoplasmic Ig in PWM-induced plasmablasts, thus suggesting that the deficiency of chain production resulted from an abnormality of terminal differentiation.

Polyclonal Gammopathies are hypergammaglobulinemias with increase in the levels of more than one immunoglobulin class. Electrophoresis of the sera of these patients shows a diffuse increase of the gamma globulin fraction and a reduction of the albumin fraction. These conditions always appear to be associated with alterations in the connective tissue such as systemic lupus erythematosus and rheumatoid arthritis, hepatopathies, chronic infections, and sarcoidosis. There can be an increase of three immunoglobulin classes (triclonal gammopathies) or of just two (diclonal gammopathies), but in any case the components of the paraproteins are homogeneous. By using idiotypic antibodies, it is possible to verify that many of the diclonal components possess identical V regions bound to different heavy chains. However, not all diclonal paraproteins exhibit the same idiotype. The paraprotein can be of the κ or λ type, even when the V regions of the heavy chains are identical, in which case the light chains would be of different allotypes.

T Cell Deficiencies

Thymus-dependent immunologic deficiencies are those that affect the thymus-dependent immune system. In general, these patients exhibit lymphopenia of variable intensity, are incapable of developing delayed-type hypersensitivity, and their lymphocytes do not undergo blast transformation when incubated with phytohemagglutinin or other plant mitogens. However, the patient possesses normal serum levels of immunoglobulins. The most important forms that have been described are DiGeorge's syndrome, Mucocutaneous Candidiasis and the immunologic deficiency associated with Hodgkin's disease.

DiGeorge's Syndrome

DiGeorge's syndrome is a diseae characterized by simultaneous agenesis of the thymus and parathyroids and consequent defects in the development of the III and IV pharyngeal bursas. In addition to the deficiencies in cellular immunity described previously, the patient exhibits symptoms of hypoparathyroidism such as tetany and hypocalcemia. The patient generally succumbs to viral or mycotic infections. Histologic examination of the peripheral lymphoid organs reveals depression of lymphocyte levels in thymus-dependent areas; the lymphoid follicles are normal and rich in plasma cells.

Mucocutaneous Candidiasis

This disorder is associated with a selective defect in cell-mediated immunity to candida in form of an absent delayed type hypersensitivity skin test response. Antibody-mediated immunity is intact, resulting in a normal antibody response to candida. The numbers of T cells in the peripheral blood are usually normal; they respond to PHA, to allogeneic cells, and to antigens others than candida. In some patients, increased numbers of suppressor T cells have been found. A familial occurrence has been reported, suggesting an autosomal-recessive inheritance. The clinical picture is characterized by persistent candida infections of skin and mucosa (respiratory and gastrointestinal tracts) and by a series of endocrine disturbances.

Hodgkin's Disease

Hodgkin's disease, a pathologic condition occurring exclusively in human, exhibits two pathognomic characteristics: it is granulomatous, and it shows accentuated cellular pleomorphism. Hodgkin's disease has some characteristics of an infectious disease, probably due to a virus, which leads to an ineffective proliferation of T cells with depletion of T cells in time combined with neoplastic monoclonal proliferation of B lymphocytes or B cell precursors (Reed-Sternberg's giant cells in granulomas). The course of the disease depends to a great extent upon the competency of the immune system, which is, in turn, threatened by the disease itself. Patients with Hodgkin's disease who are over 60 years of age tend to have disseminated lymphocyte-depleted tumors, and a relatively poor clinical prognosis. Grafts of fetal thymus tissue into such patients have been followed by a degree of immunological reconstitution. Serum immunoglobulin levels are normal or even somewhat elevated, but cellular immunity is depressed. The patients, though capable of resisting bacterial infections, are highly susceptible to viral and mycotic infections.

Combined T, B Cell Deficiencies

Combined immunodeficiency diseases are due to various causes and are of variable severity. Defective T and B cell immunity may be complete (as in severe combined immunodeficiency, SCID), or partial. The onset of symptoms in patients with combined immunodeficiency diseases, usually appears early in infancy.

Severe Combined Immunodeficiency Syndromes (SCID)

These are defined as all diseases resulting from marked and long-lasting functional impairment of both the T and B cell systems. Accordingly, the clinical symptoms and signs involve many organs and invariably lead to death. An almost constant feature is thymic dysplasia.

Immunologically, patients are lymphopenic, and B and T cells are severely diminished in absolute numbers. The severe depression of immunoglobulin synthesis becomes manifest after the age of 3 months, when maternal IgG has been exhausted; IgM deficiency might be detected earlier. All cell-mediated immune functions are absent. The architecture of the lymphatic tissue is severely disrupted. Lymph nodes are very small, and they lack germinal centers and plasma cells. The intestinal mucosa shows severe atrophy of the lymphatic system. If the thymus can be found, its architecture can barely be recognized. There are very few lymphocytes, the predominant cells being large, clear reticulum cells, and complete absence or severe diminution of Hassall's corpuscles is a constant finding. The syndrome is caused by several distinct clinical entities with different pathogenesis.

Lymphoid Stem Cell Defect. The SCID syndrome caused by a failure of maturation of bone marrow stem cells into lymphoid precursor cells was the first SCID syndrome described by Swiss authors; it was, therefore, called "Swiss-type" deficiency. The majority of these cases are hereditary; two modes of inheritance have been demonstrated: in some families the disease follows a sex-linked pattern, but in others, it is transmitted as an autosomal recessive trait. It has been claimed that this form is associated with the HLA-A 1 or HLA-B 7 types, but this is not accepted unanimously.

Adenosine-Deaminase Deficiency. In 1972, it was found that some SCID patients lacked the enzyme adenosine-deaminase (ADA). Meanwhile, it is recognized that ½ to ⅓ of

SCID patients with autosomal recessive transmission are ADA deficient; ADA deficiency without immunodeficiency has never been observed. ADA is an enzyme of the purine salvage pathway which catalyzes the deamination of both adenosine and deoxyadenosine to yield inosine and deoxyinosine, respectively. The structural gene for ADA is located on chromosome 20 in man. This low molecular weight (32,000 daltons) ADA enzyme is found free in erythrocytes, thymus cells, and spleen and lymph node cells. ADA deficiency apparently results in an accumulation of deoxyadenosine and deoxyATP; deoxyATP is a potent inhibitor of the ribonucleotide reductase activity responsible for the generation of the 2′-deoxyribonucleotides and thus for the production of the substrate for DNA synthesis.

Purine Nucleoside Phosphorylase (PNP) Deficiency. PNP is also an enzyme in the purine salvage pathway and catalyzes reversibly the phosphorolysis of guanosine, inosine, deoxyguanosine, and deoxyinosine. The human enzyme is a trimer consisting of subunits with molecular weights of 30,000. The PNP locus has been mapped to chromosome 14; the deficiency is inherited as an autosomal recessive disorder. Patients have severe T cell dysfunction but less impaired humoral immunity. The effect of PNP deficiency is similar to that of ADA deficiency only that in this case, deoxyGTP is the toxic product inhibiting ribonucleotide reductase activity and resulting in depletion of the cells for one of the necessary substrates for DNA synthesis. PNP activity – like ADA activity – is predominantly found in peripheral T cells and thymus, which might be an explanation for the T cell specific effect of PNP deficiency.

Transcobalamin II Deficiency. Transcobalamin II is the binding protein necessary for transporting vitamin B_{12} into cells. Patients deficient in this protein develop agammaglobulinemia, macrocytic anemia, leukopenia, thrombocytopenia, and severe malabsorption due to atrophy of the small intestinal mucosa. This deficiency appears to result in a block in clonal expansion and maturation of lymphocytes, but not in differentiation of antigen specific memory cells.

The lack of cobalamin impedes the production of tetrahydrofolate from N^5-methyltetrahydrofolate which is necessary for the synthesis of thymidylate and TTP, a substrate required for DNA synthesis.

Nezelof's Syndrome. This is characterized by impaired cell-mediated immune responses due to thymic dysplasia (embryonal thymus) and variable (up to normal) circulating antibodies. However, the antibody response to specific antigens is usually absent. It is not associated with endocrine dysfunctions, thus distinguishing it from DiGeorge's syndrome. The disease is transmitted as an autosomal recessive trait.

Reticular Dysgenesia. This is a particularly malignant congenital deficiency of all blood leukocytes. Presumably, it is caused by a lack of differentiation of the primitive hematopoietic stem cell into a common precursor cell.

Wiskott-Aldrich Syndrome

The Wiskott-Aldrich syndrome is characterized by thrombocytopenia, eczema, recurrent bacterial infections, and is transmitted in an X-linked pattern. Immunologically, it is characterized by normal IgG, decreased IgM, increased IgA and IgE levels, normal numbers of B cells, but an inability to respond to polysaccharide and lipopolysaccharide antigens. T cell-mediated immune responses are initially intact, but become severe with advancing age. The patients, in general, do not survive their first decade, succumbing to infections accompanied by hemorrhagic processes.

Ataxia Telangiectasia

This syndrome is transmitted in an autosomal recessive pattern. Patients exhibit progressive degeneration of the cerebellum with ataxia, multiple telangiectasia of the skin and conjunctiva, and susceptibility to

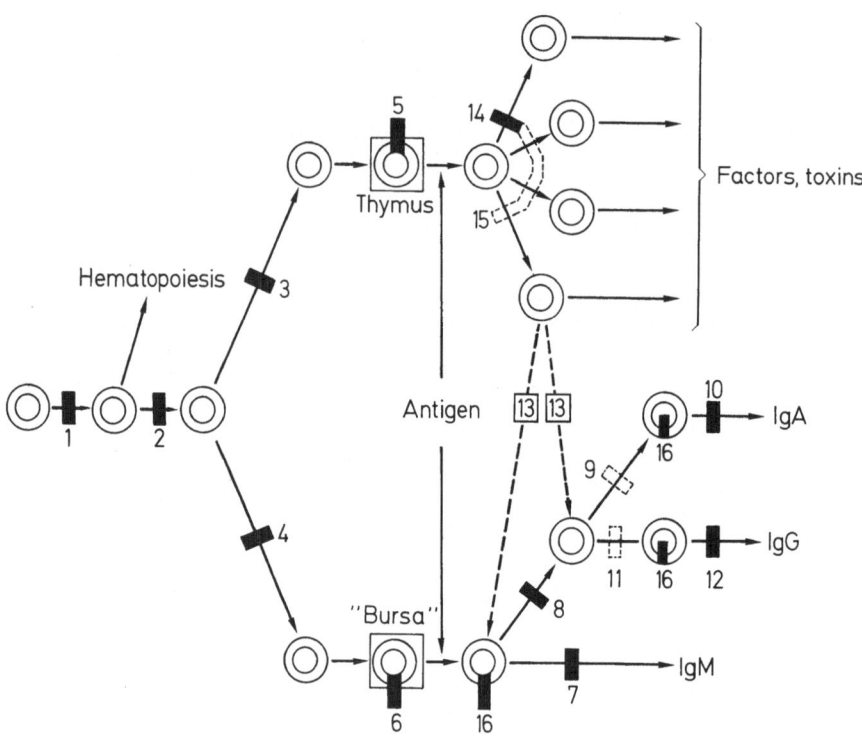

Fig. 12.4. Localization of defects along the differentiation pathways of lymphocytes. The black bars indicate positions of maturation or differentiation arrest; dashed boxes indicate conceivable block; open boxes on dashed lines regulatory (here, inhibitory) interactions. *1*, reticular dysgenesia; *2* (or *3* and *4*), severe combined immunodeficiencies, SCID; *5*, thymus dysplasia; *6*, X-linked hypogammaglobulinemia; *7*, selective IgM deficiency, Wiskott-Aldrich syndrome; *8*, selective IgG and IgA deficiency with elevated IgM (X-linked); *7* and *9*, selective IgA and IgM deficiency; *10* (and *9*), selective IgA deficiency; *12* (and *11*), selective IgG deficiency; *13*, acquired primary hypogammaglobulinemia (suppressor T cells?); *14*, mucocutaneous candidiasis (clonal T cell abortion?); *15*, Hodgkin's disease associated immunodeficiency (ineffective T cells?); *16*, gammopathies with abnormally structured immunoglobulins (deletion, translation defect?)

infections. The most common immunologic abnormality is a simultaneous deficiency of IgA and IgE in the serum and in the secretions in approximately 60% of patients. Cellular immunity is depressed in many cases and becomes more severe with advancing age.

A synopsis of the localizations of defects in the lymphocyte differentiation pathways from the primitive stem cell to the finally differentiated plasma cells and T effector cells is given in Fig. 12.4.

B and T Lymphocyte Proliferative Disorders

Lymphomas

Lymphomas are disorders of hemopoiesis associated with defects in the regulation,

maturation, and/or differentiation mechanisms of lymphocyte lineages resulting in an uncontrolled growth which eventually leads to immunologic deficiencies due to loss of functionally active cells. Non-Hodgkin lymphomas are tumors of lymphatic origin, which are characterized by infiltrative growth of abnormal lymphoblast cells, usually clonally derived from B, or B/T precursor cells, less frequently from T cells.

The classification of non-Hodgkin lymphomas follows morphological (Rappaport) or functional (Lukes and Collins), or functional and malignancy (Lennert) criteria: The classification proposed by Lukes and Collins, and that proposed by Lennert (also called "Kiel" classification) are similar and are given in Table 12.3 together with Rappa-

Table 12.3. Classification of non-Hodgkin lymphomas according to Lukes and Collins, Lennert ("Kiel" classification), and Rappaport

Lukes and Collins	Lennert (Kiel classification)
Low malignancy	
B cell-small lymphocyte, CLL	Lymphocytic lymphomas (L), e.g. CLL, Hairy cell L
B cell plasmocytoide lymphocytic	Lymphoplasmocytic L
B cell-small cleaved follicular center cell (FCC)	Centrocytic L
B cell cleaved FCC (small and large)	Centrocytic-blastic L
High malignancy	
B cell-large cleaved FCC	Centroblastic L
B cell-small non-cleaved FCC	Lymphoblastic L
Burkitt's type	Burkitt's type
Non-Burkitt's type	Non-Burkitt's type
T cell convoluted lymphocytic	convoluted or acid phosphatase type, others
0 cell-undefined, unclassifiable	
B cell immunoblastic sarcoma	Immunoblastic L
T cell immunoblastic sarcoma	
Rappaport's classification on the basis of morphology	
Nodular pattern	Diffuse pattern
NLWD Lymphocytic well differentiated	DLWD Lymphocytic well differentiated
NLPD Lymphocytic poorly differentiated	DLPD Lymphocytic poorly differentiated
NH Histiocytic	DH Histiocytic
NM Mixed histiocytic-lymphocytic	DU Undifferentiated (non-Burkitt)

port's classification which has found wide acceptance because of its practical clinical usefulness and the separation of the prognostically more favorable nodular lymphomas from diffuse lymphomas.

All forms may be histologically divided into those with nodular and those with diffuse architecture. Nodular lymphomas arise from follicular center cells and have been proven to be B cell derived malignancies with usually a high density of Ig molecules bound to the membrane of the neoplastic cells. These cells bear also C3 receptors as the predominant cell of the lymphoid follicle does.

Burkitt's Lymphoma. Two forms of Burkitt's lymphoma are distinguished. *African Burkitt's lymphoma* is endemic in some areas in Africa and New Guinea and affects predominantly small children; it is expressed as a tumor localized in the yaw and/or orbita bone as well as in the abdomen (lymph nodes, ovaries, kidney, and adrenal gland). The affected cells contain EB virus DNA or EB

virus specific nuclear antigen. *European* and *American Burkitt's lymphoma* is identical to the African form in its cytology. Cervical and abdominal lymph nodes are predominantly affected, and no EB virus can be identified. In both instances, B lymphocytes are the infected cells.

Most cases of diffuse poorly differentiated lymphocytic lymphomas in adults are malignancies of B cell origin (presence of cleaved cells). In approximately 10% of cases, the neoplastic cells have T surface characteristics, and a similar proportion of cases has not detectable surface markers (0 cells).

Childhood Lymphoblastic Lymphoma is a subgroup of childhood lymphomas of the diffuse poorly differentiated lymphocytic lymphomas that has been defined by immunologic studies. The proliferating cells may have a convoluted appearance, and in most cases, the neoplastic cells bear T lymphocytic markers [complement receptors, human T lymphocyte antigen (HuTLA), presence of acid phosphatase], and it is very likely that they are of thymus cell origin. In many of these patients, acute lymphoblastic leukemia develops rapidly, and it is probable that these two diseases are closely related. Diffuse large cell lymphomas (reticulum cell sarcomas, histiocytic lymphomas) represent a heterogeneous group of lymphomas: some of them are of monocytic origin (lysozyme synthesis); more than half originate from B cell clones; less than 10% are T cell derived; and in more than 30% of the cases, the neoplastic cells are devoid of the usual membrane markers of B or T lymphocytes.

Cutaneous T Cell Lymphomas

Mycosis fungoides is a chronic disease of the lymphoreticular system. Clinically, it is confined to the skin for a long period of time with the development of scaly, eczematous, or erythematous patches, followed by infiltrated lichenified plaques, and progressing to ulcers and tumors of lymph nodes and internal organs. The proliferating cells in cutaneous lesions have surface marker characteristics of thymus-derived lymphocytes and are morphologically similar to PHA-stimulated normal lymphoblasts.

The disease occurs more commonly in males than in females, and is less common in blacks than in whites. The disease usually appears in the fifth decade of life. In advanced stages, patients show decreased numbers of B and T cells, but increased numbers of null cells in the circulation. Skin testing reveals an impaired cell-mediated immunity; the lymphoproliferative response in vitro is also impaired. Serum levels of IgA and IgE are increased, and a high level of leukocyte-inhibition factor (MIF) as well as thymic factor has been observed in the serum.

Sézary Syndrome (SS) is characterized by generalized exfoliative erythrodermia, intensive pruritus, and the presence of atypical cells (Sézary cells) in the peripheral blood as well as the cellular infiltrate of the skin. The observed blood leukocytosis is due to an increase of lymphocytes; atypical lymphocytes account for about 10% or more of peripheral blood cells.

These abnormal cells are lymphocytes of thymus-derived origin. It is believed that the Sézary syndrome and mycosis fungoides are identical diseases with proliferation of T lymphocytes, one with a leukemic presentation (SS), and the other without it.

Leukemias

According to the clinical course, two major groups of leukemias can be distinguished, with subgroups according to the cell types involved: acute and chronic leukemias (Table 12.4).

Acute Leukemias, particularly acute lymphoblastic leukemias and acute myeloblastic

Table 12.4. Forms of leukemias (L); in parenthesis classification of the French-American-British (FAB) co-operative group

I. Acute leukemias
 Acute lymphoblastic leukemias, ALL (L_1-L_3)[a]
  B cell type approx. 4%
  T cell type approx. 26%
  0 cell type approx. 70%
 Acute myelocytic leukemias, AML
  Granulocytic
   (myeloblastic without and with maturation, M_1 and M_2; hypergranular promyelocytic, M_3) L
  Myelomonocytic L (M_4)
  Monocytic L (M_5)
  Erythroleukemia (M_6)
  Eosinophil L
  Basophil L
  Mast cell L
  Plasma cell L
  Megakaryocytic L
II. Chronic leukemias
  Chronic lymphatic leukemia (CLL)
  Chronic myeloid leukemia (CML)
  Chronic myelomonocytic leukemia (CMML)

[a] L_1-L_3 does not correspond to B, T, or 0 cell type leukemia; L_1-L_3 denote morphological characteristics: L_1, small cell type; L_2, large, heterogeneous type; L_3, large, homogeneous type

leukemias occur predominantly in children, with the highest incidence between 3 and 5 years of age. Boys are more often afflicted than girls. Chronic lymphocytic leukemia is typically a disease of the elderly; chronic myeloid leukemia is commonly observed between the third and fifth decades.

In many animal leukemias, lymphomas, and sarcomas, RNA-containing oncornaviruses with reverse transcriptase and high-molecular weight RNA have been found. In analogy, it is assumed that similar viruses play an important etiologic role in human leukemias, although direct evidence for this contention has not been unambiguously presented thus far – except for the herpes-like Epstein-Barr virus in Burkitt's lymphoma (see above) and lymphoepithelial nasopharyngeal carcinoma. However, reverse transcriptase and high-molecular weight RNA have been identified in human leukemic cells which are not present in normal cells. Genetic and environmental factors are apparently the triggers which permit the phenotypic expression of uncontrolled proliferation. Thus, a number of genetic disorders characterized by constitutional chromosomal instability and/or immunodeficiency (Fanconi's anemia, Bloom's syndrome, Chediak-Higashi syndrome) or aneuploidy (Down's syndrome) are associated with a high incidence of acute (mainly myeloid) leukemia; exposure to radiation (therapeutic; in Japan after World War II) increases particularly acute leukemias and chronic myeloid leukemia; exposure to chemicals (benzene, alkylating agents) increases the risk of acute leukemias.

Chromosomal and biochemical findings strongly suggest that leukemias are of monoclonal origin. Normal leukocytes are formed in leukemic patients; but their generation is more and more decreased, which is not only due to "lack of space," but also to a regulatory phenomenon. The leukemic lymphocytes show an increased spontaneous proliferative response, which is inhibitable by PHA, a disturbed lymphotoxin formation, and they are immunologically inactive. Leukemic granulocytes and mono-

cytes show impaired migration, phagocytosis, and bacterial killing.

Clinical symptoms are pallor, fatigue, recurrent fever with severe or without apparent infections (gram-negative bacteria, fungi, *Pneumocystis carinii*), hepatosplenomegaly, hemorrhage, ostealgia, and arthralgia. Each organ can be infiltrated and this causes additional "organ-specific" symptoms.

Cells from which lymphoblastic leukemias arise are thought to be precursor cells of T and B lymphocytes. Accordingly, acute lymphoblastic leukemias can be subdivided in respect to their membrane markers. This classification has proven invaluable for diagnosis of preleukemic stages, early recognition of relapses, and prognosis (B cell type ALL has the poorest, 0 cell type – pluripotent stem cell ALL – the best prognosis). B cell type acute leukemias may be in most instances lymphomas (see below) with leukemic presentation. 0 cells type ALL possess in the majority markers similar to thymocytes or T cells rather than B cells. It appears, therefore, that acute lymphoblastic ALLs are primarily T cell disorders, whereas acute B cell disorders manifest themselves rather in the form of lymphomas (see above).

It is generally believed that acute myeloid leukemias (M_1–M_6) have a common precursor cell, namely a cell committed to myeloid differentiation. Among the acute myelytic leukemias (AML) those with predominant granulocytic differentiation character (M_1–M_3) are more frequent than myelomonocytic and monocytic leukemias (M_4 and M_5, leukemias of the monocyte-macrophage system with elevated serum muramidase activity), or erythroleukemia; eosinophil, basophil, and mast cell leukemias are rare.

Chronic lymphatic leukemias can be divided, again, by surface markers into those with (a) B cell characteristics of a single clone (the vast majority of CLL), (b) T cell characteristics, and (c) some B cell (surface bound Ig, SmIg) and some T cell (E rosetting, reaction with anti-T serum) characteristics.

As a general rule, CLL represent B cell-derived monoclonal proliferations with expression of IgM. In rare cases, IgG or IgA are produced. In patients in whom several Ig classes are found, all have the same light chains, idiotype specificity, and antibody activity.

In most patients with CLL, the cells do not secrete monoclonal protein, but show a uniform and faint fluorescence pattern with SmIg density much lower than on normal lymphocytes, suggesting that their development is apparently "frozen" with a block in maturation along the pathway of differentiation of the B cell lineage.

In patients with CLL and a serum monoclonal Ig, the very same Ig chain with identical idiotypic determinants are found on the leukemic cell and serum monoclonal Ig. These findings indicate that such cases represent a B cell proliferation with some degree of persistent maturation of the neoplastic clone into plasma cells, a situation intermediate between that of common CLL (without serum monoclonal Ig) with a complete block in the maturation process and Waldenström's macroglobulinemia (see p. 367) with interrupted maturation of the proliferating clone up to the IgM secreting cell.

The proliferating lymphocytes of B-derived CLL are different in some respect for their markers from normal B cells: they possess a complement receptor for C3d, but lack the receptor for C3b; and they have a receptor for *Helix pomatia A* hemagglutinin, which is usually found on T lymphocytes in normal individuals.

Chronic myeloid leukemia (CML) is characterized by an increase of stem cells and myeloblasts which results in an increased production of granulocytic cells, the lifespan of which is additionally prolonged in the peripheral blood. These two mechanisms cause an excessive enlargement of the pool of myelopoietic cells (leukocyte numbers in the peripheral blood reach 100,000 per mm^3 and more). More than 90% of the cases of CML show an *acquired* chromosomal abnormality, the Philadelphia (Ph^1—) chromosome.

Chronic myelomonocytic leukemia (CMML) occurs only in adults with a predominant increase of promonocytes and monocytes. It is not clear whether or not this form represents a leukemia; it may be only an extreme and benign proliferation of monocytes.

Phagocyte Deficiency Diseases

Susceptibility to infections in phagocytic dysfunction syndromes may range from absence of clinical symptoms to mild recurrent skin infections to severe overwhelming, fatal systemic infections. Characteristically, patients are susceptible to bacterial infections and have little difficulty with viral or protozoal infectious processes.

Neutropenias

Infantile genetic agranulocytosis was described by Kostmann as an autosomal recessive disorder. It is assumed that it is caused by a defect interaction of stroma cells and granulocyte precursor cells resulting in a reduced production of granulocytes. The few granulocytes detectable are functionally normal. The disease appears within the first year of life with chronic and recurrent bacterial infections, usually leading to death. There is a marked neutropenia in the blood, occasionally accompanied by eosinophilia and monocytosis. In the bone marrow, cells after the stage of promyelocyte/myelocyte are completely absent.

Familial severe neutropenia is an autosomal dominant disorder of unknown pathogenesis. Bacterial infections occur early after birth. Patients show neutropenia accompanied by monocytosis; the bone marrow shows a deficiency in granulocytes beyond the myelocyte stage.

Cyclic neutropenia is autosomal-dominantly inherited. The pathogenic mechanism causing the cyclic variation of the number of monocytes and reticulocytes is unknown, but presumably involves a regulatory (feedback) defect. The function of granulocytes is normal. The neutropenic phases appear in intervals of 14–45 days and last 4–10 days. During this time, patients show fever, mucosal ulcerations, periodonitis, and skin infections.

Immunoneutropenias comprise at least two disease entities: (a) a transitory form caused by maternal antibodies transferred transplancentally against paternal neutrophil antigens present in the newborn; and (b) a form caused by autoantibodies to granulocyte antigens (NA1, NA2, NB1, NCVaz; see p.316).

Chemotactic Deficiencies

Chediak-Higashi syndrome (CHS) is an autosomal recessive disease. Patients show oculo-cutaneous albinism and recurrent pyogenic infections. The syndrome is characterized by giant granules in all granule-possessing cells which are abnormal primary lysosomes. It is assumed that the enlarged size of the granules causes reduction in mobility and plasticity, and slowed migration. Phagocytosis is not disturbed; however, degranulation (phagolysosome formation) is defective, which results in reduced intracellular killing of bacteria. The defective phagolysosome formation is thought to be caused by absence of induction of microtubulin formation (assembly). Cyclic GMP and cholinergic agents (carbachol and bethanechol) elevate intracellular cyclic GMP and enhance microtubule assembly; and, indeed, the function of leukocytes from CHS patients (degranulation and bactericidal activity) is partially corrected when they are incubated in vitro with cyclic GMP or cholinergic agents. Intraleukocytic concentrations of cyclic AMP are markedly elevated in CHS leukocytes; cyclic AMP has been shown to suppress neutrophil degranulation and mobility. Reduction of intracellular cyclic AMP to normal levels by treatment with high doses of ascorbic acid results

in normal chemotaxis, degranulation, and bactericidal activity.

Job's syndrome: There are a number of single case reports about severed chemotactic activity of neutrophils as the only pathologic parameter detectable, accompanied by recurrent staphylococcal infections of the dermis (pyogenic abscesses) and respiratory tract (pneumonia). Some of these patients exhibit an extremely high serum IgE level (19,000–24,000 ng per ml; normal value about 330 ng per ml). In most patients, humoral and cell-mediated responses were normal, as were phagocytosis and bactericidal activity. In some, however, there is also a reduced bactericidal activity. It might be assumed that the high IgE level is caused by the persistent presence of bacterial antigenic material in skin and mucosa (see p.342). Defective chemotactic activity has also been observed in a number of patients with epidermal disorders such as ichthyosis, eczema, and dermatitis.

Lazy leukocyte syndrome is characterized by neutropenia associated with impaired random as well as chemotactic locomotion of neutrophils. Patients show recurrent infections. All other phagocytic parameters are normal, but some patients show an elevated IgE level.

Actin polymerization deficiency is characterized by recurrent staphylococcal infections of newborns without development of pus. Infiltrations consist only of monocytes and histiocytes. The migration of neutrophils is extremely impaired, but also ingestion is retarded. It is thought, thought not proven, that the cause is a defect in actin polymerization.

Ingestion Deficiency

Tuftsin deficiency (see p.323) is an autosomal recessive disorder. Patients exhibit a generally increased susceptibility to infections of the respiratory tract and skin. Tuftsin is a tetrapeptide cleaved from a gamma

Table 12.5. Disorders of neutrophil chemotaxis

Lazy leukocyte syndrome
Wiskott-Aldrich syndrome
Chediak-Higashi syndrome
Job's syndrome
Actin dysfunction
Hyperimmunoglobulin E
Hyperimmunoglobulin A
Mucocutaneous candidiasis
Cellular immune defects
Toxic neutrophils
Measles
Hodgkin's disease
Cirrhosis
Diabetes mellitus
Rheumatoid arthritis
Malignancy
Protein-calorie malnutrition

against the action of not only antibodies but also that of antibiotics. Inside granulocytes, they spread all over the organism and cause granulomas. The clinical picture is characterized by recurrent infections (particularly pneumonia), lymphadenitis, formation of abscesses, and hepatosplenomegaly. Also typical are granulomatous, eczematoid, or lupus-like skin lesions, liver abscesses, and osteomyelitis. Histologic examination reveals typical granulomas in lymph nodes, lungs, liver, spleen, and skin with giant cell formation, central necrosis, and lymphohistiocytic inflammation.

The inheritance is X-linked recessively in patients in whom the disease is caused by a

globulin (Leukokinin; C 2 domaine, position 289–292) by the combined action of two proteolytic enzymes, one present in the spleen cleaving the carboxy-terminal part between residue 292 and 293, and the other one localized in the membrane of neutrophils (leukokininase) liberating the tetrapeptide by cleavage between position 288 and 289. The free tetrapeptide stimulates neutrophils to increased phagocytosis. The defect is probably caused by the absence of the splenic enzyme.

Bactericidal Deficiency

Chronic granulomatous disease (CGD) of childhood is characterized by a defect of granulocytic bactericidal activity of catalase-positive bacteria. The critical defect appears to be the inability of granulocytes to generate H_2O_2 (NADPH-oxidase deficiency). The increased O_2-consumption and activation of the hexose-phosphate shunt (see pp. 324–326) after phagocytosis is absent. The granulocytes are unable, therefore, to kill catalase-positive bacteria (catalase reaction: $2 H_2O_2 \rightarrow 2 H_2O + O_2$; these bacteria destroy H_2O_2 which they produce by themselves; catalase-negative bacteria – pneumococcus, β-hemolytic streptococcus – are killed by their own H_2O_2). The bacteria remain intracellularly, and are protected

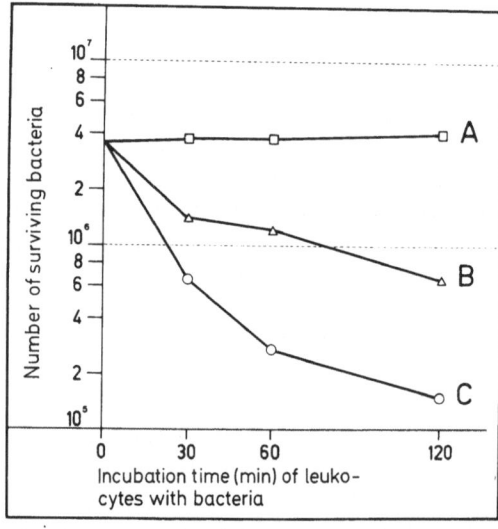

Fig. 12.5. Intracellular killing of *Staphylococcus aureus* in leukocytes of CGD patients *A*; conductors *B*; and normal, healthy individuals *C* as assessed by the intraleukocytic killing test (see p. 343). (Reproduced with kind permission from Hitzig WH, Weber Ch 1980)

Table 12.6.
Disorders of neutrophil bactericidal function

Chronic granulomatous disease (CGD)
Glucose-6-phosphate dehydrogenase deficiency
Myeloperoxidase deficiency
Chediak-Higashi syndrome
Acute leukemia
Down's syndrome
Leukocyte alkaline phosphatase deficiency
Felty's syndrome

Table 12.7. Survey of complement component deficiencies

Deficient component	Clinical symptoms	Inheritance	Laboratory findings[a]
C1q	Usually found in combination with severe combined immuno-deficiencies (SCID) like Swiss- or Bruton-type (see p. 351)	Depending on basic disease	Lack of C1q
C1r	Infections of the respiratory tract, chronic glomerulonephritis, LE-like skin lesions	Autosomal, recessive	Lack of C1r, decrease of C1s, increase of C4, C1-inhibitor; decreased bacteriocidic activity
C1s	LE-like systemic symptoms; persistent antigen-antibody complexes	Autosomal, dominant	Lack of C1s; increase of C4 and C2
C1-inhibitor	Also called Hereditary angioneurotic syndrom. Two forms exists: (a) lack of inhibitor, and (b) functionally inactive inhibitor. Symptoms are edemas of extremities, face, and respiratory tract (glottis, bronchi) and abdominal pain attacks. C1-inhibitor also physiologically blocks factor XII (Hage-mann) of the clotting system; the lack of it causes kinin liberation and, via plasmin activation, fibrinolysis. Degraded fibrin activates the complement system, and since C1s is not inactivated, a continuous consumption of C4 and C2 reduces their serum level	Autosomal, dominant	(a) Lack of C1-inhibitor, (b) increased C1-inhibitor (inactive) with abnormal electrophoretic mobility; decrease in C4 and C2, increase in C1s
C4	Most carriers are healthy; few cases have been reported to have shown a LE-like picture without LE-cells, and Ig- and C3-deposits in the skin. In some patients, the IgM to IgG switch does not occur after immunization	Autosomal, recessive; association with HLA	Lack of C4; defect in chemotaxis
C2	Usually, no symptoms; occasionally, autoimmune-like syndroms (lupus erythematodes, dermatomyositis, glomerulo-nephritis)	Autosomal, recessive; association with HLA	Lack of C2
C3	Recurrent, severe bacterial infections without (expected) leukocytosis	Autosomal, recessive	Lack of C3; deficient chemotactic activity, opsonisation, and bacteriocidic activity
C3b-inactivator	Increased susceptibility to infections. C3 catabolism is increased, this causes a high level of C3a (anaphylatoxin) and C3b. C3b activites properdin which, in turn, leads to high catabo-lism of factor B. Increased C3a activates histamin-release	Autosomal, recessive	Lack of C3b-inactivator; deficient chemotactic activity, opsonisation, particle ingestion, and bacteriocidic activity; histamine in urine
C5	Two forms are known: (a) lack of C5, and (b) dysfunction of C5. (a) Frequent and recurrent bacterial infections, and visceral LE-like symptoms. (b) Eczema, diarrhea, increased susceptibility to bacterial (staphylococcal) infections	(a) Autosomal, recessive; (b) unclear	(a) Lack of C5; decreased chemotactic activity. (b) Defect in properdin pathway?; reduced opsonizing activity;

	Clinical symptoms	Inheritance	Deficiency
C6	Usually healthy; occasionally Raynaud-like symptoms; increased susceptibility to gram-negative (meningococcal, gonococcal) infections		Lack of C6; reduced bacteriocidic activity
C7	Usually healthy; in some cases Raynaud-like symptoms with sclerodactyly and teleangiectasy	Autosomal, recessive	Lack of C7; increased levels of C8 and C9. Reduced chemotactic activity, opsonisation, and bacteriocidic activity
C8	Usually healthy; occasionally increased susceptibility to infections with N. meningococcus and N. gonorrhoea; LE-like symptoms	Autosomal, recessive	Lack of C8; reduced bacteriocidic activity
C9	Healthy	Autosomal, recessive	Lack of C9

a All deficiencies show a significant reduction of the total hemolytic activity (CH_{50}) (see p. 117)

deficiency of the NADPH-oxidase; some cases have been described, however, for whom an autosomal-recessive pattern is more likely; in these cases, glutathion-peroxidase deficiency in addition to oxidase deficiency has been demonstrated. Furthermore, the sex-linked dominantly inherited glucose-6-phosphate dehydrogenase deficiency results in the same clinical disease if the deficiency occurs not only in erythrocytes but also in leukocytes.

Some patients with X-chromosomal recessive CGD show an association to the rare McLeod phenotype of the Kell blood group ($= K_o$). The absence of K_x on leukocytes reduces their bactericidal activity.

Immunologically, humoral as well as cell-mediated immune responses are normal. The phagocytic functions of neutrophils are all normal, i.e., chemotactic migration, ingestion, degranulation, except bacterial killing (Fig. 12.5). The NBT test is always negative.

Lipochrome histiocytosis has a course similar to CGD including negative NBT, but without granuloma formation; there is a lipochrome pigmentation of histiocytes, which is pathognomonic. Lipochrome histiocytosis is autosomal-recessively transmitted.

Myeloperoxidase (MPO) deficiency in neutrophils and monocytes is autosomal-recessively inherited. Generally it does not *cause disease;* however, dissiminated candidiasis and acne vulgaris have been described.

Complement Deficiencies

Deficiencies for each complement component of the classical pathway were described by 1980. All these deficiencies are rare, the most common being a C1-inhibitor deficiency, and a lack of C2 expression. All deficiencies are inherited; C4 and C2 deficiencies are associated with HLA genotypes (see p. 154). In many patients, complement deficiencies exist without signs of disease. When symptoms do appear, they usually develop within weeks· after birth until early childhood and consist of an increased susceptibility to infections (skin, respiratory tract, joints, kidney), and sometimes they are similar to autoimmune diseases (lupus erythematosus-like but without LE cells, anti-nuclear antibodies, and Ig- and C3-deposits in the skin). In all patients, laboratory tests reveal a significantly reduced total hemolytic activity of the serum (CH_{50}), lack of the respective single complement component, and, depending upon which component is deficient, decreased chemotactic activity of polymorphonuclear cells (C4, C3b-inactivator, C5, C7), reduced opsonization (C3, C5, C7), and reduced phagocytosis (C1r, C3, C3b-inactivator, C6, C7, C8). The deficiencies are summarized in Table 12.7.

References

Agnello V (1978) Complement deficiency states. Medicine 57:1

Bernard A, Boumsell L, Dausset I, Milstein C, Schlossman SF, (eds) (1984) Leucocyte typing. Springer Berlin Heidelberg

Chandra RK, Cooper MD, Hitzig WH, Rosen FS, Seligman M, Scoothill JF, Terry RJ (1979) Immunodeficiency: Report of a WHO scientific group. Clin Immunol Immunopathol 13:296

Clinical Oncology (1978) A manual for students and doctors. Edited under the auspices of the International Union Against Cancer (2nd edition). Springer-Verlag, Heidelberg New York

Cooper MD, Seligman M (1977) B and T lymphocytes in immunodeficiency and lymphoproliferative diseases. In: Loor F, Roelants GE (eds) B and T cells in immune recognition. Wiley, p 347

Cooper MD, Lawton AR, Miescher PA, Müller-Eberhard (eds) (1979) Immunodeficiency. Springer, New York

Gallin JI, Quie PG (eds) (1978) Leukocyte chemotaxis. Raven

Güttler F, Seakins JWT, Harkness RA (eds) (1979) Inborn errors of immunity and phagocytosis. MTP Press, Falcon House, London

Hitzig WH, Weber CH (1980) Die progressive septische Granulomatose. Adv Int Med Ped 44:37

Kobayashi N (ed) (1978) Immunodeficiency. University Park Press, Baltimore

Mendes NF (1973) Technical aspects of the rosette tests used to detect human complement receptor (B) and sheep erythrocyte-binding(T) lymphocytes. J Immunol 111:860

Chapter 13   Autoimmunity

Wilmar Dias da Silva and Dietrich Götze

Contents

Autorecognition 383
Autoimmunity. 386
  Induction of Autoimmunity 386
  Factors Influencing Autoimmunity 389
Autoimmune Diseases 391
  Tissue Lesions in Autoimmune Diseases . . 391
  Some Autoimmune Diseases. 391
  Autoimmune Diseases of the Central
    Nervous System 392
  Autoimmune Diseases of Endocrine Glands . 396
  Hematologic Autoimmune Diseases 399
  Autoimmune Diseases of the Gastrointestinal
    Tract and Liver 403
  Autoimmune Disease of the Kidney 404
  Autoimmune Diseases of the Lung 406
  Autoimmune Diseases of the Heart 407
  Autoimmune Diseases of the Eye 407
  Autoimmune Disease of the Skin 408
  Systemic Autoimmune Diseases 408
References 413

Autorecognition

Paul Ehrlich introduced the term "horror autotoxicus" to circumscribe the observation that an organism would not react under normal conditions against its own constituents (containment of auto-reactivity, self-tolerance). A mechanism by which self-tolerance might be established was proposed by Burnet and became known as clonal abortion (deletion) theory: during fetal life, lymphocytes for self-determinants are eliminated (forbidden clones). First indications that this theory might not be an explanation for self-tolerance were obtained by Witebsky and Rose in 1956. These authors could demonstrate that rabbits were able to produce antibodies specific for their own thyroglobulin when immunized with thyroglobulin in complete Freund's ad-

juvant. Subsequent studies revealed that normal individuals possessed B lymphocytes able to bind specifically thyroglobulin. Elimination of these B cells by binding of highly labeled thyroglobulin (suicide) prevents the formation of antibodies and the development of an autoimmune thyroiditis. Since then numerous experiments have provided ample evidence that auto-antibodies against a large number of self-antigens are found naturally in the serum of normal, healthy individuals, and that auto-antibodies against virtually all self-constituents can be elicited when appropriately immunized or stimulated; thus, polyclonal B cell mitogens such as lipopolysaccharide can indiscriminately activate potentially auto-reactive cells in vivo, causing the production of measurable concentrations of serum auto-antibodies. This LPS-induced autoimmune state tends to be self-limiting, and the auto-antibodies disappear within a short time after the last LPS administration.

Furthermore, auto-antibodies can be demonstrated in many pathologic events, e.g., infectious diseases, which are usually only transiently present and not harmful to the individual (Table 13.1). Moreover, Cohn and Weckerle could furnish evidence that cell-mediated auto-reactivity is also present under normal conditions: They incubated lymphoid cells for 5 days on syngeneic fibroblast monolayer cultures, after which time specifically sensitized T lymphocytes were able to lyse syngeneic target cells, and to induce a graft versus host-like reaction of splenomegaly or lymph node enlargement after in vivo transfer into syngeneic hosts. Adsorption experiments on syngeneic fibroblasts, followed by transfer onto syngeneic

Table 13.1. Examples of autoantibodies in nonimmunized normal individuals and nonautoimmune diseases

Normal	Disease
Cold agglutinins, e.g. anti-I and anti-i (see p. 236)	Antibodies to:
Pan-agglutinins, react with neuraminidase-treated RBC, lymphocytes, spermatozoa	Nuclei, kidney, heart, gastric tissue, thyroglobulin, tumor tissue, cardiolipin, complement (immunoconglutinins, anti-C3, C4)
Antibodies to lung tissue, elastin, nuclear components, immunoglobulins (particularly their degradation products), myelin	Skin, tumor tissue (particular colon tumor), liver surface lipoprotein, insulin

or allogeneic sensitizing monolayers, have demonstrated that T cells endowed with specific recognition structures for self-antigens exist in the spleen prior to in vitro sensitization. The induction of autoreactive T lymphocytes could be blocked by the addition of syngeneic, but not allogeneic, serum; this inhibition is caused by soluble antigens.

Thus, auto-reactive B and T lymphocytes constitute a normal fraction of the immunologically reactive cell pool, and auto-antibodies are permanently present under normal conditions, though at low concentrations. Tolerance and (concomitant) immunity are both a continuously acquired property of the immune system, kept in an equilibrium by regulatory interactions of the immune cells, actually based on continuous self-recognition (see Chap. 6, p. 168, and Chap. 10, p. 310). Disturbances of these regulatory interactions result in autoimmunity (or allergy, or anergy). The mechanisms by which tolerance is established and maintained are thought to be (1) clonal inactivation of maturing lymphocytes by the continuous presence of small amounts of auto-antigens (e.g., thyroglobulin, peptide hormones, plasma membrane glycoproteins – HLA, H-2 –, and others); (2) antibody-mediated inhibition; and (3) T cell regulation (see also Chap. 10, pp. 309–311).

Clonal inactivation: In 1975, Nossal extending Burnet's deletion theory, proposed that at some stage during their differentiation from stem cells to mature antibody-forming cells, B lymphocytes go through a phase during which contact with antigen induces tolerance only and not immunity. Indeed, it could be demonstrated that primary B cells which start to express surface IgM are highly susceptible to induction of tolerance, and that tolerance is very rapidly induced in these cells. The underlying mechanism(s) for the preferential development of tolerance rather than stimulation to antibody-secreting cells is not known, but it might be related to the observation that immature B cells are unable to regenerate receptors once removed (e.g., by capping, see p. 157). It has been suggested that this form of tolerance induction is only possible as long as there is a deficiency of high avidity cells as in the newborn in comparison to adults. Additional mechanism(s) appear to be required, therefore, to explain self-tolerance.

Since B lymphocytes have a rather short lifespan, and there is a continuous generation of new B cells, functional inactivation has to occur over and over again whenever new lymphocytes mature that possess receptors for self-determinants. It is, therefore, conceivable that even under normal conditions, but particularly under pathologic conditions, some B cells with anti-self specificity reach the mature stage without having been inactivated (they escaped).

The same mechanism(s) may operate for tolerance induction of T lymphocytes (see p. 309, low zone tolerance).

Antibody-mediated inhibition: It has been demonstrated that antibodies can contribute to an unresponsive state by competing with lymphocyte receptors for available antigens. Furthermore, anti-idiotypic antibodies may contain the anti-self-reactivity of lymphocytes (see pp.110–113). In addition, immune complexes can act as blocking factors (see p. 350, and immunologic enhancement p.307). The effect of immune complexes might be due to (a) a free combining site of the complexed antibody binding to cell-bound antigen and thus masking it so that it can not be recognized by potential effector cells, and/or (b) free antigenic determinants which may interact with surface receptors and induce lymphocyte inactivation (see above).

T cell regulation: It is now recognized that the activity of effector cells (B/plasma cells, cytotoxic T cells) is regulated by at least two types of T lymphocytes: T helper cells and T suppressor cells (see Chap. 2, p. 41–44; Chap. 4, pp. 111–113; Chap. 6, p. 165, and Chap. 10, p. 310). Containment of autoreactivity might be achieved by two means: activation of suppressor T cells or inactivation (or nonactivation) of helper T cells. These effects might result from antigen-inactivation of T helper cells as outlined

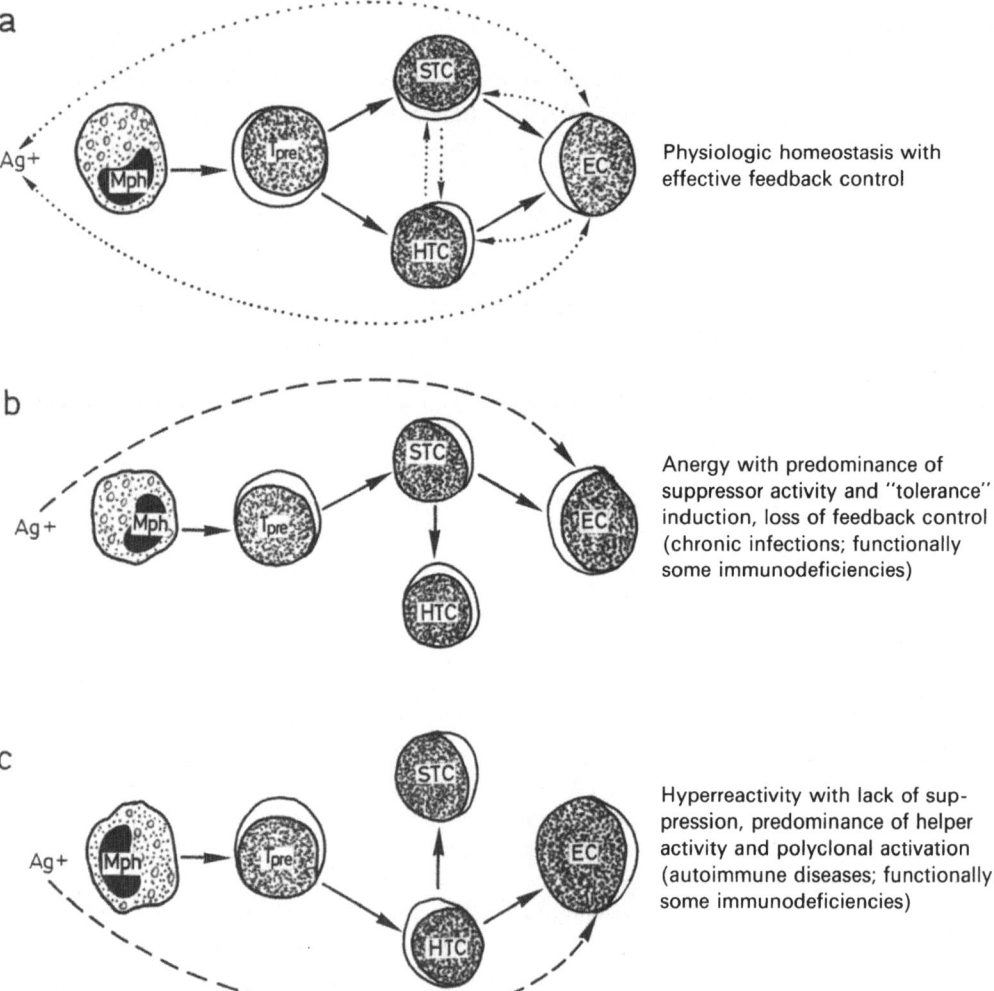

a   Physiologic homeostasis with effective feedback control

b   Anergy with predominance of suppressor activity and "tolerance" induction, loss of feedback control (chronic infections; functionally some immunodeficiencies)

c   Hyperreactivity with lack of suppression, predominance of helper activity and polyclonal activation (autoimmune diseases; functionally some immunodeficiencies)

Fig. 13.1 a–c. Homeostasis of the immune system by activating (→) and regulatory (----→) positive and negative feedback interactions of antigen (Ag), macrophages (mph), suppressor T cells (STC), helper T cells (HTC), and effector cells (EC; cytotoxic T cells or B/plasma cells and their products, antibodies). **a** System in equilibrium, physiologic condition; **b** Predominance of suppressor T cell activity with loss of stimulating helper activity resulting in antigen specific or general anergy; **c** Predominance of helper T cell activity with loss of suppressor activity resulting in antigen-specific or general hyperreactivity

above for B cells, or antigen-activation of suppressor T cells, or anti-idiotypic interactions as described in Chap. 4 (pp. 110–113), and thus, do not only include the two mechanisms described above, but also fit more the actual findings. Since B lymphocytes will react against most antigens only if helped by T lymphocytes, the inactivation of T helper cells (by antigen, by suppressor cells) would be a sufficient requirement to establish tolerance in the intact organism.

Both types of unresponsiveness, i.e., due to inactivated T helper cells and to activated suppressor cells, are transferable into "B animals" (depleted of T cells); however, responsiveness can be restored by mature T cells in case of inactivated T helper cells only. Which type of tolerance prevails for a given antigen depends upon the nature and dose of the antigen and the immunologic experience of the organism, as well as the genetic make-up of the individual with respect to the alleles of its MHC (see Chap. 6, pp. 167–177).

Autoimmunity

As outlined above, autoimmunity or better still auto-recognition, appears to be a normal feature of the immune system's reactivity, i.e., is a physiologic event far removed from the immunopathology of autoimmune diseases, and an important device for the maintenance of a state of equilibrium of the immune system (see Chap. 6, pp. 168–170). Talal has suggested, therefore, the distinction of three stages in the response to self: auto-recognition, autoimmunity, and autoimmune diseases, in order to indicate the range of reactivity from normal (regulated) to pathologic (deregulated) conditions.

Auto-recognition of membrane idiotypic receptors and MHC molecules appears to be a fundamental principle facilitating regulatory interactions between cells constituting the immune system in order to adjust their response to signals from within as well as outside. In addition, the continuous interaction of receptors with soluble self-antigens which are always present in low concentrations, is necessary in order to maintain a state of tolerance.

This state of auto-recognition as described has been interpreted by Grabar not only as a necessary means of immune system regulation, but as the essence of the immune system's physiologic function (theory of immunoglobulins as "transporters"): namely, handling and eliminating metabolic and catabolic substances regardless of their origin, self or nonself.

Autoimmunity is then characterized by enhanced auto-reactions concomitant to nonself reactions due to temporary disturbances (e.g., infections and injuries), in which the immunologic network is fundamentally intact.

Autoimmune diseases are severe derangements of the immunologic network (or a part of it) that are non-reversible from within the systems and lead to pathologic conditions. Autoimmune states might be the result of intrinsic defects of the immune system (e.g., experimental systemic lupus erythematosus (SLE) in NZB mice, see below), or the result of either an induced, inadequate immune response (active chronic hepatitis) or an antigen-specific deficient recognition (e.g., probably most autoimmune diseases associated with certain HLA types, see Chap. 6, Table 6.18, p. 176, and below) of an otherwise normally functioning immune system.

Induction of Autoimmunity

Three major mechanisms are considered to bring about the development of autoimmune disease states: (1) Antigen seclusion, (2) T cell bypass, and (3) disordered immunologic regulation.

Antigen seclusion: Antigens confined inside cells, or located at anatomical sites not in contact with the circulation are thought not to participate in the induction of tolerance of lymphocytes. Whenever those self-components come into contact with lymphocytes, for example after tissue damage due to infections or injuries, a normal immune response will follow. Such a mechanism may underlie the reactivity toward the basic protein of myelin, organ-specific microsomal antigens of the thyroid gland, the testicles, and gastric parietal cells, nuclear antigens, and the crystalline lens.

T cell bypass: As was pointed out above, tolerance appears to be maintained by the inactivation (nonactivation) of T helper cells (and/or activation of suppressor T cells) due to the continuous presence of small amounts of antigen; this resembles low zone tolerance (see p. 307–311), which affects primarily T lymphocytes but not B lymphocytes. However, since B lymphocytes need the help of T cells for activation to differentiate into antibody-secreting cells, the overall effect on the organism is tolerance. Any mechanism, therefore, which can circumvent the T cell participation-requirement (mitogens, adjuvants), or cause T helper cell activation (providing helper determinants = carrier) may lead to the activation of (non-tolerant)

B cells. Such mechanisms are: Drugs that bind to body constituents, partially degraded autoantigens, bacterial, viral, and parasitic infections, and graft-versus-host reaction (Table 13.2).

Many drugs are known today to cause autoimmune thrombocytopenia, Coombs'-positive hemolytic anemia, leukopenia, and/or immune complex syndromes. The underlying mechanisms are thought to be due to binding of the drug to proteins and/or cell surfaces (platelets, erythrocytes, leukocytes, tissue cells) so that T helper cells are activated which, in turn, activate B cells specific for the drug, but sometimes also drug-associated (self) components. Antigen-(drug)-antibody complexes activate complement which results in inflammatory reactions and cell-lysis.

Partially degraded self-components may expose antigenic determinants to which the immune system is not tolerant, and thus may elicit a regular immune response.

Many microorganisms possess or release substances such as lipopolysaccharide, tuberculin, *B. pertussis* components, *T. brucei* components, that act as polyclonal B cell (and T cell) mitogen, and are experimentally used as adjuvants. That such substances in-

Table 13.2. Mechanisms to bypass T cells in B lymphocyte activation

Mechanism	Mode of action
Drugs	provide helper determinant(= carrier) to T cells, e.g. α-methyldopa (anti-e of Rh), procainamide and hydralazine (anti-nuclear), hydantoin (anti-MHC), nitrofurantoin
Partially degraded autoantigens	Presentation of antigenic determinants to which no tolerance exists, e.g. thyreoglobulin, collagen, immunoglobulins
Bacterial infections	Polyclonal B (and T) cell activation, adjuvant effect (e.g., lipopolysaccharide, PPD, *B. pertussis*); presentation of determinants cross-reacting with self (e.g., polysaccharide antigens of E. coli 0:14 with colon antigen, basement membrane antigens (?), and group A hemolytic streptococcus antigen with cardiac muscle)
Viral infections	Viral antigens form complexes with self-antigens (MHC); polyclonal B cell stimulation (e.g. EB-virus) among them autoantibodies
Graft-versus-Host reaction	Donor T helper cells stimulated by host antigens induce proliferation of host B cells (allogenic effect)
Multiple specificities of antibodies	According to Richards et al. an antibody combining site may be able to react with several structurally completely unrelated determinants; by accident, an antibody specifically produced against an infectious agent may turn out to also react with a self-antigen (RF?)

deed induce autoimmune diseases is amply demonstrated by the fact that Freund's adjuvant (see p. 71) is widely used to induce experimental autoimmune diseases; furthermore, it has been shown that after stimulation of B cells with mitogens, large numbers of cells are found forming antibodies against autologous red cells. Well known are antibodies to cardiolipin (Wassermann) and cold auto-antibodies to erythrocytes in syphilis, auto-antibodies to the lung in tuberculosis, antibodies against thyroglobulin, immunoglobulins (rheumatoid factor, RF), cardiolipin, and nuclear components in lepromatous leprosy, cold agglutinins in *Mycoplasma* pneumonia infections, and auto-antibodies in parasitic infections.

Another effect of microorganisms is that they provide helper determinants. Thus, in rheumatic fever, streptococcal determinants cross-react with cardiac tissue antigens. Type 12 streptococcus infections are usually accompanied by glomerulonephritis, probably because they possess antigens resembling those encountered in renal glomeruli, and the antibodies produced against these antigens react with glomerular basement membrane.

In other instances, bacterial glycolipids may become inserted into host cell membranes and in this way activate T helper cells for auto-antigen specific B cells. Similarly, many viruses express viral antigens in the membrane of the infected host cell, and these antigens are recognized by immune cells; interaction of virus-infected host cells with immune cells causes destruction of the former, liberating intracellular components which might be immunogenic (e.g., active chronic hepatitis).

Lymphocytes infected by viruses might be induced to proliferate and differentiate to a certain functional stage; since this would be, in general, a polyclonal activation, severe disturbances of the immune regulation might be expected (e.g. systemic lupus erythematosus; usually not severe: infectious mononucleosis).

The production of antibodies of recipient origin (demonstrated by allotype markers)

against erythrocytes, basement membranes, and cytotoxic antibodies could be demonstrated during graft-versus-host reactions.

The concept of T cell bypass as an important mechanism for the initiation of an autoimmune disease implies that most autoimmune diseases are, indeed, caused by antibody activities. As a matter of fact, this has been demonstrated to be true in many instances.

T cell dysregulation: The immune response is controlled by the activity of T lymphocytes. Defects in these controlling elements are, therefore, expected to cause aberrant immune reactions (Table 13.3). An increase in the activity of suppressor T cells may lead to the complete absence of any detectable *specific* immune response (anergy); the concurrent presence of a polyclonal B cell mitogen leads to an elevation of (unspecific) antibodies, including auto-antibodies. Deficiency in suppressor T cell activity may cause the opposite effect: a general "unleashing" of B lymphocytes due to the overwhelming ac-

Table 13.3. T cell dysregulations

Decreased T suppressor cell activity:[a]
  Experimental allergic encephalomyelitis (?)
  Multiple sclerosis (?)
  Systemic lupus erythematosus
  Rheumatoid arthritis (?)
  Sjögren's syndrome
  Experimental autoimmune thyroiditis
  Autoimmune active chronic hepatitis
  Pemphigus vulgaris
  Progressive systemic sclerosis (scleroderma)
Increased T suppressor cell activity:
  Lepromatous leprosy
  Fulminant tuberculosis
  Candidiasis (some)
  Histoplasmosis
  Measles
  Myxo- und Paramyxo-viruses
  Infectious mononucleosis
  Mucocutaneous leishmaniasis
  Acquired hypogammaglobulinemia (some)
  Selective IgA deficiency (some)
  Hodgkin's disease
  Acute lymphatic leukemia

---

[a] An increase in T helper cell activity equals a deficiency in T suppressor cells

tivity of T helper cells, (e.g., experimental SLE, see below). Other mechanisms may involve (a) unresponsiveness of effector cells to controlling signals of regulator cells, or (b) inefficiency of effector functions with uncoupling of feedback control mechanisms. Disturbances of these latter kinds are observed in many lymphoproliferative disorders, and some infections (e.g., chronic lymphatic leukemia, lymphosarcoma, infectious mononucleosis).

Factors Influencing Autoimmunity

Factors influencing the development of autoimmune diseases are of environmental (drugs, food, dust; infections) and organism-inherent (genetic, immunodeficiency, hormonal, thymic, and age) origin.

Many drugs induce autoimmune reactions which are often asymptomatic, and/or disappear after discontinuation of exposure. Food, dust, and other agents may cause autoimmune symptoms, usually of the immediate hypersensitivity (see pp. 244–278) type I rather than of other types.

Many infections by viruses, bacteria, fungi, and parasites cause temporary autoimmune symptoms, particularly rheumatoid factor and anti-nuclear antibodies (Table 13.4). Some acute virus infections (e.g. infectious mononucleosis) and parasite infections (e.g., African trypanosomiasis) are characterized by polyclonal B cell activation. In general, these symptoms are reversible after eradication of the infectious agent. However, tissue damage caused as a result of excessive immune reactions is not always reversible. The resulting immunopathology in such cases is so similar to many "spontaneous" autoimmune diseases that an infectious cause is strongly suggested for them (Table 13.5). The infectious agents in such cases not only elude our detection so far, but they also defy elimination by the affected organism (persistent infections, slow-virus infections). In other words, many of the so-called autoimmune diseases will probably turn out to be infectious diseases, with which the infected organism cannot cope with appropriately because of some selective immunodeficiencies (see below).

Table 13.4. Examples of autoimmune symptoms associated with infections

Rheumatoid factor	Arthritis	Anti-nuclear antibodies	Coombs' positive hemolytic anemia	Immune complex nephritis	Polyclonal gammopathy
Subacute bacterial endocarditis	Gonorrhea	Leprosy	Syphilis	Streptococcus	Syphilis
Syphilis	Tuberculosis	Tuberculosis	Mycoplasma pneumoniae	S. typhi	Rubella
Lepromatous leprosy	Serum hepatitis	Cytomegalo-virus	Hepatitis	Serum hepatitis	Leishmaniasis
Tuberculosis	Yersinia infection	Infectious mononucleosis	Influenza	Infectious mononucleosis	Trypanosomiasis (T. brucei, T. cruzi)
Hepatitis B			Cytomegalovirus	Coxsackie virus	
Influenza A			Infectious mononucleosis	Varicella	
Cytomegalovirus				Measles	
Rubella				Malaria	
Herpes zoster				Toxoplasmosis (congenital)	
Infectious mononucleosis				Schistosomiasis	
Malaria				Filariasis	
Kala-Azar					
Schistosomiasis					

Table 13.5. Infectious agents suspected as inducers of autoimmune diseases

Autoimmune disease	Suspected infectious agent
Rheumatoid arthritis	EB-virus related agent
Insulin-dependent diabetes mellitus	Coxsackie B virus
Multiple sclerosis	Defective measles virus
Sclerosing panencephalitis	
Systemic lupus erythematosus (in NZB mice, in dogs)	C-type RNA virus
Equine infectious anemia	
Sjögren's syndrome	A-type virus (?)
Rheumatic fever	Group A streptococcus
Ankylosing spondylitis	Chronic infections of the bowl and genitourinary tract
Reiter's disease	Shigellae
Ulcerative colitis	Rheovirus-like agent
Crohn's disease	
IgG(warm) antibody-mediated hemolytic anemia	Mycoplasma pneumoniae
Guillain-Barré-Strohl syndrome	Viruses, e.g., influenza, cytomegalo, varicella-zoster, measles, mumps, rubella, vaccinia

Genetic factors play an important role as demonstrated by the fact that almost all autoimmune diseases show a preferential association to certain HLA alleles (see Table 6.18, p. 176). The underlying mechanisms of these associations are discussed at the end of Chap. 6 (pp. 176–177). In view of the suspicion that many of the autoimmune diseases may have been initiated by infections, the immune response theory of these associations is most likely correct, i.e., a certain allele predisposes to low responsiveness which leads to a persistent infection followed by aberrant or inadequate immune responses which are not effective in eliminating the causative agent but, to the contrary, now cause the pathology; the process of inadequate immune reactions may eventually become dissociated from the infections and perpetuate itself.

Many immunodeficiencies are genetically determined and are associated with autoimmune reactions (Table 13.6). It should be kept in mind that an existing immunodeficiency leads to the net effect that an infectious agent cannot be eliminated, thus resembling the picture of a persistent or "slow-microbe" infection, which of course will result eventually in immunopathologic lesions identical to those of "autoimmune diseases" (e.g. CGD, p. 379).

Hormonal factors, particularly sex hormones, have a critical influence on the expression, severity, and time course of many autoimmune diseases. Thus, systemic lupus erythematosus, Hashimoto's thyroiditis, Graves' disease, Addison's disease, and scleroderma show a high prevalence for females, and usually during pregnancies, the disease exacerbates. Systemic lupus erythematosus in female NZB mice appears much earlier and more severely than in males; prepubertal castration of males causes the "female-type" disease, and prepubertal castration of females with subsequent administration of androgens reverts the disease to the "male-type."

For all these influences to occur a functioning thymus is needed. Severe autoimmune diseases are not seen in nude (athymic) mice. For many autoimmune diseases, there is an age-related peak incidence; however, autoimmune diseases in general are not clearly related to older age groups.

Table 13.6. Immunodeficiencies associated with autoimmune symptoms

Immunodeficiency	Autoimmune symptoms
Hypogammaglobulinemia:	
Congenital	Rheumatoid arthritis, dermatomyositis, scleroderma, Felty's syndrome, hemolytic anemia
Acquired	Hemolytic anemia, pernicious anemia
Selective IgA deficiency	Systemic lupus erythematosus, rheumatoid arthritis, dermatomyositis, pernicious anemia, thyreoditis, celiac disease (autoantibodies to double stranded DNA, to basement membrane), Addison's disease, thrombocytopenic purpura, regional enteritis
Dysgammaglobulinemias (selective IgG, selective IgM deficiency)	Hemolytic anemia, systemic lupus erythematosus, thrombocytic purpura
Chronic mucocutaneous candidiasis	Endocrinopathies (Addison's disease), pernicious anemia
Wiskott-Aldrich syndrome	Hemolytic anemia (Coombs' positive)
Ataxia telangiectasia	Autoantibodies against thyroglobulin, immunoglobulins, parietal cells, smooth muscle, nuclear material, basement membrane
Chronic granulomatous disease (female carriers)	Discoid and systemic lupus erythematosus with autoantibodies to DNA
Complement deficiencies (C1r, C1s, C2, C4, C5, C1-inhibititor)	Systemic lupus erythematosus

Autoimmune Diseases

Tissue Lesions in Autoimmune Diseases

Tissue lesions in autoimmune diseases can be produced by humoral, by cellular, or by a combined mechanism. In the former instance, antibody-antigen complexes are deposited in the tissue, particularly if the antibody is of the IgG type, complement is activated, and these effects result in inflammatory reactions, particularly of blood vessels (vasculitis, see Chap. 9, p. 284), and lysis of cells in cases where the antigen is cellbound. Cell-mediated lesions are caused by the direct action of cytotoxic T cells as well as by antibody-dependent, cell-mediated cytotoxicity of killer cells and macrophages (see pp. 305–307; Chap. 10) (Fig. 13.2).

Some Autoimmune Diseases

The presence of auto-antibodies or even their distribution in the tissues does not necessarily imply that the cause of the lesions and of the clinical symptoms of the disease is necessarily the autoimmune process itself. For a given disease to be considered autoim-

mune, the following criteria must be fulfilled: (1) For at least some stages of the evolutionary process of the disease in question, the existence of an immune response must be demonstrated, as indicated by the presence of autoantibodies or of sensitized cells, with specificity for auto-antigens localized in the injured tissue. (2) The sensitizing agent should be identified or characterized. (3) The disease should be reproducible by the injection of purified or partially purified auto-antigens into laboratory animals. (4) The pathologic events in experimental animals should correspond to those in man. (5) It should be possible to transfer the disease produced in laboratory animals to syngeneic animals by serum or lymphocytes.

There are several possible ways of classifying autoimmune diseases; since we do not understand the underlying mechanism for all these diseases (which would probably lead to a more logical classification), the classification as organ-specific or systemic appears to have some etiologic significance. The organ-specific autoimmune diseases are possibly related to the liberation of endogenous tissue constituents or modified autoantigens. On the other hand, the systemic

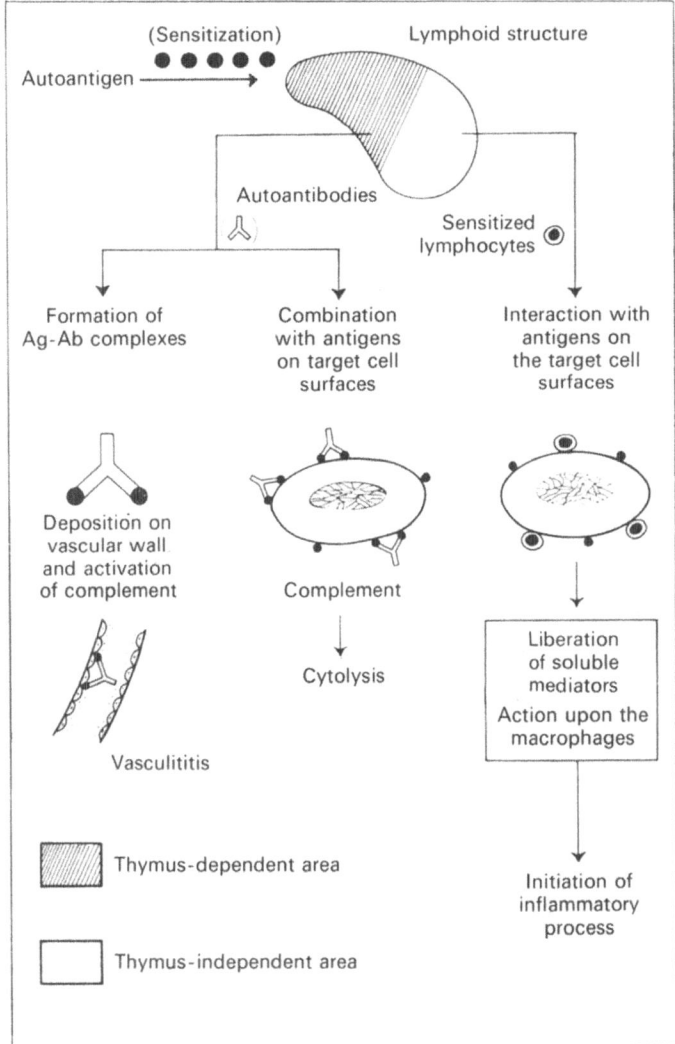

Fig. 13.2. Mechanism of tissue lesions in autoimmune processes

autoimmune diseases are probably due to alterations in the recognition mechanism of the central immune system (Table 13.7).

Autoimmune Diseases of the Central Nervous System

The diseases that affect the central nervous system and in which the autoimmune phenomena probably play an important part are: (1) experimental allergic encephalomyelitis (EAE), (2) multiple sclerosis, (3) acute disseminated encephalomyelitis, (4) acute postinfectious encephalomyelitis, and (5) postrabies vaccinal encephalomyelitis.

Experimental allergic encephalomyelitis (EAE) was first described by Rivers and his colleagues in 1933. The disease was elicited by repeated injections of brain extracts into monkeys; after 6–12 months, a demyelinating disease caused the death of some of the animals. Later, it could be demonstrated that brain extracts in complete Freund's adjuvant produced the disease with much greater regularity and in a far shorter period of time (10–30 days after the injection). The disease can also be produced in other species such as guinea-pigs, rabbits, mice, rats, and birds. In rats, the disease has been evaluated exhaustively using inbred strains: some

Table 13.7. Classification of the autoimmune diseases

Autoimmune diseases	Characteristics
Organ-specific	a) The antibodies usually are specific for one or more antigens of a particular organ b) The antigens are usually "segregated," c) The lesions can be reproduced experimentelly by injecting the antigen in complete Freund's adjuvant Examples: encephalomyelitis, thyroiditis, orchitis, epididymitis, glomerulonephritis, and autoimmune nephroses
Systemic	a) Antibodies exist for antigens of various tissues or organs; antigens react with antibodies obtained from either the same or different species b) The antigens are not "segregated"; under normal conditions the immune system is tolerant to them c) The diseases appear spontaneously in animals of the appropriate genotype (e.g., in NZB mice) Examples: lupus erythematosus, rheumatoid arthritis, some forms of acquired hemolytic anemia
Combination of both forms: organ-specific and systemic	a) Diseases that generally involve antibodies for various tissues, even though the inflammatory lesions are restricted to a small number of organs Examples: Sjögren's syndrome, ulcerative colitis, lupoid hepatitis, primary biliary cirrhosis, and some forms of acquired hemolytic anemia

strains are more susceptible to the development of the disease than others, and this susceptibility is genetically associated with certain alleles of the major histocompatibility complex. Similar results have been obtained in mice, in which susceptibility was found to be associated with the H-2^s haplotype, more precisely with the I-A^s allele.

The clinical symptoms vary from species to species but usually include paraparesis with urinary incontinence progressing to tetraplegia or death; weight loss is common.

The antigen responsible for the pathologic reactions in EAE has been identified as myelin basic protein, which is found in the myelin sheath in the white matter (it is not found in the newborns; EAE is, therefore, not induced in very young animals). Myelin basic protein has been completely characterized as a heat-stable, acid-resistant protein with a molecular weight of about 18,000 dalton with 170 residues. Residues 116–122 contain the only tryptophan in the molecule, and this part of the molecule represents the major encephalitogenic region for the guinea-pig.

66	67	68	69	70	71	72	73	74	75
Thr–	Thr–	His–	**Tyr–**	**Gly–**	Ser–	Leu–	Pro–	**Gln–**	**Lys**

113	114	115	116	117	118	119	120	121	122
Arg–	Phe–	Ser–	**Trp–**	**Gly–**	Ala–	Glu–	Gly–	**Gln–**	**Lys**

Residues 66–75 appear to be the major encephalitogenic determinant for the rabbit and the rat (the similarity of the important positions are indicated).

Histopathologically, there are two fundamental alterations: inflammatory infiltrations and demyelination. Other alterations such as vasculitis, necrosis of the nervous tissue, and hemorrhage are less frequent and appear only in the most severe cases. At first, the lesions are characterized by perivenular infiltrations of macrophages and lymphocytes, with small lymphocytes predominant. The infiltrations appear first in the white matter, from which they can spread to the meninges and choroid plexus. Within 48–72 h, macrophages become predominant; myelin destruction is accomplished by macrophages. The histopathologic aspect of EAE closely resembles that encountered in postrabies vaccinal and acute postinfectious encephaloyelitis (Fig. 13.3).

Electron microscopic studies of the lesions have revealed interesting pecularities with respect to the disposition of the cells of the inflammatory infiltrates. For example, it has been observed that in the areas where demyelination has occurred, the macrophages generally envelop the axis cylinders (Fig. 13.4) with their pseudopodia, which suggests that these cells are directly impli-

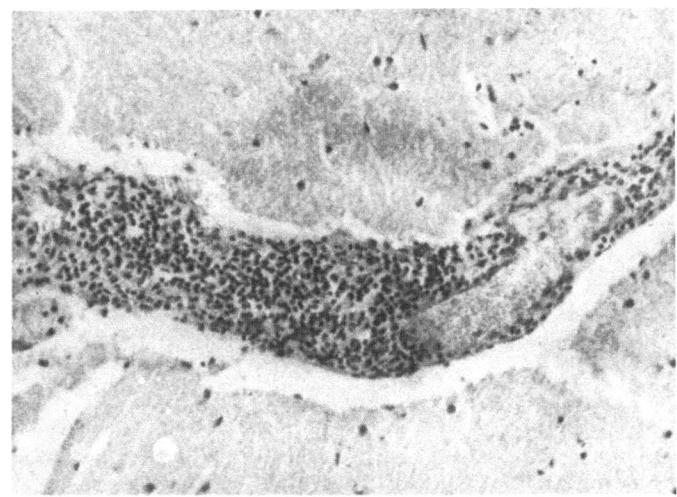

Fig. 13.3. Autoimmune encephalomyelitis. Perivenular inflammatory infiltrate of mononuclear cells. Bovine brain vaccinated with antirabies vaccine. (Courtesy of Prof. José M. Lamas da Silva, Departemento de Patologia, Escola de Veterinária, Universidade Federal de Minas Gerais)

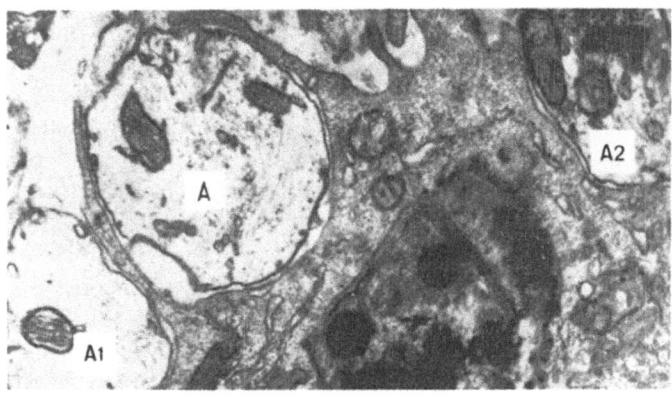

Fig. 13.4. Ultrastructure of autoimmune encephalitis. The cytoplasm of a mononuclear cell is enveloping the axons A, A_1, and A_2, which are demyelinated. Rubis JJ, Luse SA (1964) Am J Path 44:299

cated in myelinolysis. These are focal areas that correspond in general to the zones of inflammatory infiltrations. In addition to the destructive processes, areas of remyelination also exist, which could explain the remission of paralysis in some patients.

EAE is a T cell-dependent and cell-mediated disease, and antibodies are not of major importance for its development. Thus, the disease will not develop in thymectomized animals, but can be induced in bursectomized chicken. Furthermore, the disease can be passively transmitted with cells, but not with serum. Delayed-type hypersensitivity to basic protein can always be demonstrated by skin testing, and peripheral blood lymphocytes from EAE animals show a proliferative response to basic protein in vitro. Cells from EAE animals can destroy cultured myelinated nerve cells.

Animals can be protected from EAE by administration of basic protein in incomplete Freund's adjuvant, most probably because of the induction of suppressor T cell activity.

Multiple sclerosis (MS) is a demyelinating disease of the CNS in man; epidemiologic studies indicate that it occurs more commonly in regions with temperate or harsh climates and is rare in regions with warm climates. An environmental factor is, therefore, assumed to be important in the development of this disease. Immunogenetically, the HLA-D 2/DR 2 type is overrepresented in MS patients.

Histopathologically the disease shows a picture similar to EAE, and is characterized by plaques which consist of discrete regions in the white matter within which myelin and oligodendrocytes (the cells synthesizing myelin) are lost. During the acute inflammatory stage, large numbers of lymphocytes and macrophages are seen around the venules within plaques.

The etiology of the disease is still unknown, but it is suspected to be caused by immune reactions to cells infected with defective measles virus; alternatively, it might be an autoallergy. The target antigen does not appear to be the basic protein of myelin.

In the majority of MS patients, T cells in the peripheral blood are significantly reduced – however, this might be due to recruitment of T cells into the CNS. Con-A activated nonspecific T cell suppressor function is depressed in MS patients; it also has been shown that T cells (suppressor T cells) are markedly reduced in their number during active stages of the disease.

Acute disseminated encephalomyelitis appears as a sequel to infections such as measles, smallpox, chicken pox, and mumps, and is relatively similar to EAE. The lesions are found more frequently in the optic nerve, brain stem (in particular in bridges with ocular muscle nuclei), in the cerebellum and cerebellar peduncle, the pyramidal tracts, the base of the fourth ventricle, and in the posterior column of the spinal cord. It appears that the virus or viral components responsible for these lesions modify the structure of certain components of the neural tissue, possibly by the action of neuraminidase, or by the incorporation of liberated antigenic constituents of the host from the blood.

Another form of acute disseminated encephalomyelitis can occur after treatment with antirabies vaccine prepared with attenuated virus (see Fig. 13.3). In this case, the autoimmune response is unleashed by the presence of neural tissue components in the vaccine, the entire process presumably being almost analogous to that of experimental allergic encephalomyelitis.

Myasthenia gravis is characterized by weakness due to a defect in neuromuscular transmission. The disease is more frequent in women than in man; familial cases are know; the HLA-B 8 type is overrepresented in patients with myasthenia gravis. The weakness symptom is abrogated by anti-cholinergic drugs, which is a sign frequently employed as a diagnostic test. The underlying defect appears to be a depletion of acetylcholine-receptors, or a block of the receptors, in the subsynaptic region of myoneural junctions. In more than 90% of patients, antibodies to acetylcholine receptors can be demonstrated. This antibody is responsible for the disease since myasthenia gravis symptoms can be induced to occur in mice to which the antibody has been transferred.

In 60%–70% of patients, there are alterations of the thymus that vary from simple hyperlastic to thymoma (about 10%), occasionally malignant. In the hyperplasia form, numerous lymphoid follicles differentiate in the medullary zone with germinal centers rich in plasma cells. The cortex, although there are no fundamental changes, shrinks little by little to a fine layer. The medulla is proportionally enriched in lymphoid follicles with many B lymphocytes. This (and the findings of an increased incidence among myasthenia gravis patients of diseases with known or presumed autoimmune character such as thyroiditis, pernicious anemia, pemphigus, rheumatoid arthritis, systemic lupus erythematosus, insulin-dependent diabetes mellitus, and adrenalitis) have suggested an autoimmune pathogenesis of the disease.

Many myasthenics have antibodies against nuclear material, parietal cells, thyroid, and gammaglobulin (RF) in their sera. Moreover, with immunofluorescence methods, auto-antibodies can be detected which react specifically with the A and/or I band of myofibrils of normal individuals. These auto-antibodies react also with epithelial cells of the thymus, probably because of the presence of constituents common to the two types of cells; these antibodies can also be absorbed by thymus epithelial cells. These antibodies are not related to the disease, and are found in those patients in whom thymus alterations are observed.

Cellular immunity appears to be slightly abnormal, and in many patients, thymectomy apparently improves the prognosis. Although the etiology is not known, it is speculated that a viral infection (oncogenic virus?) of the thymus might be the cause.

Autoimmune Diseases of Endocrine Glands

The endocrine system is characterized by two important features: its activity is mediated by hormones via receptors, and the activity is regulates via feedback control. Therefore, immune reactions may play an important role at different levels: affecting the endocrine gland (e.g. Hashimoto's thyroiditis, Addison's disease, and insulin-dependent diabetes mellitus), intercepting circulating hormones (e.g., hypothyroidism, diabetes due to antibodies against insulin), and/or interfering with the receptor of the (hormone) target cell and thus disturbing the regulation (e.g., Graves' disease and insulin-resistant diabetes mellitus).

Experimental autoimmune thyroiditis. Witebsky and Rose demonstrated first that injection of thyroid lobe extracts in Freund's adjuvant into rabbits produced thyroiditis; since then, this model and other animal models (guinea-pig, dog, rat, mouse, chicken, and monkey) have been used to study this disease. Thyroiditis induced with thyroid extract in Freund's adjuvant is characterized by lymphocytic infiltrations of the thyroid gland and circulating antibodies to thyroglobulin. Although this disease is in some aspects similar to Hashimoto's thyroiditis in man (see below), it differs in that no germinal centers are found in the thyroid gland, and in that the antibodies produced are almost only anti-thyroglobulins. More similar to Hashimoto's thyroiditis are the thyroid disorders which occur spontaneously in the obese chicken strain and in buf-

falo (BUF) rats. It appears from studies in these animals that the production of antibodies is necessary for the development of the disease, but that T cells play an important part in controlling this development: thymectomy increases the incidence of the disease, whereas bursectomy inhibits the production of antibodies and decreases the incidence of the disorder. From these and other studies, it is assumed that a decrease in functionally active suppressor T cells (the same effect would be achieved by hyperreactive helper T cells!) may be the cause of the occurrence of the disease.

Hashimoto's thyroiditis or chronic lymphocytic thyroiditis represents a form of goiter occuring more frequently in women than in men, and is always associated with hypothyroidism.

Histopathologically, the first observed alterations appear as centers of perivascular inflammatory infiltrations, rich in lymphocytes and macrophages, and irregularly distributed but predominating in the capsule. As the process advances, the infiltrates spread out in the parenchyma between the thyroid vesicles. As revealed by electronmicroscopy, the mononuclear cells can penetrate the cells of the epithelium; in these areas, one encounters ruptures of the follicles and spreading of the colloid into the interstitial tissue (Fig. 13.5).

A variety of antibodies to different components of thyroid tissue has been found in the circulation of patients (Table 13.8). The role of these antibodies in relation to the disease is uncertain; the disease is not transferable to monkeys by serum of Hashimoto patients, and there is no correlation between the levels of circulating auto-antibodies and the intensity of lesions. On the other hand, cutaneous delayed-type hypersensitivity turns positive at the same time that lesions appear, whether or not circulating antibodies are detectable in the serum. From the histologic point of view the degenerative alterations occur only in thyroid follicles that are in contact with mononuclear cell infiltrates, the intensity of the alterations being

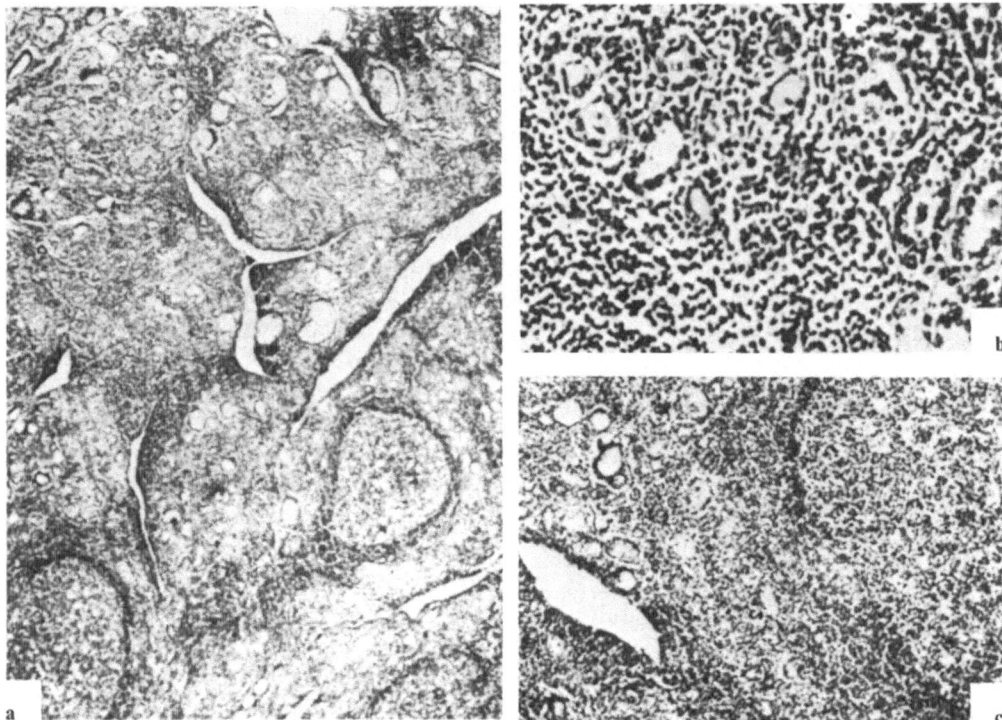

Fig. 13.5 a–c. Hashimoto's Thyroiditis. **a** Intense infiltration of lymphocytes in the glandular parenchyma with formation of lymphoid follicles exhibiting germinal centers. **b** Detail showing lymphocytic infiltration among the glandular follicles, with destruction of the same. **c** Lymphoid follicle in the interior of the glandular parenchyma, with distinct germinal center. (Courtesy of Prof. Fausto E. Lima Pereira, Departemento de Anatomia Patologica, Faculdade de Medicina, Universidade Federal de Espirito Santo)

proportional to the quantity of the infiltrate. More importantly, autoimmune thyroiditis can be transferred to normal guinea-pigs using suspensions of lymphoid cells of diseased animals. Furthermore, lymphocytes from patients show a proliferative response to thyroid antigens in vitro, and their lymphocytes are cytotoxic to thyroid cells in culture. Moreover, antibody-dependent cell-mediated cytotoxicity might be involved in the pathologic process: thus, cytotoxicity has been demonstrated using patients' lymphocytes and normal serum (i.e., activated "armed" K cells).

Table 13.8. Antibodies found in Hashimoto's thyroiditis

Antigen	Nature	Antibody	Detection[a]
Thyroglobulin (TG)	Glycoprotein, m.w. of 660,000, organ-specific	IgG, complement fixing	AG, CF, RIA
Microsomes	Membrane lipoprotein, organ-specific	IgG, complement fixing	CF, FAT, RIA
Antigen$_2$. colloid	Colloid protein, organ-specific	IgG, noncomplement fixing	FAT
Surface membrane	Organ-specific	IgM, IgG	FAT
TSH receptor	Glycoprotein, 200,00 mol. w.	IgG	RIA

[a] AG, agglutination of TG-coated latex particle; CF, complement fixation; FAT, fluorescence antibody technique; RIA, radioimmune assay

Graves' disease is a disorder characterized by hyperthyroidism, infiltrative ophthalmopathy, and pretibial myxedema. The thyroid hyperfunction is the result of stimulation of the thyroid gland by an auto-antibody with specificity for the TSH (thyroid stimulating hormone) receptor (long-acting thyroid stimulator, LATS). As a result, nearly all patients have elevated serum T_3 and T_4 concentrations, and show an increased thyroidal uptake of radioiodine.

An association of the disease occurrence with the HLA-D 3 type (and HLA-B 8 which is linkage disequilibrium with HLA-D 3) has been found.

Some circumstantial evidence suggests that Graves' disease is an autoimmune disorder: there is an incidence of thymic hyperplasia, lymphadenopathy, splenomegaly, peripheral lymphocytosis, and diffuse lymphocytic infiltrates in the thyroid gland. However, nothing is known about the etiology and pathogenesis.

Addison's disease is, in the majority of patients, caused by adrenal tuberculosis; the remaining cases result from amyloid degeneration, from Waterhouse-Friderichsen syndrome or its sequelae, or from prolonged administration of corticosteroids. In rare cases, Addison's disease is idiopathic; this form is more common in females than in males, and appears to be associated with an increased incidence of HLA-B 8.

The underlying pathogenic mechanism appears to be an autoimmune reaction to adrenal tissue. This is suggested by (a) its association with other autoimmune diseases (e.g., Hashimoto's thyroiditis); (b) its histology, characterized by atrophy and diffuse lymphocytic infiltration, particularly in the cortex, the structure of which is completely disrupted whereas the medulla is often preserved; (c) the presence of anti-adrenal antibodies, the antigen to which they are produced being unknown; (d) evidence for the presence of cell-mediated immunity, since patients show delayed-type hypersensitivity skin reactions to adrenal extracts; and (e) the production of experimental autoimmune adrenalitis after injection of adrenal gland extracts in Freund's adjuvant into rabbits or guinea-pigs. In these animals, the disease cannot be transferred by serum, but by cells.

Autoimmune pancreatitis: Diabetes mellitus is a symptom (sweet urine) and comprises a variety of different etiologic and pathogenic disease entities. Of the different forms of diabetes mellitus, a classification into insulin-dependent and insulin-independent has been suggested in recent years, providing a better understanding of the pathophysiology and genetics of diabetes than a classification based on the age of onset. Of these two groups, the insulin-dependent forms are those in which autoimmune phenomena play an important role.

Insulin-dependent diabetes mellitus is characterized by an early (usually less than 30 years of age) and rapid onset, a male predominance, severely reduced islet mass with inflammatory reactions in the islets, an association with HLA-D 3/D 4 types and other endocrinopathies (e.g. autoimmune adrenal or autoimmune thyroid diseases), and immunologic symptoms (cell-mediated immunity and auto-antibodies to endocrine pancreas, but also a high prevalence of auto-antibodies to nonpancreatic antigens).

Histologically, the islets are infiltrated by lymphocytes and large mononuclear cells (insulitis) with a reduction in the number of islets and gross atrophy of those which remain.

Insulitis can be induced in experimental animals by injection of endocrine pancreas homogenates; it is also seen in animals infected with encephalomyocarditis virus, suggesting a possible etiology of insulin-dependent diabetes in man (see Table 13.5).

Two types of auto-antibodies are found in the serum of patients: early after onset of the disease, an auto-antibody with specificity for cytoplasmic or microsomal membrane fractions can be detected with the fluorescence antibody technique; this antibody is usually of IgG type and fixes complement; it is organ-specific, but not species-specific. A second antibody is found reacting specifically with the surface membrane of islet cells, usually of the IgM or IgG type. It is not clear, whether or not these antibodies are important for the generation of the disease. The fact that a diabetic syndrome can be provoked in nude mice after transfer of lymphocytes from insulin-dependent diabetes mellitus patients strongly suggests that the disease is mediated by cellular immune mechanisms. It can be shown that lymphocytes of patients possess a specific cytotoxic activity to cultured insuloma cells; this cytotoxicity could be enhanced by addition of serum from diabetes mellitus patients, perhaps indicating that T cell-mediated as well as antibody-dependent cell-mediated reactions are important.

Acanthosis nigricans is a rare disease of the skin with a wart-like hyperplasia of the stratum spinosum of the epithelium with pigment deposits. In some of these patients, a severe impairment of insulin binding to lymphocyte receptors has been diagnosed. This impairment is caused by anti-receptor antibodies competing with insulin. In those patients, an increase in serum gammaglobulin, leukopenia, the presence of anti-nuclear antibodies and arthralgia has been observed.

Hematologic Autoimmune Diseases

Autoimmune hemolytic anemia: The hemolytic anemias comprise a group of diseases in which the life of the red blood cells is abnormally short, even though all the conditions for erythropoiesis are normal.

In the congenital forms (congenital hemolytic anemia), cellular fragility is due to defects in the erythrocytes themselves and is genetically controlled. In the acquired forms, however, the defect appears to have no familial distribution, nor does it relate to the structure of the erythrocyte. These differences can be demonstrated through cross-transfusion, by studying the survival of erythrocytes transferred to normal persons or

to persons with acquired hemolytic anemia. Red blood cells of patients with congenital hemolytic anemia are short-lived even when transferred to normal individuals. On the other hand, the red blood cells obtained from patients with acquired hemolytic anemia reveal normal longevity when transferred to normal individuals. For these reasons, the congenital forms are called "intraerythrocytic" or "intracorpuscular", and the acquired forms "extraerythrocytic" or "extracorpuscular".

In 50%–60% of all cases, the acquired hemolytic anemias are not associated with any particular disease, and are termed idiopathic. In the remaining cases, they appear to be associated with other processes such as neoplasias of the lymphoreticular tissue, diseases of the "collagen", and with viral or chronic inflammatory diseases; they are then referred to as "symptomatic".

It was long suspected that the acquired hemolytic anemias were autoimmune in origin, especially after the demonstration by Donath and Landsteiner of the presence of autohemolysins in the sera of patients with paroxysmal nocturnal hemoglobulinemia. With the development of the antiglobulin test by Coombs, it could be shown that in the majority of acquired hemolytic anemias, the destruction of the red blood cells was always associated with the presence of autoantibodies on their surfaces.

Antierythrocytic auto-antibodies were classified in two groups: those that were active at body temperature (36°–37 °C), called "warm antibodies," and those that reacted optimally only at low temperatures (4°–10 °C), called "cold antibodies."

Antigens: In more than one-third of autoimmune anemia cases, the antigens correspond to the Rh system, and within this group the "e" antigen appears with the greatest frequency (98% of Rh positive individuals). In addition to these Rh system antigens that stimulate the formation of warm antibodies, other antigens have been described that stimulate the appearance of cold antibodies. The latter are designated by the letter "I."

The erythrocytes that react with the cold antibodies are designated "I-positive" whereas the nonreacting red blood cells are designated "I-negative" or simply "i." The I antigens are genetically controlled and are absent in neonates, whose erythrocytes react only with anti-i antisera; they appear only between 18 months and 2 years of age, at which time the I-positive or i character becomes definitely established.

Antibodies: In addition to the warm and cold antibodies mentioned previously, a third type of autohemolysin is encountered in paroxysmal nocturnal hemoglobinuria, known as the "Donath-Landsteiner antibody," or D–L antibody.

Warm auto-antibodies are immunoglobulins with 7S sedimentation coefficients; the majority are incomplete and do not activate complement. Their presence on the erythrocyte membrane can be disclosed either by the Coombs test (most commonly, see Fig. 13.6a) or by the direct agglutination test using erythrocytes treated with trypsin.

The cold auto-antibodies belong to the IgM immunoglobulin class (sedimentation coefficient, 19S). They function as complete antibodies, i.e., they can be revealed by methods for direct agglutination of normal red blood cells; they bind complement and easily lyse erythrocytes treated with trypsin or erythrocytes from patients with paroxysmal nocturnal hemoglobinuria. Cold antibodies aggregate on erythrocyte membranes at lower temperatures and dissociate when the temperature is raised to 37 °C. Nevertheless, Coombs' test is positive even when care

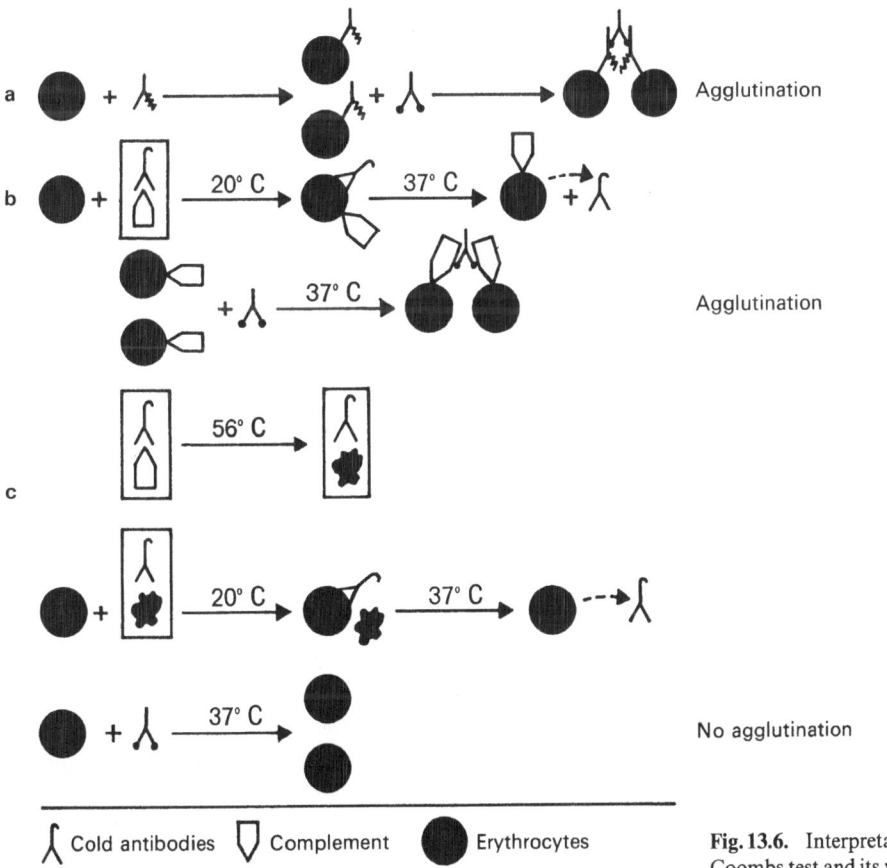

a   Agglutination

b

                                                                     Agglutination

c

                                                                     No agglutination

⋀ Cold antibodies   ⋁ Complement   ● Erythrocytes

⋀ᵥ Warm antibodies   ⋀ Antiglobulin antibodies (Coombs' serum)

Fig. 13.6. Interpretation of the Coombs test and its variants in the identification of the principal autohemolysins

is taken that the blood is not cooled lower than 37 °C, whereby cold agglutinins become disaggregated and are bound to the erythrocyte membranes (Fig. 13.6).

When the indirect Coombs test is performed (Fig. 13.6), one must take care to warm the serum to be tested to 56 °C to inactivate the complement. The addition of anti-gamma-globulin serum to the mixture does not produce agglutination of the red blood cells. This indicates that the agglutination of the red blood cells by the Coombs serum at 37 °C is not due to cold antibody reaction, but rather to components of complement bound to the red blood cell in the event that there is an erythrocyte–cold antigen reaction. These data suggest that complement, in addition to serving as a "bridge" in the antibody–antiglobulin and erythrocyte reaction, also fosters the binding of the cold antibodies to the erythrocyte membrane.

The D–L antibodies are hemolysins encountered in the sera of patients with paroxysmal nocturnal hemoglobinuria; they possess a sedimentation coefficient of the order of 7S, and require lower temperatures than do cold antibodies to affix to erythrocyte membranes. They do not require complement (C) to attach to the erythrocytes, but lytic properties are acquired only when the temperature reaches 18°–20 °C – thus the name "diphasic cold antibodies."

Hemolysis mechanisms: The destruction of red blood cells in the different forms of "autoimmune" anemias can occur in two ways: In the first mechanism, the erythrocytes carrying acquired autoantibodies adhering to their surfaces reveal spherocytosis and are retained in the macrophage system, principally in the spleen, where they are ultimately destroyed. In the second mechanism, most commonly observed in paroxysmal nocturnal hemoglobinuria and in the forms of anemia due to cold antibodies, hemolysis of erythrocytes results from the activity of complement. In this case, the autohemolysins attach to the red blood cells and fix complement when in transit through the peripheral vessels of the regions most subject to low temperature (face, ears, nose, and hands), with hemolysis occurring when the erythrocytes reach warmer regions.

There are three experimental models of autoimmune anemias: (1) homologous disease, produced by introduction of immunocompetent cells into a recipient animal that cannot eliminate them; (2) spontaneous autoimmune anemia observed in NZB mice; and (3) spontaneous autoimmune hemolytic anemia of the dog, with or without disseminated LE syndrome.

Homologous disease (Secondary or Graft-vs-Host Disease): Homologous disease occurs as a consequence of the proliferation of allogeneic immunocompetent cells in a recipient animal incapable of rejecting them, either because it has been rendered immunoincompetent (irradiation, ALS treatment) or because it is tolerant to the transfused cells, or because it is an F_1 hybrid, that has received transplanted immunocompetent cells from one of its parents. These transplanted cells proliferate and react immunologically with tissue components of the host. Among other alterations, destruction of the red blood cells, leukopenia, and sometimes thrombocytopenia are observed. The antibodies eluted from the red blood cells of the F_1 hybrid with homologous disease agglutinate the red blood cells from that parent that did not furnish the immunocompetent cells. The antigens responsible for the establishment of homologous disease belong to the group of histocompatibility antigens and the AB0 blood group antigens.

Spontaneous autoimmune anemia of the NZB mouse: This strain of mice was originally selected for cancer research. In the meantime, it was ascertained that from the third month of life these animals exhibited an autoimmune hemolytic anemia characterized by a positive Coombs test, reticulocytosis, jaundice, glomerulonephritis, and hepatosplenomegaly. Contemporaneously with the appearance of the hemolytic-antibodies – unusually warm antibodies – histologic alterations develop in the thymus, characterized by proliferation of lymph cells, with occasional formation of lymphoid follicles. The autoimmune nature of this syndrome was confirmed by transferring lymphocytes during the active phase of the disease to young mice of the same strain.

The renal alterations resemble those encountered in human lupus erythematosus. This form of autoimmune hemolytic anemia constitutes an example of the emergence of "forbidden clones" genetically conditioned for the formation of auto-antibodies directed against the animal's own erythrocyte cell membrane components.

Spontaneous autoimmune hemolytic anemia of the dog: This form of autoimmune anemia appears either alone or accompanied by symptomatology similar to that observed in lupus erythematosus. In the first case, anemia, jaundice, generalized lymphadenopathy, and splenomegaly are observed. The anemia observed is of the macrocytic type, with low hemoglobin levels (about 2.5 g/ 100 ml). Reticulocytosis, hyperplasia of the bone marrow, and thrombocytopenia are also observed in the majority of cases. The Coombs test is always positive; the antibodies can be eluted from erythrocytes, and they react with red blood cells of normal animals. In the symptomatic form, one encounters, in addition to the alterations just described, diffuse glomerulonephritis characterized by thickening and hyalinization of the basement membrane of Bowman's capsule, as well as by sclerosis of the afferent glomerular arterioles. In the majority of cases, one also encounters rheumatoid factor and LE-cells.

Thrombocytopenias: Thrombocytopenic purpura occurs as a primary disease, or as a secondary disease associated with other diseases such as lupus erythematosus or leukemia. In addition to hemorrhagic phenomena, there are alterations in the structure of platelets in the blood and of the megakaryocytes in the bone marrow. The acute forms are usually encountered in children under 8 years of age, of both sexes, whereas the chronic forms occur more often in adults – mostly in women – and persist for months or even years.

A factor exists in the serum of those afflicted with thrombocytopenic purpura that can produce thrombocytopenia when injected into normal individuals. The nature of this factor has not yet been adequately determined; however, it does exhibit characteristics of an antibody: It is adsorbed by platelets, is species-specific, and is a 7 S globulin. During purpuric crises, an increase is observed in the level of β-glycerol-phosphatase (an enzyme found in the platelets), always coinciding with thrombocytopenia, which suggests intense platelet destruction. Since it is much easier to determine glycerol-phosphatase levels than those of anti-platelet factor, testing for the former is preferred in differential diagnostics. The destruction of the platelets appears to occur either by direct action of the antiplatelet factor, agglutinating and lysing them, or by opsonizing them to facilitate their destruction by the macrophages of the reticuloendothelial system, principally those of the spleen.

The use of drugs such as sulfonamides, chlorothiazides, chlorpropamide, meprobamate, phenylbutazone, quinidine, and the sedative Sedormid can produce thrombocytopenia.

It is presumed that the drug, functioning as a foreign hapten, combines with certain components of the platelet membranes to form autoimmunogenic complexes. These complexes generate antibodies that react with the membrane-drug complex of the platelets.

Autoimmune leukopenias: Some forms of leukopenias appear to be associated with the presence of autoantibodies. Data indicating that these auto-leukoagglutinins are related to destruction of the leukocytes are summarized as follows: (1) auto-agglutinins exist in many cases of neutropenias; (2) when the neutropenia recedes either naturally or upon treatment, the auto-antibodies also disappear; and (3) in some cases of neutropenia, there is no history of transfusions, thus eliminating the possibility of formation of alloantibodies.

Autoimmune Diseases of the Gastrointestinal Tract and Liver

Gastric atrophy and pernicious anemia: Gastric atrophy is the endstage inflammatory process which begins as superficial gastritis, progresses to atrophic gastritis, and ends in atrophy. Histologically, these three phases are characterized by: first, lymphocytic, plasmocytic, and monocytic infiltrates of the superficial epithelium and lamina propria of the gastric mucosa; in the more advanced phase, mononuclear infiltrates extend more deeply and surround the tubular acini of gastric glands with partial loss of parietal and chief cells; the atrophic phase is characterized by complete loss of gastric glands.

Two types of antibodies are found: one reacting with the Vitamin B_{12}-binding glycoprotein, intrinsic factor, and the other with a lipoprotein antigen present on the microvilli of gastric parietal cells. Anti-intrinsic factor antibodies react either with the Vitamin-B_{12} binding site and compete with the binding of Vitamin B_{12}, or with a determinant away from the binding site. Usually, both antibodies are present; in the serum, they are IgG antibodies, in the stomach often IgA. These antibodies interfere with the uptake of Vitamin B_{12}.

The antiparietal antibody detects an organ-specific, but not species-specific antigen, and it may not be detected in the serum, only in the gastric juice. A high degree of correlation exists between the presence of this antibody and the extent of gastritis and gastric mucosal atrophy.

The histopathologic alterations are assumed to be the result, at least in part, of cell-mediated immunity to gastric mucosa cells. Lymphocytes of patients show an enhanced proliferative response and release leukocyte-migration inhibition factor upon stimulation with gastric mucosa homogenates.

The etiology is not known; a strong familial association exists. There is an association in a few cases between pernicious anemia and thyrotoxicosis; thyroid microsomal and thyroglobulin antibodies are also found in some patients with pernicious anemia.

Ulcerative colitis and Crohn's disease are two inflammatory diseases affecting the mucosa of rectum and colon (ulcerative colitis), and terminal ileum (Crohn's disease); they might be two expressions of a single disease. The diseases are slightly more common in females than in males. The cause is not known, although in recent years some indications have suggested a viral etiology: electron microscopic studies revealed some evidence for virus-like particles, and intestinal lesions have been demonstrated to occur after transfer of mucosa homogenate from patients' colon into laboratory animals.

Antibodies with specificity for colonic mucosal epithelial cell antigen, which is present in sterile, fetal colonic mucosa, and with specificity for polysaccharide antigens of E. coli 0:14 cross-reacting with colon antigen, have been found in patients with ulcerative colitis. These antibodies are of the IgG class, and are not cytotoxic for colon epithelial cells; moreover, neither the presence nor the titer correlates with extent or severity of the disease.

Some indications for cell-mediated immunity have been found: lymphocytes of patients are specifically cytotoxic to allogenic colonnic epithelial cells; this cytotoxicity is inhibited by preincubation with E. coli lipopolysaccharide, is complement-independent, and is mediated by K cells.

Chronic active hepatitis is characterized by periportal inflammation and liver cell injury. As etiologic agents have been identified: hepatitis B virus, drugs, and alcohol. Two groups of patients can be distinguished: one is HB_sAg negative and presents autoimmune-like symptoms; in these cases, the etiology is not always clear. Women are more frequently affected than men, and there is an overrepresentation of the HLA-B 8 type. In addition, these patients usually have high-titer of antibodies to hepatocyte-actin and smooth muscle. The other group consists of HB_sAg-positive patients with males predominant, and an overrepresentation of the HLA-B 35 type.

An antibody to hepatocyte-specific antigen, liver-surface protein (LSP), can be detected in the serum of all patients with acute hepatitis. This antibody usually disappears in patients recovering from this disease, but remains in those who develop chronic active hepatitis (the reason for this is not known). It has been shown that when injected into rabbits, LPS induces chronic aggressive hepatitis, and that the killing of liver cells in culture by lymphocytes of patients can be prevented by adding LSP to the culture.

The pathogenic mechanism leading to chronic disease is assumed to involve virus antigens on the surface of hepatocytes that stimulate T helper cells which, in turn, induce B cells to produce antibodies; this antibody response includes the formation of anti-LSP. The infected cells are killed either by complement-dependent antibody lysis, or by antibody-mediated cell lysis (which has been demonstrated to occur in vitro by K cells). In cases where the infection is controlled, stimulation of T helper cells and antibody production ceases. In persistent virus infections (HB_sAg^+), the antibody production continues; in "autoimmune" hepatitis it is assumed that the anti-LSP antibody formation has become autonomous, most probably as a result of deficient suppressor T-cell function (for which there are some hints from in vitro studies).

Autoimmune Diseases of the Kidney

Glomerulonephritis: Two immunologic mechanisms may be distinguished in the production of experimental glomerulonephritis: (a) Antibody-antigen complex deposition in the glomeruli with activation of inflammatory processes due to complement and subsequent polymorphonuclear and mononuclear cell activation (see Chap. 9. p. 284 f.), and (b) nephrotoxic glomerulonephritis (Masugi's nephritis,

glomerular basement membrane antibody glomerulonephritis) induced by antibodies specific for xenogeneic or allogeneic (autoimmune) basement membrane antigen.

Anti-glomerular basement membrane antibody-induced glomerulonephritis: Antikidney or nephrotoxic sera (NS) are produced by injecting kidney extract, emulsified in complete Freund's adjuvant, into animals of different species. Usually, rat kidney extracts have been used to immunize rabbits or, occasionally, ducks.

Intravenous injection of NS into the appropriate species induces a biphasic glomerulonephritis. Application of large amounts of antibasement antibody produces an immediate injury with proteinuria. A second phase appears 8–12 days later, when the host has mounted an immune response to the foreign antibody (see also below).

In the first hours after injection, the capillaries in the affected glomeruli dilate and are invaded by an infiltrate rich in neutrophils. Subsequently, the endothelial cells swell, proliferate, and reduce the capillary lumen, terminating in tubular hemorrhages (Fig. 13.7). The electron microscope reveals that the basal lamina becomes thickened on the capillary side from the deposition of dense material composed of xenogeneic antikidney antibodies and of complement components, among them C 3 and C 4. Continuous deposition of antibodies and complement components can result in the complete obliteration of the capillary (Fig. 13.8). In immunofluorescence staining of kidney sections, a linear configuration appears. When the lesions are focal, they tend to disappear; however, when they are diffuse, the animals either die in the first few days, or the lesions evolve to a chronic state, persisting for months or even years. In this case, the histopathologic picture closely resembles human glomerulonephritis.

The nephritogenic antigen is localized in the glomerular basement membrane, and appears to be a glycoprotein. A similar antigen is encountered in the lung, probably associ-

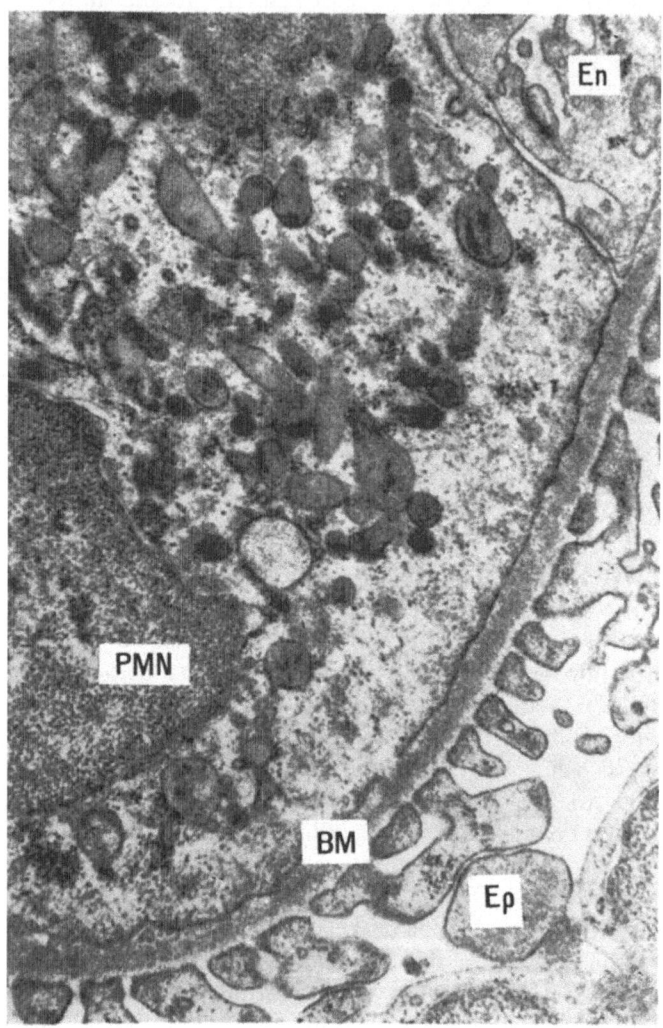

Fig. 13.7. Electron microscopic appearance of a capillary of the glomerulus of a rat killed 2.5 h after injection of nephrotoxic serum. A polymorphonuclear leukocyte is shown in intimate contact with the basement membrane of the capillary. *BM*, basement membrane; *En*, endothelial cell; *Ep*, epithelial cell; *PMN*, polymorphonuclear leukocyte

ated with the wall of the alveolar capillaries (see below, Goodpasture's syndrome).

The nephrotoxic sera contain IgG and IgM antibodies; in addition to the anti-basement membrane antibodies two other factors may be responsible for the occurrence of the glomerular lesions: complement components and polymorphonuclear cells. The injection of NS into rats decomplementized by prior administration of human IgG aggregates, antigen-antibody complexes, cobra venom, zymosan, a. o., only produces lesions of slight intensity. The same reaction occurs if the animal has been rendered leukopenic by previous administration of nitrogen mustard or similar agents. It appears, therefore, that lesions are formed only after the antibody-antigen complex on the basement membrane has activated the complement system, with the production of anaphylatoxins and chemotactic factors, followed by the accumulation of neutrophils. Electron microscopic studies show that, in many areas, the polymorphonuclear cells displace the cytoplasm of the endothelial cells and enter into contact with the basement membrane (Figs. 13.7 and 13.8).

The necessity of complement activation for the pathogenesis of the lesions has been elegantly demonstrated by using duck antibodies to basement membrane antigen of the rabbit. Duck antibodies do not activate

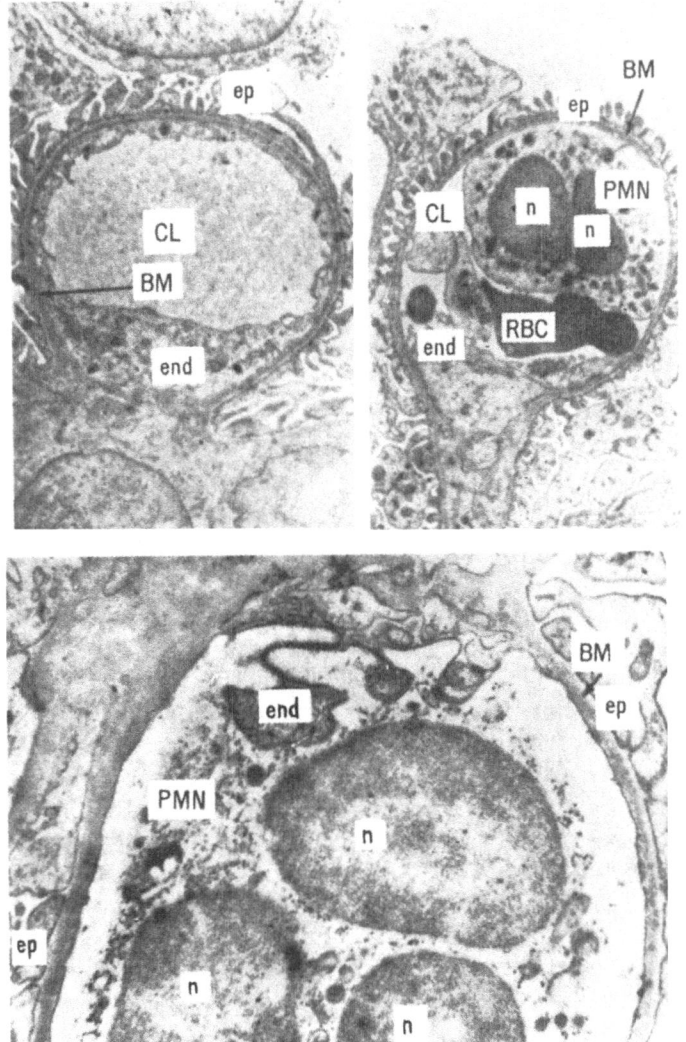

Fig. 13.8. Electron microscopic appearance of glomerular capillaries of a rat. In **a** (control), infiltration by polymorphonuclear leukocytes (*PMN*) is not observed, and the endothelial cells (*end*) are normally distributed over the surface of the basement membrane (*BM*). In **b** is shown a section of kidney obtained from a rat 2.5 h after the injection of nephrotoxic serum. The endothelial cell (*end*) was forced from its position by the polymorphonuclear (*PMN*) cells, leaving the basement membrane denuded. In **c**, the pseudopodia of the polymorphonuclear leukocyte are extended beneath the cytoplasm of the endothelial cell (*end*), entering into intimate contact with the basement membrane. This contact continues for some hours, with disappearance of the leukocytes about 6 h after the injection of the nephrotoxic serum. Cochrane CG et al. (1965) J Exp Med 122:99

mammalian complement: the clinical manifestations and histologic alterations only appear after 7–12 days. The duck antibody combines with the antigen in the basement membrane, yet does not activate complement, and is therefore unable to damage the glomeruli. However, since the duck antibody is foreign, it stimulates the formation of host antibodies, which then, after binding to the duck antibody, activate complement and produce lesions.

The pathogenesis of (isogeneic) basement-membrane antibody-induced glomerulonephritis in humans parallels the ex-perimental disease; however, nothing is known about the cause inducing the formation of auto-antibasement antibodies. It is assumed that cross-reacting antigens of infectious microorganisms (e.g., influenza) and noxious agents such as hydrocarbon solvents (inhaled) may induce the formation of this antibody.

Autoimmune Diseases of the Lung

Goodpasture's syndrome is a disease characterized by focal pulmonary hemorrhages always associated with a rapidly evolving

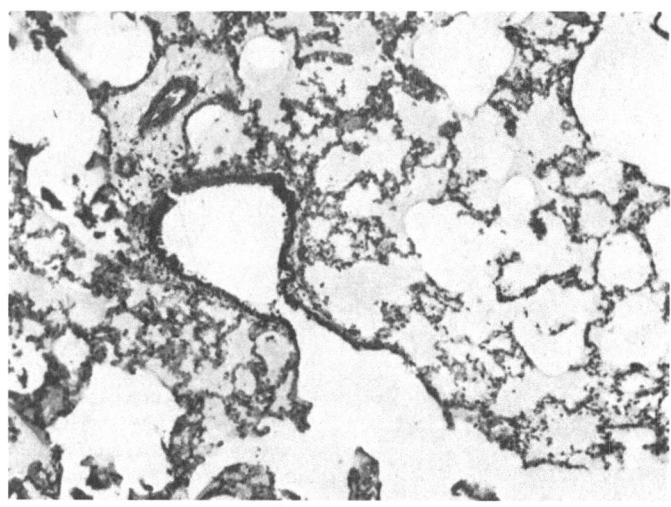

Fig. 13.9. Histologic appearance of rat lung with acute pulmonary edema produced by injection of nephrotoxic serum

membranous or proliferative glomerulonephritis. Immunofluorescence staining reveals homogeneous deposits of immunoglobulins and of complement along the basement membrane. The auto-antibodies appear to be directed against antigens shared by the lung and kidney. The same syndrome can be induced experimentally when nephrotoxic serum (anti-basement membrane antibodies) is injected into rats (Fig. 13.9).

Autoimmune Diseases of the Heart

Rheumatic fever: Auto-antibodies against antigens of the cardiac muscle appear to be a major pathogenic factor in the pathogenesis of heart disease subsequent to rheumatic fever. The antibody can be detected by complement fixation, antiglobulin consumption test, passive hemagglutination with tanned red blood cells coated with cardiac antigen, and immunofluorescence. With the latter method, it has been demonstrated that IgG and IgM auto-antibodies adhere to the sarcolemma, on the periphery of the sarcoplasm, and on the walls of the heart blood vessels of individuals with rheumatic fever. In addition, the serum of these patients contains antibodies that react with fragments of normal hearts; these antibodies are de-

posited in the same structures in which they were encountered in the hearts of afflicted individuals. Moreover, these antibodies cross-react with protein antigens in the capsular wall of group A hemolytic streptococci. On the other hand, when rabbits are injected with these streptococci causes them to produce antibodies which cross-react with human heart extract.

These observations suggest that the initial immunogenic stimulus is provided by the antigens of the streptococcus wall and that the progression of these lesions is due to the autoantigens liberated as a consequence of the tissue lesions.

Autoimmune Diseases of the Eye

It is recognized that the eye is the site of two autoimmune processes, one affecting the lens, and the other affecting the uveal tract.

Lens: The human lens contains at least nine or ten organ-specific antigens. Some of these antigens form early on in embryonic development, so that when the immune system is differentiated, these antigens are already isolated from other structures and, therefore, are potential autoantigens.
Endophthalmitis phaco-anaphylactica (greek phakos, lens) results primarily from

the liberation of crystalline lens substances due to the rupture of the lens capsule. The inflammatory process is initiated several weeks after the injury and progresses rapidly. The histologic alterations appear around the ruptured lens or its fragments in the form of three characteristic concentric layers: In the center is found the disintegrating crystalline fragment, infiltrated by polymorphonuclear leukocytes; more toward the periphery there is a layer of epithelioid cells with some multinucleated giant cells. Externally, there is granulation tissue of variable thickness, infiltrated by leukocytes and plasma cells. The experimental disease induced in rabbits exhibits, generally, the same sequence of events.

Uveal Tract. Sympathetic ophthalmia is a bilateral ocular disease that appears some weeks after a perforation injury of the eyeball, especially when the iris or the ciliary body is involved. In the beginning, there is infiltration by lymphatic cells that is particularly pronounced around the venules of the uveal tract. Later, epithelioid cells and giant cells appear which extend to the choroid and the iris. Coinciding with the disease – principally during the aggravation phase of the lesions – one observes delayed skin reactions following the injection of uveal-tract extracts. This fact, along with the lack of circulating antibodies during the active state of the disease, suggests that the lesions are mediated by cellular hypersensitivity. This disease can be produced experimentally in the guinea pig by the injection of uveal tract extracts in complete Freund's adjuvant. Studies with albino and pigmented guinea pigs indicate that at least two antigens exist in the uveal tracts that are responsible for sympathetic ophthalmia – one of them probably associated with uveal pigment.

Autoimmune Disease of the Skin

Pemphigus vulgaris is a rare blistering disorder; there is an increased frequency of HLA-A 10 and HLA-B 13. The etiology is un-known; an almost identical, but less severe disease which is endemic in south central Brazil, Pemphigus foliaceus, is assumed to be caused by an arthropod-borne infection. Histologically, there is an intraepidermal blister formation with acantholysis; electron microscopic studies show a dissolution of intercellular "cement" followed by desmosome destruction. These lesions are caused by an autoantibody with specificity for intercellular substances of the skin and mucosa; the antibody can be detected in the serum of most patients. Immunofluorescence staining reveals deposits of Ig (predominantly IgG) and complement (C 1, C 4, C 3, and properdin factor B) in the skin lesions. Identical lesions can be observed in a culture of epidermis cells to which this antibody is added.

It is assumed that in these patients a T-cell deficiency exists.

Systemic Autoimmune Diseases

Systemic lupus erythematosus (SLE) is characterized by inflammatory and destructive processes in a variety of organs such as skin, joints, kidney, heart, lungs, due to pathologic alterations of arteries and arterioles as a result of multiple immune abnormalities. The disease is more common in females than in males, and has a peak incidence between 25 and 29 years of age. Family studies, particularly of twins, have yielded evidence of a genetic susceptibility to SLE, and there appears to be a slight association of susceptibility to SLE with HLA-DR2/DR3 types. The acute condition frequently occurs after exposure to sunlight or drugs. A careful examination almost always reveals autoimmune phenomena which were in existence for some years prior to the time of diagnosis. Clinical manifestations are extremely pleiomorphic: dermatologic lesions such as erythemas (facial butterfly-shaped rash, Fig. 13.10), maculae, bullous and ulcerous lesions; polyserositis causing arthralgia, abdominal and chest pain, myalgia, Raynaud's syndrome due to lesions in arteries and arterioles, lesions of the lacrimal (keratocon-

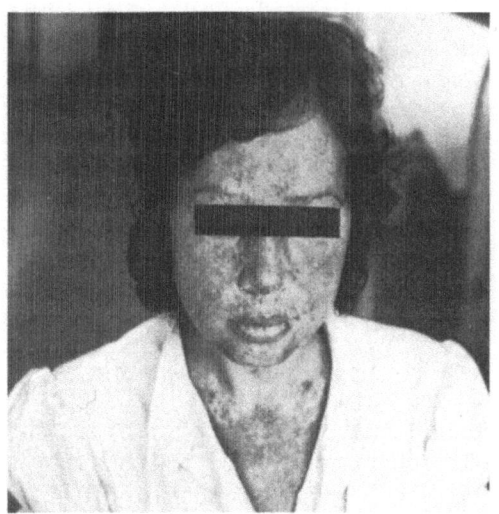

Fig. 13.10. Cutaneous lesions in SLE. Dermatologic lesions in the areas exposed to the light of a patient with SLE. The involvement of the scalp caused alopecia visible in the photograph. (Courtesy of Dr. Roberto Dias, Hosp. Clinicas, UFMG)

junctivitis sicca) and salivary glands, otitis media, pericarditis, and myocarditis, interstitial pneumonia, vascular lesions of the intestinal tract, glomerulonephritis, hemolytic anemia, thrombocytopenia, and leukopenia.

Histologically, fibrosis, lymphocyto-plasmocytic infiltrations and immune complex depositions prevail.

The etiology of the disease is unknown, but it is assumed that its occurrence is brought about by environmental factors such as UV-light, drugs, and/or viral infections, in genetically predisposed individuals.

Thus, paramyxovirus-like structures have been found in kidney, skin, and circulating lymphocytes of SLE patients; sera from patients contain a high number of antibodies to measles and other RNA and DNA viruses, and antibodies to double-stranded RNA, which is found in viruses but not in mammalian cells. Xenotropic C-type viral antigens (gp 30 and gp 70) in renal and lymphoid tissue have been identified. However, none of these possible agents has been shown to be responsible for the disease in humans.

Among the drugs which have been demonstrated to induce autoantibodies and a clinical SLE-like syndrome are procainamide, hydralazine, chloropromazine, isoniazid, hydantoins, trimethadione and α-methyldopa. These substances are able to interact with DNA or nucleoproteins (in vitro), and they induce anti-nuclear antibodies in individuals receiving them.

Sex hormones are important, as already indicated by the female to male ratio; furthermore, during pregnancy, an exacerbation of the disease is common, which extends to the postpartum period.

The most prominent abnormality in patients with SLE is their ability to produce antibodies to a wide array of self-antigens (Table 13.9). Many of these antibodies, particularly anti-nuclear antibodies (ANA), have been implicated in the pathogenesis of the disease, and SLE has been considered as a prototype of immune-complex disorders.

Table 13.9. Autoantibodies in SLE

To cells (ACA, anti-cell ab):
  Lymphocytes (ALA)
  Erythrocytes
  Platelets
  Neutrophils
To tissue (ATA, anti-tissue ab):
  Heart
  Neurons (brain)
  Collagen
  Muscle
To cytoplasm:
  Ribosomes
  Mitochondria
  Lysosomes
To nuclei:
  Nucleoprotein (NP)   ⎫
  DNA   ⎪
  Histones   ⎪
  Ribonucleoprotein ⎬ ANA
  RNA-nucleoli   ⎪
To nucleic acid: ⎪
  DNA, double- and single-stranded ⎪
  RNA, double- and single-stranded ⎭
To others:
  Immunoglobulins (RF)
  Coagulans (prothrombin converter)
  Cardiolipin
  Thyroglobulin

The observation that the antibody response to most microorganisms tested (influenza vaccine, Newcastle disease virus, respiratory syncytial virus, adenovirus, Herpes simplex, cytomegalovirus, papovavirus, hepatitis B virus, rubella; Brucella, proteus OX-2-agglutinins, tetanus toxoid, streptolysin 0) is normal, may indicate that the defect of the immune system in SLE is not a general B-cell hyperactivity, but a failure to make a distinction between self and non-self; the result is a "normal" immune response to everything which comes into contact with immune cells, including, and most prominently, auto-antigens. There appears to be a specific defect to maintain and induce self-tolerance. Indeed, numerous studies have shown that SLE patients exhibit a reduced T-cell response in vivo (delayed-type hypersensitivity reaction to common antigens such as PPD) as well as in vitro (mitogenic and antigen-specific lymphocyte proliferation), and their number of T cells in the circulation is reduced, particularly those with CD8 marker (=suppressor T cells). It has been demonstrated that T cells from SLE patients with active disease are unable to suppress the synthesis of immunoglobulins by SLE-B cells (for test, see p. 361). It is not clear whether or not antilymphocytic antibodies (ALA) specifically reacting with T cells and present in SLE patients are responsible for the reduced T-cell number or activity; however, ALA titers correlate positively with disease activity.

In addition to T-lymphocyte impairments, null-(non-T, non-B) and K-cell abnormalities have also been reported to exist during active phases of the disease. Since all of these abnormalities are much less expressed in phases of remission, it might be suspected that the defects are not intrinsic but induced, and once pathogenic antibodies (ANA, ALA, ACA-anti-cellular antibodies-, ATA-anti-tissue antibodies) are formed, which reduce T cells and cause tissue damage, a vicious self-perpetuating cycle is established:

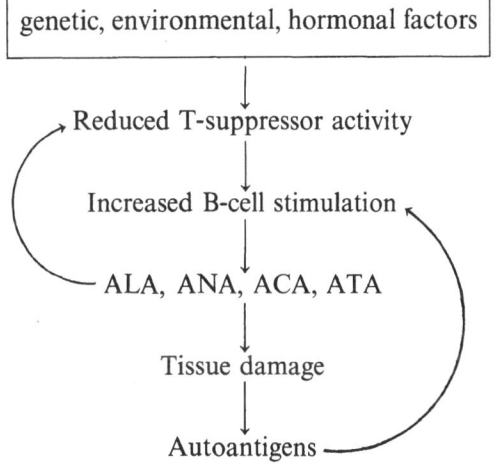

Thus far, there is no evidence for an enhanced cell-mediated reactivity to self-constituents in SLE patients.

For the pathogenesis of the disease, the most important factors appear to be antibodies to DNA (double- and single-stranded), soluble

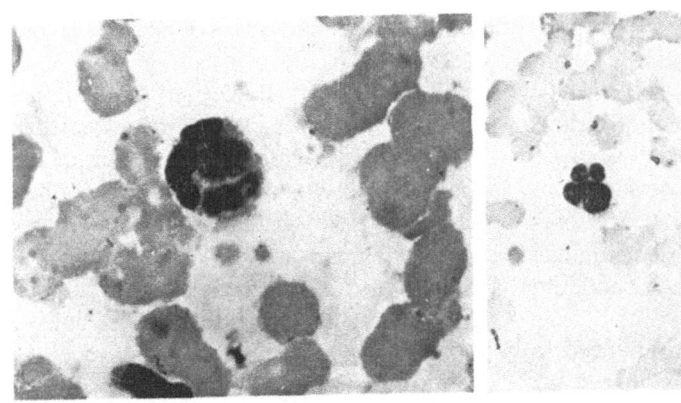

Fig. 13.11. Blood smear of patient with SLE showing LE cells

and insoluble (iNP) nucleoproteins, saline-extractable nuclear antigens, and RNA (all being anti-nuclear antibodies, ANA). Anti-iNP (also called LE factor) causes the LE phenomenon, in which phagocytic cells ingest nuclear material to which anti-iNP is bound (Fig. 13.11).

ANA and DNA-antigens are found by immunofluorescence technique as immune complexes (without or with fixed complement) deposited in the dermis, serosa, walls of blood vessels, glomeruli, synovia, lung, and heart; in addition, immune complexes formed by tissue-antigen specific antibodies are found in the respective tissue, and usually the kidney. Cell-specific antibodies lyse their target cells in a complement dependent fashion. The immunopathology develops according to type II and III hypersensitivity reactions as described in Chap. 9 (see pp. 278–284).

Experimental systemic lupus erythematosus in New Zealand Black (NZB) mice has been extensively analyzed, and has provided a clear picture of the genesis of the disease.

In NZB mice the disease occurs spontaneously and has a very fixed course: The mice are born with an immune system as mature as that of adults; they produce adult-like levels of antibodies to sheep red blood cells, and they have a very active cellular immunity. By the age of 2 months, they are highly resistant to tolerance induction, and rapidly lose tolerance induced at 3 weeks of age. Suppressor T-cell activity declines simultaneously with a decrease of thymic factors at the age of about 6–8 weeks. Auto-antibodies start to occur concurrently and rise progressively; at the age of 5 months, immune-complex nephritis, Coombs'-positive hemolytic anemia, and lymphocytic tissue infiltrations have developed. Mice which survive these disorders are susceptible to the development of malignant lymphomas, and are profoundly deficient in cell-mediated immune functions, but also in humoral immunity (exhaustion?).

This course of events is less pronounced in males, which do not show an immune-complex glomerulonephritis as severely and early as do females. Thymectomy significantly prolongs survival of females, but increases mortality of males as does neonatal splenectomy, which has no effect on female survival. In both instances, the males show the female-type course of the disease. Castration of males gives the same result, whereas females castrated and subsequently treated with androgens produce the male-type of disease.

These findings indicate that sex hormones have a profound influence on the thymus and T-cell maturation, and that T cells are important for the containment of the disease.

NZB mice carry and produce a xenotropic C-type virus in all of their cells, and the destruction (directly or indirectly due to stimulation of cytotoxic T cells specific for virus antigen on T cells) of thymus and T cells concomitant with immune stimulation by viral antigens might be the cause of the disease.

Rheumatoid arthritis is a systemic, chronic inflammatory disease, which manifests itself more dominantly in the joints as synovitis, causing progressive destruction and deformation. Extra articular features are rheumatoid nodules, arteritis, sclerosis, neuropathy, pericarditis, lymphadenopathy, and splenomegaly, which occur rather frequently. The disease occurs more frequently in women than in men; although there is an increasing incidence between 30 and 50 years of age, it also can affect children, usually older than 4 years of age (Still's disease).

Clinically, it is characterized by painful, symmetric, progressive polyarthritis that first affects the smaller, more peripheral joints (hands, wrists, knees, and feet), but later spreads to the larger joints (elbow, shoulder, hips, ankles, cervical articulations). Morning stiffness is highly characteristic of rheumatoid arthritis. The course of the disease is variable with alternating periods of activity and remission.

The pathology is characterized by synovitis, vasculitis, and granuloma formation, densely infiltrated by lymphocytes, plasmacells, mono- and polymorphonuclear cells. The thin synovial membrane thickens and develops to a chronic granulation tissue, pannus. This rheumatoid pannus inflicts severe tissue damage with erosions of the cartilage. The cartilage atrophies and the neighboring bone tissue suffers osteoporosis and erosions, which yield characteristic radiologic images.

Vasculitis involves arteries as well as veins, and is characterized by histiocytic infiltrations that can, at times, assume the appearance of giant cells.

The subcutaneous nodules found in the areas exposed to pressure (elbow, wrists, a. o.) exhibit a central zone of fibrinoid necrosis, surrounded by epithelioid and lymphoid cells.

In 1940, Waaler demonstrated that the sera of patients with rheumatoid arthritis agglutinated sheep erythrocytes coated with rabbit anti-sheep immunoglobulins (Rose-Waaler hemagglutination test). The factor(s) responsible for this agglutination is known as the "rheumatoid factor" (RF). Today, instead of erythrocytes, latex particles coated with human gamma globulin are employed for the agglutination test. The RF has been identified as IgM and/or IgG immunoglobulins reacting with IgG and thus forming IgM/IgG-IgG complexes. Exhaustive studies by many groups have shown that IgG and IgM anti-gammaglobulins with reactivity for IgA, IgE, L-chains, certain genetically determined sites on H-chains of IgG, are produced in rheumatoid arthritis. These anti-Ig antibodies are not only found in sera and synovial fluid of RA patients, but are the predominant or even only kind of immunoglobulins produced by the plasma cells within the inflammatory site (synovia). These findings suggest an intimate association of the production of rheumatoid factor with the pathogenesis of the disease. And indeed there exists a definite correlation between presence and titer of rheumatoid factor and severity of disease. How RF participates in the tissue lesions is not clear. However, RF are capable of complement activation, and thus do enhance inflammatory processes; in addition, immunoglobulin complexes and immunoglobulin-complement complexes (Ig-Ig and Ig-Ig-C) have been demonstrated in vessel walls, synovial fluid and synovia; moreover, it has been shown that immunoglobulin complexes are ingested by phagocytic synovial cells, which then release their lysosomal set of inflammatory digestive substances, including tissue cathepsin, proteases, and collagenase, the latter being able to destroy the skeleton of cartilage.

Most of the lymphocytes detected in synovial tissue inflammatory sites are Tμ cells (T helper cells); this, and the detection of lymphokines in synovial fluid may imply a role for cell-mediated immunity, but might be also a mere reflection of the activity of helper T cells.

The etiology of the disease is unknown as is the cause of the production of the anti-gamma antibodies. It is conceivable that the whole process starts with an infection, and that the initial antigens elicit the formation of antibodies which happen to cross-react with immunoglobulins. It has indeed been shown that rabbits hyperimmunized with streptococcal peptidoglycan antigens occasionally produce monoclonal IgG rheumatoid factor which shows specificity to the immunizing antigen as well. One frequently observed characteristic of cross-reactive antibodies is that they have a low association constant for the cross-reacting antigen; most rheumatoid factor antibodies have, indeed, a low affinity to Ig compared to anti-Ig antibodies produced against Ig. One may even conceive the increased formation of allotype (and idiotype?) specific antibodies to be a sign of decontrolled immune response or "frustrated allotype suppression."

In support of an infectious cause as etiology of the disease is the fact that rheumatoid factors are found in other chronic infections (see Table 13.4).

Progressive systemic sclerosis (PSS, scleroderma) is a generalized disorder of connective tissue of vessels with fibrosis and degenerative changes in the skin, synovia, digital arteries, and the parenchyma and small arteries of internal organs.

The etiology is unknown; familial association is evident, and a prevalence of the HLA-B 8 type exists. Women are more often affected than men.

The most striking feature of PSS is the widespread overgrowth of collagenous connective tissue, and often consider able inflammatory and vascular changes with lymphocyte and plasma cell infiltrates.

Most patients show hypergammaglobulinemia, predominantly IgG, small amounts of immune complexes, and about one-third have rheumatoid factors in their serum; anti-nuclear antibodies (and LE cell phenomenon), but no antibodies against native DNA are observed.

The number of T cells is reduced in the peripheral blood; however, the lymphocytes in tissue infiltrates are predominantly T cells. Patients' lymphocytes are sensitized against skin antigens, particularly human collagen type I, as measured in the migration inhibition assay. There is an increased production of lymphokines in tissue lesions, which may account for the observed significantly increased activity of fibroblasts, with an accumulation of collagen. The stimulating antigen is, however, not known.

References

Cohen S, Ward PA, McCluskey RT (1979) Mechanisms of immunopathology. John Wiley and Sons, New York

Cunningham AJ (1976) Self-tolerance maintained by active suppressor mechanisms. Transplant Rev 31:23

Gell PGH, Coombs RRA, Lachman PJ (eds) (1975) Clinical aspects of immunology. Blackwell, Oxford, England

Gershon RK, Kondo K (1971) Immunology 21:903

Grabar P (1975) Hypothesis: Auto-antibodies and immunological theories: an analytical review. Clin Immunol Immunopathol 4:453

Hughes GRU (1976) Connective Tissue diseases. Blackwell, Oxford, England

Miescher PA, Müller-Eberhard H (eds) (1976) Textbook of immunopathology. Grune and Stratton, New York

Möller G (1978) Role of macrophages in the immune response. Immunol Rev 40:3. Munksgaard, Copenhagen

Nossal GJV, Pike BL, Teale JM, Layton JE, Kay TW, Battey FL (1979) Immunol Rev 43:18

Parker CW (ed) (1980) Clinical immunology. WB Saunders, Philadelphia

Rose NR, Witebsky E (1956) Studies on organ specificity. V. Changes in the thyroid glands of rabbits following active immunization with rabbit thyroid extracts. J Immunol 76:417

Rosen NR, Bigazzi PE, Warner NL (eds) (1978) Genetic control of autoimmune diseases. Elsevier-North-Holland, New York

Stuart FP, Fitch FW (eds) (1979) Immunologic tolerance and enhancement. MTP Press, Falcon House, Lancaster, England

Talal N (ed) (1977) Autoimmunity: Genetic, immunologic, virologic, and clinical aspects. Academic, New York

Tiwari Jl, Terasaki PI (1985) HLA and disease associations. Springer, New York

Williams jr RC (1980) Immune complexes in clinical and experimental medicine. Harvard University Press, Cambridge, Mass.

Chapter 14 Immunomodulation

Wilmar Dias da Silva

Contents

Abbreviations 415
Introduction 416
Immunostimulation 416
  Adjuvants 417
  Thymic Hormones and Related
    Synthetic Analogs 420
  Lymphokines and Monokines 421
  Tuftsin 421
  Levamisole 421
  Isoprinosine 421
  Bestatin 421
  Cimetidine 421
  Cyclosporin A 421
  Adriamycin 422
  Cyclophosphamide 422
  Interferons 423
Immunosuppressors 424
  General Operative Mechanisms 424
  Thymectomy, Bursectomy, and Injection of
    Monoclonal Anti-μ Antibodies 425
  Ionizing Radiation 426
  Antilymphocytic Sera 427
  Corticosteroids 428
  Mechanisms of Actions 429
  Inhibition of Biosynthesis of Nucleic Acids
    and Proteins 431
  Specific Suppression 436
  Rules for Immunosuppression 436
References 437

Abbreviations

ALG, antilymphocytic immunoglobulins
ALS, antilymphocytic serum
AMP, adenosine monophosphate
BAF, B cell activating factor
BCG, Bacillus Calmette-Guerin
BLGF, B lymphocyte growth factor
cFA, complete Freund's adjuvant
ConA, concanavalin A
CSF, colony-stimulating factor
CY, cyclophosphamide
Cy-A, cyclosporin A
$DNBSO_3$, dinitrobenzoarsonate
DNCB, dinitrochlorbenzene
DNP, dinitrophenyl
DTH, delayed-type hypersensitivity
E, sheep erythrocytes
FCS, fetal calf serum
GRF, growth reticular cell factor
GVH, graft-versus-host reactions
iFA, incomplete Freund's adjuvant
Il-1, interleukin 1
Il-2, interleukin 2
K, killer cells
LAF, lymphocyte-activating factor
LPS, lipopolysaccharides
MAF, macrophage-activating factor
MDP, muramyl dipeptide
MHC, major histocompatibility complex
MIF, macrophage inhibitor factor
MLC, mixed leukocyte culture
MLR, mixed leukocyte reaction
NAD, niconamide adenine dinuclease
NHS, normal human serum
NK, natural killer cells
OVA, ovalbumin
PCA, passive cutaneous anaphylaxis
PFC, plaque-forming cells
PHA, passive hemagglutination
PHA, phytohemagglutinin
PPD, purified protein derivative
SDS-PAGE, sodium dodecyl sulphate–
polyacrylamide gel electrophoresis
SRBC, sheep red blood cells
TCGF, T cell growth factor
TDF, T cell depressor factor
Th, helper T cells
THAF, T helper auxiliary factor
TKCGF, T killer cell growth factor
Ts, suppressor T cells
WSA, water-soluble adjuvant

Introduction

A great deal has been learned in recent years about the mechanisms underlying the immune response. Identification of subsets of cells involved following the contact with the antigen, the cell surface components governing the interaction of these cells, and the induction and secretion of soluble factors driving the immunocompetent cells to multiply and to differentiate to secretor or effector cells are the most important achivements. Briefly, T lymphocyte activation, by soluble antigens, particulate alloantigens, or mitogens, can be summarized as follows: The sequence of events culminating in T cell proliferation starts with antigen binding to accessory cells and the subsequent presentation of foreign antigen in association with MHC products to T lymphocytes. Alternatively, T cell mitogens such as ConA and PHA can interact directly with T cells.

The details of these events have been described in other chapters of this book (Chaps. 2 and 6). This chapter reviews and integrates the accumulated information concerning the agents potentially able to be used in the treatment of a broad spectrum of disorders, including immunodeficiency, chronic infection, and autoimmunity. Particular attention is paid to the cellular targets of immunotherapy and to some intracellular mechanisms involved in the actions of the various therapeutic agents. The chapter begins with an outline of the most common adjuvants used in basic immunology, including the crude bacterial preparations such as BCG and *C. parvum,* some of their chemically defined products – LPS, MDP, etc. – and other bacterial synthetic constituents. Next comes a discussion on immunostimulators produced by the immune system, such as lymphokines, monokines, interferons, and the thymic factors (thymosine, thymopoietin, serum thymic factor, etc.); the tripeptide tuftsin; and the chemicals levamisole, isoprinosine, tilerone, SM 1213, BM 12531, and lynestrenol, bestatin, cimetidine, and phorbol. Finally, there is a survey of immunosuppressiv agents used and measures taken to suppress the immune response.

Immunostimulation

In normal individuals the immune system is in an actively proliferating state. In order to provide adequate amounts of lymphoid cells to ensure such high rates of turnover, the bone marrow and the thymus contain a large number of precursor cells. Generation of diversity and selection of repertoires are certainly facilitated by this process (see Chaps. 1, 2, 4, and 6). In the thymus – the central T cell compartment – the precursor cells are actively selected and induced to proliferation and maturation. During this process most of the selected cells (95%) die in the organ, while the peripheral turnover of mature cells is very limited. In the bone marrow – probably the most important central compartment of B cells in mammals – up to 20%–25% of all nucleated cells provide a daily output of differentiated, competent cells that accounts for 5%–10% of the whole B cells.

These cells, however, die very rapidly in the periphery, with a decay rate of 50% a day. These considerations lead to the suggestion that T cell selection operates at a stage of immunoincompetence, while the selection of B cells operates when these cells have acquired their full competence.

The activation of lymphocytes is initiated by epitope recognition clonally distributed receptors on their surface and further sustained and directed by growth factors produced by other cells. Although the receptors for the specific signal are expressed during the selection of the diversity, the receptors for the growth factors *are only functionally expressed* by cycling lymphocytes. Apparently each lymphocyte type, namely cytotoxic T cells, B lymphocytes, and Th cells, responds to distinct growth factors. These growth factors, *TCGF* or Il-1 and Il-2 for cytotoxic T cells, *BLGF* Il-2 for B lymphocytes, and *THAF* Il-3 for their helper T cells, although specific for the cell type, are devoid of immunological specificity.

In the mature immunocompetent animal the T cell sets comprise: (a) the regulatory cells characterized by the cell surface marker Lyt-1$^+$, 2$^+$, 3$^+$, corresponding to 50% of the T lymphocytes and probably representing a store of antigen-receptor positive intermediary cells that regulate the supply and function of more mature Lyt-1$^+$ and Lyt-2$^+$, 3$^+$, cells; (b) the inducer cells characterized by the cell surface marker Lyt-1$^+$, corresponding to 30% of the T lymphocytes and genetically programmed to amplify the activity of other cells after stimulation by the antigen; and (c) the mature cytotoxic and suppressor cells characterized by the phenotype Lyt-2$^+$, 3$^+$, corresponding to 5%–10% of the T cells and equipped both to develop *alloreactive* cytotoxic activity and to suppress the humoral and cell-mediated immune response. With respect to the last subset of T cells, it is still unknown whether cytotoxic and antigen-induced suppression are two manifestations of one genetic program or whether they represent the phenotype of two separate genetic programs.

The regulation of the immune response is highly complex, involving interaction of different lymphocyte populations and their subsets and collaboration of lymphocytes and macrophages, either through direct cell-to-cell contact or through the release of soluble mediators such as lymphokines and monokines.

Recent progress in the understanding of the intractions between idiotypes and anti-idiotypes, as proposed by N. K. Jerne in 1974 in his network theory, indicates that the immune system is in a dynamic steady state resulting from paratope-idiotype interaction within the system (see Chap. 4).

Adjuvants

According to Waksman (1980) the use of tapioca to form a particulate antigen depot, aiming to produce a persistent and slow-releasing pool of the antigen and to increase the immune response to it. A long and still increasing list of "adjuvants" has been introduced in basic and practical immunology. These range from simple chemicals such as Al(OH)$_3$ and AlPO$_4$ through complex bacterial and parasite products to the still more complex mixtures as the iFA and cFA adjuvants. The adjuvant activity can be ascribed to a group of events occurring both at cellular and molecular levels of the immune response. Table 14.1 lists probable mechanisms of action for the most common adjuvants (see also pp. 70–72).

Effects on the Deposition and Dissemination of Antigen. The first effect of adjuvants is to form a depot and cause a slow dissemination of the antigen in adequate conditions to be processed and recognized by the cells attracted to the site of injection or localized in the appropriate site of the immune system.

Mineral oils remain at the injection site for months and oil droplets are widely disseminated to metastatic sites in lungs, liver and LN. The transport of the antigen on the oil droplets probably accounts for the finding that the inoculation site can be removed within a half hour without reducing the later immune response to the injected material. Oil alone, as in iFA, although inducing a rapid uptake of the antigen attached to droplets, preferentially promotes antibody formation.

Antigen adsorbed on solid particles such as bentonite or latex particles is taken up much more efficiently than soluble antigens, and its immunogenicity is correspondingly enhanced. Adsorption of nonimmunogenic substances (i.e., small peptides or poor immunogenic proteins (i.e., thyreoglobulin) on acrylic particles markedly enhances the production of specific antibodies. Al(OH)$_3$ adsorbed with small amounts of antigen induces high titers of IgE in mice.

Some cationic surface active substances, chemically characterized by the presence of long alkyl side chains, are extremely potent adjuvants. Included in this group are octadecylamine and dioctadecyl-dimethyl-

Table 14.1. Targets of adjuvant action[a]

Function of adjuvant	Examples
Depot, dissemination of antigen	Mineral oil
Selective antigen localization in TDA	Alkylamines, nonpolar cationic detergents
Particles bearing antigen	$AL(OH)_3$, $AlPO_4$, immune complexes, latex,
Depot function	bentonite, polymethyl methacrylate
Enhanced macrophage uptake	
Direct B-cell triggering	
Stimulation of accessory cells	Triolein, zymosan, carbonyl iron, BCG, CP, LPS,
Increased antigen uptake	retinol, polyanions, polyelectrolytes, mineral oil
Production of helper factors	
Production of factors affecting lymphocyte	
recirculation	
Production of colony-stimulating activity	
Production of complement components	
Enhanced lymphocyte flux into TDA	Pertussis, cFA, iFA, CP, retinol
Nonspecific stimulation of T-lymphocytes	pA:U, MDP
Carrier-specific stimulation of T-lymphocytes	CFA, allogenic effects, some viruses
Nonspecific stimulation of B-lymphocytes	LPS, NWSM
IgE switch of B-cells	Nippostrongylus, other helminths
Enhanced maturation of T and B precursors	LPS, pA:U
Direct stimulation of NK-cells	Arenaviruses, interferon, tilorone, statolon, lentinan?
Direct stimulation of K-cells	cFA
Cell damage and release of nucleotides	PHA, Con A, repeated 6MP, colchine, silica
Elimination of suppressor cells	X-ray, cyclophosphamide, some viruses?

[a] From Waksman BH (1979) Adjuvants and immune regulation by lymphoid cells. Springer Ser Immunop thol 2:5–33. Immunostimulation I

ammonium chloride or octadecyl-tri-methyl-ammonium bromide. It is probable that these substances enhance the uptake of the immunogens by the lymph node sinus macrophages directing them to the thymus-dependent-areas and preferentially inducing cell-mediated immunity. cFA (mannide monooleate, paraffin oil, and killed *Mycobacterium butyricum*) and iFA (mannide monooleate and paraffin oil) are the traditional experimental adjuvants. Antigen in aqueous solution mixed with one of Freund's adjuvants and dispersed as a stable emulsion has its immunogenicity considerably increased.

Both cFA and iFA produce local and disseminated granulomas, and both, being lipophilic, penetrate the thymus-dependent-areas. iFA stimulates macrophages and promotes uptake of the antigen with a marked enhancement of antibody formation. cFA, due to the presence of mycobac-teria stimulates blast transformation of T cells, macrophage transformation into epithelioid cells, and subsequent formation of granuloma. As a result, cFA stimulates both antibody formation and cell-mediated immune response.

The mycobacteria and corynebacteria constituents with immunologic adjuvant activity include: the cell wall skeleton (insoluble peptidoglycolipid), MER (methanol extraction residue), cord factor (trehalose-6,6'-dimycolate), Wax D, WSA (water soluble adjuvant, a muramic acid glycopeptide linked to arabinogalactan), and MDP (muramyl dipeptide, i.e., *N*-acetylmuramyl-L-alanyl-D-isoglutamine). Wax D, WSA, and MDP induce the T cell blast response and granuloma formation seen with cFA. The term "cord factor" designates glycolipids produced by *Mycobacteria, Nocardiae, Corynebacteriae,* and strains of *Arthrobacter* and *Brevibacterium.* Chemically they are 6,6 diesters of α,α-D-trehalose and they can be synthesized by various methods. Despite its toxicity, partly due to a stimulation of the activity of NAD, leading to a depression of NAD, cord factor increases the antibody response. Cord factor also exerts a nonspecific protective effect on *S. typhi, K. pneumoniae, L. monocytogenes,* and *S. mansoni* infection. An antitumor action of cord factor has been also documented in induced tumors in mice and in rats.

Effects on Auxiliary Cells: Macrophages, Langerhans, Cells and Dendritic Cells. Stimulation of macrophages is accepted as the most important activity of the adjuvants. Several agents which increase either the number of macrophages or their level of activity also enhance the immune response (see Table 14.1). Some of these agents may act directly, for instance LPS or phagocytozable particles (carbonyl iron, zymosan and other glucans, polyanions, and polyacrylic acids), others indirectly through the release of T cell factors (BCG or cFA, CP, Be, LPS, pertussis, or retimol). In the later case no adjuvant effect is observed in the absence of T cells.

The activated macrophages may exert their adjuvanticity simply by virtue of having an increased surface area, an increase or redistribution of their set of Ia or other surface receptors, or a more elaborate mechanism involving the release of "helper" factors such as GRF, LAF, TAF, BAF, TDF, and CSF. An increased production of complement components, plasminogen activator factor, or other inflammatory mediator factors should be also considered. It has been shown, for instance, that complement potentiates localization of antigen-antibody aggregates in germinal centers invivo and enhances the T cell–B cell cooperation with macrophages in vitro.

There are, however, two distinct modes of action of the adjuvants on macrophages: one involves phagocytosis and induces an increase in the antigen presentation capacity and an enhanced release of LAF, whereas in the other, agents acting on the macrophage surface stimulates T cells. The circuit may be turned on by cell-soluble factors through an adjuvant agent, for instance NDP, as follows: MDP stimulates T cells to produce MAF(s), which leads to enhanced production of LAF, TAF, BAF, etc., which in turn recruit additional T cells to the local site and stimulate these to further production of T cell factors.

Effects on Lymphocytes. As a rule, the adjuvants induce a marked increase in the number of lymphocytes into the lymph nodes draining an inoculation site. This accumulation of cells is probably due to the combined increased flux of lymphocytes and to a local blast transformation of these cells. *B. pertussis* is an adjuvant affecting the lymphocyte capacity to recirculate and to respond to the antigen. The organisms contain a "lymphocytosis promoting factor" responsible for a shift of the total lymphocyte pool from the lymph nodes and spleen to the peripheral blood. This effect is due to an inhibition of the lymphocyte recirculation from the blood to these organs. In addition, the organisms contain component(s) capable to enhance the Ige antibody response markedly.

Synthetic polynucleotides, as compounds with defined structures, represent an important tool in establishing the structure-function relationship. Their adjuvant properties have been defined during the past decade following the observation that nucleic-acid-rich tissue had a restorative effect in animals rendered deficient in antibody-forming capacity.

Double-helix polyadenylic:polyuridylic acid (pA:U) and polyinosinic:polycytidylic acid (pI:C) are prepared by mixing polymerized single strands from opposite base pairs. Double-helix form and high molecular weight are two important characteristics for the polynucleotides to exert their adjuvant actions. Their potentiation of antibody synthesis is effective in very low doses and they need not be given together with the antigen. In addition to the adjuvant activity of pA:U or pI:C on macrophages, the effect of pA:U on the T cell compartment are unequivocal: Generation of Th, Ts, and both nonspecific and specific precursor cells is induced with this adjuvant. Its effect at the level of T cell precursors appears to be mediated by the cyclic AMP-GMP system, adenyl cyclase probably being the membrane target activated after union of pA:U with its receptor. This contention is supported by the observation that theophylline, an inhibitor of the enzyme phosphodiesterase, produces both elevation of cellular cyclic AMP and potentiation of the pA:U effect on the T cells.

The components Wax D and MDP of mycobacteria probably also stimulate T cells, although there is a suggestion that MDP may stimulate macrophages and B cells directly. Activation of helper T cells following the so-called allogeneic effect greatly increases antibody formation to unrelated antigens. This is particularly important since such "polyclonal activation" results from recognition of Ia allogeneic cell surface antigens by a T cell population. Certain viruses, i.e., influenza, certain arboviruses, lactic dehydrogenase virus, and Venezuelan equine encephalomyelitis virus, also exert powerful adjuvant action on Th cells as measured by the increase in antibody formation. The Th cell effect appears to be mediated through the release of soluble substances which act on B cells, stimulating them to proliferate and differentiate.

Effects on B Cells. Lipopolysaccharide (LPS) endotoxins from gram-negative bacteria have been identified as powerful adjuvants in the immune response, although under certain circumstances they can suppress such responses. These molecules are constituted by three regions: (1) The O-polysaccharide moiety specific for the immune specificity, (2) the core polysaccharide region which is common to a number of bacteria which in turn is bound to (3) lipid A responsible for the majority of their biological effects, including toxicity, pyrogenicity, leukopenia, induction of the Schwartzman phenomenon, a necrotizing

action on tumors, polyclonal activation of B cells, and an adjuvant effect.

LPS activate B cells, but not T cells, as measured by an increased DNA synthesis and increased secretion of immunoglobulins. Although IgM is the predominant immunoglobulin secreted, secretion of IgG and IgD is also stimulated. Since the stimulated B cells also secrete antibodies specific for antigens unrelated to LPS, both stimulation and differentiation are triggered. This polyclonal activation of B cells occurs directly, the signal being delivered following the interaction between the lipid of LPS and the "mitogen receptors" on the B cell membrane. These receptors can be blocked with antibodies raised in rabbits immunized with C3H/Ti (LPS high-responder) B cells and rendered specific for the receptors by prior adsorption with C3H/HeJ (non-responder) cells.

LPS exerts a specific enhancement in the production of antibody, upon simultaneous administration of the antigen. When, however, LPS is administered a few days prior to the injection of an antigen, an opposite effect is observed, i.e., suppression of the antibody response.

The cellular mode of action by which LPS stimulate the antibody production is controversial. According to some data, such effects do not require the activation of helper T cells. Other data have, however, clearly implicated these cells in the mechanisms of the LPS adjuvanticity.

Thymic Hormones and Related Synthetic Analogs

Several peptides capable of correcting some of the immunologic deficiencies resulting from the lack of thymic function in animal models, as well as in humans with immunodeficiency diseases, have been isolated from the thymus. Among these are thymosine α_1 (3,108 M.W.) and its synthetic analog; thymic humoral factor (3,000 M.W.); and serum thymic factor (857 M.W.).

Thymosine has been obtained in purified form and its sequence determined. It improves the immunologic functions in thymus-deficient animals, i.e., the capacity of athymic (nu/nu) mice and adult thymectomized irradiated bone-marrow-restored mice to reconstitute a normal IgM and IgG response to DNP haptenized antigen. It is also effective, in in vitro assays, in modulating the production of MIF, differentiating Lyt-1^+, 2^+ cells to form E rosette, and responding mixed lymphocyte culture. Thymopoietin is a peptide that induces impairment of neuromuscular transmission in vivo and promotes the appearance of T cell markers in their cell precursors.

The serum thymic factor has also been purified and its amino acid sequence determined. It enhances mitogen response in cells of nude mice in vitro, induces Ts cells in NZM mice, and corrects the abnormally high level of autologous erythrocyte-binding cells in adult thymectomized mice.

Lymphokines and Monokines

See Chaps. 2, 11, and 12

Tuftsin

Tuftsin is a basic tetrapeptide (L-threonyl-L-lysyl-L-prolyl-L-arginine) derived from the CH2 domain of the immunoglobulin molecules which, when introduced simultaneously with the antigen to macrophages, increases the response against thymus-dependent antigens (see Chap. 12, p. 378).

It is believed that the immunostimulating effect of tuftsin is based on a magnification of a normal in vivo regulatory process exerted on macrophages by immunoglobulin via the cell surface Fc receptors. The generation of tuftsin is described on p. 323 and 378. There are indications that tuftsin activates the immune response not by stimulating phagocytosis, but rather by increasing the capacity of macrophages pulsed simultaneously with antigen and tuftsin to recruit effector T lymphocytes.

Levamisole

Levamisole is a simple synthetic chemical, introduced into therapeutics because of its antihelminthic activity; it appears also to restore the effector functions of both peripheral T lymphocytes and phagocytes. Evidence has accumulated during the past few years that levamisole has cholinergic properties, i.e., increases the cell levels of cyclic GMP and/or reduces cyclic AMP in mouse T lymphocytes and macrophages.

Isoprinosine

This substance stimulates various metabolic parameters of peritoneal macrophages of the rat: level of lysosomal acidhydrolases, secretion of neutral proteases, and generation of superoxide anions. The macrophages become cytostatic for the DHD/K_{12} intestinal cell line in vitro and improve the acquired immunity to schistosome parasites in vivo. On the other hand, this compound reduces the in vitro synthesis of IgE by lymphocytes from patients with allergic bronchopulmonary aspergillosis. It also increases the response in MLC.

Bestatin

Bestatin is an immunomodulating dipeptide of actinomycete origin therapeutically effective in various experimental tumor systems, including the metastasing *Esb* lymphoma system. Peritoneal macrophages obtained from mice treated i.p. with bestatin (50–200 µg/mouse) became cytotoxic for various tumor cells used in vitro. As macrophages from athymic nude mice were also stimulated by bestatin, the dipeptide activates macrophages through a T cell independent process. It has also been demonstrated that bestatin produces an enhancement of the macrophage respiratory burst.

Cimetidine

At the dose level of 100 mg/kg/12 h s.c. for 3 days cimetidine blocks the development of suppressor nonadherent spleen cells.

Cyclosporin A

Cy-A is an eleven-amino acid cyclic peptide with seven of the amino acids methylated, making the molecule extremely hydrophobic. Studies performed in experimental models with Cy-A administered in a dose of 25 µg/kg yielded the following information regarding the immune response: (a) IgM antibody response is not influenzed by Cy-A; (b) both the stimulated and unstimulated precursors of Th cells are sensitive to the drug; (c) cells involved in GVH reactivity are, in contrast to their precursors, affected by this agent; and (d) skin allograft survival time is markedly abolished when Cy-A is given after grafting. In clinical trials the drug has been used with considerable success, largely with renal allografts, but also with a few pancreas and liver grafts. Its lack of myelotoxicity and the reduction it effects in need for steroid therapy render Cy-A a promising immunosuppressant for clinical use.

Although the intimal mechanisms underlying the Cy-A effect are unknown, the following observations have been described: T cells treated with Cy-A do not express receptors for Il-2 under the stimulus of either antigens or mitogens. In addition, Cy-A causes the Il-2 producer T cells to become unresponsive to Il-1 and unable to produce Il-2. Cy-A suppresses the synthesis of Il-1 by acting on Th cells and not on macrophages. In summary, Cy-A abrogates proliferation of T lymphocytes induced by either antigens or mitogens acting at three distinct but related stages in the process of activation of T cells: (a) by inhibiting the action of Th cells on accessory cells for the synthesis of Il-1; (b) by preventing the Il-2 producer T cell from expressing receptors for Il-1 and suppressing the synthesis of Il-2; and (c) by rendering T cells unresponsive to Il-2.

Adriamycin

Adriamycin, an antitumor drug, exerts its effects by modulating the host defense mechanisms. This statement derives from a number of experiments showing that adriamycin treatment results in significantly elevated cell-mediated cytotoxicity. The cells which appear to be stimulated by adriamycin treatment are immature macrophages and "sticky" T cells. Humoral respnoses and NK activity are, in general, inhibited by adriamycin.

Cyclophosphamide

Cyclophosphamide (CY; 200–300 mg/kg) enhances DTH to a number of antigens, the maximum potentiation being achieved when the drug is given between the 3rd day before immunization and the 1st day after. If the drug is given between the 3rd and 5th days after immunization, the response is depressed. T cell proliferation is maximally depressed on days 4 and 5 after sensitization by CY given on days 2 and 3 respectively. The effector T cells are therefore maximally sensitive to CY during their proliferating phase.

In contrast, treatment with CY causes a pronounced depression of the antibody production to a number of antigens. Thus, in guinea pigs pretreated with CY (250 mg/kg) and immunized with OVA in iFA, the production of both IgG_1 (measured by PCA reaction) and IgG_2 (measured by PH) was strongly depressed. Coinciding with these findings, a depletion of B lymphocytes was observed in draining lymph nodes.

The above effects of CY on the immuno-regulatory mechanisms were detected by identifying the population(s) of cells that can be transferred from normally sensitized animals and which are able to reconstitute the normal immune response in CY-treated animals. The cells capable of doing so have been identified as the precursors of Ts cells.

The capacity of CY to eliminate Ts cells has been used to reverse the immunological tolerance induced by the intravenous injection or feeding administration of some synthetic haptens, e.g., DNCB and $DNBSO_3$, or induced by antigenic competition. Partial or complete restoration has been achieved by administration of CY at the dose of 250–300 mg/kg.

Animals injected with an antigen in Freund's adjuvant and later reinjected with large amounts of the antigen alone become temporarily anergic. These animals fail to respond to an intradermal challenge with either the antigen used for the desensitization (specific) or another antigen (nonspecific). This state of desensitization can be prevented if CY is given 1 day after immunization with the specific antigen or either 3 days before or 1 day after immunization with the nonspecific antigen. In summary, CY is the most effective of the "immunosuppressive" agents capable of "potentiating" the immune response.

Interferons

At least two types of interferons are presently known: Type I or standard interferons have been discovered by Isaacs and Lindemann in chick chorioallantoic membranes exposed to heat-inactivated influenza virus. They are produced by both nonlymphoid and lymphoid cells in response to viruses, polynucleotides, and endotoxin. Type II or immune interferons were first described by Wheelock, and are lymphokines produced either by nonimmune lymphoid cells in response to PHA or by immunized lymphocytes after contact with specific antigens such as PPD, diphtheria, or pertussis toxoid. In contrast to the Type I interferons, Type II interferons are destroyed by treatment for 24 h at pH 2.0. At cells of the organism are probably capable of producing Type I interferons upon stimulation by diffrent species of viruses. In humans, lymphocyte-made interferons consist of sevral molecular species, called leukocyte (le-type) interferons, antigenically distinct from nonleukocyte interferons or so-called fibroblast (F-type) interferons. Le-type interferons are sensitive to 2-mercaptoethanol and their activity is distributed in analysis by SDS-PAGE into 21,000 (20%) and 15,000 (80%) M.W. In contrast, F-type interferon, which is antigenically distinct from the Le-type, reveals on SDS-PAGE analysis a single molecular species with M.W. of 20,000 (see also p. 336). In the mouse, two species of Type I interferons have been also identified by the same method, one with a molecular weight of 35,000–38,000 and the other with a molecular weight of 22,000. By N-terminal amino acid analysis the latter showed some homology with human Le-type 22,000 M.W. Type I interferons modulate both in vivo and in vitro the IgM response to SRBC. When administered prior to the antigen, mouse interferon preparations consisting of a mixture of 35,000 and 22,000 M.W. forms exert a pronounced suppressive effect, but when administered after the antigen, they produce an opposite effect. This type of interferons has been also implicated as stimulator of lymphocytotoxicity against allogeneic tumor cells and as activator of resident macrophages. Also, at the dose of 2×10^4 units per mouse the interferons produce a marked increase of NK cell activity within 3 h after inoculation.

The NK cell activity remains high for 16 h and returns to normal levels by 24 h. Human interferons of both Le- and F-type also significantly enhance NK cell activity of mononuclear cells obtained from normal donors. They appear to act not by enhancing the activity of "mature" NK cells, but rather by recruitment of "pre-NK" cells. In allograft transplantation, Type I interferons at very low doses may accelerate graft rejection, whereas at higher doses they produce an opposite effect, i.e., prolongation of the skin graft survival. Delayed-type hypersensitivity is also inhibited, in a dose-effect fashion, by administration of interferons. Type II interferons are produced by lymphoid cells either stimulated by mitogens or, specifically, when these cells are obtained from primed animals and brought in contact with the antigen. T cells produce type II interferons in response to ConA and PHA, and B cells produce it in response to pokeweed mitogen. Lymphocytes obtained from individuals previously immunized with PPD, diphtheria, or pertussis toxoid and challenged in vitro with the correspondent antigen release into the supernatants detectable amounts of interferons. In the case of lymphocytes obtained from individuals infected with some viruses, e.g., vaccinia and *Herpesvirus hominis*, the production of interferons depends both on the addition of the antigen and on the presence of macrophages in the lymphocyte cell suspension. The amount of interferon production is a reflection of the immune status of the cell donor, and in the absence of macrophages, only Type I interferons are produced. Mice previously infected with *Mycobacterium tuberculosis* make large amounts of circulating interferons and MIF when challenged with PPD. Protozoa parasites have also been implicated as inducers of interferons in in vivo experiments. Thus, mice infected with *T. cruzi* produce large amounts of circulating interferons at the

peak of parasitemia when an immune response has already been established.

Recent findings have raised the possibility that Type II interferons play a role in the modulation of the immune response and that they are natural immune regulator substances.

Immunosuppressors

General Operative Mechanisms

The immunosuppressive agents listed in Table 14.2 can act upon the immune response in one of the following ways:

Table 14.2. Classification of the most frequently used immunosuppressive agents

Group	Immunosuppressive agents
Surgery	Neonatal thymectomy
	Hormonal bursectomy
	Neonatal surgical bursectomy
	Ductus thoracicus drainage of lymphocytes
	Diabetes
Irradiation	X-rays
	Gamma rays
Hormone	Adrenocorticotropic hormone
	Corticosteroids (cortisone, hydrocortisone, prednisone, prednisolone, etc.)
Antimetabolites	Purine analogs:
	6-Mercaptopurine
	Azathioprine (Imuran)
	6-Thioguanine
	Pyrimidine analogs:
	5-Fluorouracil
	Folic acid antagonists:
	Aminopterine
	Methotrexate
Plant alkaloids	Vinblastine
	Vincristine
	Colchicine
Antibiotics	Actinomycin D
	Mitomycin C
	Puromycin
	Chloramphenicol
	Azaserine
Amino-acid antagonists	Glutamine
	Diazomycin A
	Asparagine
	L-Asparaginase[a]

[a] Works via the catalytic hydrolysis of L-asparagine, which is split into L-asparaginic acid and ammonia

1. Inhibition of formation of precursor cells.
2. Repression of production of immunocompetent cells: thymectomy and bursectomy, either pre- or neonatal, which may or may not be associated with sublethal irradiation. These immunosuppressive measures block the immune response by impeding the formation of B and T lymphocytes.
3. Destroying or blocking the immunocompetent cells: irradiation with γ- or X-rays, treatment with antilymphocytic serum (ALS) and alkylating agents.
4. Preventing effective contact between the antigenic determinants of the immunogens and the immunocompetent cells: blockage of antigens by passively transferred specific antibodies, repression of recognition of antigens through receptor blockage with anti-idiotypic antibodies.
5. Blocking the phagocytic functions to inhibit the "processing" of antigens: irradiation and corticosteroid hormones.
6. Inhibiting the biosynthesis of nucleic acids (DNA and RNA) and of proteins that respond to stimulation of the immunocompetent cells by the immunogen: antimetabolites, analogs of amino acids; antibiotics, antagonists of folic acid and some plant alkaloids.
7. Blocking the mulitplication and differentiation of cells already stimulated to impede the formation of sensitized lymphocytes (effector cells), plasma cells, and memory cells: irradiation, alkylating agents, and antimetabolites.
8. Specific paralysis. The induction of a specific suppression for the antigenic determinant is an alternative form of the immunocompetent cells.

The activity of immunosuppressive agents is evaluated primarily by assays similar to those employed in experimental chemotherapy. The laboratory animals and the antigens are chosen according to the type of immune response for which the effects of a particular immunosuppressive are to be investigated. For example, if one wishes to study the effect of an agent on the production of reaginic antibodies, the preferred animals are the mouse and the rat; the antigen is injected in small quantities together with an appropriate adjuvant such as $Al(OH)_3$ or $B. pertussis$ suspension. The immune response can be evaluated either by testing for cutaneous anaphylaxis or for the liberation of histamine from tissue in vitro, or by IgE radioimmunoasssay. The rabbit is the animal of choice for analysis of the effects upon the production of precipitating antibodies, and the antigen injected should be in Freund's adjuvant. In contrast, the guinea pig is often used to study effects upon delayed hypersensitivity of the tuberculin type; and allogeneic strains of mice are used when the test system is that of skin-graft rejection. The immunosuppressive agents included in Table 14.2 have been or are being tested in almost all forms of immune response.

Thymectomy, Bursectomy, and Injection of Monoclonal Anti-μ Antibodies

Pre- or neonatal thymectomy produces a clear reduction in the number of circulating lymphocytes, along with a depopulation of the paracortical regions of the lymph nodes and the periarteriolar sheaths of the spleen (thymus-dependent areas). The lymph follicles and the germinal centers (thymus-independent areas) are not affected, their populations of plasma cells remaining intact.

Thymectomy essentially affects specific cellular immunity: depending upon the antigen, it produces only slight alterations in humoral immunity. The extent to which it influences the immune response depends upon the developmental state which the lymphoid system has attained up to birth. In such terms, the less developed the lymphoid system, the more intense are the effects. Mice thymectomized in the first days of life accept skin transplants from donors that differ in strong H-2 antigens. The effects of thymectomy in adult animals are observed only when sufficient time has passed for the disappearance of "long-lived lymphocytes" located in the thymus-dependent areas. Immediate effects are obtained by accompanying thymectomy with total body irradition of the animal. Bursectomy (in birds), unlike thymectomy, does not reduce the circulating lymphocyte population, nor does it modify the thymus-dependent structures. The principal modifications are encountered in the thymus-independent regions of the lymph nodes and spleen, which do not exhibit germinal centers and in which there are practically no plasma cells. The level of circulating immunoglobulins is low, and the animal's capacity to produce antibodies is diminished considerably.

"Hormonal bursectomy," performed by inoculating chicken eggs with 19-nortestosterone, is much more efficient than surgical bursectomy. Thymectomy and bursectomy have been important in experimental immunology for the resolution of problems related to the cytophysiology of immunocompetent cells. However, the use of thymectomy in clinical immunology is limited: it is restricted to situations in which the immune disease is primarily dependent on thymus hyperplasia or in which thymus hpyerplasia leads to secondary clinical events.

Neonatal injection of monoclonal anti-μ antibodies induces a profound inhibition of IgM production as detected by PFC assay.

Ionizing Radiation

Radiation damages hemopoietic and intestinal tissues, leading to leukopenia and increasing permeability of the intestinal mucosa for bacteria of the normal flora. Resistance to infectious diseases is therefore decreased due to impairment of both nonspecific and specific immune defense mechanisms. These alterations include break-up of the blood-tissue barriers, reduction of the number of phagocytes and of their ability to kill ingested organisms, reduction of the serum complement levels, and pronounced disturbance of the immune response. In this case, the effect of radiation is stronger on the antibody response than on cellular immunity, i.e., DTH.

Radiation doses from 200 to 700 rad depress the antibody response when the antigen is injected shortly before or immediately after the irradiation. Recovery of the immune response starts after about a week and may be complete 2 months after radiation exposure. With lower radiation dosage, i.e., 25–100 rad, prolonged production and a transiently higher antibody peak titer may be observed in irradiated as compared to unirradiated animals. This enhancement in the antibody production by the combined action of a low dose of radiation and time of introduction of the antigen amy be explained by a disproportionate repopulation of the depleted lymphoid tissues by rapidly dividing antigen-activated cells, by the adjuvant effect of bacteria or endotoxins entering the bloodstream from the radiation-damaged intestinal mucosa, or by a preferential inactivation of suppressor T cells.

Secondary antibody response is more radioresistant than the primary response, an observation that has been explained in terms of a greater number of potentially responsive immunocompetent cells in primed animals rather than by more radiosensitivity of the nonprimed immunocompetent cells. It has been also demonstrated that the antibody affinity, i.e., the binding energy of the antibody sites for specific antigenic epitopes, is remarkably higher in sublethally irradiated mice (450 rad) primed immediately or 30 days after irradiation than in unirradiated controls.

Irradiation causes profound depression in the production of polymorphs and of the macrophage precursors, but does not affect phagocytosis. Nevertheless, the bactericidal activity of polymorphs is decreased when they are irradiated before phagocytosis. Antigen retention in lymphatic follicles is strongly affected by sublethal X-irradiation due to radiation damage either of the reticular cell expression of Fc receptor or of impairment of opsonin production. Macrophage migration, phagocytosis, and intracellular catabolism of ingested antigen are not appreciably affected by radiation. It is therefore difficult to evaluate the overall influence of radiation on the antibody response through its action on auxiliary cells or antigen-presenting cells. Thus, radiation-induced dysfunction of antibody responses is likely to depend mainly on lymphocyte radiosensitivity.

The lymphocytes are markedly radiosensitive; circulating lymphocytes are reduced to 25% of control upon exposure of the animal to 100 rad. They are damaged even when irradiated at the interphase. B lymphocytes are more radiosensitive than T lymphocytes, 8% of the latter cells being radioresistant to 800 rad.

As already explained in preceding chapters the antibody response of B cells requires the participation of Th cells (Lyt 1^+, 2^-) which are characterized by membrane phenotype, presence of anti-idiotype receptors, MHC restriction, and mode of action.

One Th cell type recognizes carrier epitopes of the antigen molecule in association with MHC determinants on antigen processing and presenting auxiliary cells, and interacts with B cells through an antigen bridge between the carrier and the hapten determinants. The other Th cell type recognizes idiotypic and allotypic determinants present on B cells, is not MHC restricted, and does not require physical linkage of carrier and hapten determinants for effective T cell–B cell cooperation. X-irradiation has selective effects on the Th cell population, leading to inactivation of some but not other subpopulations.

The preferential selection of the Th subpopulation for higher affinity receptor B cells, may also result in selection of B cells responsible for the production of antibodies with average higher affinity, as observed in irradiated primed animals.

Suppressor T cells (Ts), one of the major cellular components of the immune regulating network, exert their functions by reducing the amplification signals provided by Th cells or by acting on effector B cells. Current work on this field has indicated

that at least three phenotypically different cells types are involved in this regulatory network: Ts_1 (LyT 1^+) cells produce the TSF 1 soluble factor which induces the differentiation of the Ts_2 (Lyt $1^+ 2^+$) cells, which in turn secrete the soluble factor TSF2 responsible for the stimulation of Ts_3 (Lyt 2^+) cells which dampen Th or B cell activity. This cell-soluble factor circuit has been detected out through the relative radiosensitivity of its cellular components.

Results obtained from both in vitro and in vivo experiments indicate, however, that the Ts cells are more radiosensitive than Th cells, their suppressing activity being reduced by 200 rad and abolished by 400 rad.

Antilymphocytic Sera

Antilymphocytic sera (ALS) are prepared by injecting into the appropriate animals – generally rabbits or horses – preparations of lymphoid cells from the thymus, spleen, lymph nodes, or even the lymph (obtained by cannulation of the thoracic duct).

The lymphoid cell suspensions are usually injected intravenously without Freund's adjuvant. Additional injections are administered either intravenously or subcutaneously. The antisera obtained are absorbed with washed red cells to remove traces of antierythrocytic antibodies, then the γ-globulin fractions are isolated from the absorbed serum. The antilymphocytic immunoglobulins (ALG) can agglutinate lymphocytes or lyse them in the presence of complement. ALG contain almost exclusively antibodies for antigens of the cell surface.

There is evidence that ALS administration can reduce the number of peripheral blood lymphocytes. The lymphocytes forming spontaneous E rosettes with SRBC constitute the subset population of lymphocytes most affected, followed by the K cells. With respect to B lymphocytes the reports are controversial, some indicating a fall in the number in circulation while others suggest no effect at all.

The mechanism by which ALS deplets circulating T lymphocytes in human subjects is not yet known. Some evidence indicates that ALS deplets these cells by coating and opsonizing them, thus promoting their phagocytosis by macrophages within the liver and in lymphoid organs. Heterologous IgG have, however, been demonstrated by IF test on lymphocytes from human subjects receiving ALS in comparable percentages of T and non-T lymphocytes. The presence of ALG on other cell types than T lymphocytes can be explained either by the presence of a ALS-binding glycoprotein on the surface membranes of different subpopulations of lymphocytes or by a nonspecific adsorption of the Ig through their FC moiety by the correspondent receptors.

With respect to the clinical use of ALS or of its correspondent Ig-rich preparation, the 15 years experience has failed to provide convincing support for their claimed effect in prolonging renal and cardiac allograft survival. Their use in aplastic anemia is promising in view of the observations of bone marrow regeneration in a number of patients treated with ALS.

The growing interest in monoclonal antilymphocytic antibodies indicates the urgent need for the development of studies to determine their clinical use fulness in prolonging the survival of transplanted organs, in preventing or treating GVH disease, and in treating lymphoma, leukemia, and aplastic anemia.

Mechanisms of Immunosuppression with ALG. The mechanisms by which ALG suppresses the immune response are not yet completely understood. One may be its cytolytic action upon lymphocytes. Numerous investigations have shown, however, that the immunosuppressive potency of ALG is not entirely dependent upon lysing of lymphocytes, a fact that suggests the participation of other mechanisms. Among these, an antigen-receptor blockade could play a role. The principal objection to this hypothesis is that the immunosuppressive effects upon the lymphocytes are perma-

nent, being transmitted to the descendant cells even beyond two generations. It is thus possible that we are dealing with biochemical alternations much more complicated than those of simple blockage of chemical groupings on the cellular surface. Observations suggest that the ALG acts upon the auxiliary cells of the immune response, blocking them and facilitating the action of suppressor cells.

Prevention of Contact Between the Antigen Determinants and Receptors of Immunocompentent Cells. The prior injection of antibodies specific for a particular antigen can impede the production of antibodies against this antigen. A possible mechanism is that of blockage of antigenic determinants, thus preventing them from contacting the receptors localized on the membranes of immunocompetent cells. This type of immunosuppression is used for the prophylaxis of fetal erythroblastosis induced by Th incomaptibility.

Corticosteroids

Corticosteroids (cortisone, dihydrocorticosterone, and similar agents) have been used extensively as immunosuppressive agents. They have been shown to have a wide range of effects on virtually every phase and component of the immune and inflammatory response in both animals and man. Although the precise mechanism(s) of these agents as anti-inflammatories and immunosuppressors have not been clearly defined, they have been used in pharmacologic doses in a number of diseases, particularly those with an inflammatory or immune-mediated component.

Extensive studies of the effects, both in vitro and in vivo, of corticosteroids on different stages of the immune response in various animals models have contributed greatly to the understanding of their mechanisms of action. In view of the facts that in the in vitro studies the corticosteroids are frequently used in suprapharmacologic doses and that the in vivo studies are usually done in the so-called steroid-sensitive species, extrapolation of the results to man, a so-called steroid-resistant species, should be undertaken cautiously.

Mechanisms of Action

At Subcellular Level. Recent findings indicate that the corticosteroids combine with specific intracytoplasmatic receptors, leading the target cell genome to produce RNA. In cause quence, the tanget cells, after transcription of mRNA, produce and express the steroid-stimulated proteins.

These intracytoplasmatic receptors have been identified in leukocytes, their density, however, varying according to the type of cell or to its functional state. Thus, cells from lymphoid neoplasms, normal T lymphocytes isolatd by E rosette, and mitogen-stimulated lymphocytes in the S or post-S phase of the cell cycle possess greater numbers of corticosteroid receptors than other cells. The increased number of such receptors appears, however, not to correlate with the cell sensitivity to corticosteroids. Thus, while $T\mu$ and $T\delta$ have quantitatively similar intracytoplasmatic corticosteroid receptors with similar binding activities and dissociation constants, the former subset of cells is the most susceptible to the corticosteroid effect. It can be suggested, therefore, that the corticosteroid receptor-related parameters such as densitiy, affinity, or binding constants do not account for the range of heterogenous response of immunoreactive cells to corticosteroids. Other parameters, e.g., differences in the rate of metabolism of cortisol, the capacity of the cell to respond to the corticosteroids with an elevation of the intracellular levels of cAMP, and changes in the density of some cell surface components (β_2-microglobulin, MHC antigens, etc.) may be relevant to understanding the corticoid effects.

At Cellular Level in General. Some lymphoid cell subsets from rodents are very susceptible to the lytic effects of corticoids at pharmacologic concentrations. In contrast, normal lymphoid cells from man, guinea pig, etc. are quite resistants to such effects. Despite this, single doses of corticosteroids administered in man result in a rapid (within 4 h) but transient lymphopenia with a return to normal lymphocyte count in 24 h. Such lymphopenia results from a redistribution of circulating lymphocytes to other lymphoid compartments. Moreover, certain activated T cells, e.g., those activated in MLC or obtained from arthritic joints, are susceptible to lysis by physiologic doses of corticoids. Corticoids have been also implicated as inhibitors of the release of some soluble factors in absence of cell lysis. These include inhibition of Il-2 production through a process apparently involving a direct interference with Il-1 stimulation of Il-2 production by T cells, rather than suppressing the proliferative response to Il-2. Corticosteroids also suppress production of plasminogen activator by human monocytes, inhibit histamine release from human basophils but not from guinea pig mast cells, inhibit the production of lymphotoxin and of monocyte chemotactic factor, and potentiate the Sendai-virus-induced interferon production in human tumor lines.

Following a pharmacologic dose of glucocorticoids in man, shifts of the circulating peripheral leukocytes are observed. This includes an increase both in the number and in proportion of neutrophils, the period of peak being around 4–6 h after the injection of the drug, the number of circulating neutrophils returning to the normal values by 24 h. With respect to the other leukocytes, the number of circulating cells is depressed or unaltered, and in the case of eosinophils and basophils, the peak of the steroid effect appears several hours later and returns to normal at 72 h. The circulating T lymphocytes are depressed following steroid administration to a greater degree than monocytes and B cells. Within the T cell population, the cell subsets $T\mu$ and $T\varepsilon$ are depleted to a greater extent than are $T\delta$ cells. With the exception of the T cells in which the expression of the receptors for IgE can be inhibited by corticosteroids, the circulating depression of the other cell types is thought to be a consequence of the redistribution effect of corticosteroids.

The site of redistribution of lymphocytes following administration of glucocorticoids is probably the bone marrow. The precise mechanisms governing this redistribution phenomenon induced by glucocorticoids are not yet known.

Alterations of the molecular configurations on lymphocyte surface membrane and changes in the endothelium of small vessels resulting from corticosteroids effects are, obviously, the plausible suggested mechanisms.

Effects on Monocytes. Among the immune cell components, the monocytes appear to be particularly sensitive to glucocorticoid-induced changes. Pharmacologic doses of glocucorticoids inhibit the response of monocytes to the action of several chemotactic agents in in vitro experiments.

Probably correlated with this is the higher sensitivity of monocytes than lymphocytes to the in vivo redistribution effect of lower doses of glucocorticoids.

In addition, the following in vitro effects of glucocorticoids on monocytes have been observed: (a) monocyte depletion potentiates the corticosteroid-induced suppression of lectin-induced blastogenesis, an effect partially reconstituted by the addition of normal autologous monocytes to the cultures; (b) monocyte bactericidal action is suppressed by glucocorticoids; (c) monocyte IgG and C 3 fragments receptor functions are suppressed by suprapharmacologic doses of glucocorticoids; and (d) secretion of soluble factors such as Il-1 and plasminogen activator by monocytes is suppressed, as noted above, by glucocorticoids.

Effect on T Lymphocytes. Induced blastogenesis of T lymphocytes by ConA or PHA is suppressed by corticosteroids. While the effect induced by ConA is attained with pharmacologic doses of corticosteroids, the action of these agents on PHA-induced blastogenesis is dependent upon both the relative PHA – corticosteroids dose and the corticosteroid preparation employed. Lymphocyte blastogenesis induced by specific antigens, i.e., T lymphocytes obtained from subjects sensitized to tetanus toxoid and previously treated in vivo with corticosteroids, fail to proliferate in vitro upon incubation with the corrspondent antigen. MLR, both allogeneic and autologous, are also inhibited by corticosteroids.

Effects on B Lymphocytes. Glucocorticosteroids anministered in vivo suppress the production of IgG and IgA and to a lesser extent that of IgM. Such effects, detected by measuring serum levels of these immunoglobulins, follow a brief course of split-dose daily corticosteroid administration, and appear 2–4 weeks after treatment.

In contrast, total IgE and specific IgE increase 1 week after completion of corticoid therapy for an acute asthmatic attack. The explanation for this observation may be provided by the decrease in T cell-mediated suppressor activity induced by corticosteroids, as noted previously.

Pharmacologic concentrations of glucocorticoids added to the lymphocyte cultures induce marked increases in the production of IgG, IgA, and IgM in in vitro experiments. Such effects depend upon the presence of FCS in the culture medium as a background mitogenic signal. On substituting FCS by NHS, which possesses smaller mitogenic stimulatory activity, the potentiation of Ig production by corticoids is not observed. Since, however, the immunoregulation of the B cell response is modulated by soluble factors and multiple accessory cells at different phases of the activation and expression of B cell activity, it is difficult to define the precise immunoregulatory role of the glucocorticoids. Even so, the following statements can be made: (a) glucocorticoids may exert their effects at the beginning of the stimulation of the B cells; (b) traffic and proliferation activities of B cells are relatively resistant to the effects of glucocorticoids as compared with other lymphocyte subsets; (c) Ig production is usually suppressed by pharmacologic doses of glucocorticoids in vivo and generally unaffected or potentiated by the addition of corticosteroids into the lymphocyte cultures. The effect of glucocorticoids on both NK and K cells is controversial. Observations indicating either potentiation or suppression of the cytotoxic activity of these cells have been reported.

Inhibition of Biosynthesis of Nucleic Acids and Proteins

Antigenic stimulation induces cellular multiplication and differentiation processes that involve the syntheses of nucleic acids

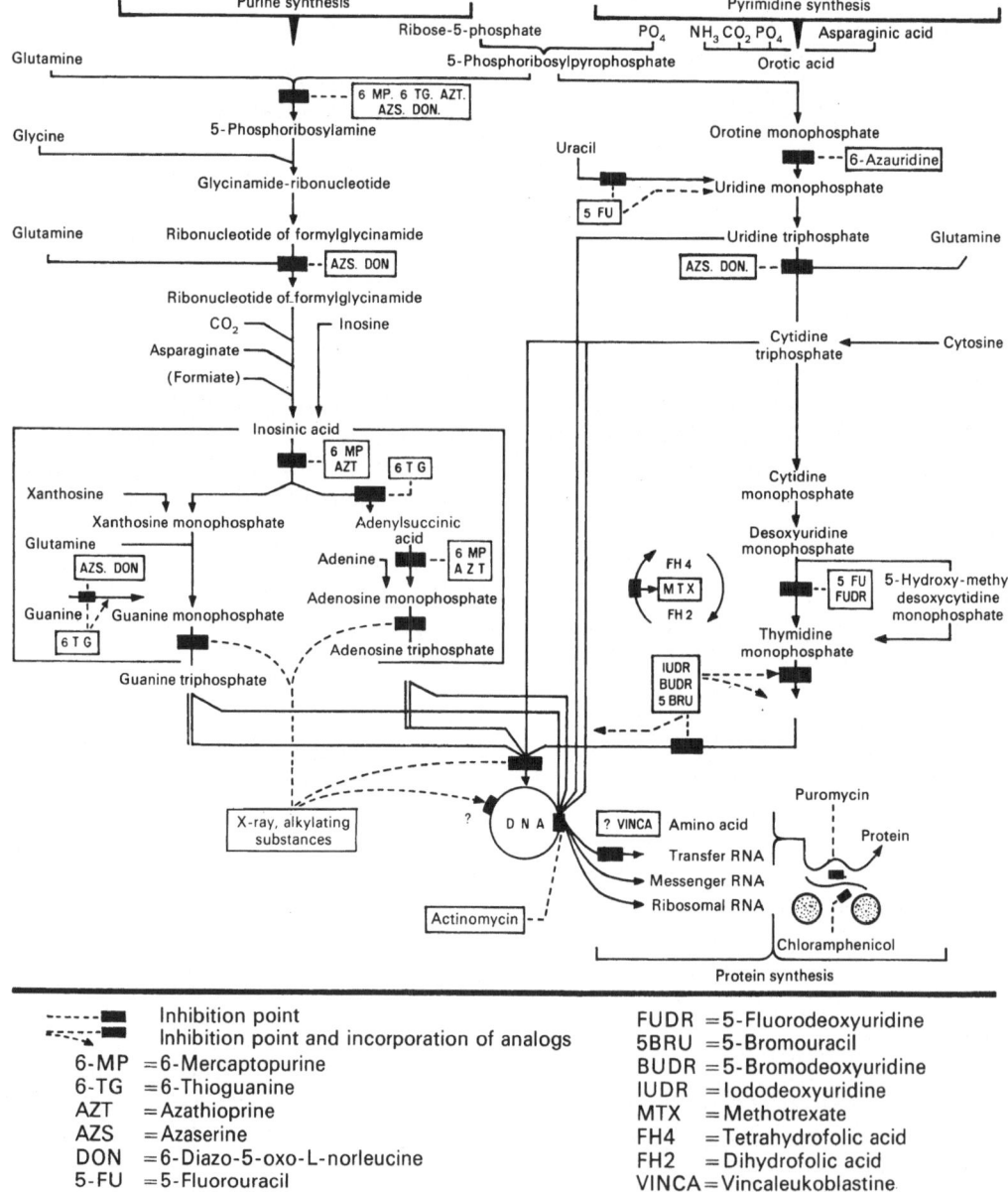

Fig. 14.1. Effect of immunosuppressive agents on biochemical reaction paths

(DNA, RNA) and proteins, and involve the participation of different enzymatic systems. At each stage of synthesis intermediate products are formed, some of fundamental importance for the continuation of the synthesis process. Consequently, numerous facets of the metabolic process are exposed, thus making the cells much more vulnerable to the blocking action of numerous drugs. As a result of the search for agents capable of inhibiting the growth of neoplasms (especially leukemias), a great variety of substances have been investigated for properties inhibiting the synthesis of DNA, RNA, or proteins.

Most of the substances tested are selectively toxic for cells in the process of multiplication. Since the immune response exhibits stages during which intense mitotic activity is observed – principally just after induction by the immunogen – many of these substances have been tested in relation to this response. It should be emphasized that the results, though encouraging, vary depending upon the animal species utilized for testing; this has hampered the formation of definitive conclusions regarding the operative modes of the individual substances tested.

An empirical classification of the immunosuppressive drugs is given in Table 14.1, while Fig. 14.1 presents the chemical reaction steps at which these substances might act. It is beyond the scope of this book to describe all the numerous immunosuppressive drugs that have been tested thus far; however, an important example from each group is described in some detail.

Alkylating Agents. Alkylating agents have been used in experimental immunology for more than 40 years, but only since an association was established between their immunosuppressive properties and their properties toxic for cancerous cells have they been more intensely investigated.

Alkylating agents probably act upon DNA, blocking cellular mitosis. These agents have high affinity for negtively charged proteins of chromatin, establishing bonds between

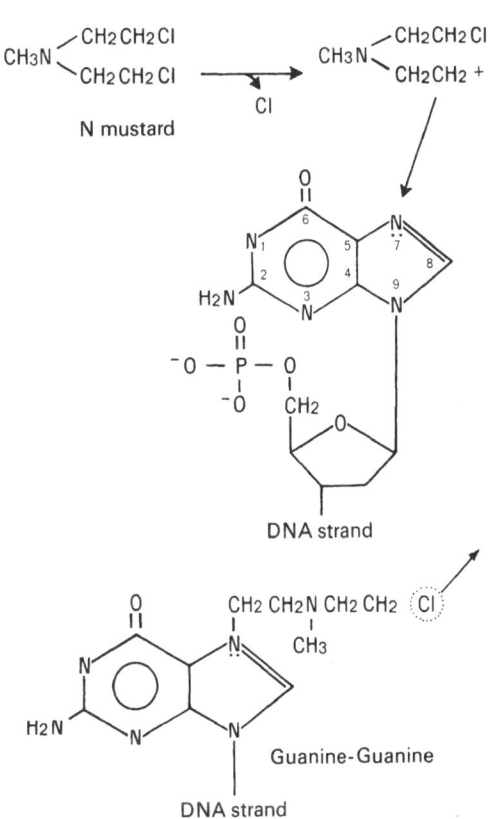

Fig. 14.2. Mechanism of alkylating substances

the chromatids and inhibiting separation of the DNA strands in mitosis (Fig. 14.2). Guanine is the primary base for such action, which leads to (1) an altered transcription of DNA to mRNA, and (2) rupture of the glycosidic linkages of deoxyribose liberating alkylated guanine. The fact that these agents can also act upon other cellular constituents cannot be excluded: for example, they can alkylate RNA or certain proteins important for cellular multiplication (mitotic fusion proteins). These agents act selectively upon the cells that are in the process of rapid multiplication, as occurs with the T and B lymphocytes stimulated by the antigens.

The compounds called nitrogen mustards (mechlorethamine) suppress the production of antibodies for a series of antigens in various animals species when administered prior to, or at least simultaneously with, injection of the antigen. They have only a weak effect on the secondary response.

Cyclophosphamide (CY) is the transport form of nitrogen mustard. The active molecule is liberated after its enzymatic degradation in the liver. It is much more active upon the production of antibodies and upon graft rejection than are other nitrogen mustards, having the additional capability of blocking an immune response that has already been initiated.

Interesting information about the effects of CY at the cellular level has been obtained through comparative studies of this drug and methotrexate. It has been verified that these two drugs inhibit the development of hypersensitivity of oxazolone in guinea pigs, but that they act upon different segments of the immune response. Histologic preparations of regional lymph nodes of guinea pigs sensitized with oxazolone 2 days after the initiation of treatment with CY in daily 10 mg doses reveal that there is no formation of so-called reveal that there is no formation of so-called large pyroninophilic cells or lymphoblasts; in contrast, in animals treated with methotrexate, blockage of the immune response appears to occur in the maturation phase of the small lymphocytes. Nitrogen mustards have an inhibitory effect on the cellular elements of bone marrow (inhibition of the formation of polymorphonuclear leukocytes). CY is usually used in a dose of 5 mg/kg body weight, with its toxic effect upon the bone marrow being controlled by periodic counts of polymorphonuclear leukocytes.

Antimetabolites. The diagrams in Fig. 14.2 show the possible biochemical sites for the action of the antimetabolites cited in Table 14.2. Generally speaking, the antimetabolites are more efficient as immunosuppressives when applied after the injection of the antigen (after about 2 weeks), probably because in this period the antigen-induced cellular proliferation already has begun.

6-Mercaptopurine (6-MP). This purine analog blocks the formation of circulating antibodies for a series of antigens in the rabbit, the dog, the mouse, and in man. Doses effective in blocking the primary immune response are about 6 mg/kg of body weight, administered daily and intravenously; larger doses, 12–15 mg/kg body weight, usually are necessary to block the secondary response. Doses of this order also are efficient in prolonging the time required for rejection of skin transplants in the rabbit and kidney transplants in the dog. However, at this level the doses are much more toxic, which prevents more prolonged treatment.

The injection of an antigen such as bovine serum albumin into an animal under treatment with 6-MP can induce tolerance to this antigen. In experiments of this type, the proportion of animals that become tolerant rises with increasing doses of the antigen.

The immunosuppressive activities of 6-MP are due to its antimetabolic action upon purines. This can occur at various biochemical levels, including that of competitive inhibition and, probably, that of being incorporated into the nucleic acid molecules, thus being able to form, for example, a messenger RNA with an incomplete or distorted message.

Azathioprine (Imuran) is an imidazole derivative of 6-MP that is less toxic for the intestinal epithelium and for the bone marrow than the original compound, yet somehow retains its original immunosuppressive properties. Azathioprine is transformed in the liver into its active immunosuppressive form (Fig. 14.3); currently it is included in the majority of immunosuppressive protocols for the treatment of autoimmune diseases and the prevention of graft rejection. This drug must be administered in several daily doses to facilitate the regular liberation of the active form (6-MP) by the liver. Despite its low toxicity in relation to 6-MP, azathioprine can produce collateral effects such as gastrointestinal disturbances and leukopenia.

6-Thioguanine (6-TG). 6-Thioguanine is similar to 6-MP, but it acts more directly through the formation of abnormal DNA.

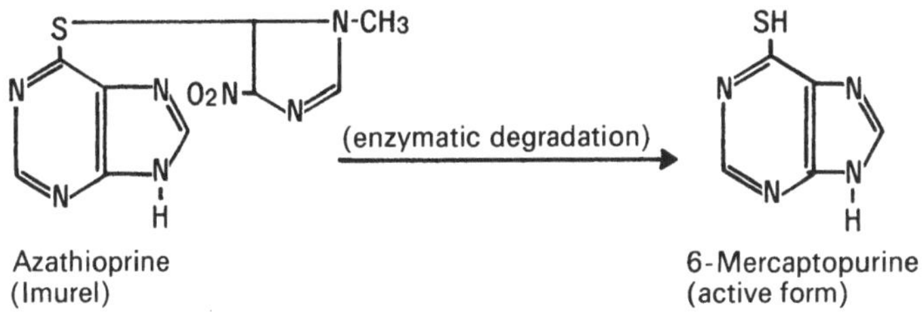

N-CH3
O2N
(enzymatic degradation)
SH
Azathioprine
(Imurel)
6-Mercaptopurine
(active form)

Fig. 14.4. Mechanism of folic acid antagonists

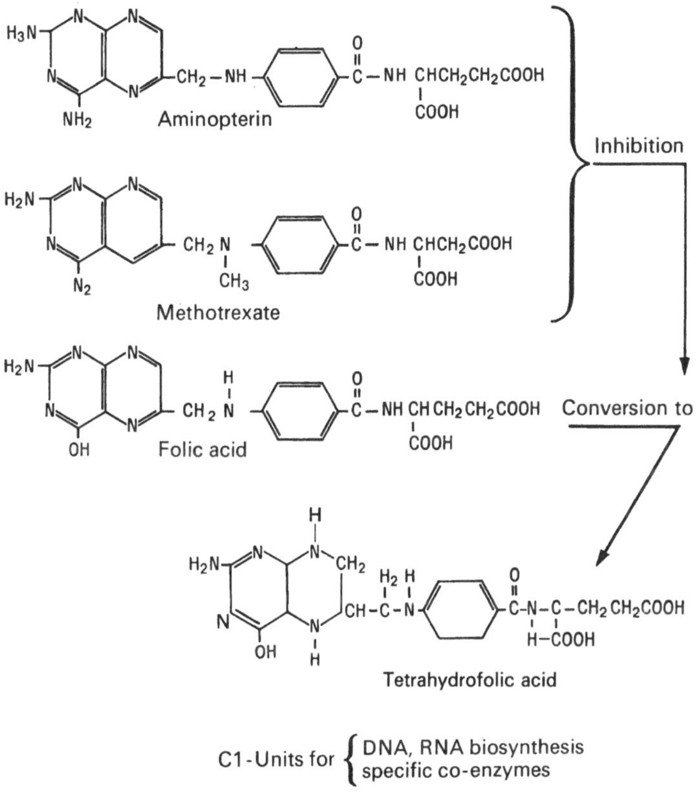

Aminopterin
Methotrexate
Folic acid
Inhibition
Conversion to
Tetrahydrofolic acid
C1-Units for
DNA, RNA biosynthesis
specific co-enzymes

Fig. 14.3 Conversion of azathioprine to 6-mercaptopurine

As is the case with its congener, 6-TG also blocks the formation of circulating antibodies and has been used with relative success in the treatment of some autoimmune diseases, including hemolytic anemia, lupus erythematosus, chronic hepatitis, and hyperglobulinemic purpura. This drug has the drawback of cumulative toxic side effects, which to some extent limit its use in the prolonged immunosuppressive protocols usual in transplantation.

5-Fluorouracil (5-FU) and Analogs. Analogs of the pyrimidine bases are not often used in immunosuppression because doses that are effective in vivo are poorly tolerated. However, they have frequently been used in studies in vitro on the production of antibodies, and have given rise to important observations clarifying the cellular processes that occur during the secondary response. These compounds inhibit the production of antibodies. The fact that their effects are reversed by thymidine indicates that they are acting upon the DNA.

Antagonists of Folic Acid. Aminopterin, and particularly its methylated analog methotrexate, are highly potent immunosuppressive agents that act on cellular metabolism, interfering with the conversion of folic acid to its active form, tetrahydrofolic acid (Fig. 14.4). Despite the fact that this conversion of folic acid is an essential step for many biochemical processes, including the synthesis of DNA and RNA and that of coenzymes containing purines, it still is not known whether or not this is the exclusive means by which antagonists of folic acid block the immune response. It appears, however, that the principal site of inhibition is in the interphase during the synthesis of DNA. Methotrexate acts by inhibiting the formation of large pyrininophilic cells into plasma cells or into sensitized lymphocytes.

As usually occurs with immunosuppressive drugs, the antagonists of folic acid exhibit greater efficiency in blocking the primary response and the production of IgG. Because of its high toxicity, the use of methotrexate is severely restricted in clinical immunology.

Plant Alkaloids. Some plant alkaloids are being investigated in immunosuppression experiments. Notable, among others, are colchicine (from *Colchicum autumnale*) and the vinca alkaloids, vincristine and vinblastine (from *Vinca rosacea* and *Vinca rosea*, respectively). These three alkaloids are mitotic inhibitors that block the formation of the mitotic spindle, paralyzing cell division in metaphase. In addition, they possess lymphotoxic activity: Colchicine acts as a powerful inhibitor of phagocytosis. These pharmacologic properties could explain their immunosuppressive activities upon delayed-type hypersensitivity reactions as well as upon the production of circulating antibodies.

Antibiotics. Almost all antibiotics, even the more common ones, interfere to a lesser or greater extent with the immune response; here we consider briefly those five cited in Table 14.2.

Actinomycins C and D. Actinomycins C and D are used principally in the study of the production of antibodies in vitro; however, due to their excessive toxicity, their use in vivo is limited. Studies of the operative mechanism of the actinomycins indicate that they form complexes with the guanine residues of the DNA molecules, impeding the subsequent formation of RNA molecules. This inhibition includes not only the formation of ribosomal RNA, but also the synthesis of messenger and transfer RNA; thus such inhibition obviously affects the synthesis of proteins.

Studies of the effects of actinomycin D upon the formation of antibodies have shown that the production of 19S immunoglobulins is much more affected than is the production of 7S immunoglobulins. These observations suggest that the RNA destined for 19S antibody synthesis is especially susceptible to the action of actinomycin.

Puromycin. Puromycin was isolated from *Streptomyces alboniger* and appears to act in cellular metabolism, inhibiting the transfer of amino acids of soluble RNA to the ribosomal protein. Whereas its use in vivo is limited because of its high toxicity, it has been used in some systems in vitro, behaving as a powerful blocker of antibody production. Puromycin is also efficacious in systems in which the formation of antibodies is underway, having the further advantage of not killing the cells.

Chloramphenicol. Chloramphenicol was originally isolated from *Stréptomyces venezuelae;* later it became the first antibiotic to be synthesized. It impedes the transfer of amino acids to the ribosomes by competing, preferentially, for the sites that receive the amino acids.

In relatively high doses, chloramphenicol inhibits the primary response in vivo. Used in cell cultures, it also impedes the secondary response when it has been placed in the culture medium together with the immunogen, but little or no effect is observed if the cells have already begun producing immunoglobulins.

Azaserine. Azaserine is an antibiotic produced by *Streptomyces fragilis* that functions as an analog of glutamine for bacteria and probably as an alkylating agent for animal cells. When used alone, it has almost no immunosuppressive effect, but it has been often used in transplants in association with azathioprine.

Amino Acid Antagonists. The antagonists of amino acids have only recently been used in immunosuppression. L-Asparaginase, for example, catalyzes the hydrolysis of the L-asparagine in aspartic acid and ammonia, thereby indirectly inhibiting the production of antibodies in the mouse for antigens on the surfaces of sheep erythrocytes, blocking the blastogenic response of the lymphocytes to phytohemagglutinin. In doses of 25,000–50,000 IU per day, it suppresses in man the production of antibodies against hemocyanin.

Niridazole. Is a anti-schistosomal drug which markedly suppresses granulomatous inflammation against schistosome eggs and suppresses DTH in previously sensitized animals. In addition, it causes marked prolongation of skin allograft survival in mice across H-2 barriers. In contrast, in therapeutic doses, niridazole produces only a moderate and transient suppression of the antibody response to several antigens.

Diabetes. Streptozotocin- and alloxan-induced diabetes in mice produces the following effects: (a) partial suppression of inflammation around *S. mansoni* eggs, an effect reversed by the administration of insulin; and (b) DTH inhibition and prolongation of skin graft survival for incompatible H-2 transplants.

Specific Suppression

Suppression of the immune response by a feedback mechanism and by induction of tolerance represent two specific immunosuppressive courses of action. By these methods, one can determine which antibodies can be inhibited. The basic mechanism involved in these forms of immunosuppression is not yet understood.

The immunosuppressive agents described thus far act, as we have seen, indiscriminately, blocking or damaging all cells that happen to be in mitosis, i.e., including normally functioning cells that are particularly important to the organism's survival.

The immune response, characterized at the cellular level by a sequence of divisions and by specifically oriented cellular differentiations, must possess some strategically located mechanism that brings the cell either to a state of immunologic activity (production of antibodies, development of sensitized lymphocytes), or to a state of specific nonreactivity (tolerance). It is probable that once the biochemical events involved in this mechanism are understood, agents will be developed that can specifically paralyze it or cause it to induce tolerance.

Rules for Immunosuppression

Immunosuppressive experiments in laboratory animals have permitted the formulation of generalizations that can provide orientation for the use of immunosuppressive agents in clinical immunology:

1. When the proper doses of the immunosuppressive agent are used and applied at the optimum time with respect to the introduction of the antigen, one can obtain:

a) Prevention of the primary and secondary humoral immune responses
b) Induction of immunologic tolerance
c) Prolongation of the period of IgM production, thereby inhibiting the formation of IgG
d) An increase in the formation of antibodies
e) Suppression of delayed-type hypersensitivity

2. The nearer the dosage of the drug comes to its toxic limit, the greater its immunosuppressive action becomes.

3. Antimetabolites are more active when employed in the induction period of the im-

mune response, whereas alkylating substances function better in the preinduction phase.

4. After the formation of antibodies has begun, much higher immunosuppressive doses, generally toxic, are required for its suppression.

5. The primary response is more sensitive to the action of immunosuppressive drugs than is the secondary response.

6. It is much easier to block the development of a delayed immune response than it is to alter the manifestation of an already established lesion.

7. Any time the administration of the immunosuppressive is stopped before the antigen is totally catabolized, a subsequent immune response can occur.

References

Abstracts of the Second International Conference on Immunopharmacology, Washington, USA, 5–9 July, 1982

Bach JF (1975) The mode of action of immunosuppressive agents. North-Holland, Amsterdam

Chedid L, Miescher PA, Müller-Eberhard HJ (1980) Immunostimulation. Springer, Berlin Heidelberg New York (Springer Series in Immunopathology, vol p2)

Cortesini R (ed) (1979) Modulation of immunologic responsiveness. Transplant Proc 11:839

Fauci AS, Dale DC, Balow JE (1976) Glucocorticosteroid therapy: mechanisms of action and clinical considerations. Ann Intern Med 84:304

Gerber NL, Steinberg AD (1976) Clinical use of immunosuppressive drugs (2 parts). Drugs 11:14, 90

Jerne NK (1974) Towards a network theory of the immune system. In: La genétique des immunoglobines et de la réponse immunitaire. Ann Immunol (Inst Pasteur), 125 C:309–37

Kaplan SR, Calabresi P (1973) Immunosuppressive agents (2 parts). N Engl J Med 289:952, 1234

Lance EM, Medawar PB, Taub RN (1973) Antilymphocytic serum. Adv Immunol 17:2

Möller G (ed) (1982) Immunosuppressive agents. Immunol Rev 65:5–155. Munksgaard, Copenhagen, Denmark

Oudin J (1974) L'idiotype des anticorps. In: La genétique des immunoglobulines et de la réponse immunitaire. Ann Immunol (Inst Pasteur) 125 C:309–37

Parker CW, Vaura JD (1974) Immunosuppression. Prog Hematol 6:1

Schein PS, Winokur SH (1975) Immunosuppressive and cytotoxic chemotherapy: long-term complications. Ann Intern Med 82:84

Vilcek J, Gresser I, Merigan TC (eds) (1980) Regulatory functions of interferons. Ann NY Acad Sci 350:1–641

Waksman BH (1980) Adjuvants and immune regulation by lymphoid cells. In: Chedid L, Miescher PA, Müller-Eberhard HJ (eds) Immunostimulation. Springer, Berlin Heidelberg New York, pp 5–33 (Springer Series in Immunopathology, vol p2)

Winkelstein A (1977) Effects of immunosuppressive drugs on T and B lymphocytes. Blood 50:81

Brief History of Important Immunologic Discoveries and Developments

Year	Event	Author(s)
1798	Cowpox vaccination	Edward Jenner
1866	Wound disinfection	Joseph Lister
1876	Discovery of *B. antracis*, foundation of bacteriology	Robert Koch
1880	Discovery of attenuated vaccine by invitro passages	Louis Pasteur
1883	Phagocytosis, cellular immunity theory	Elie I. I. Metchnikoff
1888	Discovery of bacterial toxins	P. P. Emile Roux and Alexandre E. J. Yersin
1890	Discovery of antitoxins, foundation of serotherapy	Emil A. von Behring and Shibasaburo Kitasato
1894	Immunologic bacteriolysis	Richard F. J. Pfeiffer and Vasily I. Isaeff
1894	Discovery of antibody and complement activity as the active factors in bacteriolysis	Jules J. B. V. Bordet
1896	Discovery of specific agglutination	Herbert E. Durham and Max von Gruber
1896	Agglutination test for the diagnosis of typhoid (Widal test)	Georges F. I. Widal and Arthur Sicard
1900	Formulation of side-chain theory of antibody formation	Paul Ehrlich
1900	Discovery of A, B, 0 blood groups	Karl Landsteiner
1900	Development of complement fixation reaction	Jules J. B. V. Bordet and Octave Gengou
1902	Discovery of anaphylaxis	Charles R. Richet and Paul Portier
1903	Local anaphylaxis due to antibody-antigen complex: Arthus reaction	Nicholas M. Arthus
1903	Discovery of opsonization	Almroth E. Wright and Steward R. Douglas

Year	Event	Author(s)
1905	Description of serum sickness	Clemens von Pirquet and Bela Schick
1910	Introduction of salvarsan, later neo-salvarsan, foundation of chemotherapy of infections	Paul Ehrlich and Sahachiro Hata
1910	Development of anaphylaxis test (Schultz-Dale)	William Schultz
1914	Formulation of genetic theory of tumor transplantation	Clarence C. Little
1921	Experimental trial with BCG vaccine	Albert L. C. Calmette and Camille Guérin
1921	Development of cutaneous anaphylactic reaction	Carl W. Prausnitz and Heinz Küstner
1923	Production of anatoxin (toxoid) by formaldehyde treatment	Ramon Gaston
1928	Discovery of penicillin, the first antibiotic	Alexander Fleming
1935	Discovery of sulfonamides for chemotherapy of infections	Gerhard Domagk
1935	Discovery of local immunity; oral vaccination	Alexandre Besredka
1935–36	Purification of antibodies, quantitative precipitation reaction	Michael Heidelberger and Forrest E. Kendall
1937	Evidence for identity of the gene for blood group antigen II with one gene for tumor resistance in the mouse (H–2)	Peter A. Gorer
1938	Evidence that antibodies are γ-globulins	Arne Tiselius and Elvin A. Kabat
1942	Discovery of cellular transfer of delayed type hypersensitivity in guinea pigs	Karl Landsteiner and Merrill W. Chase
1942	Fluorescence labeling of antibodies and antigens	Albert H. Coons
1942	Introduction of adjuvants	Jules T. Freund
1943–44	Establishment of immunologic basis of rejection of normal tissue transplants	Peter B. Medawar
1946–48	Theory of congenic mouse lines formulated, first congenic lines initiated, and the term histocompatibility introduced	George D. Snell
1945	Development of antiglobulin test for incomplete Rh antibodies	Robin R. A. Coombs, R. R. Race, and A. E. Mourant

Year	Event	Author(s)
1945	Description of tolerance (chimerism) in dizygotic cattle twins	Ray D. Owen
1946	Development of precipitin test in gels	Jaques Oudin
1947	Immunoglobulins as "transporteurs"	Pierre Grabar
1948	Development of double immunodiffusion test in gels	Örjan Ouchterlony and Stephen D. Elek
1948	Discovery of plasma cells as antibody producing cells	Astrid E. Fagraeus
1949	Elucidation of the structure of A, B, 0 blood group antigens	Elvin A. Kabat, W. T. J. Morgan, and W. M. Watkins
1952	Description of agammaglobulinemia in human	Ogdon Carr Bruton
1952	Discovery of histamine in mast cells	James F. Riley and Geoffrey B. West
1953	Development of immunoelectrophoresis	Pierre Grabar
1953	Experimental evidence of acquired immunologic tolerance	Milan Hašek
1956	Major histocompatibility (H–2) complex in the mouse defined	George D. Snell
1956	Discovery of human leukocyte antigen, later be shown to belong to the major histocompatibility complex of man (HLA)	Jean Dausset
1956	Experimental induction of autoimmunity	Ernest Witebsky and Noel R. Rose
1956	Discovery of allotypes	Rune Grubb and Jaques Oudin
1957	Discovery of interferon	Jean Lindemann and Alick Isaacs
1957	Discovery of macroglobulins with antibody activity	H. Hugh Fudenberg and Henry G. Kunkel
1957	Discovery of Australia antigen, later shown to be Hepatitis B antigen	Baruch Blumberg
1957	Discovery of human slow virus infection (Kuru)	Carleton Gajdusek
1959	Introduction of the radioimmune assay	Rosalyn Yalow and Solomon A. Berson
1960	Antibody structure	Alfred Nisonoff, Gerald Edelman, Rodney P. Porter, Henry G. Kunkel
1961	Discovery of the thymus as part of the immune system	Jaques F. A. P. Miller, Robert A. Good

Year	Event	Author(s)
1963	Development of the plaque formation test	Nils K. Jerne, Richard J. Henry, Albert A. Nordin
1963	Ss Locus in the H–2 complex discovered coding for the C4-complement component	Donald C. Shreffler
1963 (1953)	Histamine release by mast cells in anaphylaxis	Ivan Mota
1964	Development of rosette-test	G. Biozzi
1965	Discovery of the variable region of antibody molecules	Norbert Hilschmann
1965	Linkage of MLR reactivity to the HLA complex discovered	Fritz Bach, Kurt Hirschhorn
1965	Immune response-1 (Ir-1) locus in the mouse discovered	Hugh O. McDevitt and Michael Sela
1966	Enzyme labeling of antibodies and antigens	S. Avremeas
1966	Discovery of IgE as reaginic antibody	Kimishige Ishizaka
1969	Thymus function defined, dichotomy of the immune system discovered	Jaques F. A. P. Miller and Graham Mitchell
1969	H–2 antigen isolated	Stanley G. Nathenson and Akira Shimada
1969	T helper function in antibody formation described (T-B Collaboration)	N. Avrion Mitchison
1969	B lymphocytes as cells with surface-bound Ig discovered	Benvenuto Pernis
1969	Discovery of idiotypes	Jaques Oudin
1971–72	Cytotoxic T cells described	Jean-Charles Cerrotini, K. Theodor Brunner, Peter Perlmann, Hermann Wagner
1971	Discovery of *MLR* locus linked to *HLA* in man	Edmond J. Yunis and Bernhard Amos
1971	Two-locus model of the mouse *MHC* (*H–2*) formulated	George D. Snell, Jan Klein, Donald C. Shreffler, Jack Stimpfling
1971	T and B cell tolerance defined	Jaques Chiller
1972	T suppressor cells described	Richard K. Gershon
1972	Discovery of *MHC*-restriction of T cell dependent immune responses	Berenice Kindred and Donald C. Shreffler
1973	Discovery of Ia antigens	Chella S. David, Donald C. Shreffler, Jan Klein, Dietrich Götze, David H. Sachs

Year	Event	Author(s)
1973	T-B cell collaboration *I* region restricted	David H. Katz and Baruch Benacerraf
1974	Idiotypic network theory formulated	Nils K. Jerne
1974	K,D-restriction of cytotoxic T cells discovered	Peter Doherty and Rolf Zinkernagel
1975	Fusion of myeloma cells with normal, specific antibody-producing plasma cells (hybridoma)	George Köhler and Cesar Milstein
1978	Structure of MHC (H–2 and HLA) antigens defined	Stanley G. Nathenson, Jack Strominger
1978	Macrophage-T cell collaboration *I*-region restricted	Jonathan Sprent
1978–80	Elucidation of immunoglobulin genes; generation of diversity is (almost) solved	Suzuma Tonegawa
1980	Smallpox worldwide eradicated	World Health Organization (WHO)
1982	CD antigens defined by monoclonal antibodies	Leukocyte antigen workshop, Paris (Reinharz)
1983–85	T cell antigen receptor genes elucidated	Marrack, Allison

Glossary of Immunologic Terms

Accessory cells. Lymphoid cells predominantly of the monocyte and macrophage lineage which cooperate with T and B lymphocytes in immune reactions

Acquired immunity. Immunity that develops as a result of exposure to a foreigne substrate

Activated lymphocytes. Lymphocytes that have been stimulated by specific antigen or nonspecific mitogen

Adoptive transfer. Transfer of immunity by immunocompetent cells from one animal to another

Affinity. Binding strength between antibody and antigen in an antibody-antigen reaction

Agglutination. An antibody-antigen reaction in which a solid or particulate antigen forms a lattice with a soluble antibody

Allelic exclusion. The phenotypic expression of a single allele in cells containing 2 different alleles for that genetic locus

Allergens. Antigens which give rise to allergic sensitization by IgE antibodies

Allergy. An overshouting hypersensitivity reaction

Allogeneic. Denotes the relationship which exists between genetically dissimilar members of the same species

Allograft. A tissue or organ graft between two genetically dissimilar members of the same species

Allotype. The genetically determined antigenic difference on molecules, varying in different members of the same species

Anamnesis (immunologic memory). A heightened responsiveness to the second or subsequent administration of antigen to an immune animal

Anaphylatoxin. A substance produced by complement activation which causes an increased vascular permeability through the release of pharmacologically active mediators from mast cells

Anaphylaxis. A reaction of immediate hypersensitivity present in nearly all vertebrates which results from sensitization of tissue-fixed mast cells by cytotropic antibodies following exposure to antigen

Anergy. The inability to react to an antigen (microorganism)

Antibody. A protein that is produced as a result of the introduction of an antigen and which has the ability to combine with the antigen that stimulated its production

Antibody combining site. That configuration present on an antibody molecule which links with a corresponding antigenic determinant

Antibody-dependent cell-mediated cytotoxicity (ADCC). A form of lymphocyte-mediated cytotoxicity in which an effector cell kills an antibody-coated target cell

Anticomplementarity. Unspecific complement activation, i.e., not due to antibody-antigen reaction

Antigen. A substance which can induce a detectable immune response when introduced into an animal

Antigenic determinant (epitope). That area of an antigen which determines the specificity of the antigen-antibody reaction

Antigenicity. Property of a substance to react with an antibody, but not necessarily to induce its formation

Antigen processing. The series of events which occurs following antigen administration until antibody production

Antiglobulin test (Coombs' test). A technic to detect cell-bound immunoglobulin. In the direct Coombs' test, red blood cells taken directly from a sensitized individual are agglutinated by antigammaglobulin antibodies. In the indirect Coombs' test, a patient's serum is incubated with test red blood cells and the sensitized cells are then agglutinated with an antiimmunoglobulin or with Coombs reagent

Antitoxins. Protective antibodies which inactivate soluble toxic proteins of bacteria

Atopy. A genetically determined abnormal state of hypersensitivity as distinguished from hypersensitivity responses in normal individuals

Attenuated. Rendered less virulent

Autoantibody. Antibody to self antigen

Autoantigens. Self antigens

Autograft. A tissue graft between genetically identical members of the same species

Avidity. Refers broadly to the ability of antibodies to bind to antigens. (Affinity is a more precisely used term referring to activity per antibody-combining site)

Basement membrane. A sheet of material up to 0.2 μ thick lying immediately below epithelial (and endothelial) cells and supporting them. Contains glycoproteins and collagen and to some extent acts as a diffusion barrier for microorganisms. Thickness and structure varies in different parts of the body

B cell (B lymphocyte). Strictly a bursa-derived cell in avian species and, by analogy, bursa-equivalent derived cells in nonavian species. B cells are the precursors of plasma cells that produce antibody

BCG (bacillus Calmette-Guérin). A viable attenuated strain of *Mycobacterium bovis* which has been obtained by progressive reduction of virulence and which confers immunitiy to mycobacterial infection and possibly possesses anticancer activity in selected diseases

Bence-Jones proteins. Monoclonal light chains present in the urine of patients with paraproteinemic disorders

Blast cell. A large lymphocyte or other immature cell containing a nucleus with loosely packed chromatin, a large nucleolus, and a large amount of cytoplasm with numerous polyribosomes

Blocking factors (antibody). Substances that are present in the serum of tumor-bearing animals and are capable of blocking the ability of immune lymphocytes to kill tumor cells

Blood groups. Antigens present at the surface of red blood cells which may vary between individuals of the same species. The most important blood groups in man are the ABO and the Rh blood groups

Bone marrow. Soft connective tissue located in the cavities of the bones

Bone marrow-derived cell. A lymphoid cell present in one of the lymphoid organs which originated in the bone marrow and escaped the influence of the thymus

Bursa of Fabricius. The hindgut organ located in the cloaca of birds which controls the ontogeny of B lymphocytes

Bursal equivalent. Hypothetical organ or organs analogous to the bursa of Fabricius in nonavian species

C. The abbreviation for serum complement

Capping. The movement of cell surface antigens toward one pole of a cell after the antigens are cross-linked by specific antibody

Cardiolipin. A substance derived from beef heart, probably a component of mitochondrial membranes, which serves as an antigenic substrate for reagin or antitreponemal antibody

Carrier. An immunogenic substance which, when coupled to a hapten, renders the hapten immunogenic

Cell-mediated immunity. Immunity in which the participation of lymphocytes and macrophages is predominant

Cell-mediated lymphocytolysis. An in vitro assay for cellular immunity in which a standard mixed lymphocyte reaction is followed by destruction of target cells which are used to sensitize allogeneic cells during the MLC

CH$_{50}$ unit. The quantity or dilution of serum required to lyse 50% of the red blood cells in a standard hemolytic complement assay

Chemotaxis. A process whereby phagocytic cells are attracted to the vicinity of invading pathogens

Classical complement pathway. A series of enzyme-substrate and protein-protein interactions which ultimately leads to biologically active complement enzymes. It proceeds sequentially C 1, 423, 567, 89

Clonal selection theory. The theory of antibody synthesis proposed by Burnet which predicts that the individual carries a complement of clones of lymphoid cells which are capable of reacting with all possible antigenic determinants. The antigens which actually come in contact with the organism select "their" clones; these clones differentiate and expand

Clone. A group of cells all of which are the progeny of a single cell

Cold agglutinins. Antibodies which agglutinate bacteria or erythrocytes more efficiently at temperatures below 37 °C than at 37 °C

Committed cell. Antigen-specifically sensitized lymphocytes

Complement. A system of serum proteins which is the primary humoral mediator of antigen-antibody reactions

Complement fixation. A standard serologic assay used for the detection of an antigen-antibody reaction in which complement is fixed as a result of the formation of an immune complex. The subsequent failure of lysis of sensitized red blood cells by complement which has been fixed indicates the degree of antigen-antibody reaction

Concanavalin A (ConA). A lectin which is derived from the jack bean and which stimulates predominantly T lymphocytes

Congenic. (originally called **congenic resistant**) Denotes a line of mice identical or nearly identical with other inbred strains except for the substitution at one locus of a foreign allele introduced by appropriate crosses with a second inbred strain

Coombs' test. See antiglobulin test

C region (constant region). The carboxyl terminal portion of the H or L chain which is identical in immunoglobulin molecules of a given class and subclass apart from genetic polymorphisms

Cross-reaction. The reaction of an antibody with an antigen other than the one which induced its formation

Cytotoxic antibody. Antibody which reacts with antigens present on a cell surface and which produces damage to that cell or its surface

Cytotoxic T lymphocytes (CTL). Thymus-derived lymphocytes with the ability to lyse complement-independently target cells against which they have been specifically sensitized

Cytotropic antibodies. Antibodies of the IgG and IgE classes which sensitize cells for subsequent anaphylaxis

Defective virus replication. Incomplete virus replication, with production only of viral nucleic acid, proteins or non-infectious virus particles

Degranulation. A process whereby cytoplasmic granules of phagocytic cells fuse with phagosomes and discharge their contents into the phagolysosome thus formed

Delayed hypersensitivity. A cell-mediated immune reaction which can be elicited by subcutaneous injection of antigen, with a subsequent cellular infiltrate and edema which are maximal between 24 and 28 h after antigen challenge

Diapedesis. The outward passage of cells through intact vessel walls

Direct immunofluorescence. The detection of antigens by fluorescently labeled antibody

Diversity. Multitude of different antigen-specific combining sites (V_H and V_L regions)

Domains. Segments of H or L chains that are folded 3-dimensionally and stabilized with disulfide bonds

EAC rosette. Formation of a cluster of red cells (erythrocytes) sensitized with antibody and complement around human B lymphocytes

Eczema. A skin eruption common to atopic persons, with characteristic itching, inflammation and swelling

Effector cells. Usually denotes T cells capable of mediating cytotoxicity, suppression, or helper function

Encapsulation. A quasi-immunologic phenomenon in which foreign material is walled off within the tissues of invertebrates

Endocytosis. The process whereby material external to a cell is internalized within a particular cell. It consists of pinocytosis and phagocytosis

Endotoxins. Lipopolysaccharides which are derived from the cell walls of gram-negative microorganisms and have toxic and pyrogenic effects when injected in vivo

Enhancement. Improved survival of tumor cells in animals which have been previously immunized to the antigens of a given tumor

Epitope. The simplest form of an antigenic determinant present on a complex antigenic molecule

Equivalence. A ratio of antigen-antibody concentration where maximal precipitation occurs

E rosette. Formation of a cluster (rosette) of cells consisting of sheep erythrocytes surrounded by bound human T lymphocytes

Erythroblastosis fetalis. The medical term for Rh incompatibility disease of the newborn

Euglobulin. Class of globulins which are insoluble in water, but soluble in salt solution

Exotoxins. Diffusible toxins produced by certain gram-positive and gram-negative microorganisms

Fab. Antigen-binding fragment produced by enzymatic digestion of an IgG molecule with papain

F(ab')$_2$. Fragment obtained by pepsin digestion of immunoglobulin molecules containing the 2 H and 2 L chains linked by disulfide bonds. It contains antigen-binding activity. An F(ab')$_2$ fragment and an Fc fragment comprise an entire monomeric immunoglobulin molecule

Fc fragment. Crystallizable fragment obtained by papain digestion of IgG molecules. Fc fragment consists of the C-terminal half of 2 H chains linked by disulfide bonds. Contains no antigen-binding capability but determines important biologic characteristics of the intact molecule

Fc receptor. A receptor present on various subclasses of lymphocytes for the Fc fragment of immunoglobulins

F_1 generation. The first generation of offspring after a designated mating

F_2 generation. The second generation of offspring after a designated mating

Fluorescence. The emission of light of one color while a substance is irradiated with a light of a different color

Forssman-antigen, -antibody. So-called heterophil antigen that can be demonstrated on tissue cells of different species, e.g., horse, sheep, mouse a.o., but is absent from tissue of human and rabbit. Forssman-antibodies are present as "natural antibodies" in the serum of man, and agglutinate red blood cells, e.g., of sheep

Freund's complete adjuvant (FCA). An oil-water emulsion which contains killed mycobacteria and enhances immune responses when mixed in an emulsion with antigen

Freund's incomplete adjuvant. Contains all of the elements of Freund's complete adjuvant with the exception of killed mycobacteria

Gamma globulins. Serum proteins with gamma mobility in electrophoresis which comprise the majority of immunoglobulins

Gammopathy. Paraprotein disorder involving abnormalities of immunoglobulins

Genetic switch hypothesis. A hypothesis which postulates that there is a switch in the gene controlling heavy chain synthesis in plasma cells during the development of an immune response

Germinal centers. A collection of metabolically active lymphoblasts, macrophages, and plasma cells which appears within the primary follicle of lymphoid tissues following antigenic stimulation

Glomerulonephritis. An autoimmune disease in which the major damage is to the glomeruli of the kidney

Gm marker. Allotypic determinant on the heavy chain of human IgG

Graft rejection. A cell-mediated immune reaction elicited by the grafting of genetically dissimilar tissue onto a recipient. The reaction leads to destruction and ultimate rejection of the transplanted tissue

Graft-versus-host (GVH reaction). The clinical and phatologic sequelae of the reactions of immunocompetent cells in a graft against the cells of the histoincompatible and immunodeficient recipient

Gram-negative. Losing the primary violet or blue during decolorization in Gram's staining method

Gram-positive. Retaining the primary violet or blue stain in Gram's method

Granuloma. A local accumulation of densely packed macrophages, often fusing to form giant cells and sometimes together with lymphocytes and plasma cells. Seen in chronic infections such as tuberculosis and syphilis

Granulopoietin (Colony-stimulating factor). A glycoprotein with a molecular weight of 45,000 derived from monocytes which controls the production of granulocytes by the bone marrow

H-2 locus. The major histocompatibility complex (MHC) in the mouse

Haplotype. That portion of the phenotype determined by closely linked genes of a single chromosome inherited from one parent

Hapten. A substance which is not immunogenic but can react with an antibody of appropriate specificity

Hassall's corpuscles. Whorls of thymic epithelial cells whose function is unknown

HB antigen. Hepatitis B virus antigen detectable in serum of infected though not necessarily sick individuals

Hay fever. A seasonal allergic disease causing inflammation of the eyes and nasal passages

H chain (heavy chain). One pair of identical polypeptide chains making up an immunoglobulin molecule. The heavy chain contains approximately twice the number of amino acids and is twice the molecular weight of the light chain

Heavy chain diseases. A heterogeneous group of paraprotein disorders characterized by the presence of monoclonal but incomplete heavy chains without light chains in serum or urine

Helper T cells. A subtype of T lymphocytes which cooperate with B cells in antibody formation

Hemagglutination inhibition. A technic for detecting small amounts of antigen in which homologous antigen inhibits the agglutination of red cells or other particles coated with antigen by specific antibody

Hematopoietic system. All tissues responsible for production of the cellular elements of peripheral blood

Hemolysin. Antibody or other substance capable of lysing red blood cells

Heterocytotropic antibodies. Antibody which can passively sensitize tissues of species other than those in which the antibody is present

Heterologous antigen. An antigen which participates in a cross-reaction

High dose (high zone) tolerance. Classical immunologic unresponsiveness produced by repeated injections of large amounts of antigen

Hinge region. The area of the H chains between the first and second C region domains. It is the site of enzymatic cleavage into F(ab')$_2$ and Fc fragments

Histocompatible. Sharing transplantation antigens

HLA (human leukocyte antigen). The major histocompatibility complex in man

Homocytotropic antibody. Antibody which attaches to cells of animals of the same species

Homologous antigen. An antigen which induces an antibody and reacts specifically with it

Homozygous typing cells (HTC). Cells that carry the same allele at their two HLA-D loci (homozygous) which are used as stimulating cells in mixed lymphocyte cultures for the typing of HLA-D phenotypes

Horizontal transmission. The transmission of infection from individual to individual in a population rather than from parent to offspring

Hot antigen suicide. A technic in which an antigen is labeled with high-specific-activity radioisotope (^{131}I). Used either in vivo or in vitro to inhibit specific lymphocyte function by attachment to an antigen-binding lymphocyte, subsequently killing it by radiolysis

Humoral. Pertaining to molecules in solution in a body fluid, particularly antibody and complement

Hybridoma. Specific antibodies secreting *hybrid* cells obtained by fusion of plasma cells with myeloma cells

Hypersensitivity. The state, existing in a previously immunized individual, in which tissue damage results from the immune reaction to a further dose of antigen. If tissue damage is severe, the condition may be referred to as one form of allergy

Hypervariable regions. At least 4 regions of extreme variability which occur throughout the V region of H and L chains and which determine the antibody combining site of an antibody molecule

Hypogammaglobulinemia (agammaglobulinemia). Deficiency of all major classes of serum immunoglobulins

Ia antigens (I region-associated antigens). Antigens which are controlled by Ir genes and are present on lymphocytes and macrophages

Idiotope. An epitope of the antigen-binding site of an antibody

Idiotype. Unique antigenic determinants present on homogeneous antibody or myeloma protein. The idiotype appears to represent the antigenicity of the antigen-binding site of an antibody and is therefore located in the V region

IgA. Predominant immunoglobulin class present in secretions

IgD. Predominant immunoglobulin class present on human B lymphocytes

IgE. Reaginic antibody involved in immediate hypersensitivity reactions

IgG. Predominant immunoglobulin class present in human serum

IgM. A pentameric immunoglobulin comprising approximately 10% of normal human serum immunoglobulins, with a molecular weight of 900,000 and a sedimentation coefficient of 19 S

7S IgM. A monomeric IgM consisting of one monomer of 5 identical subunits

Immediate hypersensitivity. An immunologic sensitivity to antigens that manifests itself by tissue reactions occurring within minutes after the antigen combines with its appropriate antibody

Immune complexes. Antigen-antibody complexes

Immune elimination. The enhanced clearance of an injected antigen from the circulation as a result of immunity to that antigen brought about by enhanced phagocytosis of the reticuloendothelial system

Immune response genes (Ir genes). Genes which control immune responses to specific antigens

Immune surveillance. A theory which holds that the immune system destroys tumor cells, which are constantly arising during the life of the individual

Immunodominant. That antigenic determinant of an antigen which is dominant in eliciting antibody formation

Immunoelectrophoresis. A technic combining an initial electrophoretic separation of proteins followed by immunodiffusion with resultant precipitation arcs

Immunofluorescence. A histo- or cytochemical technic for the detection and localization of antigens in which specific antibody is conjugated with fluorescent compounds, resulting in a sensitive tracer which can be detected by fluorometric measurements

Immunogen. A substance which, when introduced into an animal, stimulates the immune response

Immunogenicity. Property of a substance making it capable of inducing a detectable immune response

Immunoglobulin. A glycoprotein composed of H and L chains which functions as antibody. All antibodies are immunoglobulins, but it is not certain that all immunoglobulins have antibody function

Imunoglobulin class. A subdivision of immunoglobulin molecules based on structural and unique antigenic differences in the C regions of the H chains. In man there are 5 classes of immunoglobulins designated IgG, IgA, IgM, IgD, and IgE

Immunoglobulin subclass. A subdivision of the classes of immunoglobulins based on structural and antigenic differences in the H chains. For human IgG there are 4 subclasses: IgG 1, IgG 2, IgG 3, and IgG 4

Immunopathology. Pathological changes partly or completely caused by the immune response

Immunosuppression. Suppression of immune responsiveness by irradiation, drugs, or microbial toxins

Immune tolerance. An immunologically specific reduction in immune responsiveness to a given antigen

Interferon. A heterogeneous group of low-molecular-weight proteins elaborated by infected host cells which protect noninfected cells from viral infection

Inv marker. See Km marker

I region. That portion of the major histocompatibility complex which contains genes that control immune responses

Ir genes. See Immune response genes

J chain. A glycopeptide chain which is normally found in polymeric immunoglobulins, particularly IgA and IgM

Joining. Linking together DNA segments (introns) of genes in somatic cells which are separated by non-translated DNA sequences (exons) in the germ line

Kappa (κ) chains. One of 2 major types of L chains

K cell. Killer cell responsible for antibody-dependent cell-mediated cytotoxicity

K and D regions. Genetic loci in the major histocompatibility complex of the mouse, coding for H-2 molecules which are the restricting elements of cytotoxic T cells

Kinin. A peptide that increases vascular permeability and is formed by the action of esterases on kallikreins, which then act as vasodilators

Km marker (also called **Inv**). Allotypic marker on the κ L chain of human immunoglobulins

Koch phenomenon. Delayed hypersensitivity reaction by tuberculin in the skin of a guinea pig following infection with *Mycobacterium tuberculosis*

Kupffer cells. Fixed mononuclear phagocytes of the reticuloendothelial system that are present within the sinusoids of the liver

Lambda (λ) chain. One of 2 major types of L chains

Latency. Stage of persistent infection in which microorganism causes no disease, but remains capable of activation and disease production

Latex fixation test. An agglutination reaction in which latex particles are used to passively adsorb soluble protein and polysaccharide antigens

LATS (long-acting thyroid stimulator). An antibody reacting with the thyroid stimulating hormone (TSH) receptor in the thyroid gland; this antibody is present in about 45% of patients with hyperthyroidism and causes delayed uptake of iodine in an animal assay system

LE cell phenomenon. Phagocytic leukocytes that have engulfed DNA, immunoglobulin, and complement and are present as a large homogeneous mass which is extruded from a damaged lymphocyte in systemic lupus erythematosus and other rheumatoid diseases

Lectin. A substance that is derived from a plant and has panagglutinating activity for red blood cells. Lectins are commonly mitogens as well

Leishmaniasis. Disease caused by protozoa of genus *Leishmania*, e.g. cutaneous leishmaniasis (oriental sore) or generalized leishmaniasis (kala-azar)

Leukocyte inhibitory factor (LIF). A lymphokine which inhibits the migration of polymorphonuclear leukocytes

Leukocyte mitogenic factor (LMF). A lymphokine that will induce normal lymphocytes to undergo blast transformation and DNA synthesis

Leucocytes. Circulating white blood cells. There are about 9,000/mm^3 in human blood, divided into granulocytes (polymorphs 68%–70% eosinophils 3% basophils 0.5%) and mononuclear cells (monocytes 4% lymphocytes 23–25%)

Light chain (L chain). Polypeptide chain present in all immunoglobulin molecules. Two types exist in most species and are termed kappa (κ) and lambda (λ)

Linkage disequilibrium. When alleles of two closely linked loci are found together more frequently than predicted by their individual gene frequencies

Lipopolysaccharide (also called endotoxin). A compound derived from a variety of gram-negative enteric bacteria which have various biologic functions including mitogenic activity for B lymphocytes

Low dose (low zone) tolerance. A state of tolerance induced with small subimmunogenic doses of soluble antigen

Lupus erythematosus. A fatal autoimmune disease, characterized by certain antinuclear antibodies

Ly antigens. Differentiation antigens present on thymocytes and peripheral T cells

Lymph nodes. Small pea-sized organs distributed widely throughout the body which are composed mostly of lymphoid cells

Lymphocyte. A mononuclear cell 7–12 µm in diameter containing a nucleus with densely packed chromatin and a small rim of cytoplasm

Lymphocyte activation (lymphocyte stimulation, lymphocyte transformation, or blastogenesis). An in vitro technic in which lymphocytes are stimulatedto become metabolically active by antigen or mitogen

Lymphocyte defined (LD) antigens. A series of histocompatibility antigens that are present on the majority of mammalian cells and detectable primarily by reactivity in the mixed lymphocyte reaction (MLR)

Lymphokine. Soluble factor released by primed lymphocyte on contact with specific antigen

Lysosome. Cytoplasmic sac present in many cells, bounded by a lipoprotein membrane and containing various enzymes. Plays an important part in intracellular digestion

Lysostrip. Removal of one kind of surface antigen by capping with subsequent reaction of the same cells with antibodies and complement to another kind of surface antigen. Employed for the demonstration of antigenic determinants on the same or different molecules

Lysozyme. An enzyme present in the granules of polymorphs, in macrophages, in tears, mucus and saliva. It lyses certain bacteria, especially gram-positive cocci, splitting the muramic acid-β (1-4)-N-acetylglucosamine linkage in the bacterial cell wall. It potentiates the action of complement on these bacteria

Macrophage activation factor (MAF). A lymphokine which will activate macrophages to become avid phagocytic cells

Macrophage chemotactic factor (MCF). A lymphokine which selectively attracts monocytes or macrophages to the area of its release

Macrophages. Phagocytic mononuclear cells that derive from bone marrow monocytes and subserve accessory roles in cellular immunity

Macrophage processing. Uptake of antigens by macrophages, especially in the form of large particles or microorganisms, and preparation of antigen or antigens for delivery to adjacent immunocompetent lymphoytes

Major histocompatibility complex (MHC). An as yet undetermined number of genes located in close proximity which determine histocompatibility antigens of members of a species

Mast cell. A tissue cell which resembles a peripheral blood basophil and contains granules with serotonin and histamine present

Memory cells. Sensitized cells generated during an immune response, and surviving in large enough numbers to give an accelerated immune response on challenge

β_2 Microglobulin. A protein (MW 11,600) that is associated with the outer membrane of many cells, including lymphocytes, and which may function as a structural part of the histocompatibility antigens on cells

Migration inhibitory factor (MIF). A lymphokine which is capable of inhibiting the migration of macrophages

Mitogens (also called **phytomitogens**). Substances which cause DNA synthesis, blast transformation, and ultimately division of lymphocytes

Mixed lymphocyte culture (mixed leukocyte culture) (MLC). An in vitro test for cellular immunity in which lymphocytes or leukocytes from different individuals are mixed and mutually stimulate DNA synthesis

Mixed lymphocyte reaction (MLR). See Mixed lymphocyte culture

Monoclonal immunoglobulin molecules. Identical copies of antibody which consist of one H chain class and one L chain type

Monoclonal protein. A protein produced from the progeny of a single cell called a clone

Monokines. Soluble factors released by activated macrophages/monocytes

Multiple myeloma. A paraproteinemic disorder consisting typically of the presence of serum paraprotein, anemia, and lytic bone lesions

Myeloma protein. Either an intact monoclonal immunoglobulin molecule or a portion of one produced by malignant plasma cells

Myeloperoxidase. An enzyme that is present within granules of phagocytic cells and catalyzes peroxidation of a variety of microorganisms

Natural antibody. Antibody present in the serum produced against unknown antigens, primarily antigenic structures of the intestinal microorganism flora

Neutralization. The process by which antibody or antibody and complement neutralizes the infectivity of microorganisms, particularly viruses

NK cells (natural killer cells). Cytotoxic cells of undefined lineage, responsible for cellular cytotoxicity without prior sensitization

Nonresponder. An animal unable to respond to an antigen, usually because of genetic factors

Nude mouse. A hairless mouse which congenitally lacks a thymus and has a marked deficiency of thymus-derived lymphocytes

Null cells. Cells lacking the specific identifying surface markers for either T or B lymphocytes

NZB mouse. A genetically inbred strain of mice in which autoimmune disease resembling systemic lupus erythematosus develops spontaneously

Ontogeny. The developmental history of an individual organism within a group of animals

Opsonin. A substance capable of enhancing phagocytosis. Antibodies and complement are the 2 main opsonins

Paralysis. The pseudotolerant condition in which an ongoing immune response is masked by the presence of overwhelming amounts of antigen

Paraproteinemia. A heterogeneous group of diseases characterized by the presence in serum or urine of a monoclonal immunoglobulin

Paratope. An antibody combining site for epitope, the simplest form of an antigenic determinant

Passive cutaneous anaphylaxis (PCA). An in vivo passive transfer test for recognizing cytotropic antibody responsible for immediate hypersensitivity reactions

Passive immunity. Transfer of preformed antibodies to non-immune individual by means of blood, serum components, etc. e.g. maternal antibodies transferred to fetus via placenta or milk, or immunoglobulins injected to prevent or modify infections

Patching. The reorganization of a cell surface membrane component into discrete patches over the entire cell surface

Pathogenic. Producing disease or pathological changes

Persistent infection. An infection in which the microorganism persists in the body, not necessarily in a fully infectious form, but often for long periods or throughout life

Peyer's patches. Collections of lymphoid tissue in the submucosa of the small intestine which contain lymphocytes, plasma cells, germinal centers, and T cell-dependent areas

Pfeiffer phenomenon. Demonstration that cholera vibrios introduced into the peritoneal cavity of an immune guinea pig lose their mobility and are lysed regardless of the presence of cells

Phagocytes. Cells which are capable of ingesting particulate matter

Phagocytosis. The engulfment of microorganisms or other particles by leukocytes

Phagolysosome. A cellular organelle which is the product of the fusion of a phagosome and a lysosome

Phagosome. A phagocytic vesicle bounded by inverted plasma membrane

Phylogeny. The developmental and evolutionary history of a group of animals

Phytohemagglutinin (PHA). A lectin which is derived from the red kidney bean *(Phaseolus vulgaris)* and which stimulates predominantly T lymphocytes

Pinocytosis. The ingestion of soluble materials by cells

Plaque-forming cells (PFC). Antibody producing cell capable of forming a hemolytic plaque in the presence of complement and antigenic erythrocytes

Plasma cells. Fully differentiated antibody-synthesizing cells which are derived from B lymphocytes

Pokeweed mitogen (PWM). A lectin that is derived from pokeweed *(Phytolacca americana)* and stimulates both B and T lymphocytes

Polyclonal mitogens. Mitogens which activate large subpopulations of lymphocytes

Polyethylenglycol (PEG). Substance used as fusion reagent for the production of somatic cell hybrids

Pre-B cells. Large immature lymphoid cells with diffuse cytoplasmic IgM which eventually develop into cells

Precipitation. A reaction between a soluble antigen and soluble antibody in which a complex lattice of interlocking aggregates forms

Primary follicles. Tightly packed aggregates of lymphocytes found in the cortex of the lymph node or in the white pulp of the spleen after antigenic stimulation. Primary follicles develop into germinal centers

Primary lymphoid organs. Lymphoid organs that are essential to the development of the immune response, i.e., the thymus and the bursa of Fabricius

Private antigen. A composition of antigenic determinants on MHC molecules characteristic of an allele

Properdin system (or alternate pathway of complement activation). A group of proteins which after activation by microbial substances (e.g. zymosan, complex polysaccharides a. o.) activate C 3 of the classical complement pathway independently of antibody-antigen reactions

Prostaglandins. A variety of naturally occurring aliphatic acids with various biologic activities, including increased vascular permeability, smooth muscle contraction, bronchial constriction, and alteration in the pain threshold

Prothymocytes. Immature precursors of mature thymocytes which develop within the thymus gland

Prozone phenomenon. Suboptimal immune reaction in vitro (precipitation, cytolysis, agglutination) which occurs in the region of antibody excess during immune reactions

Pyogenic microorganisms. Microorganisms whose presence in tissues stimulates an outpouring of polymorphonuclear leukocytes

Pyrogens. Substances released either endogenously from leukocytes or administered exogenously, usually from bacteria, and which produce fever in susceptible hosts

Reagin. Synonymous with IgE antibody. Also denotes a complement-fixing antibody which reacts in the Wassermann reaction with cardiolipin

Receptor. A chemical structure on the surface of any immunologically competent cell

Recombinant. An animal which has experienced a recombinational event during meiosis, consisting of cross-over and recombination of parts of 2 chromosomes

Rejection response. Immune response with both humoral and cellular components directed against transplanted tissue

Reservoir. Animal (bird, mammal, mosquito, etc.) or animals in which microorganism maintains itself independently of human infection

Restriction. Stimulation and activation of cooperating cells in the immune response occurs only if the reacting cells share either K, D molecules (cytotoxic T cells) or Ia molecules (helper/suppressor T cells), i.e. the recognition of antigens is restricted to the concomitant presence of antigen and the own MHC molecules

Reticuloendothelial system. A system of cells that take up particles and certain dyes injected into the body. Comprises Kupffer cells of liver, tissue, histocytes, monocytes, and the lymph node, splenic, alveolar, peritoneal, and pleural macrophages

Rh incompatibility. Incompatibility between certain blood group antigens of a mother and her baby or between donor and recipient in blood transfusions

Rheumatoid factor (RF). An anti-immunoglobulin antibody directed against denatured IgG present in the serum of patients with rheumatoid arthritis and other rheumatoid diseases

Rocket electrophoresis (Laurell technic). An electroimmunodiffusion technic in which antigen is electrophoresed into agar containing specific antibody and precipitates in a tapered rocket-shaped pattern. This technic is used for quantitation of antigens

Rose-Waaler test. A type of passive hemagglutination test for the detection of rheumatoid factor which employs tanned red blood cells coated with rabbit 7S IgG antibodies specific for sheep red blood cells

Schistosomiasis (= bilharzia). Disease with urinary symptoms common in many parts of Africa. Caused by the fluke (trematode) *Schistosoma haematobium;* larvae from infected snails enter water and penetrate human skin

Secondary lymphoid organs. Lymphoid organs not essential to the ontogeny of immune responses, i.e., the spleen, lymph nodes, tonsils, and Peyer's patches

Secretory IgA. A dimer of IgA molecules with a sedimentation coefficient of 11 S, linked by J chain and secretory component

Secretory immune system. A distinct immune system that is common to external secretions and consists predominantly of IgA

Secretory piece (T piece). A molecule of MW 70,000 produced in epithelial cells and associated with secretory immunoglobulins, particularly IgA and IgM

Self-recognition. Recognition of self-antigens by one's own immunologic system

Sensitized. Synonymous with immunized

Serologically defined (SD) antigens. Antigens that are present on membranes of nearly all mammalian cells and are controlled by genes present in the major histocompatibility complex. They can be easily detected with antibodies

Serology. Literally, the study of serum. Refers to the determination of antibodies to infectious agents important in clinical medicine

Serum (pl. sera). The liquid part of the blood remaining after cells and fibrin have been removed

Serum sickness. An adverse immunologic response to a foreign antigen, usually a heterologous protein

Shedding. The liberation of microorganisms from the infected host

Side chain theory. Theory of antibody synthesis proposed by Ehrlich in 1900 suggesting that specific side chains which form antigen receptors are present on the surface membranes of antibody-producing cells

Slow virus. A virus which produces disease with a greatly delayed onset and protracted course

Specificity. A term referring to the selective reaction which occurs between an antigen and its corresponding antibody or lymphocyte

Spleen. An organ in the abdominal cavity, composed largely of lymphocytes and macrophages. It is an important site of antibody production

S region. The chromosomal region in the H-2 complex containing the gene for a serum β-globulin (C4 complement component)

Streptococci. Classified into groups A–H by antigenic properties of carbohydrate extracted from cell wall. Important human pathogens belong to Group A ($=Streptococcus\ pyogenes$), which is divided into 47 types according to antigenic properties of M protein present on outermost surface of bacteria

Streptolysin O. Exotoxin produced by *Streptococcus pyogenes*. Oxygen-labile, haemolytic, and a powerful antigen

Streptolysin S. Exotoxin produced by *Streptococcus pyogenes*. Oxygen-stable, causing β haemolysis on blood agar plates, but not demonstrably antigenic

Suppressor T cells. A subset of T lymphocytes which suppress antibody synthesis by B cells or inhibit other cellular immune reactions by effector T cells

Surveillance. The process by which an intact immune system monitors both self and foreign antigens

S value. Svedberg unit. Denotes the sedimentation coefficient of a protein, determined usually by analytic ultracentrifugation

Syngeneic. Denotes the relationship which exists between genetically identical members of the same species

Systemic infection. Infection that spreads throughout the body

T cell (T lymphocyte). A thymus-derived cell which participates in a variety of cell-mediated immune reactions

T cell rosette. See E rosette

Teleology. Doctrine that biological phenomena generally have a purpose, serving some function

Thy-1 antigen (theta antigen). An alloantigen present on the surface of most thymocytes and peripheral T lymphocytes

Thymopoietin (originally termed thymin). A protein of MW 7,000 that is dervied originally from the thymus of animals with autoimmune thymitis and myasthenia gravis and which can impair neuromuscular transmission

Thymosin. A thymic hormone protein of MW 12,000 which can restore T cell immunity in rhymectomized animals

Thymus. The central lymphoid organ which is present in the thorax and controls the ontogeny of T lymphocytes

Thymus-dependent antigen. Antigen which depends on T cell interaction with B cells for antibody synthesis, e.g., erythrocytes, serum proteins, and hapten-carrier complexes

Thymus-derived lymphocytes (T lymphocyte). Small lymphocytes which on (or after) residence in the thymus attain new immunologic capabilities

Thymus-independent antigen. Antigen which can induce an immune response without the apparent participation of T lymphocytes

Tissue typing. The processes of identifying and matching antigens on prospective donor and recipient tissues

Titre (1). A measure of units of antibody per unit volume of serum, usually quoted as reciprocal of last serum dilution giving antibody-mediated reaction e.g. 120. (2) Measure of units of virus per unit volume of fluid or tissue. Usually given in log 10 units per ml or G e.g. $10^{5.5}$ pfu/ml

TL antigen. A membrane antigen that is present on prothymocytes in mice with a TL+ gene, but which is lost during thymic maturation

Tolerance. Traditionally denotes that condition in which responsive cell clones have been inactivated by prior contact with antigen, with the result that no immune response occurs on administration of antigen

Toxoids. Antigenic but nontoxic derivatives of toxins

T piece. See Secretory piece

Transfer factor. A dialyzable extract of immune lymphocytes that is capable of transferring cell-mediated immunity in humans and possibly in other animal species

Translocon. Stretch of chromosome containing gene sequences coding for heavy, kappa or lambda polypeptide chains of immunoglobulins

Transplantation antigens. Those antigens which are expressed on the surface of virtually all cells and which induce rejection of tissues transplanted from one individual to a genetically disparate individual

Tuberculin test. A skin test for delayed hypersensitivity to antigens from *Mycobacterium tuberculosis*. In man the antigen is introduced into the skin by intradermal injection (Mantoux test)

Tuftsin. A γ-globulin which is capable of stimulating endocytosis by neutrophils

Vaccination. Immunization with antigens administered for the prevention of infectious diseases (term originally coined to denote immunization against vaccinia or cowpox virus)

V antigens. Virally induced antigens which are expressed on viruses and virus-infected cells

Vertical transmission. The transmission of infection directly from parent to offspring. This can take place *in utero* via egg, sperm, placenta, or postnatally via milk, blood, contact, etc.

Viremia. Presence of virus in blood stream. Virus may be associated with leucocytes (leucocyte viraemia), or free in the plasma (plasma viraemia), or occasionally associated with erythrocytes or platelets

Virion. The complete virus particle

V (variable) region. The amino terminal portion of the H or L chain of an immunoglobulin molecule, containing considerable heterogeneity in the amino acid residues compared to the constant region

V region subgroups. Subdivisions of V regions of kappa chains based on substantial homology in sequences of amino acids

Wasting disease (runt disease). A chronic, ultimately fatal illness associated with lymphoid atrophy in mice who are neonatally thymectomized

Xenogeneic. Denotes the relationship which exists between members of genetically different species

Xenograft. A tissue or organ graft between members of 2 distinct or different species

References

Fudenberg HH, Stites DP, Caldwell JL, Wells JV (1980) Basic and clinical immunology, 4th ed. Lange Medical Publications, Los Altos/Calif.

Mims CA (1977) The pathogenesis of infectious diseases. Academic Press, New York

Amos DB (ed) (1976) Immunology: Its role in disease and health. US DHEW publication No. (NIH) 75–940

Subject and Author Index

Page numbers in *italics* refer to the principle discussion of each subject.

AAME (N-acetyl-arginine-methyl ester) 121
ABC (antigen binding capacity),
  inhibition of 219
  method 218
ABO blood group
  alloantibodies 229
  biochemistry 231
  genetics 229
  serology 227
  typing 311
abortion, clonal 310, 350, 383
acanthosis nigricans 399
actin polymerization deficiency,
  phagocyte deficiencies 378
actinomycin 435
acute leukemias 375–376
  B,T cell proliferative disorders
  375–376
  bone marrow transplantation
  314
acute respiratory distress syndrome, ARDS 129
adaptive immunity 330
ADCC, antibody-dependent cell-
  mediated cytolysis 292, 346
Addison's disease 398
adenosine-deaminase, ADA,
  deficiency 371
adenosine-deaminase deficiency,
  T,B cell combined deficiencies
  371
adherence, white blood cells 323,
  362
adherent cells 60
adjuvants 70, 417–420
  depot effect 71
  effect on cells 419
  immunostimulation 417
  mitogenicity 71
  tapioca 417
  target of action 418
adoptive immunization 243
adoptive transfer 355
adrenal 21-hydroxylase, 21-OH
  154
adrenogenitale syndrome, AGS
  176

adriamycin, immunostimulation
  422
affinity labeling technique 92
agammaglobulinemia 365
age, influence of immune response 108
agglutination 187, 332
  passive 191
agnates 32
agranulocystosis, infantile genetic
  377
Aldrich 271
alexin 115
alginate of calcium 70
alkaloids 435
alkylating agents 432
alleles, MHC 144
allelic exclusion 53, 101
alloantibodies
  ABO blood groups 229
  H-2 molecules 143–146
  HLA molecules 148–150
  Rh antigens 234
alloantigen 139
  B cells 54, 55
  erythrocytes 227, 297
  Gv 41
  histocompatibility 45, 143, 148
  leukocytes 143, 148, 297
  Lyt antigens 11, 41, 45, 55, 59
  Qa antigens 11
  T cells 11, 47, 55, 173
  TL antigen 12, 19, 41
  Thy-1 antigen 11, 19, 39, 41
  thymocytes 12, 19, 20
alloantiserum 73
  effect 61
  reactive cells 304
allogeneic 140, 297
alloreactivity 170
allotransplant 140
allotypes 98, 99
allotypic restriction 98
alpha chain
  T cell receptor 172
alpha chain disease 369
alpha method of precipitation 181
alpha-naphtyl acetate 363

alternative complement pathway
  133, 135
  properties of components 134
alum 71
aluminium hydroxide 70
aluminium phosphate 70
am, human Ig allotype 98
amebiasis 343
amino acid antagonists 436
aminopterine 79, 436
amphibians 32
ANA, anti-nuclear-antibodies in
  LE 409
anaphylactic shock, after serotherapy 352
anaphylatoxin 116, 128
anaphylaxis
  acute 267
  atopy 268
  basophils 259
  bradykinin 253
  cAMP 265, 272
  calcium influx 265
  cells involved 255–257
  eosinophil chemotactic factor
  252, 254
  eosinophils 260
  Forssman shock 266
  in guinea pigs 245–267
  heparin 255
  leukotriens 254
  local 267
  in man 267–278
  mechanism 244
  mediators 244, 252
  neutrophil chemotactic factor
  254
  passive 246
  platelet activating factor 252,
  255
  platelets 259
ancylosing spondylitis 176
ancylostoma duodenale 345
anemia
  aplastic 315
  autoimmune hemolytic 399
  autoimmune in NZB mice 401
  autoimmune in dogs 402
  pernicious 173, 403

anergy   388
aneuploidy   376
animal
  Ig   97
  MHC   156
annelids   32
anti-idiotype antibody   271
antibacterial sera
  protective action of   212
antibiotics   435
antibodies *see also* immunoglobulin
  affinity labeling technique   92
  agglutination   187, 332
  allotypes   98
  anti-basement   404
  antigen combining site   91
  antigen complexes, type III hy-
    persensitivity   279
  binding site   67
  blocking   270, 297
  catabolism   89
  chromatography   82, 87
  classes human   92
  classes of horse Ig   97
  classes of rodent Ig   97
  clonal selection theory   100, 105
  Cohn fractination   83
  cold   399
  dependent cell-mediated lym-
    pholysis, ADCC   292, 302,
    305, *306*
  detection in infectious diseases
    332
  differentiation of   78
  differentiation of antibody form-
    ing cells   78
  domains   89
  Donath-Landsteiner   400
  dynamics of formation   74
  electronmicroscopy   100
  enzymatic fragmentation   87
  feedback control of synthesis
    109
  forming cells   78
  Forssmann   74
  frame work region   91
  generation of diversity   101, 105
  H chain translocon   103
  heavy chain, gene structure   102
  heavy chain, protein structure
    86
  heterocytotropic   248
  heterogeneity   84, 89
  hinge region   88
  homocytotropic   248
  hypervariable region   91
  idiotypes   99
  IgA   94
  IgD   95
  IgE   96
  IgG   93

IgM   93
J(unction) chain   94
kappa chain   90
kappa chain translocon   103
lambda chain   90
mediated inhibition   384
monoclonal   79
nomenclature of animal Ig   97
physicochemical properties   93,
    94
precipitation   83, 180, 332
preformed (natural)   318, 320
primary response   74
production   39
purification   81
regulation of formation   105
regulatory cell circuits of anti-
    body formation   111
secondary response   75
secretion piece of IgA   95
sedimentation constant   84
serologic reactions   179
structure   85, 94
subclasses human   92
subclasses of rodent Ig   97
synthesis of IgA   95
translocons   101
transport piece of IgA   95
variable region   90
warm   399
antibody-antigen complexes   350
antibody-dependent cell-mediated
    cytotoxicity, ADCC   45, 292,
    302, 305, 306
antibody-mediated inhibition   384
antibody reactions
  agglutination   187, 332
  complement fixation   196, 332
  conglutination   203
  immunoadherence   202
  immunocytolysis   21
  immunocytotoxicity   201
  immunofluorescence   194, 332
  neutralization, toxin   209
  opsonization   206
  precipitation   180, 332
  serologic reactions   179
antigen   63
  antibody formation related to
    105
  CD   361
  cluster of differentiation   55
  combining site, structure   91
  competition   348
  determinants   67
  E 271
  Forssman   67, 74
  leukocyte specific   315
  lipid   64
  loss   349
  natural   65

neutrophil specific   316
particulate   75
phylogenic distance   106
platelet specific   316
polar groups   65
polylysine, PLL   69
polysaccharide   66, 75
protein   64, 68, 75
protein, molecular weight   106
recall   361
recognition by antibodies   89
recognition by T cells   162
seclusion   348, 386
species-specific   67
synthetic   64
T cell receptor   56
thymus-independent   72
variation   348
antigen-antibody complex reaction,
    hypersensitivity type III   279
antigenic determinants   1, 64
antigenic drift, influenza virus
    338
antigenic shift, influenza virus
    339
antilymphocyte serum (globulin)
    427
  immunosuppressors   427
  mechanism of action   428
antimetabolites, immunosup-
    pressors   433
antitoxin, avidity   211
antiviral effector molecules,
    AVEMs   337
aquafor   71
arachidonic acid in anaphylaxis
    254
arlacel   71
arthritis, rheumatoid   176
Arthus   131, 283
Arthus reaction   131, 279, 283
ascaris lumbricoides   345
Aschoff   205
Askenase   294
asparaginase   436
ataxia teleangiectasia, T,B cell
    combined deficiencies   372
ATEE, n-acetyl-L-tyrosine-ethyl
    ester   121
athymic mice   41
atopy   109, 268
Austen   263
Australia antigen   187
autoantibodies   383, 384
autogenic   140
autoimmune disease
  acanthosis nigricans   399
  Addison's disease   398
  anemia, autoimmune
    hemolytic   399
  blood   399

central nervous system 392
classification 393
endocrine glands 396
erythrocytes 399
experimental allergic encephalo-
    myelitis 392
eye 407
factors influencing 389
gastrointestinal tract 403
Graves disease 398
Hashimoto thyreoiditis 396
heart 407
induction 386
infectious agents in 390
insulin-dependant diabetes melli-
    tus 398
kidney 404
liver 403
lung 406
lupus erythematosus, systemic
    408
mechanisms 392
multiple sclerosis 394
myasthenia gravis 395
pancreatitis, autoimmune 398
progressive systemic sclerosis,
    PSS 413
rheumatoid arthritis 411
skin 408
specific 391–413
systemic 408–413
thyreoiditis, experimental
    autoimmune 396
tissue lesions 391
autoimmune symptoms,
    associated with immunodeficien-
        cies 391
    associated with infections 389
autoimmunity 384, 386
autorecognition 63, 383, 386
autotransplant 140
auxiliary regulatory circuits 113
avidity, antitoxin 211
azathioprine (Imuran) 433

B animals 303
B cell
    alloantigen 54, 55
    differentiation factor 49
    immunodeficiencies 364–370
    tolerance 310
B complex, chicken major his-
    tocompatibility complex 140
B factor B 134
B factor, man 154
B lymphocytes 12, 48
    activation 49
    anti serum 39
    clonal expansion 50
    differences from T 54
    differentiation of 13

evaluation of function 360
IgE producing, ontogeny 263
marker 55
B,T cell, immunodeficiencies
    371–373
B,T cell proliferative disorder
    acute leukemias 375–376
    Burkitt's lymphoma 374
    childhood lymphoblastic lym-
        phoma 374
    chronic lymphatic leukemia
        376
    classification 374
    cutaneous lymphoma, mucosis
        fungoides 375
    immunodeficiencies 373–377
    leukemias 375
    lymphomas 373–375
    Sezary syndrome 375
    T cell lymphoma 375
    babesia 349
Bach 152
backcross system 141
bacterial infections 334
bacterial toxins 335
bactericidal deficiencies 379
bactericidy
    oxygen-dependent 324
    oxygen-independent 326
bacteriolysis, complement-medi-
    ated 116, 127
Baroni 311
basophils 8, 344
    in anaphylaxis 259
Basten 77
Bayol F 71
BCG 355
    vaccine 209
Becker 263
Behrendt 257
Behring 209
Benaceraff 20, 97, 109, 165
Bence-Jones protein 89
Bennich 262
Bert 311
beryllium sulfate 70
bestatin, immunostimulation 421
beta method of precipitation 181
Binz 56
Biozzi 76, 203
birds
    immune system 22, 23
Bittner virus 176
Bjorneboe 52
Black 253
Blaser 271
blast 39
    transformation 49, 150
blocking antibodies 270, 297
Bloom's syndrome 376
Blundell 227

Bombay type, erythrocyte blood
    group 228
bone marrow transplantation
    indications 314
    prognosis 314
booster 75, 109
Bordet 115, 116, 187, 196, 199
Boyden chamber 130, 362
Boyden's technique 192
Boyse 11, 303
bradykinin in anaphylaxis 253
Bruton-type hypogammaglobu-
    linemia 365
Burkitt's lymphoma, B,T cell pro-
    liferative disorders 374
Burnet 100, 163, 308, 383
bursa of Fabricius 2, 22
bursectomy in chicken 365
bursectomy, immunosuppressors
    426
C genes 102
C reactive protein 320
C1 120
C1-esterase 121, 131
C1-esterase deficiency 121, 380
C1q solid phase radioimmune as-
    say 282
C1R, C3b-receptor 134
C2 123
C3 123
C3-convertase 124, 164, 174
C3 gene, man 124
C3 gene, mouse 147
C3b-inactivator 124
C3b receptor 54
C4 122
C4 gene, man 154
C4, man 154, 164
C4, mouse 146, 164
C5 124
C6 124
C7 124
C8 124
C9 125
cAMP, in anaphylaxis 265, 272
CD, see cluster of differentiation
CD antigens 361
    on T cells 173
CD8 antigen, structure 161
calcium alginate 70
calcium influx, anaphylaxis 265
Campbell 84
Cantor 11, 112, 303
capillary tube migration test 362
capping 51, 157
Capron 259
caps 51
Carrel 311
carrier 64
cartwheel picture 13
Castellani's test 191

Catty   262
celiac disease   176
cell mediated hypersensitivity   284
cell-mediated cytotoxicity   305,
   333
   genetics   305
cell-mediated immunity, assay systems   333
cellular immunity, macrophages
   61
cellular typing, human   150
cestodes   339, 345
chagas disease   343
Chediak-Higashi syndrome, phagocyte deficiencies   376, 378
chemiluminescence   324
chemotactic deficiencies   378
chemotactic factors   116, 129, 322
   eosinophils   291
   lymphocytes   291
   macrophages   291
   neutrophils   291
chemotactic substances,
   generation   321, 331
chemotaxis   320, 321, 333
Chen   277
Chido, complement marker   137,
   154
childhood lymphoblastic lymphoma, B,T cell proliferative
   disorders   37
chimerism   314
chloramines   325
chloramphenicol   435
cholera vaccine   356
Christiansen   197
chromoglycate   272
chromosomal location of Ig genes
   101
chronic granulomatous disease,
   CGD of childhood   379
chronic lymphatic leukemia, B,T
   cell proliferative disorders
   376
chronic lymphatic leukemias,
   CLL   376–377
chronic myeloid leukemia, CML
   377
chronic myelomonocytic
   leukemia   377
cimetidine, immunostimulation
   421
Cinader   211
Cinader index   211
cistrons of Ig   101
class I genes, mouse   143
class I molecules, structure   159
class II genes, mouse   144
class II molecules, structure   161
class III molecules, structure   162
classes of animal Ig   97

classes of human antibodies   92
classification
   autoimmune disease   393
   B,T cell proliferative disorders
      374
   hypersensitivity   244
   immunodeficiencies   364
   immunosuppressors   424
   lymphomas   374
clonal (T cell) abortion   373
clonal deletion   310
clonal expansion   50, 105
clonal inactivation   384
clonal selection   78, 105
   theory of antibody formation
      100
clone, B lymphocyte   13
cloning, monoclonal antibodies
   79
clonotypic determinant   171
cluster of differentiation, CD   47,
   55
Cobra venom factor   128, 136
Cohn   83, 383
Cohn fractionation of antibodies
   83
Cohn's fractionation   352
colchicine   435
colitis, ulcerative   403
Collins   373
colony stimulating factor, CSF   5
complement   118
   alternative pathway   133
   biologic activities   127
   biosynthesis   137
   C1   123
   C1-esterase   121, 131
   C2   123
   C3   123
   C3-convertase   124, 164, 174
   C4   122
   C5   124
   C6   124
   C7   124
   C8   124
   C9   125
   cascade   119
   deficiencies   177, 380–382
   dependent liberation of hista-
      mine   130
   fixation   89, 196, 332
   fixation, mechanism   199
   formation of kinines   131
   hereditary deficiencies   137, 380
   in host defense against infec-
      tion   132
   MHC linked components   174
   nomenclature   118
   properties of human   118
   quantitative determination   126

solubilization of immune complexes   137
tissue injuries   131
titration of hemolytic   116
concanavalin A, Con A   60
configuration, protein   192
   spatial   65
conformational determinants   68
congenic mouse strains   142
   nomenclature   142
   production   141
congenital (passive) immunity
   350
conglutinin activating factor   124,
   203
conglutinin radioimmune assay
   282
connective tissue mast cells   8
contingency table   149
Coombs   399
Coomb's test   400
Coons   52, 75, 195
cooperation between T and B lymphocyte   57–59
cord factor   418
core regulatory circuits   112
correlation coefficient test   149
corticosteroids   428
   effects on lymphocytes   430
   immunosuppressors   428–430
   mechanism of action   429
Cosenza   110
counter-immunoelectrophoresis
   186
Crohn's disease   403
cross-absorption   143
cross-reaction   65
   agglutination   190
   precipitation   218
51Cr-release assay   165
cutaneous basophil hypersensitivity   294, 342
cutaneous delayed
   hypersensitivity   61
cutaneous lymphoma, mucosis fungoides, B,T cell proliferative
   disorders   375
cyclophosphamide, immunostimulation   422
cyclosporin A,
   immunostimulation   421
cysticercosis   345
cytolysis, complement-mediated
   116, 125
cytoreductive treatment   314
cytotoxic lymphocyte   45
cytotoxic reaction, hypersensitivity
   type II   278
cytotoxicity
   cell-mediated   333

eosinophil-IgG   347
  macrophage-IgE   347
cytotropy   89

D, C3-proactivator convertase
  134
Dale   246, 269
Dausset   148
Dean   181
degranulation   362
  phagocytosis   323
delayed hypersensitivity   39, 61,
  71, 284 ff.
  contact sensitivity   287
  effector cells   289
  mast cells   294
  pathogenesis   285, 293
  protein   287
  transfer   288
  transfer factor   288
  tuberculin   286
deletion   383
depot effect   71
dermatitis, contact   287
dermatitis herpetiformis   176
Deutsch   83
Deutsch's paraproteinemia   369
de Weck   271
DFP, diisoporyl fluorophosphate
  121
diGeorge's syndrome   370
diabetes, juvenile   176
dialysis, equilibrium   222
diazotization   65
dichotomy of lymphatic system   4,
  22
differences between T and B lymphocytes   54
differentiation of antibody forming
  cells   78
  differentiation, antigen-depen-
    dent   111
  cluster of, CD   47, 55
  human T lymphocytes   47
  lymphoid cells   2
  mouse T lymphocytes   10, 20,
    40 ff.
  plasma cells   53
  thymic cells   19
digestion, intracellular   208
diphyllobothrium latum   345
disease association, to MHC   176
diversity of antibodies,
  generation   101, 105
diversity, D segment, Ig genes
  104
DLA, dog leukocyte antigen   140
Doherty   164
domains of antibodies   89
Donath   399

Donath-Landsteiner antibodies
  400
DP antigens, HLA   152
dracunculus medinensis   345
DTH skin test   333
DTP, diphteria-tetanus-pertussis
  vaccine   355
Durham   187

E, antigen   154, 271
ECF-A
  eosinophil chemotactic factor-A,
    in anaphylaxis   252, 254
  metazoal infection   346
  eosinophil chemotactic factor
    133, 322
  enhancing factor of allergy   277
echinococcus granulosis   343, 345
echinococcus multilocularis   342,
  345
ecotaxis   36
Edelman   85, 86
Ehrlich   100, 199, 210, 256, 307,
  383
ELISA, enzyme-linked immunosorbent assay   221, 332
encephalomyelitis
  acute disseminated   395
  experimental allergic   392
endophthalmitis phaco-anaphylactica   407
end-point dilution   189
enhancement   297, 307, 385
enzyme-linked immunosorbent assay, ELISA   221, 332
eosinophil stimulation promotor,
  ESP   346
eosinophilia   344, 346
eosinophils   8
  in anaphylaxis   260
  chemotactic factors   291
epitopes   1, 64, 110
equilibrium dialysis   222
erythroblastosis fetalis   110
erythrocytes, alloantigen   297
euglobulin   81, 203
eurotransplant   312
exotoxins   334
external image of the idiotype   63

fab, antigen-binding fragment   87
Falba   71
Fanconi's anemia   376
Farr   217
fasciola hepatica   342, 345
Fc, crystallizable fragment   87
Fe-receptor   46, 55
feedback control of antibody synthesis   109
feedback inhibition of antibody
  synthesis   109

Feldman   77
Feldman and Basten chamber   77
Fenner   308
Ferrata   116
fetal erythroblastosis   353
fibrinopeptide B   132
Fick's law   181
filopodia   350
Fisher   234
Fisher-Race nomenclature   235
Fleischman   86
flocculation   211, 332
fluorescence microscopy   194
fluorescent quenching   222, 223
5-fluorouracil   434
folic acid antagonists   434
Foreman   265
Forssman   266
Forssman antigen   67
Forssman shock   266
Fragraeus   52
frame work, regions of, FR   91 ff
Franklin's disease   368
Freund's adjuvant   71
Friedburger   128
Friend virus   176
Fudenberg   98, 365
Fulthrope   182

GAT, glutamine-alanine-tyrosine
  42
gametic association, HLA   153
gamma chain disease   368
gammopathies
  alpha chain disease   369
  Deutsch's paraproteinemia   369
  heavy chain disease   368
  light chain abnormalities   370
  mu chain disease   369
  polyclonal   370
gastric atrophy   403
Gauss's function   222
gel precipitation   181
genetics, HLA   152
  complement   124
  immune response   109
Gengou   196
germinal centers   26
Gershon   42, 112
Giemsa staining   9
Glo gene
  man   154
  mouse   147
glomerulonephritis   131, 279, 283,
  404
  experimental   202
glucose-6-phosphate dehydrogenase deficiency   381
glutathion peroxidase deficiency
  381
glyoxalase genes   147, 154

Gm, human Ig allotype 98
Good 315
Goodpasture syndrome 131, 176, 405, 406
Gorer 139, 311
GPLA, guinea pig leukocyte antigen 140
Grabar 84, 184, 386
graft
    heterotopic 297
    orthotopic 297
graft rejection
    genetics 299, 300, 304
    hyperacute 313
    mechanism 301
graft versus host reaction 297, 299
    disease 401
    genetics 300
granulocytopoiesis 6
granulopoietin 5
Graves' disease 176, 398
Gross virus 176
growth factors, immunostimulation 416
Grubb 98
Gruber 187
guanidine silica 70
Guthrie 311

H agglutinogen 228
H chain translocon 103
H-2 recombinant strains 147
    linkage analysis 146
    mouse major histocompatibility complex 140
H-2A,E molecules, structure 161
H-2K,D molecules, structure 159
Haber-Weiss cycle 326
Hacek 308
Hageman factor 322
hagfish 32
Haldane 139
haplotypes, HLA 153
hapten 64
hapten-antibody reaction, thermodynamics 223
Hardy-Weinberg theorem 152
Hashimoto thyreoiditis 396
    antibodies in 397
Hassal's corpuscle 15
HAT medium 79
hay-fever 270, 275
heat labile serum factor, HLF 204
heavy chain disease 368
heavy chain of Ig 86
heavy chain switch 104
Heidelberger 84, 214, 217
Heidelberger-Kendall method 217

helper lymphocytes 41
hemagglutination 187, 332
hemodialysis 312
hemoglobinuria, paroxysmal nocturnal 400
hemolysis 179, 332
    immune 116, 127
hemopoietic-inducing microenvironment, HIM 1
heparin in anaphylaxis 255
hepatitis HBs antigen 187
    chronic active 176, 403
Herzenberg 112
HETE, 12-L-hydroxy-5,8,10,14-eicosatetraenoic acid 133, 321
heterocytotropic antibodies 248
heterotopic graft 297
hetrazan 272
hexosemonophosphate shunt 324
HHT, 12-L-hydroxy-5,8,10-heptadecatrienoic acid 133, 321
HIM, see hemopoietic-inducing microenvironment 1
hinge region 88
histamine in anaphylaxis 252, 253
    complement-dependent release 130
    receptors 253
    released from mast cells 132
histamine-sensitizing factor, HSF 71
histiocytes 9
histocompatibility,
    alloantigen 143, 148
    antigens 45
    major complex,
    allele frequency 144
        alloreactivity 170
        cellular typing, HLA 150
        cytogenetics of mouse 147
        disease association 176
        genes 140
        genetic map, man 155
        genetic map, mouse MHC 148
        H-2K,D genes mouse 143
        H-2K,D molecules 145
        human (HLA) 148
        Ia antigens 145, 146
        I-A locus 145
        I-E locus 146
        immune response genes, mouse 144
        L locus 146
        linkage analysis, man 154
        linkage analysis, mouse 148
        mouse 141
        mouse recombinant strains 147
        polymophism 144, 170
        restriction 164, 168, 169

serology, human 148
serology, mouse 13
tissue distribution of molecules 1
histogenesis of immun system 1
histology of immune system 1
    thymus dependent region 17, 23
    thymus independent regions 23
HLA disease association 176
    DP genes 152
    HLA-D gene(s) 151
    genetics 152
    human leukocyte antigen complex 148
HLA-A 149
HLA-A,B,C molecules, structure 159
HLA-B 149
HLA-C 149
HLA-D molecules, structure 161, 162
HLA-DQ 149
HLA-DR 149
HLA-DZ 149
Hockley 349
Hodgkin's disease 371
homing receptor of lymphocytes 37
homochromatosis, idiopathic 176
homocytotropic antibodies 248
homologous disease 401
Honjo 104
horse Ig 97
host versus graft reaction 297, 298
    genetics 299
Hozumi 102
HTC, homozygous typing cells, HLA 152
Hudack 51
human alloantigens
    cluster of differentiation 47, 55
    T lymphocytes 47
human gamma globulin, in serotherapy 352
hybridoma 78
hydrogen peroxide 61
hyperacute rejection, kidney 313
hypersensitivity 243–296
    anaphylaxis in guinea pigs 245
    anaphylaxis in man 267–278
    antibody-antigen complexes (type III) 279
    Arthus reaction 279, 283
    cell-mediated 284
    classification 244
    contact dermatitis 287
    cytotoxic reactions (type II) 278
    delayed type 284–294

immediate type 244–284
  mediators of 252
  serum sickness 285
  tuberculin reaction 286
hypervariable region of antibodies 91
hypogammaglobulinemia
  aquired primary 365
  aquired secondary 365
  Bruton-type 365
  in infants 364
  macroglobulinemia Walden-
    ström 367
  monoclonal gammopathies 367
  multiple myeloma 367
  polyclonal 370
  selective, variable 366–367
hypoxanthin-guanine-phosphoryl-
  transferase, HGPRT 79
hytatide cyst 345

I, C3b-inactivator 134
I region, mouse, molecule structure 161
I-A locus, mouse MHC 146
Ia molecule 61
idiotope 110
idiotype 42, 112
  external image of 63
idiotype-anti-idiotype network
  44, 63
idiotypic determinants, T cell receptor 56
idiotypic network 110
Ig genes 101
Ig superfamily 174
IgA 94
  and IgG selective deficiency 366
  and IgM selective deficiency 367
  selective deficiency 366
  synthesis 95
IgD 95
IgE 96
  dependent mediator secretion
    264
  macrophage cytotoxicity 347
  ontogeny of producing lympho-
    cytes 263
  reaginic antibody 249, 262
  receptor, structure 250–277
  response, metazoal infections
    342
IgG 93
  and IgA selective deficiency
    366
  selective deficiency 366
IgM 93
  and IgA selective deficiency
    367
  secrete 12
  selective deficiency 366

I-J antigen 43
image
  external of antibody 63
  internal of antibody 110
immobilization (TPI) test 202
immune complexes
  diseases associated with 280
  hypersensitivity type III 279
  methods of detection 282
immune response
  bacterial infections 334
  control by MHC 175
  escape from 348
    anatomical inaccessibility 347
    antigenic variation 348
    immunosuppression 349
    MHC antigen loss 349
    molecular masking 349
    seclusion 348
    soluble antigen 348
  evaluation of function 359
  genes (Ir-genes), mouse 144,
    145, 162, 166
  genetic factors 109
  in guinea pigs 107
  infections 331
  influence of age 108
  influence of antigen 106
  in LE patients 410
  macrophages in 59
  mapping 166
  maturation 53
  metazoal infections 342
  to parasites 340
  PLL gene 109
  primary 53, 63, 74
  protozoal infections 340, 343
  restriction 164, 168
  secondary 63, 75
  viral infections 334
immune serum
  with adjuvant 74
  monoclonal 79
  polyclonal 78
  preparation 73
immune system
  dichotomy 4, 22
  histogenesis 1
  histology 1
  homeostasis 385
  ontogeny 32
  phylogeny 32
immunity
  active 355
  adaptive 330
  aquisition 350
  concomitant 340
  escape 337
  natural 317
  nonsterilizing 340
  passive 350

sequence of events in 319
immunization, scheme 355, 356
immunoadherence 202
immunocompetence
  lymphocytes 38
  ontogeny of 108
immunocytoadherence 76
immunocytolysis 201
immunocytotoxicity 201
immunodeficiencies
  B cell 364–370
  B and T cell 371–373
  B and T cell proliferative dis-
    orders 373–377
  classification 364
  complement deficiencies 380–
    382
  phagocytic dysfunctions 377–
    381
  severe 315
  T cell 370–371
immunodiffusion 180 ff., 332
immunoelectrophoresis 184, 186,
  332
immunofluorescence 194
immunogen
  polysaccharides 106
immunogenicity 68
Immunoglobulin
  allotypes 98
  on B cell membrane 51
  binding factor, IBF 331
  catabolic elimination 360
  evaluation of function 359
  gene organisation 101
  genetic markers 97
  idiotypes 99
  maternal-fetal transfer 351
  secretion 53
  serotherapy 352
  structure of IgE 96
  synthesis 53
immunologic memory 38
immuno-osmophoresis 186
immunostimulants, thymic hormones 420
immunostimulation 416–424
  adjuvants 417
  adriamycin 422
  bestatin 421
  cimetidine 421
  cyclophosphamide 422
  cyclosporin A 421
  growth factors 416
  interferons 423
  isoprinosine 421
  levamisol 421
  lymphokines 421
  monokines 421
  thymic hormones 420
  tuftsin 421

immunosuppression 349
immunosuppressive agents 72
immunosuppressive therapy 314
immunosuppressors
  alkylating agents 432
  amino acid antagonists 436
  antibiotics 435
  antilymphocytic serum 427
  antimetabolites 433
  bursectomy 426
  classification 424
  corticosteroids 428–430
  folic acid antagonists 434
  irridation 426
  mechanism 424
  niridazole 436
  nucleic acid, inhibition of bio-
    synthesis 431
  plant alkaloids 435
  proteins, inhibition of biosynthe-
    sis 431
  rules 437
  specific 436
  thymectomy 425
immunotherapy 352
  mechanism in atopic diseases
    270
inbred strains, mouse 141
infections
  complement in 132
inflammatory lesions,
  pathogenesis 279
influenza vaccine 356
influenza virus
  antigenic drift 338
  antigenic shift 339
  pandemic strains 339
ingestion 323, 362
ingestion deficiencies, phagocyte
  deficiencies 378–379
inhibition of precipitation 219
instructive theory of antibody formation 100
insulin-dependent diabetes
  mellitus 398
insulitis 398
interferon 327, 330, 333, *336*
interferons, immunostimulation
  423
interleukin-1, IL-1 49, 327, 330
  properties 170
interleukin-2, IL-2 49, 330
  properties 170
internal image 110
intraleukocyte killing test 379
intrinsic factor 403
In V, human Ig allotype 98
IPCA, inverse passive cutaneous
  anaphylaxis 247
Ir gene 109, 275
  mouse 144, 145, *162*, 167

irradiation
  immunosuppressors 426
  lethal 19
Isaacs 336
ISF, human IG allotype 98
Iskizaka 96, 199, 276
isofixation curve, antibody-antigen
  reaction 199
isogenic 140
isoprinosine, immunostimulation
  421
isothiocyanate 194
isotransplant 140
Issaeff 115

Jenner 355
Jerne 44, 63, 100, 105, 110, 417
Jerne plaque technique 76
Job's syndrome, phagocyte
  deficiencies 378
Johansson 262
joining, J segment 103, 104
Jones-Mota reaction 294
j(unction) chain of IgM 94

Kabat 67, 84, 92, 105, 219
KAF 134
Kala-Azar 343
Kaposi sarkom 176
Kapp 42
kappa chain 90
kappa chain translocon 103
Kataoka 104
Katz 271, 277
Kendall 217
Kendrew 68
Kern, isotype of human lambda
  chain 98
kidney transplantation 312
  complications 313
  pregnancy 313
  survival 313
Kiel classification of lymphomas
  374
killer cells 45
Kindred 168
Kishimoto 276
Kitasato 209
Kline test 191
ko, platelet specific antigen 316
Koch 286
Koch's phenomenon 286
Köhler 78, 110
Korngold 90
Kostmann 377
Küstner 247, 268
Kupffer cells 9
Kwashiorkor 108

L locus, mouse MHC 146
lactoferrin 326

lactoperoxidase 317
lambda chain 90
lambda chain translocon 102
lamprey 32
Landsteiner 64, 100, 227, 399
Landsteiner's rule 228
Langerhans cells 61
Lapresle 66
latency 328
latex test 332
Laurell 186
Lawrence 288
lazy leukocyte syndrome, phagocyte deficiencies 378
leader, L segment, Ig genes 103
leishmania 327, 340, 343
Lennert 373
leukemias, B,T cell proliferative
  disorders 375
leukin 208
leukoaggressin 132
leukocidin 329
leukocytes, alloantigen 297
leukokininase 323
leukopenia, autoimmune 402
leukotrienes in anaphylaxis 254
Leung 290
levanisol, immunostimulation
  421
levine 227, 234, 275
Lewis, blood group system 230
life span
  lymphocytes 37, 109
  monocytes 9
  polymorphnuclear cells 5
light chain abnormalities 370
light chain of Ig 86
Lindemann 336
lingual tonsil 30
linkage analysis
  animals 156
  H-2 148
  HLA 154
linkage disequilibrium 152
Lipari 90
lipochrome histiocytosis 381
lipomodulin 276
lipopolysaccharides 71
Little 139, 311
liver surface protein, LSP 404
loa loa 345
local lymph node weight test 299
locomotion of polymorphnuclear
  cells 7
Loeb 139, 311
Lukes 373
Lukes and Collins classification of
  lymphomas 374
lupus erythematosus,
  experimental 411
  systemic 408

Lutheran, blood group system 230
lymph nodes 23
  autoradiograph of 31
lymph vessels 2
lymphatic cells 5, 9, 35
  B lymphocytes 12
  differentiation 2
  origin 2
  stem cell 21
  subpopulations 42
  T lymphocytes 10, 41
lymphatic system
  dichotomy 4
  primary organs 3
  secondary organs 23
lymphochoriomeningitis virus, LCM 176
lymphocyte mitogenic factor, LMF 331
  stimulation 333
  typing, primary 149
lymphocytes 9, 35
  chemotactic factors 291
  homing receptors 37
  immunocompetence 38
  life-span 37
  migration 35
  mitotic activity 15
  thymus-dependent 39
  thymus-independent 39
  trapping 30
lymphocytotoxicity 202
lymphoid follicles 26
  nodules 23
  stem cell defect, T,B cell combined deficiencies 371
lymphokines 132, 330, 331
  immunostimulation 421
  properties 291
lymphomas, B,T cell proliferative disorders 373–375
lymphotoxins 291, 330, 331, 333
lysosomes 9
lysozyme 201, 208, 317, 324, 326, 327
Lyt antigens 11, 41, 55, 59

M protein, streptococcal 177
macrophage activating factor 291
  inhibition factor, MIF 302
  inhibition test 282, 290
macrophage-T cell cooperation 303
macrophages 9, 59
  chemotactic factors 291
  in immunity 326
  marker 55
major histocompatiblity complex, MHC 20, 139 ff
malaria 343

Malpighian bodies 28
Maltaner 197
Mancini 181, 269
Mancini test 181, 360
Mantoux test 287
Mantovani 280
Marbrook culture 77
Marx 51
mast cell 8, 344
  anaphylaxis 255
  delayed hypersensitivity 294
  eosinophil cooperation 346
mastocytes in anaphylaxis 255
Masugi nephritis 404
maternal-fetal transfer, immunity 340, 350
maturation, immune response 53, 108
Maximow 35
Mayer 116, 197
MBP, major basic protein 133
McDevitt 165
McLeod phenotype, Kell blood group 381
McMaster 51
measle vaccine 355
Medawar 140, 308, 311
mediator secretion, IgE dependent 264
mediators, liberation 274
mediterranean lymphoma 369
megakaryocytes 14
memory, cells 39, 75, 109
  immunologic 38
meningitis 106
6-Mercaptopurine 433
Merril 311
metazoa
  human pathogenic 345
  vectors 345
metazoal infections 342
Metchnikoff 5, 204
methotrexate 79, 435
Meyer 126
MHC see major histocompatibility complex
  antigen loss 349
  genetic organisation, BoLA, cattle 156
  ChLA, chimpanzee 156
  DLA, dog 156
  ELA, horse 156
  GPLA, guinea pig 156
  H-2, mouse 156
  H-B, chicken 156
  HLA, man 156
  OLA, sheep 156
  RhLA, rhesus monkey 156
  RLA, rabbit 156
  RT1, rat 156
  SLA, swine 156

  linked complement components 174
  restriction 165, 169
MHC molecules
  biochemistry 158
  class I, structure 159
  class II, structure 161
  class III, structure 162
  tissue distribution 156
micro-dye exclusion test 202
microcomplement consumption test 282
microdrop, technique 78
microfilaria 349
β_2-microglobulin 160
microorganisms 328
MIF 375
  macrophage inhibition test 290
migration
  current 36
  inhibition 333
  inhibition factor 330, 331
  leukocytes 320, 321
  lymphocytes 35
Milstein 78
mineral oil emulsion 70
minimum lethal dose, MLD 209, 210
minimum reactive dose, MRD 209
mitogenic factor 291
mitogenicity of adjuvants 71
mitogens 60
mixed lymphocyte culture, MLC 45, 150, 302, 311
MNSs blood group system 232
mobility, white blood cells 362
molecular mimicry 177
Mongar 265
monoclonal antibodies
  cloning 79
  to HLA 149
  production 79
monocytes 9
monokines 327
  immunostimulation 421
Mota 256, 262, 276
mouse alloantigens
  T lymphocytes 11
mu chain disease 369
mucocutaneous candidiasis 370
Müller-Eberhard 124
multiple sclerosis 176, 394
mumps vaccine 355
Murray 311
myasthenia gravis 176, 395
myelin basic protein 393
myeloperoxidase deficiency 381
myoglobin 68

NA, neutrophil antigen 316
NADPH-oxidase deficiency 381

Nakagawa 271
α-Naphtyl acetate 363
narcolepsy 176
Nash 290
Nathenson 158
natural killer cells 46
NB, neutrophil antigen 316
NBT, nitroblue tetrazolium dye 324
NBT test 381
necator americanus 345
nematodes 339, 345
    human pathogenic 345
neutralization
    mechanism 212
    toxin 209, 332
    of virions 335
neutropenia, cyclic 377
    familial severe 377
    immuno 378
    phagocyte deficiencies 377–378
neutrophil chemotactic factor in anaphylaxis 254
neutrophils 5
    chemotactic factors 291
Newhauser's space 365
Nezelof's syndrome, T,B cell combined deficiencies 372
Nicholson 157
niridazole 436
Nisonoff 110
nitroblue tetrazolium dye 324
nitrogen mustard 432
nomenclature
    animal Ig 97
    congenic mouse strains 142
    histocompatibility 140
    human Ig 97
    inbred strains 141
    transplantation 140
Nossal 78, 384
NP40, non-ionic detergent 159
nucleic acids, inhibition of biosynthesis 431
Nussenzweig 281

Oakley 182
Oakley's technique 183
Obermayer 65
onchocerca volvulus 345
onchocercosis 345
oncogenic virus 176
one-hit-theory, complement 126
one way reaction 151
one way stimulation 151
ontogeny
    IgE producing B lymphocytes 263
    immune system 30
    immunocompetent cells 108
    immunologic capacity 351

ophthalmia, sympathetic 408
oppossum 33
opsonization 116, 130, 204, 206, 322, 362
oriental sore 343
orthotopic graft 297
osteoclasts 9
Ouchterlony 183
Ouchterlony test 183
Oudin 98, 181
Oudin's test 181
Owen 308
oxygen, singlet 325
Oz, isotype of human lambda chain 98

P, properdin 134
PAF, platelet activating factor, in anaphylaxis 252, 255
    structure 260
Pain 86
palatine tonsil 30
papain digestion of antibodies 88
parabiosis 308
paracortical region 24
paragonimus 342, 345
paratope 110
Parfentjev 83
PAS reaction 363
patch test 287
pathogenesis
    Arthus reaction 284
    serum sickness 285
Paul-Bunnell reaction 191
PCA, passive cutaneous anaphylaxis 247
Pedersen 84
pemphigus vulgaris 176, 408
pepsin digestion of antibodies 88
perfect fit, antibody-antigen reaction 108, 113
periarteriolar sheath 28
Perini 262
periodic acid Schiff reaction 363
permeability 320
Peyer's patches 3, 30, 318
Pfeiffer 51, 115
Pfeiffer's phenomenon 115, 201, 213
Pg-5 gene, mouse 147
    urine-pepsinogen-5, man 154
Pgk gene, mouse 147
PGm, phosphoglucomutase-3, man 154
phagocyte deficiencies
    actin polymerization deficiency 378
    Chediak-Higashi syndrome 378
    chemotactic deficiencies 378
    ingestion deficiencies 378–379

Job's syndrome 378
    lazy leukocyte syndrome 378
    neutropenias 377–378
    tuftsin deficiency 378
phagocyte dysfunctions, immunodeficiencies 377–381
phagocytic index 205
phagocytin 208
phagocytosis 59, 204
    complement-mediated 166, 322
    evaluation of function 362
    stimulation 71
phagolysosome 324, 328
phagosome 207, 323
pharyngeal tonsil 30
phylogenic distance of antigen 106
phylogenicity of immune system 30
physicochemical properties of human Ig 93
phythemagglutinin, PHA 60
Pick 65
Pillemer 136
PK reaction 247, 268
    inverse 270
PK test 96
plaque forming cells, PFC 77
    plaque technique, Jerne 76
    vaccine 356
plasma cell 13, 49, 51
    differentiation 54
plasmocytosis 52
platelet aggregation test 282
    factor 4 15
    lytic factor 347
    specific antigen 316
platelets 13
    in anaphylaxis 259
Plᵉ, platelet specific antigen 316
PLT gene 109
PLL, see polylysine
PLT, primary lymphocyte typing 152, 312
pokeweed mitogen stimulation 360
poliomyelitis vaccine 355
polyclonal gammopathies 370
polyethylenglycol 79
polylysine, PLL 69
polymorphism, genetic of MHC 144
polymorphnuclear cells
    characteristics 5
    in immunity 320
    locomotion 7
polynucleic acids 70
Pope 83
Porter 85, 86
Portier 244
postcapillary venules 25
PPD, purified protein derivative 286

Prausnitz 247, 268
Prausnitz-Küstner (PK) reaction
    247, 268
precipitation, antibody reaction
    180
precipitation reactions
    ABC method 218
    Heidelberger-Kendall method
        217
    immunodiffusion, double 182
        double radial (Ouchterlony)
            183, 332
        radial (Mancini) 181
        simple (Oudin) 181
    immunoelectrophoresis 184
    inhibition of 219
    in liquid media 180
    neutralization, toxin 209
    P-80 method 217
    quantitative 214
    rocket i-e 186
    two dimensional 186
Preer 183
preformed antibodies 318, 320
premunition 340
prepatency 345
primary lymphocyte typing 149
primary lymphoid organs
    activity 15
    function 4
    origin 3
primordial cell, immune system 41
private antigen 143
properdin 201
properdin syndrom, see alternative
    complement pathway
prostaglandins 327
    in anaphylaxis 252, 254
protective action of antibacterial
    sera 203
protein A, staphylococcus aureus
    159
protein elimination
    syngeneic 285
    xenogeneic 285
proteins, inhibition of bio-
    synthesis 431
protopod 7
protozoa 339
protozoal infections 340
protracted shock 246
prozone 188
pseudoglobulin 81
psoriasis vulgaris 176
public antigen 143
pulmonary edema 131
pulmonate fishes 32
purine nucleoside phosphorylase
    deficiency, T,B cell combined
    deficiency 372
puromycin 435

Qa antigens 11
Qa loci 147
quenching, fluorescent 222, 223

rabies vaccine 356
Race 234
radiation-induced leukemia virus
    176
radioallergosorbent test, RAST
    221, 268
radioimmunoassay 220, 332, 360
radioimmunodiffusion (Mancini)
    269
Raji cell assay 282
Ramon 70, 181
Ramon flocculation 181
Rappaport 373
Rappaport classification of lym-
    phomas 374
RAST, radioallergosorbent test
    221
Raynaud's syndrome 408
Rays 32
rearrangement of Ig genes 102
Rebuck skin test 363
recognition of antigen 162
red pulp, spleen 27
regulatory cell circuits 111
    regulatory circuits 44
Reisfeld 158
Reiter's disease 176
reptiles 32
respiratory burst 208, 323, 324
respiratory distress syndrom,
    acute 129
restriction, genetic of immune re-
    sponse 164, 168
reticular cells 61
reticular dysgenesia, T,B cell com-
    bined deficiencies 372
reticuloendothelial system, RES
    205
Rh blood group system 234
    genetics 235
    nomenclature 235
rheumatic fever 407
rheumatoid agglutinins 98
    arthritis 411
    factor 412
RhLA, rhesus monkey leukocyte
    antigen 140
rhodmine B 194
Richet 244
Rieckenberg reaction 202
Riley 256
ring test 180
Rivers 392
rocket immunoelectrophoresis 186
rodents, Ig 97
Rodgers, complement marker
    137, 154

Römer 210
Ropartz 98
Rose 383, 396, 412
Rose-Waaler test 412
Rosenthal 168
rosette formation 203
    technique 77
rosettes, erythrocytes 361
RT1, rat transplantation locus
    140
rubella vaccine 355
runt disease 299

S region, mouse MHC 146, 164
Sabin 355
Saito 57
sandwich technique, immuno-
    fluorescence 195
SA-P, sialic acid rich polysac-
    charide 134
saponin 70
Scatchard's equation 221
Schick reaction 360
Schild 253, 265
schistosoma hematobium 328,
    342, 345, 346
    japonicum 345
    mansoni 345
schlepper 64
Schultz 269
Schultz-Dale reaction 269
Schulze venules 26
SCID, severe combined immuno-
    deficiencies, T,B cell combined
    deficiencies 371
scleroderma 413
sclerosis, progressive systemic 413
seclusion, of antigen 348
secondary disease 299, 401
secondary lymphoid organs 23,
    36
secretion piece of IgA 95
Sedormid 279, 402
Sela 69
selection
    negative 303
    positive 303
self-recognition 384
self-tolerance 165, 383
Sercarz 75
serine esterase 263
serodiagnostic tests 197
serotherapy 352
serotonin in anaphylaxis 252, 253
serum sickness 280
Sezary cell 375
Sezary syndrome, B,T cell prolifer-
    ative disorders 375
SFA, suppressive factor of
    allergy 277
sharks 32

Shaw 152
Shevach 168
shock organ, in hypersensitivity
    246
Shreffler 168
side-chain theory of antibodies
    100
silica guanidine 70
Singer 157
Sip's function 221
skin reactive factor 291
sleeping sickness 343
slow reacting substance, SRS
    252, 254
slow virus 339
    infections 390
Slp gene, mouse MHC 146, 164
Smithers 349
Snell 140, 143, 311
solubilization of immune com-
    plexes by complement 137
species-specific antigens 67
spectrophotometry 179
spermine 318
spleen 27
spleen index 299
splenomegaly test 299
SRS 347
Ss gene, mouse MHC 146
Stein 197
stem cell 21, 41
Still's disease 411
stimulation index 299
Stokes' law 194
streptolysine 329
strongyloides stercoralis 342, 345
subclasses of animal Ig 97
    of human antibodies 92
superoxide anion 61, 324
    dismutase 324
suppressor lymphocytes 42
susceptibility to tumors 139
syngenic 140, 297
syphilis 191, 196

T cell antigen receptor 56, 171
    genes 172
    structure 161
T cell
    alloantigen 11, 47, 55, 173
    bypass 387
    deficiencies 370–371
    dysregulation 388
    immunodeficiencies 370–371
    lymphoma, B,T cell proliferative
        disorders 375
    regulation, immunity 385
    replacing factor 49
    tolerance 310
T component, IgG T horse 97
T cytolytic cells 11

marker 55
T helper cells 11, 41
    marker 55
T lymphocyte 10, 40
    activity in toads 32
    clones 170
    cytotoxic 45, 47
    differences from B 54
    differentiation 20, 47
    evaluation of function 361
    helper 41, 47
    interaction with antigen 169
    marker 55
    regulatory 44
    specificity 20
    subpopulations 42
    suppressor 42, 47
T,B cell combined deficiencies
    adenosine-deaminase
        deficiency 371
    ataxia telangiectasia 372
    lymphoid stem cell defect 371
    Nezelof's syndrome 372
    purine nucleoside phosphorylase
        deficiency 372
    reticular dysgenesia 372
    SCID, severe combined immu-
        nodeficiencies 371
    transcobalamin II deficiency
        372
    Wiskott-Aldrich syndrome 372
tadpoles 33
taenia saginata 342, 345
taenia solium 345
Tagliacozzi 311
Takatsy microtitrator 192
Talal 386
TAME, N-p-toluenesulfonyl-
    methyl ester 121
tanning 192
tapioca, adjuvant 417
teleosts 32
Tennant virus 176
Terry 349
thermodynamics of hapten-anti-
    body reaction 223
6-thioguanine 433
thoracic duct 3, 54
thrombin 136
thrombin-arachidonic acid path-
    way 136
thrombocytes 13
thrombocytopenia 202
    autoimmune 402
thrombopoiesis 14
thromboxane A2 255
thy-1 antigen 11, 41
thymectomy 16, 40
    immunosuppressors 425
thymic hormones, immunostimu-
    lants 420

thymidinkinase 79
thymocytes, alloantigen 12, 19,
    20
thymoma 395
thymopoietin 4, 21, 41
thymosine 21
    fraction 21
    thymic hormones 420
thymus 2, 5
    aplasia 315
    cells
        destiny 16
        differentiation 19
        mitotic activity 15
    graft 18
    hormonal activity 21
thymus-dependent, lymphocytes
    39
    regions in lymphnodes 24, 41
    regions in spleen 28, 41
thymus-dependent regions 17
    antigen 72
    lymphnodes 24
    spleen 28
thymus-independent region
    antigen 72
    lymphnodes 24
    spleen 28
thyphoid vaccine 356
thyphus vaccine 356
thyreoiditis, subacute Quervain
    176
Tiselius 84
TL antigen 12, 41
TLa locus 147
toads 32
Todd 98
Todd phenomenon 98
tolerance 297, 303, *307*
    adaptive 340
    low zone 111, 387
    mechanism 310
    self 165
Tomasi 95
Tonegawa 102
total body irradiation 314
toxid infections
    serotherapy 353
toxin neutralization by antibodies
    209
toxins, bacterial 335
toxocarna canis 345
toxoplasmosis 343
TPI, trepanoma pallidum immobil-
    isation test 202
transcobalamin II deficiency, T,B
    cell combined deficiencies 372
transfer factor 291
    delayed hypersensitivity 288
transferrin gene 154
translocons of Ig 101

transmission, virus   334
transplantation
   blood transfusion   315
   bone marrow   314
   kidney   312
   nomenclature   140
   organ   311–316
   thymus   315
   tumor   139
transport piece of IgA   95
trematodes   339, 345
triad, antibody formation   111
trichinella spiralis   345
trichuris trichiura   342, 345
trypan blue   202
trypanosomiasis   343
tryptophol   349
T-T lymphocyte cooperation   58
t/t complex   147
tuftsin   323
   deficiency, phagocyte deficien-
      cies   378
   immunostimulation   421
tumor susceptibility   139
   transplantation   139
two-dimensional immunoelectro-
      phoresis   186
typhoid fever   191
typing, cellular, human   150, 311
   homozygous cells   151
   primed lymphocyte   149, *152*
   serologic, human   148, 311

serologic, mouse   143
Tyzzer   139

uropod   7

V genes   102
vaccines   354–357
vaccinia virus   176
van Bekkum   314
van Krogh's equation   116
van Ngú   197
van Rood   149
variable region   90
vasculitis, hypersensitivity type
      III   279
vasectomy   280
Vaz   275
V-C joining   103
VDRL test   191
vinblastine   435
vincristine   435
viral infections   334
   serotherapy   353
vitamin B12-binding protein   403

Waaler   412
Wagner   303
Waldeyer, ring of   318
Wassermann   196
Wassermann reaction   196
wasting disease   21
   syndrome   299

wax D   418
Webb   181
Webster   338
Weckerle   383
West   256
white blood cell, evaluation of
      function   363–363
white graft rejection   299
white pulp, spleen   27
White-Kaufman table   191
Widal's test   191
Wiener   234
Wigzell   56
Wilander   256
Williams   184
Wiscott   271
Wiscott-Aldrich syndrome   271
Witebsky   383, 396
Wright staining   9
wucheria bancrofti   345

χ^2-test   149
xenoantiserum   73
xenogenic   140, 297
xenotransplant   140

yellow fever vaccine   356
Yodoi   277
Yoffey   36

Zinkernagel   164
Zw, platelet specific antigen   316